An Introduction to
Principles and Practice of

Respiratory Medicine

Theory to Bedside

An Introduction to Principles and Practice of

Respiratory Medicine

Theory to Bedside

Editors

PA Mahesh
JSS Medical College, Mysore, India

RS Bhatia
Adesh Medical College and Hospital, Ludhiana, India

BS Jayaraj
JSS Medical College, Mysore, India

Basappa
University of Mysore, India

Gautam Sethi
National University of Singapore, Singapore

World Scientific

NEW JERSEY • LONDON • SINGAPORE • BEIJING • SHANGHAI • HONG KONG • TAIPEI • CHENNAI • TOKYO

Published by

World Scientific Publishing Co. Pte. Ltd.
5 Toh Tuck Link, Singapore 596224
USA office: 27 Warren Street, Suite 401-402, Hackensack, NJ 07601
UK office: 57 Shelton Street, Covent Garden, London WC2H 9HE

British Library Cataloguing-in-Publication Data
A catalogue record for this book is available from the British Library.

AN INTRODUCTION TO PRINCIPLES AND PRACTICE OF RESPIRATORY MEDICINE
Theory to Bedside

ISBN 978-981-127-140-3 (hardcover)
ISBN 978-981-127-141-0 (ebook for institutions)
ISBN 978-981-127-142-7 (ebook for individuals)

For any available supplementary material, please visit
https://www.worldscientific.com/worldscibooks/10.1142/13281#t=suppl

Typeset by Stallion Press
Email: enquiries@stallionpress.com

https://doi.org/10.1142/9789811271410_fmatter

Acknowledgements

P.A. Mahesh

I would like to acknowledge my wife Dr. Amrutha D Holla and son Chirag for their patience. My parents Dr. P. Anand Rao and P. Neerada Rao for their encouragement, spirit of never giving up, and positive inputs. My father is a general practitioner and has been an important influence on me in understanding how to relate to patients and develop the important skill of patient communication. As a medical student, I was amazed at the dedication and commitment of my uncle, Dr. P. Laxminarayan Rao, professor in physiology and former Dean of Kasturba College, Manipal (only the second Indian to complete 50 years of teaching in physiology), who also instilled in me a desire to be a teacher. I am also greatly indebted to my mentor, Prof. P. Ravindran, for helping me to develop both the attitude and aptitude in academics, clinical medicine, and research. He remains my main role model and has guided my career decisions and has always led by example.

R.S. Bhatia

With the grace of God and blessings of my parents, the knowledge imparted to me from my teachers as well as the scientific enrichment by my colleagues, this humble collection, in a concise and updated manner to disseminate knowledge of pulmonary medicine has become possible. I am also indebted to my patients for stimulating me to follow a humane approach to serve the community.

Jayaraj Biligere

With the blessings of my parents M. Siddaiah and Sundaramma for their encouragement. I would like to gratefully acknowledge my beloved teachers from PGI Chandigarh Prof. Dr. S.K. Jindal, Prof. Dr. D. Behera, and late Prof. Dr. Dheeraj Gupta for their support and have taught me all that I know in pulmonary medicine and their continued encouragement over the last three decades. I would like to acknowledge my wife K.M. Uma Mangala and daughter J.M. Sanjana. I would also like to thank my colleagues at PGI Chandigarh, constant interaction with whom improved my understanding of my subject.

Basappa

This book would not have been possible without the dedication and time of Prof. Peter E. Lobie. In this regard, I would like to acknowledge my daughter Shreeja Basappa, and my son Dhiganth Basappa. Thank you to my mother Nagamma and my wife M.P. Latha, who encouraged me to keep going, never giving up, and provided positive perspectives. In my years as a medicinal chemist, Prof. K.S. Rangappa has inspired me to strive to be a teacher, which I attribute to his dedication and commitment. The passion for academics, and aptitude for innovative research, that I developed in the late Prof. Kazuyuki Sugahara is also much indebted to him. In addition to being my main role model, he has led by example and guided my career decisions.

Gautam Sethi

This book would not have been possible without the initiative taken by Dr. Basappa who encouraged all the contributors to compile a comprehensive book related to respiratory medicine. I would also like to thank all the coeditor and contributors for their enormous efforts in successfully completing this entire project and delivering vast information that will be useful for clinicians and researchers working in this field.

List of Contributors

Editors

Editor I: Dr. P.A. Mahesh, Professor and Former Head, Department of Respiratory Medicine, JSS Medical College, JSS Academy of Higher Education & Research, Mysore, Karnataka, India.

E-mail: mahesh1971in@yahoo.com

Tel: +91-9448044003

Editor II: Dr. R.S. Bhatia, Honorary visiting Professor, Department of Respiratory Medicine, Adesh Medical College and Hospital, Shahbad, India.

E-mail: rajbirsingh533@gmail.com

Tel: +91-9815574610

Editor III: Dr. B.S. Jayaraj, Professor and Head, Department of Respiratory Medicine, JSS Medical College, JSS Academy of Higher Education & Research, Mysore, Karnataka, India.

E-mail: drjayarajbs@yahoo.com

Tel: +91-9945671286

Editor IV: Dr. Basappa, Chairman (Wrangler DC Pavate Fellow), Department of Studies in Organic Chemistry, University of Mysore, Manasagangotri, Mysore Karnataka, India.

E-mail: salundibasappa@gmail.com

Tel:: +91-9481200076; +91-821-2419323

Editor V: Dr. Gautam Sethi, Professor, Department of Pharmacology, NUS Centre for Cancer Research(N2CR), Yong Loo Lin School of Medicine, National University of Singapore, 117600, Singapore.
E-mail: phcgs@nus.edu.sg

Senior contributors

Dr. Vikram Patil, MBBS, MD
Associate Professor, Department of Radiology
JSS Medical College, JSSAHER, Mysore, Karnataka, India.

Dr. Sumalatha Arunachala, MBBS, MD, DM (critical care medicine), (PhD), EDIC
Consultant and Head, Department of Critical Care Medicine
Clearmedi multispecialty hospital, Mysore, Karnataka, India.
PhD Scholar, JSS Academy of Higher Education & Research, Mysore, Researcher, PHRII, Mysore, Karnataka, India.

Dr. Ranganath Ramananjaneya, DTCD, DNB — Resp Dis
Senior Consultant Pulmonologist, Head of the Department
Department of Pulmonology and Internal Medicine
NH-Majumdar Shaw Medical Center
Bangalore, Karnataka, India.

Dr. R. Subramanian, MD PDF (Clinical Immunology & Rheumatology)
Professor
Department of Clinical Immunology & Rheumatology
JSS Medical College
JSS Academy of Higher Education and Research, Mysuru, Karnataka, India.

Dr. S.K. Chaya, DTCD, DNB
Associate Professor, Department of Respiratory Medicine
JSS Medical College, JSSAHER, Mysore, Karnataka, India.

Dr. K.S. Lokesh, MBBS, DNB
Assistant Professor, Department of Respiratory Medicine
JSS Medical College, JSSAHER, Mysore, Karnataka, India.

Dr. M. Ramesh, MPharm, PhD, Dip Clin Pharm
Professor, Department of Pharmacy Practice
JSS College of Pharmacy, JSSAHER, Mysore, Karnataka, India.

Ms. Shilpa Palaksha, MPharm (PhD)
Associate Professor, Department of Pharmacy Practice
JSS College of Pharmacy, JSS AHER, Mysore, Karnataka, India.

Dr. Rajbir Singh, BDS, MDS
Associate Professor
Genesis Institute of Dental Sciences & Research
Ferozepur, Punjab, India.

Dr. Prabhpreet Kaur, BDS, MDS
Associate Professor
Genesis Institute of Dental Sciences & Research
Ferozepur, Punjab, India.

Dr. Vaibhav C. Padashetti, MBBS, MD
Senior Resident, Department of Respiratory Medicine
Gulbarga Institute of Medical Sciences, Kalaburagi, Karnataka, India.

Dr. K. Vishwa Vijeth, MBBS, MD
Senior Resident, Department of Respiratory Medicine
East Point College of Medical Sciences, Bengaluru, Karnataka, India.

Dr. Mikash Mohan
Senior Resident, Department of Respiratory Medicine
JSS Medical College, JSSAHER, Mysore, Karnataka, India.

Dr. Mohd Akram Qureshi
Consultant, Respiratory Medicine
Hope Chest Hospital, Bidar, Karnataka, India.

Dr. Meghna Rai Prasad
Senior Resident, Department of Respiratory Medicine
Rajiv Gandhi Institute of Chest Diseases, Bengaluru, Karnataka, India.

Dr. Athira Satheesh
Consultant, Respiratory Medicine.

Early career contributors

Ms. K. Greeshma (PhD), JSS Medical College, JSSAHER.
Mr. M. Kaleem (PhD), JSS Medical College, JSSAHER, GID fellow, university of Berkeley.
Dr. V.S. Rekha (MD), JSS Medical College, JSSAHER.
Dr. Nidhi Bansal (MD), JSS Medical College, JSSAHER.
Dr. R . Sukanya (MD), JSS Medical College, JSSAHER.
Dr. Shreedhar Kulkarni (MD), JSS Medical College, JSSAHER.
Mr. Sunag Padukudru (graduate student), Yenepoya Medical College, Manglore.
Mr. R. Akshay (PhD), University of Mysore.

Department of Pharmacy Practice JSS College of Pharmacy, JSSAHER, Mysore.
Dr. Kanchi Dhakan, Pharm D
Dr. Monisha Manoharan Pharm D
Dr. Mahima Ray, Pharm D
Dr. Jehath Syed, Pharm D
Dr. Abaka Mohith Kumar, Pharm D
Dr. Elechi Emelda Chinemerem, Pharm D
Dr. Nnachi Ezinne Perpetua, Pharm D

Contents

https://doi.org/10.1142/9789811271410_0001

1 Anatomy of the lung

Lungs are the organs of respiration. Less was known about them, until nearly 200 years ago, because they did not seem important. The chest and lungs are both critical for respiration necessary for survival. Respiration is needed for an adequate supply of oxygen and provides protection from an excess accumulation of carbon dioxide. The chest is a composite structure comprising bones, cartilages, and muscles involved in the movement of the chest. Anteriorly it is bound by the sternum, manubrium, and costal cartilages; laterally, by the ribs which are 12 in number and posteriorly by the thoracic vertebrae and the ribs. While the 12 pairs of ribs are connected to the thoracic vertebrae, only the upper seven are attached to the sternum by costal cartilages. Ribs 11 and 12 (floating ribs) attach only posteriorly. The lateral diameter of the chest usually exceeds the anterior-posterior (AP) diameter.

The main muscles of respiration are the diaphragm and the intercostal muscles of which the diaphragm is the most important as it does not get fatigued. When it contracts, it moves downward during inspiration and increases the intrathoracic space. The external intercostal muscles increase the AP diameter during inspiration. The other important group of muscles is the internal intercostal muscles, which are expiratory muscles.

Fissures of the lungs

Each lung is divided into lobes by the oblique and/or horizontal fissure(s). The right lung has both fissures and hence divided into three lobes, while the left lung has only one fissure and hence divided into two lobes. The surface marking of the major (oblique) fissure starts at the sixth costochondral junction anteriorly, extending along the sixth rib, to meet the spinous process of the third thoracic vertebra. The horizontal fissure in the right lung starts at the fourth costal cartilage and extends horizontally toward the oblique fissure, which intersects at the fifth rib in the midaxillary line.

Segments of the lung

The segments of the lung are also known as bronchopulmonary segments. Their significance is as follows:

1. They are more or less uniformly distributed.
2. The infections of the lung are generally localized to one or more neighboring segments.
3. Lung tissue is thus often preserved in the resection of the diseased areas.

The right lung

The right lung, as stated above, is divided into three lobes by the two fissures. The lobes are upper lobe, middle lobe, and lower lobe. The upper lobe extends from the apex to the horizontal fissure. The middle lobe lies in between the two fissures. The lower lobe extends from the oblique fissure to the diaphragmatic surface of the lung.

Upper lobe: It consists of three among the 10 segments, namely, apical, anterior, and posterior.

Apical segment: This segment forms the dome of the lung. It is pyramidal in shape. It has anterior, posterior, medial, and lateral surfaces.

Anterior segment: This segment lies below, anteromedially to the apical segment. It has anterior, lateral, and inferior surfaces.

Posterior segment: The segment itself presents laterally and posteriorly. This also has an inferior surface. The inferior surface of the posterior segment and that of the anterior segment together are separated from the middle lobe by the horizontal fissure. The posterior segment of these segments is separated from the superior segment of the lower lobe by the oblique/vertical fissure.

The posterior segment of the upper lobe of the right lung is a common site of aspiration abscess, septic pneumonitis, and tuberculosis. The lesions of the anterior segment of the upper lobe tend to be cancerous in nature.

Middle lobe: This lobe consists of two segments, namely, medial and lateral segments, which lie anteromedially and anterolaterally, respectively. Its anterior surface is the largest. This lobe does not reach the chest wall posteriorly. The triangular surfaces are bounded by fourth and fifth ribs laterally and by the pericardium of the heart, on its medial aspect. The middle lobe bronchus is long and has the longest intrapulmonary course and lies along the course of the lymphatics that drain the right lower lobe and is surrounded by multiple lymph nodes. It is also the narrowest of all the lobar bronchi and originates at right angles from the intermediate bronchus. Consequently, as the middle lobar bronchus is surrounded by the lymph nodes, which on enlargement, may compress the bronchus, thus causing a lung collapse. Lymph nodes are present in between the bronchial branching; hence, calcified nodes are often clearly visible, in X-ray images, near the hilum of the lung in cases of severe lymphadenitis.

Lower lobe: This lobe consists of superior and inferior segments.

Superior segment: It is also often called the apical segment of the lower lobe. It is related to the fourth and eighth ribs posteriorly. The medial and lateral aspects meet the posterior segment of the upper lobe by extending around to the fissure. Hence, this segment, which is prone to aspiration sequelae, has a surface that is in contact with the lateral chest wall and another one that is in contact with the mediastinum.

Inferior portion: It consists of four basal segments, each of which lies on the diaphragm. Together, the inferior surfaces of each of the lobes form the diaphragmatic surface of the right lung. The medial segment is entirely medial and diaphragmatic and comes in contact with the right atrium of the heart. The posterior segment of this lobe contributes to the mediastinal surface of the right lung. The lateral segment also has a posterior aspect, while the anterior segment also presents laterally.

Azygos lobes: Accessory lobes like the azygos lobe, although rarely, could be present in the right lung in some people. This may appear in one of the three situations:

1. Lobe of the azygos vein: due to the abnormality of the azygos vein.
2. Upper azygos lobe: does not involve any abnormality of the azygos vein.
3. Lower azygos lobe: does not involve any abnormality of the azygos vein.

The first one is of importance to a clinician while the other two are not practically important as they are associated with no abnormalities. The lobe of the azygos vein may be the site of a pulmonary disease or may show up as an unusual appearance on X-ray imaging of the patient's lungs.

A double pleural septum, called the meso-azygos, cuts off a portion of the inner surface of the upper right lobe. At the apex of this invagination, there lies the upper part of the azygos vein. Thus, the right pleural cavity is divided by the meso-azygos into an upper compartment and a lower compartment which contain in them, the accessory lobe and the remainder of the lung, respectively. This accessory lobe is variable in size. The invagination containing the azygos vein with the meso-azygos appears as a line extending nearly up to the root of the lung and the vein itself will appear as a dark shadow at the end of the fissure/invagination.

The left lung

It consists of two lobes, each of which consists of five bronchopulmonary segments.

Upper lobe: This lobe is made up of five segments. The lower two segments among them are called superior and inferior lingual segments respectively. The inferior lingular segment, in its lower part, extends downward to reach the diaphragm as well as the pericardium covering the left ventricle. The arrangement of segments on the upper lobe above these two is very much like the right lung. It has apical, anterior, and posterior segments. The apical and posterior segments are ventilated by a single bronchus and hence they are often collectively called the apicoposterior segment.

Lower lobe: The lower lobe of the left lung is much smaller than its right counterpart. It is, however, divided into five segments in the same manner as the right lower lobe, thus giving rise to one superior lobe and four basal segments.

The bronchial tree:

Right lung: The right main bronchus is more vertical, shorter in length, and has a wider diameter than its left counterpart. The upper lobe bronchus passes laterally and slightly upwards for about 1 cm and then branches into three divisions: apical, anterior, and posterior. On the anterior aspect of the main bronchus, just beyond the origin of the upper lobe branches, there is a groove for the pulmonary artery. Just distal to this groove, the middle lobe bronchus arises from the anterolateral aspects and divides into medial and lateral segments. All the remaining bronchi, that lie distal to the middle lobe bronchus, are designated to the lower lobe segments. The bronchus to the superior segment of the right lower lobe is given off posteriorly and runs rearward horizontally. Although this bronchus is given off distal to the bronchus of the middle lobe, it may be given off in front of or even proximally to it. This anatomical immediacy of the two lobes implies that the middle lobe should also be resected along with the lower one in case of a neoplastic or an inflammatory infection of the lower lobe. Also, the size, thickness of the lumen, and the vertical position of the right main bronchus heavily favor lodging of aspirated foreign bodies, more so in children. The risk of lodging is high in the right middle lobe.

Left lung: The left main bronchus is longer and more angulated than its right counterpart. After bifurcation, 5 cm away from the carina, the left main bronchus branches into an upper lobe stem bronchus and a branch to the lower lobe. The upper lobe stem bronchus curves laterally and the lingular lobar bronchus branches from the upper stem bronchus nearly 1 cm from its origin and then the lingular bronchus further divides into superior and inferior segmental bronchi. Subsequent to this bifurcation, the upper lobe stem bronchus immediately divides into a branch for the anterior segment and one for the posterior and apical segments, which then bifurcate into separate bronchi for each segment. The superior segmental bronchus, which comes from the posterior aspect of the left lower lobe, is the first one to be given off by the lower lobe branch. More often than not, there are three bronchi, which are meant one each for the posterior and lateral segments and one for the anterior and medial segments combined, which will later divide into individual segmental bronchi. In around 30% of the radiographs, an additional bronchus appears, just distal to the lower lobe bronchus. It may occur in both lungs and is sometimes known as subsuperior bronchus. It is important to note this during the interpretations of bronchograms.

Blood supply and lymphatic drainage of the lungs

Right pulmonary artery: It travels horizontally for a short length in front of the right main bronchus and reaches the anterior aspect of the upper lobe bronchus, where it gives off its first upper lobe branch. This branch divides into an apical and an anterior vessel. The main pulmonary artery travels downward within a groove in the anterior aspect of the bronchus in front of its upper lobe branch. It then enters the lobe well beneath the fissure and hence can only be revealed by deep dissection of the fissure. The middle lobe is always supplied by two branches of the pulmonary artery, which arise at the base of the meeting point of the fissures distal to the posterior segmental branch of the upper lobe. They are closely related to the bronchus when they enter the middle lobe. The pulmonary artery terminates after supplying the lower lobe of the lung. The first vessel to take birth is the superior lobe vessel that passes downward and backward. The other segments are supplied by a collection of vessels.

Left pulmonary artery: The main trunk of this artery is longer than its right counterpart. The artery curves upwards and over the bronchus. Then the first branch arises and supplies the apical and posterior segments. It then arches behind the upper lobe bronchus, where it gives birth to the branches of the upper three segments of the lobe. The artery gives off a lingular artery in the interlobar fissure, which then divides into an artery for each of the lingular segments. Sometimes, there may be a single artery to the lingula. The interlobar part of the main arteries gives rise to the lower lobe arteries.

Venous system: The venous system of both lungs is similar. The convergence of the segmental veins to form large trunks leads to the formation of superior and inferior pulmonary veins at the hilum of the lung. The apical, anterior, and posterior segments of the upper lobe along with two segments of the middle lobe drain into the superior pulmonary vein. The veins from the segments of the lower lobe drain into the inferior pulmonary vein. The most anterior structures at the hilum are the veins.

Bronchial vessels: Bronchial arteries are nutritive vessels of the lungs. Commonly, each lung is supplied by a single main artery, which may arise from the aorta, just beyond the birth of the left subclavian artery or from one of the upper aortic intercostal arteries. One or more smaller arteries may arise from the thoracic aorta.

Bronchopulmonary circulation: The arteries and veins belonging to the pulmonary and bronchial circulation communicate freely with each other and hence form an open circuit and allow for the mixing of arterial and venous blood. The uniqueness of bronchial circulation lies in the fact that the bronchial artery arises from systemic circulation and the vein drains into the pulmonary circulation. This accounts for the physiological decrease in the partial pressure difference of oxygen between alveoli and capillaries leaving the lungs. This phenomenon is called arteriovenous shunt or anatomical shunt. Multiple anastomoses between bronchial and pulmonary arterial systems are of prime importance in cases of inflammatory

pulmonary disease. Thrombosis of the bronchial vessels occurs in cases of inflammatory pulmonary diseases, which in turn leads to enlargement of the bronchial arterial systems. This is almost certainly followed by massive hemoptysis. The embolization techniques of bronchial arteries demand thorough knowledge of these anastomoses and their variants. The fact that the interaction between intercostal and bronchial blood vessels gives off branches to the spinal cord at the midthoracic section is of utmost importance as paraplegia follows the embolization of spinal branches of bronchial vessels, thus conferring the inflammatory pulmonary disorders a prime place in the list of pulmonary disorders.

Azygos and hemiazygos interruption of inferior vena cava (IVC): It is quite rare but worth discussing. The patient presents with symptoms of cough and breathlessness. Physical examination reveals bilateral crackling sound on auscultation, with remainder of the examinations usually being normal. Computed tomography (CT) of the chest reveals peripheral, subpleural peribronchovascular opacities, and consolidations without honeycomb changes in bilateral lungs. The lung functions are below normal. An IVC angiography clearly indicates the continuation of IVC by azygos or hemiazygos veins. The common site of occurrence is at the hepatic part of the IVC. This may also be an indicator of situs inversus or splenic anomalies like polysplenia and asplenia. It is also associated with dextrocardia (3),(2).

Lymph nodes and lymphatics of the lungs: The lymph from the lungs are drained mostly by peritracheobronchial lymph nodes, belonging to the visceral lymph node group of the thoracic lymph nodes. The lymph that accumulates on the hila is not drained in a strictly lobar manner. The right lung lymphatics drain directly or indirectly into intratracheobronchial or pretracheobronchial lymph nodes, which are in turn related to the tracheal bifurcation.

The left lung lymphatics drains into three lymph regions. Superior part of the upper lobe drains into the left pretracheobronchial lymph nodes.

Lymph from the upper part of the lower lobe and the lower part of the upper lobe also drains into these nodes along with the right pretracheobronchial nodes via the subcranial nodes. The remaining parts of the left lower lobe drain also into the right pretracheobronchial lymph nodes via the nodes at the tracheal bifurcation. The lymph nodes related to the sides of the trachea drain into the jugular lymph trunk through the inferior deep cervical lymph nodes.

The bronchomediastinal trunk, an efferent lymph trunk that drains the superior mediastinal group of lymph nodes, is joined by the lymphatic trunk formed by the tracheobronchial lymph nodes. This commonly enters the junction between the jugular vein and the subclavian vein; however, it is also possible that they enter the right lymphatic trunk or the thoracic duct, according to the side.

thoracic lymph nodes
visceral lymph nodes
superior mediastinal nodes

peritracheobronchial lymph nodes

parietal lymph nodes
internal mammary lymph nodes

posterior mediastinal lymph nodes

intercostal lymph nodes

diaphragmatic lymph nodes

Flowchart: hierarchy of thoracic lymph nodes

Applied anatomy for lymphatics

Metastatic lung cancer is associated with Warthin's tumor: Warthin's tumor is a tumor-like lesion of the salivary gland that affects males predominantly, in their mid-50s or 60s. Diagnosis can be made with a regular

magnetic resonance imaging scan, which is usually inadequate. Hence, 18F-fluorodeoxy-D-glucose positron emission tomography/CT scans are advisable, as they show the increased glucose metabolism by the tumor cells (4).

Lymphatic impairment of the lungs leads to the formation of tertiary lymphoid organs and alveolar damage. In an experiment conducted in mice, it is found that impairment of lymphatic drainage of the lungs chronically leads to the formation of tertiary lymphoid organs and produces hypoxic symptoms similar to that found in emphysema (5).

Pleura

Definition: Pleura is the double-layered serous sac that encloses each of the lungs.

Layers: The pleura has two layers: outer parietal pleura and inner visceral pleura. Between the two layers, there is a narrow space filled with fluid called the pleural cavity or pleural space. It is, however, important to note that the space between the two layers is only potential and only a small volume of fluid exists between the two layers. Excess fluid accumulation in the pleural cavity is called pleural effusion, which is discussed later in the chapter. The parietal pleura is closely related to the relations of the lungs. In contrast, the visceral pleura is adherent to the lung tissue in the entire extent of the lung except at its root, where it is continuous with the parietal pleura. The visceral pleura lines the major and minor fissures of the lungs. There are anatomical variations of the pleura based on the organ that it covers. On the visceral surface, the pleura is thin with flattened mesothelial cells and sparse microvilli. On the parietal surface, the pleura may be dense and fuse with the periosteum of the underlying rib. There are ~1,500–4,500 cells in 1 mL of pleural fluid normally. These are mononuclear cells with occasional lymphocytes. The mononuclear cells are mostly macrophage-like.

Contents of pleural space	Amount (approx. values)
Pleural fluid (mL)	8.4 ± 4.3
Protein (g/100 mL)	1–2
Cells/mL	1,500–4,500

To understand the arrangement of the two pleural layers completely, a little embryology of the lung and pleura is necessary, which is discussed in the following text.

The lung develops from the lung bud. There are two primitive pleurae lateral to each of the lung bud. As the lungs develop, they invaginate the pleural cavities from their medial aspects. The "medial wall" of the primitive pleural cavity, now comes in close contact with the developing lung and becomes the visceral pleura by closely investing the lung. The "lateral wall" now becomes the parietal pleura. The pleural cavity between the two layers is reduced to a narrow, slit-like space. The point at the medial surface of the lung has the root of the lung, where the bronchi, vessels, and nerves enter or leave the lung. This prevents complete covering of the lung by the pleura at the root of the lung and thus the two pleurae are continuous at the root of the lung.

Parts of the pleura

The parietal pleura has the following parts:

1. Costal pleura: It is the part that is in close contact with the thoracic cage and the respiratory muscles. The costal pleura is attached to the thoracic cage by a loose areolar connective tissue called endothoracic fascia.
2. Diaphragmatic pleura: It is the part that covers the upper surface of the dome of the thoracic diaphragm inferior to the inferior surface (diaphragmatic surface) of the lung.

3. Mediastinal pleura: It is the part that covers the mediastinal surface of the lung. It is related to the structures in the mediastinum like the heart, great vessels, thymus, phrenic nerves, and vagi.
4. Dome of the pleura: It is also known as cervical pleura. It extends 5 cm above the costal cartilage of the first rib, into the root of the neck. It is about 1.2 cm above the middle one-third of the clavicle. It is related anteriorly to the subclavian artery, posteriorly to the neck of the first rib, the sympathetic chain and the stellate ganglion, the supreme intercostal vein, the first intercostal artery, and the nerve root of T1.

The costal pleura is continuous with the mediastinal pleura at the anterior and posterior borders of the lung and with the diaphragmatic pleura at the inferior border of the lung. The mediastinal pleura is continuous with the cervical pleura, the costal, and diaphragmatic pleurae.

Pulmonary ligament: The parietal pleura, at the root of the lung, extends downward like a shirt sleeve, below the root as a loose fold called the pulmonary ligament. This fold is filled with loose areolar connective tissue. This provides free space into which the pulmonary veins can expand in times of increased venous return and also for the upward and downward movement of the root of the lung during breathing. It is created during the invagination of the lung into the thoracic cavity (vide supra), pulling along the ventral and dorsal aspects of the visceral pleura.

Recesses of the pleura: The areas of reflection of the parietal pleura on the diaphragm and the mediastinum, due to which the pleural cavity has increased space in those areas are called the pleural recesses. It is quite important to study the pleural recesses in detail as they hold importance in cases of pleural effusion and pneumonia.

There are two pleural recesses:

1. Costodiaphragmatic recess
2. Costomediastinal recess

Costodiaphragmatic recess: It is the area of reflection of the parietal pleura over the diaphragm. It lies in between the costal and the diaphragmatic pleura. In the midaxillary line, this recess spans the area between the 8th and the 10th rib. Its vertical measurement is about 5 cm. The sharp lower lung margins move into costodiaphragmatic recesses during complete inspiration, wherein both the lungs and pleura are over the structures of the upper abdomen. In the junction where the diaphragmatic and the costal sections of the pleura meet, they are attached to the costal cartilages via the endothoracic fascia (phrenicopleural fascia).

In a posteroanterior chest X-ray it appears just above the domes of the diaphragm as a more or less triangular space of air density in normal individuals. The junction between the thoracic cage and the diaphragm presents an angle called the costodiaphragmatic angle.

Costomediastinal recess: It lies anteriorly behind the sternum and is formed between the costal and mediastinal pleurae. On the right side, it is usually obliterated by the right lung; however on the left side, it is more obvious because of the deep cardiac notch of the left lung.

The costodiaphragmatic recess, however, is the most dependent of the two recesses.

Blood supply, nerve supply, and lymphatics of the pleurae:

The development of the pleurae, in brief, will make it more convenient to understand the nerve supply of the pleurae. Pleura develops from the layers of the lateral plate mesoderm. The parietal pleura develops from the somatopleuric layer, and the visceral pleura develops from the splanchnopleuric layer of the lateral plate mesoderm. Hence, the parietal pleura has a somatic nerve supply by the intercostal and phrenic nerves, while the visceral pleura has an autonomic nerve supply consisting of parasympathetic fibers from the vagi and the sympathetic fibers derived from the second to fifth sympathetic ganglia. The bronchial vessels accompany the nerves. The intercostal nerves supply the costal pleura and the outer parts of the diaphragmatic pleura, and the rest is supplied by the phrenic nerve.

The blood supply of the parietal pleura is the same as the thoracic wall, with the intercostal, internal mammary, and musculophrenic arteries providing the arterial blood supply. The veins that drain the parietal pleura flow into azygos and internal thoracic veins. The pleural lymphatics drain into several groups of lymph nodes: intercostal, internal mammary, posterior mediastinal, and diaphragmatic nodes. The bronchial arteries supply the visceral pleura similar to the lung, while the veins draining the visceral pleura flow into bronchial veins. The lymphatic drainage of the visceral pleura is by the bronchopulmonary lymph nodes.

Ultrastructure of pleura

The pleura has a single layer of mesothelial cells. These cells become important in cases of malignant and infectious disorders of the pleura. Below the mesothelial cell layer, the pleura has four other layers; they are basal lamina, elastic layer, loose connective tissue, and a fibroelastic layer. The connective tissue layer contains the nerves, blood vessels, and lymphatics. Hence, in case of pleural inflammation, the cells have to pass through the connective tissue, the basal lamina, out of the mesothelial layer and later into the pleural space. Along with the mesothelial cells, dendritic cells have also been found in the human visceral pleura. The dendritic cells function similarly to other dendritic cells in the airways and predominantly work as antigen-presenting cells and can trigger an immune response. Extensive cytoplasmic processes are observed in these dendritic cells, which appear elongated and two to three cytoplasmic processes are placed parallel to the mesothelial cells. The pleural dendritic cells unlike those present in the airways that are constantly exposed to noxious stimuli are observed to not contain any ingested particles. The lymphatic vessels in the costal pleura form funnel-like projections called stomata (singular: stoma). However, these are found to be absent in diaphragmatic pleurae. These stomata open directly into the pleural cavity. They help drain the pleural fluid thereby maintaining a constant volume of the fluid in the pleural cavity.

References and suggested reading

1. McGregor AL, Decker GAG. Lee McGregor's synopsis of surgical anatomy [Internet]. Bristol: John Wright; 1986 [cited 2019 May 1]. Available from: http://www.tandfonline.com/toc/rwhi20
2. Liu Y, Guo D, Li J, Zhang X, He J, Huang M, et al. Radiological features of azygos and hemiazygos continuation of inferior vena cava: a case report. Medicine (Baltimore). 2018 Apr;97(17):e0546.
3. Sheley RC, Nyberg DA, Kapur R. Azygous continuation of the interrupted inferior vena cava: a clue to prenatal diagnosis of the cardiosplenic syndromes. J Ultrasound Med Off J Am Inst Ultrasound Med. 1995 May;14(5):381–387.
4. Haberal M, Akar E, Dikis O. Metastatic lung cancer associated with Warthin's tumour. Niger J Clin Pract. 2019;22(4):585.
5. Outtz Reed H, Wang L, Sonett J, Chen M, Yang J, Li L, et al. Lymphatic impairment leads to pulmonary tertiary lymphoid organ formation and alveolar damage. J Clin Invest. 2019 Apr 4;130.
6. Sertl K, Takemura T, Tschachler E, Ferrans VJ, Kaliner MA, Shevach EM. Dendritic cells with antigen-presenting capability reside in airway epithelium, lung parenchyma, and visceral pleura. J Exp Med. 1986 Feb 1;163(2):436–451.
7. Oshiro H, Miura M, Iobe H, Kudo T, Shimazu Y, Aoba T, et al. Lymphatic stomata in the adult human pulmonary ligament. Lymphat Res Biol. 2015 Jun;13(2):137–145.
8. Aspal M, Zemans RL. Mechanisms of ATII-to-ATI cell differentiation during lung regeneration. Int J Mol Sci. 2020 Apr 30;21(9):3188. doi: 10.3390/ijms21093188. PMID: 32366033; PMCID: PMC7246911.
9. Cho SJ, Stout-Delgado HW. Aging and lung disease. Annu Rev Physiol. 2020 Feb 10;82:433–459. doi: 10.1146/annurev-physiol-021119-034610. Epub 2019 Nov 15. PMID: 31730381; PMCID: PMC7998901.
10. Ruaro B, Salton F, Braga L, Wade B, Confalonieri P, Volpe MC, Baratella E, Maiocchi S, Confalonieri M. The history and mystery of alveolar epithelial type II cells: focus on their physiologic and pathologic role in lung. Int J Mol Sci. 2021 Mar 4;22(5):2566. doi: 10.3390/ijms22052566. PMID: 33806395; PMCID: PMC7961977.
11. Sun X, Perl AK, Li R, Bell SM, Sajti E, Kalinichenko VV, Kalin TV, Misra RS, Deshmukh H, Clair G, Kyle J, Crotty Alexander LE, Masso-Silva JA, Kitzmiller

JA, Wikenheiser-Brokamp KA, Deutsch G, Guo M, Du Y, Morley MP, Valdez MJ, Yu HV, Jin K, Bardes EE, Zepp JA, Neithamer T, Basil MC, Zacharias WJ, Verheyden J, Young R, Bandyopadhyay G, Lin S, Ansong C, Adkins J, Salomonis N, Aronow BJ, Xu Y, Pryhuber G, Whitsett J, Morrisey EE. NHLBI LungMAP Consortium. A census of the lung: CellCards from LungMAP. Dev Cell. 2022 Jan 10;57(1):112–145.e2. doi: 10.1016/j.devcel.2021.11.007. Epub 2021 Dec 21. PMID: 34936882; PMCID: PMC9202574.

12. Hai J, Zhang H, Zhou J, Wu Z, Chen T, Papadopoulos E, Dowling CM, Pyon V, Pan Y, Liu JB, Bronson RT, Silver H, Lizotte PH, Deng J, Campbell JD, Sholl LM, Ng C, Tsao MS, Thakurdin C, Bass AJ, Wong KK. Generation of genetically engineered mouse lung organoid models for squamous cell lung cancers allows for the study of combinatorial immunotherapy. Clin Cancer Res. 2020 Jul 1;26(13):3431–3442. doi: 10.1158/1078-0432.CCR-19-1627. Epub 2020 Mar 24. PMID: 32209571; PMCID: PMC7334092.
13. Archer F, Bobet-Erny A, Gomes M. State of the art on lung organoids in mammals. Vet Res. 2021 Jun 2;52(1):77. doi: 10.1186/s13567-021-00946-6. PMID: 34078444; PMCID: PMC8170649.
14. Li X, Zhao F, Wang A, Cheng P, Chen H. Role and mechanisms of autophagy in lung metabolism and repair. Cell Mol Life Sci. 2021 Jun;78(12):5051–5068. doi: 10.1007/s00018-021-03841-7. Epub 2021 Apr 17. PMID: 33864479.
15. Weibel ER. Lung morphometry: the link between structure and function. Cell Tissue Res. 2017 Mar;367(3):413–426. doi: 10.1007/s00441-016-2541-4. Epub 2016 Dec 16. PMID: 27981379.

https://doi.org/10.1142/9789811271410_0002

2 Cough

One of the most common symptoms in respiratory medicine is cough with or without sputum production. Cough is not a disease per say, but a marker for one or more diseases. Cough is an important reflex, impairment of which can lead to a multitude of complications. Cough is an explosive expiration that provides a normal protective mechanism for clearing the tracheobronchial tree of secretions and foreign material. Coughing may be initiated either voluntarily or reflexively.

As with any symptom, the first task for the clinician is to identify the site of disease that has led to the cough. This is important since specialists do not treat cough as a symptom, but treat the cause for cough leading to the amelioration of the symptom. For this, one has to carefully evaluate all the sites that have cough receptors. It is important to remember that in many patients, especially those with long-standing cough usually have more than one cause/site of disease for their symptoms.

Where are the cough receptors situated? They are present both in pulmonary and extrapulmonary sites. In the lungs, they are present in the upper airways, lower airways, parenchyma, interstitium, and pleura. The extrapulmonary sites of cough receptors include esophagus, stomach, pericardium, and external auditory canal. From most of these sites, vagus is the key afferent nerve and recurrent laryngeal nerve and spinal nerve form the efferent pathway (Figure 1).

The density of cough receptors varies from site to site and determines the severity of cough. Unlike dyspnoea, a severe cough may not be related to a severe disease. Trivial diseases such as pharyngitis can cause severe cough and a severe disease such as a malignant pleural effusion may only

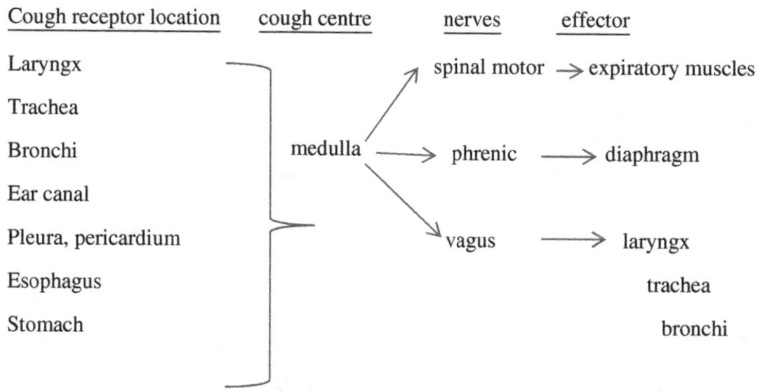

Figure 1: Cough reflex pathway.

cause minimal cough. The highest densities of cough receptors in the lungs are present in the upper airways and major airways. The density reduces towards the periphery of the airways and onwards towards the pleura, which has the least density of cough receptors. This information is clinically relevant as one suspects an underlying lung lesion in a patient with pleural effusion who has cough as a dominant symptom. The pleural effusion otherwise masks both the clinical and radiological signs of an underlying lung disease. Among extrapulmonary sites, esophagus has one of the highest density and the pericardium the least. External auditory canal involvement can lead to severe cough in a few cases, especially in children and needs to be kept in mind, especially if they are not responding to usual treatment for common causes.

Mechanism of cough reflex

Cough reflex can be initiated by mechanical stimuli via the rapidly adapting receptors (RARs), slowly adapting stretch receptors (SARs), or by chemical stimuli via the C-fibers. Cough essentially has four phases, namely, Inspiratory, Compressive, Expiratory, and Relaxation. Cough begins with a rapid inspiration followed by the closure of epiglottis, and vocal cords shut tightly to entrap air within the lungs. There is a forceful contraction of the abdominal muscles, pushing against the diaphragm. Intrathoracic pressure raises to 100 mm Hg or more and causes narrowing of the trachea. During

the expiratory phase, the vocal cord and epiglottis suddenly open and the large pressure difference between airways and atmosphere in addition to tracheal narrowing produces rapid expiratory flow rates. Air is expelled at very high velocities of 75–100 miles per hour.

Sputum

Sputum is one of the most important symptoms that should be asked about in every patient with a cough. The reason it is so important is the fact that it confirms pulmonary involvement. Cough can be present entirely due to extrapulmonary causes, but when sputum is present, the clinician can be sure that there is pulmonary involvement. The type of sputum can give a clue to the site of disease within the lungs. There are serous and mucous glands in the upper respiratory tract and lower respiratory tract and the concentration reduces towards smaller airways. There are no serous and mucous glands in the alveoli. A patient with serous or mucoid secretions has either an upper or lower airway disease. Only in the case of a bronchioloalveolar carcinoma, there can be watery secretions from an alveolar pathology. If there are purulent secretions, usually indicating infections and can be from upper airways, lower airways, lung parenchyma, or even pleural diseases such as empyema which has ruptured into the airways causing a bronchopleural fistula. Interstitial lung diseases usually present with dry cough since there are no serous and mucous glands in the interstitium. Pleural diseases usually do not communicate with the airways and can have minimal dry cough except when there is a purulent collection that erodes into the airways. A copious, foul-smelling purulent expectoration with postural variation almost always means a large collection of pus in the airways (bronchiectasis), lung parenchyma (lung abscess), or pleura (bronchopleural fistula).

Though the presence of sputum is very useful to the clinician and confirms pulmonary involvement, the absence of sputum does not rule out pulmonary involvement. Pathologies in any part of the lung can still present as dry cough. For example, patients with rhinosinusitis or asthma

commonly present with dry cough. It is important to note that some patients, very young children or very old or debilitated patients, or those with neuromuscular weakness may not be able to expectorate due to the lack of strength in their cough, which is ineffective to push out the secretions. In addition, in some of these cases, the secretions can be very thick and tenacious with difficulty in expectorating them. Severe bronchospasm is another reason for dry cough, and patients report plenty of sputum expectoration after treatment. Early stages of pneumonia in the stage of hepatization may not have any sputum. Sometimes, sputum is characteristic of certain conditions: black-colored sputum (melanoptysis) in aspergillosis and coal workers pneumoconiosis, red currant jelly sputum in *Klebsiella pneumonia*, anchovy sauce sputum in amoebiasis, pista green sputum in *Pseudomonas* infection, and pseudohempotysis due to the red-colored pigment in *Serratia marcescens* infection (Figure 2).

Most common cause of impaired cough is due to altered sensorium due to a variety of iatrogenic (anesthesia, narcotics, sedatives, endotracheal or tracheostomy tubes) and non-iatrogenic causes (alcohol, coma, stroke, seizure). Other causes include laryngeal and upper airway disorders, neuromuscular diseases, chronic debilitating diseases, and chronically bedridden patients. Consequences of impaired cough are many ranging from mild impairment to life-threatening. Macroaspiration of oropharyngeal or stomach contents or an acute airway obstruction can be immediately life-threatening. Microaspirations can lead to pneumonias or lung abscesses in the dependent regions of the lung. There is also a risk for bronchiectasis, pulmonary fibrosis, respiratory failure, and acute respiratory distress syndrome (ARDS) due to impaired cough reflex.

In addition to the usual history of onset; duration; progression; aggravating and relieving factors; diurnal, seasonal, and postural variations of cough and sputum, it is important to collect information on the severity of cough as well as complications of cough. Severity of cough is assessed by its impact on day-to-day activities such as school or work and sleep. A significant organic disease usually has a cough at the night. A mother/spouse may

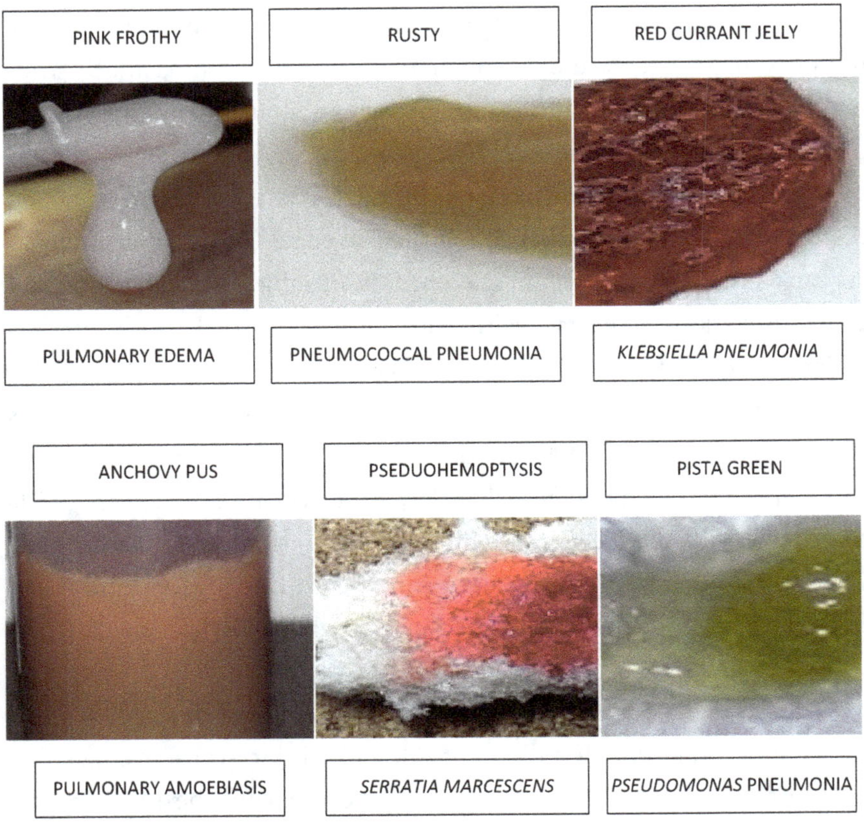

Figure 2: The color of the sputum as an indicator of disease etiology.

observe that the subject coughs during sleep that does not wake them up (mild cough), or it can be so severe that the subject is coughing throughout the night and cannot sleep at all. A psychogenic cough on the other hand is characterized by the absence of any cough on any night after the subject falls asleep.

A drug history is critical, especially in subjects above the age of 40 years. The common drugs that need to be asked for are aspirin, beta-blockers, and angiotensin-converting enzyme (ACE) inhibitors. Newer drugs such as sitagliptin are also known to be associated with cough. Aspirin sensitivity, along with another non-steroidal anti-inflammatory drug (NSAID)

sensitivity is known to be prevalent in around 4% of asthmatics, and the response may range from mild cough to a very severe asthma attack needing intensive care unit admission. Aspirin inhibits the cyclooxygenase pathway which in some cases leads to an increase in leukotrienes as well as the reduction of protective prostanoids. Studies have confirmed increased LTC4 in serum and urine after an aspirin challenge. The use of beta-blockers can cause bronchospasm in selected 11% of subjects, which can lead to cough. Bradykinins and tachykinins are released regularly in the airways which are degraded by the ACE released from the airway epithelium. Inhibition of this enzyme due to the use of ACE inhibitors can stimulate RARs and cause cough in 5%–30% of patients. Sitagliptin is a dipeptidyl peptidase-4 inhibitor, used in type II diabetes, that can cause cough in about 5% of patients with allergic rhinitis with or without asthma. The mechanism is similar to ACE inhibitor–induced cough with inadequate degradation of the neuropeptides and cytokines causing both rhinorrhea and cough.

Environmental and occupational history should never be ignored in the evaluation of cough. If these are not recognized and managed (avoided or treated), cough may never be controlled. The injury-causing cough due to these environmental and occupational exposures could be direct or indirect. Construction dust, other particulate matter, and gaseous vapor exposure are common examples of direct exposures causing cough. Increasing inflammation or increasing neurogenic sensitivity (vagal and trigeminal nerves, cough receptors such as C-fibers and RARs) causing cough are common indirect mechanisms.

Environmental triggers can be indoors or outdoors, allergic or irritant. Important indoor triggers for cough that many patients do not realize include burning of mosquito coils (in all forms: electric and non-electric), incense sticks, dhoop sticks, biomass fuel burning for both cooking and heating purposes, renovation of houses with new paints, cleaning solutions, solvents, glues, insecticides, pesticides among others. Particulate matter during construction is a big hazard with many subjects having recalcitrant cough that resolves only after the construction/renovation is

completed. During renovation, there is also a risk of heavy exposure to house dust mites and molds. Pigeon or bird feathers in pillows and blankets are another important source to be considered. Outdoor triggers could be related to construction/demolition activity or road-building activities in the neighborhood or due to various pollens such as weeds, grasses, and trees.

Many occupations are known to be associated with cough and need careful history to unravel the temporal association between the onset of cough and work. In many cases, subjects work for many years before they develop sensitization and clinical symptoms. Absence of symptoms when away from work on holidays and recurrence of symptoms on reporting back to work are important clues that can lead to more objective testing with serial peak flow meter readings, spirometry before and after exposure at work, or an actual challenge of the offending agent in the subject's occupation in the laboratory. A few common occupations that cause cough are construction work, exposure to silk moths and boiling of cocoons, brick kilns, curing of tobacco, harvesting, agriculture, welding, metal and gas exposures, garbage collectors, sugar factory, and cotton and textile mill workers.

Cough is induced mainly by the sensory receptors (RARs) and the C-fibers that cause neurogenic inflammation. The most common cause of cough is airway diseases that include both the upper and lower airways. Infections both in the upper airways and lower airways caused by both viruses and bacteria may damage the airway epithelium. There may be an increase in the endogenous tachykinins due to the reduction in endopeptidases. This reduces the threshold for triggering the RARs and C-fibers by various irritants causing cough. Postnasal drip syndrome, a common outcome of both infective and allergic rhinosinusitis, causes cough due to the entry of the inflammatory secretions into the larynx. Pharyngeal irritation as such does not cause cough as it is innervated by the glossopharyngeal nerve and not the vagus. In asthma and chronic bronchitis, various allergens and noxious particles directly (tobacco smoke, biomass

smoke) or indirectly (inflammatory mediators, mucus secretion) activate the RARs and C-fibers inducing cough. Gastroesophageal reflux, another common cause of cough is due to the activation of sensory receptors in the distal esophagus. Other pathologies causing cough include inflammatory and neoplastic diseases, dealt with in detail elsewhere.

The common types of cough and their causes are enumerated in Table 1.

Table 1

Type of cough	Common causes
Dry cough	Early LRTI, URTI, asthma, bronchiolitis, ILD, drug induced (ACEI, aspirin, beta-blockers, sitagliptin)
Productive cough	URTI, LRTI, suppurative lung disease, asthma, COPD, PTB
Brassy cough	Cough with a metallic sound produced by compression of the trachea
Bovine cough	Cough with the absence of phonation-recurrent laryngeal nerve palsy
Barking cough	Acute or chronic laryngitis, tracheomalacia, somatic cough
Postural cough	Lung abscess, bronchiectasis, bronchopleural fistula
Whooping cough	Prolonged bouts of cough followed by long inspiratory whoop
Nocturnal cough	Asthma, tropical pulmonary eosinophilia, postnasal drip

Common complications of violent cough include short-term complications such as chest pain, cough syncope, cough micturition, cough vomiting, cough defecation, rib fractures, pneumothorax, sleep disturbances, and long-term complications such as hernias. Chest pain is usually in the infraaxillary region on one or both sides and follows a few days of intense cough and is due to microtear of the muscle fibers. It is important to elucidate in the history, the temporal relationship between the onset of cough

and the onset of chest pain. If the time of onset of chest pain is simultaneous or soon after the onset of cough, then the chest pain is likely to be due to other causes. Cough syncope is observed in patients with violent bouts of continuous cough that prevent the return of vena caval blood into the right side of the heart, thus decreasing blood to the left side of the heart. Reduced left ventricular output causes reduced blood flow to the brain causing syncope. The transient loss of consciousness due to cough syncope itself does not cause any harm to the brain, as the cough immediately stops as well. But the situation that the subject is in can lead to life-threatening insults. Cough syncope when on a flight of stairs, while driving, while cooking with hot oil, or crossing a busy road can put the subject at great risk of serious injury. Increased intra-abdominal pressure can lead to cough micturition, especially in women with prolapse of the uterus. Cough syncope can be associated with both cough micturition and cough defecation. Many subjects due to the increased intra-abdominal pressure on a full stomach complain of cough-induced vomiting while eating or soon after. Elderly subjects with osteoporosis can have rib fractures after a violent bout of cough. Blebs and bulla can rupture or a sharp end of rib fracture can puncture the lung causing pneumothorax. Chronic cough especially in elderly subjects with poor anterior abdominal muscle tone is at risk for direct or indirect hernias due to repetitive instances of raised intra-abdominal pressure.

Approach to a patient with a cough

The expert group from the American College of Chest Physicians (ACCP, 2018) has recommended that the patients be classified into three groups based on the duration of cough that may give a clue to the etiologies and thus the investigations that need to be undertaken. Acute cough are those that are less than 3 weeks of duration, subacute cough are of 3–8 weeks of duration, and chronic coughs are those that are lasting for more than 8 weeks (Figure 3). The list of causes in Figure 3 is only indicative and not exhaustive and may fit into multiple categories at different time points. For example, non-infective causes such as bronchiectasis due to ciliary

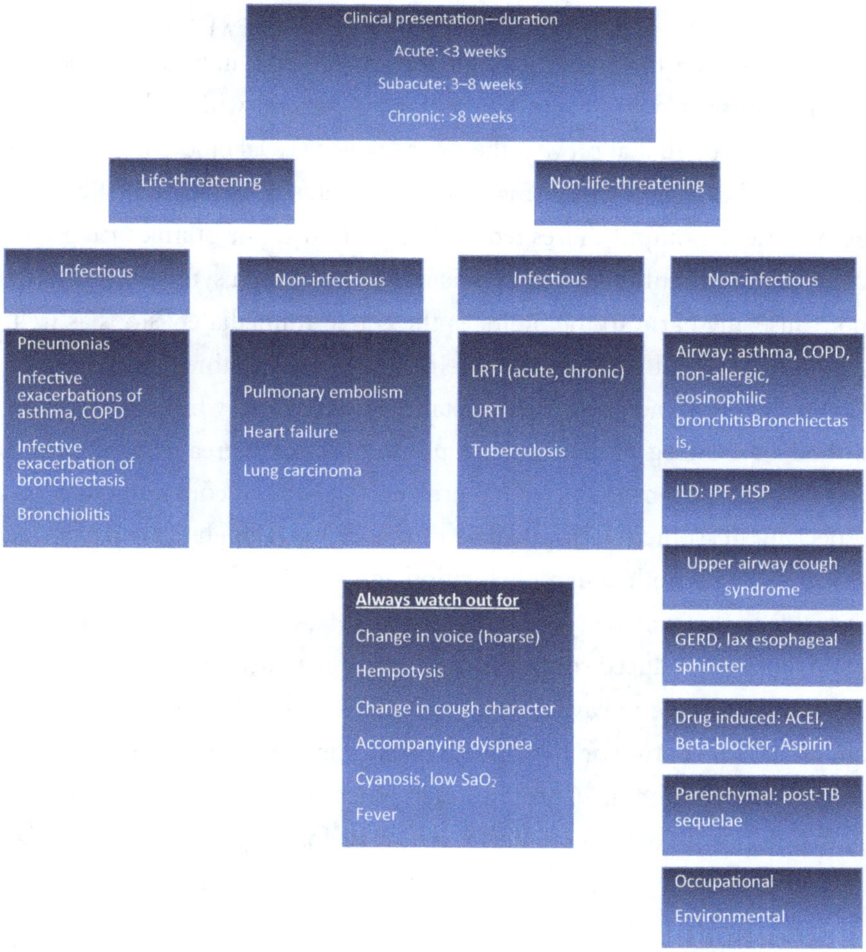

Figure 3: Approach to cough (adapted from ACCP Cough Guidelines, 2018).

dyskinesias may have an infective exacerbation, which may or may not be life-threatening.

The investigations for the confirmation of diagnosis and management of each of the conditions listed in Figure 3 are discussed in their respective chapters. In brief, some specific investigations include CT PNS, HRCT thorax (both inspiratory and expiratory films), CT pulmonary angiogram, 24-hour esophageal pH monitoring, Barium swallow, esophageal motility studies, spirometry, DLCO, arterial blood gases, bronchoscopy, nasopharyngeal endoscopy, sputum eosinophilia, FENO, allergy testing, and

occupational and environmental assessments. Common treatments used depending on the diagnosis include antihistamines, decongestants, inhaled corticosteroids, inhaled beta-agonists, inhaled anticholinergics, avoidance of the drugs causing cough, avoidance of environmental and occupational allergens and irritants, parental steroids, antifibrotic agents for IPF, postural drainage, antibiotics when indicated, leukotrienes, acid suppression and antireflux measures (both pharmacological and non-pharmacological), and aids to quitting smoking.

Problem-based learning

Case 1

A 50-year-old obese woman presented with a history of intractable cough, first triggered by an upper respiratory infection, for the last 2 years, not responding to treatment by multiple physicians. Initially, there was partial relief from her symptoms, but there was no response in the last 10 months, when cough was present every day. Cough was debilitating with severe impairment of sleep and daily activities. Cough was worst at night and early morning and worse during rainy and winter seasons. She complained of mild heartburn. She was on treatment almost daily for the last 9 months with various cough syrups, multiple courses of antibiotics, pantoprazole, multiple short courses of oral steroids, and daily oral bronchodilators. She was a diabetic on oral hypoglycemics and hypertensive on antihypertensive drugs and both were under good control. Her physician changed her antihypertensives (ACE inhibitors) after the onset of cough, which did not give her much relief. Her chest X-ray and HRCT thorax were normal.

What would be your approach in this case?

As discussed earlier in the text, there are many cases with multiple causes of cough and non-responsiveness needs to be carefully re-evaluated. Subjects who are obese are particularly prone to such severe unresponsive cough. On careful evaluation, these are the additional findings of clinical relevance that were observed. Managing these issues led to the amelioration of her cough.

a. She used mosquito coils (liquidators) and at least 10 incense sticks every day. Studies have shown that these are equivalent to burning more than 100 cigarettes within the house per day. These exposures in allergic subjects can change the eosinophilic inflammation to neutrophilic inflammation, which then does not respond to steroids. Stopping these environmental insults can help the inflammation to revert back to steroid-responsive eosinophilic inflammation.
b. Additional drug that needed to be asked was sitagliptin. ACE inhibitors were changed but not sitagliptin, which also can cause cough.
c. On clinical evaluation, she had throat clearing during interview and postnasal drip on examination, which needed intranasal steroids and leukotriene antagonists.
d. Her spirometry, which was not done earlier, revealed moderate obstruction with reversibility of more than 12%, needing regular ICS + LABA. Short courses of oral steroids may not help.
e. Her GERD needs additional measures (pharmacological and non-pharmacological) to PPIs. Oral bronchodilators (beta-agonists) also cause relaxation of the lower esophageal sphincter and needs to be avoided.
f. Obstructive sleep apneas (OSAs) are also associated with intractable cough. She had excessive daytime sleepiness and an Epworth's sleepiness score of 15. Her neck circumference was 22, and her sleep study showed severe OSA. Studies have confirmed the usefulness of treating OSA with CPAP with additional benefits in improving chronic cough in these subjects.

Case 2

A 70-year-old man who has been suffering from asthma for the last 30 years presents to the clinic with non-responsive cough for 3 months. He is on regular inhaled medications (ICS+LABA) for his asthma for the last 20 years, and his asthma has been under good control. He does not have any upper respiratory symptoms, and his cough which started 3 months ago was not triggered by a upper respiratory infection. He has no wheeze and feels tired only on severe exertion, which he has noticed recently. He is not

on any drugs that can cause cough. There are no environmental or occupational triggers. He has never smoked. His cardiovascular status has been evaluated by electrocardiography (ECG) and echocardiography (ECHO) and is found to be normal. There is no anemia and no other comorbidities. His chest X-ray is normal. Pre- and postbronchodilator spirometry is normal.

How do you approach this case?

New onset of cough in a well-controlled asthmatic who is adherent to medications and also has normal spirometry points towards a different pathology. In the elderly, two possibilities in this situation are important. Malignancy and interstitial lung disease (ILD). In this case, on inching auscultation (every inch of the chest has to be auscultated), a 1 cm bibasal fine end-inspiratory velcro crepitations were heard. This can indicate either interstitial lung disease or in the elderly small airway disease or chronic heart failure, which can have similar velcro crepitations. A high-resolution CT scan with supine and prone films to rule out gravitation as a cause of minimal subpleural interstitial shadows and inspiratory and expiratory films would help differentiate between ILD and small airway disease. An elevated BNP can indicate chronic heart failure even when ECG and ECHO are normal (heart failure with normal or preserved ejection fraction). This case had a new-onset IPF and that was the reason for the unresponsive cough for asthma medications.

Hemoptysis

One of the dreaded symptoms in respiratory medicine is hemoptysis, which is the coughing of blood from the respiratory tract. Patients may wait for months or years before seeking medical attention for cough but will usually seek a doctor quickly if they have hemoptysis. Hemoptysis is from the Greek words "haima" meaning "blood" and "ptysis," which means "spitting." Hemoptysis can range from blood-streaking of sputum to a more serious expectoration of gross blood or blood clots in the absence of any accompanying sputum. Hemoptysis is classified as "massive" if the

subject coughs out blood more than 600 mL per day or 150 mL per episode. The mortality rates vary from 25% to 83%.

Vascular origin of hemoptysis

Blood flowing through the pulmonary system comes from the pulmonary or bronchial circulation. Most of the cardiac output flows through the low-pressure pulmonary circulation while a small portion of the cardiac output (1%–3%) flows through the bronchial arteries under much higher (systemic) pressure. Bronchial circulation supplies the bronchi up to terminal bronchioles. Though blood flowing through the bronchial circulation is much less, it is the most important source of clinically important hemoptysis. Bronchial arteries supply the airways and in subjects with hemoptysis, develop hypervascularity, tortuousness, and aneurysms. Bronchial arteries are responsible for around 90% of hemoptysis, whereas pulmonary arteries are responsible for around 10% of the cases. In rare cases, intercostal arteries can be involved.

Differential diagnosis of hemoptysis

One of the important tasks before the clinician deals with hemoptysis is to confirm whether the source of bleeding is from the pulmonary system or whether there is a possibility that blood may be coming from a non-pulmonary source, such as the upper airway including paranasal sinuses, oral cavity including gingival bleeding, or the gastrointestinal (GI) tract (esophagus, stomach, duodenum).

These are important differences for the clinician to suspect whether the source of the bleeding is pulmonary or non-pulmonary, but most of these are not confirmatory. In an emergency one can differentiate hemoptysis from hematemesis by inserting a Ryle's tube and lavage with saline, in case of hematemesis bloody lavage is seen while in case of hemoptysis it is usually clear. However, this is not a confirmatory test and only helps in situations where there is a time constraint. The clinician should always

Table 2: Difference between hemoptysis and hematemesis

Characteristic	Hemoptysis	Hematemesis
Definition	Coughing of blood	Vomiting of blood
Colour	Bright red	Coffee ground
pH	Alkaline pH	Acidic pH
Appearance	May be frothy	Food particles
Associated symptoms	Usually no nausea and vomiting	Nausea and vomiting
Associated symptoms	Cough usually dominant	Cough may be present
Previous disease	Respiratory	Gastrointestinal (GI)
Melena	Absent	Seen in large upper GI bleed
Sputum mixed blood	Can be present (when present confirms upper or lower respiratory source)	Always absent
Diagnosis	Bronchoscopy Bronchial arteriography	Endoscopy Stool for occult blood

carefully consider both sources. For example, though hematemesis is coffee ground in color when it comes from the stomach, it will be bright red if it comes out directly from the esophagus in a patient with esophageal varices in portal hypertension. A subject with hemoptysis may swallow the blood and due to gastric irritation from the iron in the blood can then vomit it out. When endoscopy does not show any evidence of injury in the upper GI tract, then pulmonary source has to be suspected. Fallacies of measuring the pH are much the same as evaluating the color. Many risk factors for pulmonary and GI disease are similar. Many alcoholics may also smoke, and liver disease (cirrhosis) may increase the risk of developing tuberculosis, which then may cause hemoptysis. Similarly, smoking is an important risk factor for pulmonary diseases associated with hemoptysis such as tuberculosis, and lung cancer is also a risk factor for duodenal ulcer. Assessing risk factors, thus, though of value has to be viewed with all the other factors (the whole clinical picture).

Some factors have more value in differentiating between hemoptysis and hematemesis. The presence of melena has a much stronger relevance favoring hematemesis and indicates a fairly large upper GI bleed. It is very difficult for the subject with hemoptysis to swallow so much blood as to cause melena and is more likely to vomit what they have swallowed. For the pulmonary source of bleeding, the presence of sputum streaked with blood is 100% confirmatory that blood is coming from a pulmonary source that includes the upper airways.

Causes of hemoptysis

The most common causes of hemoptysis are infective, neoplastic, and inflammatory causes. Cardiac causes including drugs should be kept in mind especially in the elderly, and foreign bodies in children should always be kept in mind. Table 3 lists some common and rare causes of hemoptysis and is by no means complete.

The initial history and clinical examination should give rise to appropriate suspicion of the source of bleeding so that relevant investigations can be undertaken to confirm the final diagnosis. In many countries, infections such as tuberculosis are the most common cause of hemoptysis, which can be less severe (50 mL/day or less) due to vascular granulation tissue, mucosal ulceration, bronchiolar erosion during active tubercular pneumonitis, scar carcinoma, or massive hemoptysis (>200 mL/day) due to the rupture of Rasmussen's aneurysm, post-tubercular bronchiectasis, mycetoma, usually aspergilloma causing vasculitis and vascular erosions in a preexisting cavity or a calcified lymph node eroding the airway and bronchial arteries.

In patients with bronchiectasis, there will be a development of peribronchial and submucosal arteriolar anastomosis, bronchial and pulmonary vascular anastomosis, and hypertrophy of the bronchial arteries. In patients with mycetoma (aspergillosis), additionally vascular injury can occur due to proteases and endotoxin from *Aspergillus* or an immune complex–mediated reaction. In patients with malignant pulmonary tumors, necrosis of the tumors and inflammation of the vessels can lead to hemoptysis.

Table 3: Common and rare causes of hemoptysis

Source	Common causes	Rare causes
Airways	Bronchiectasis, cystic fibrosis, acute bronchitis, chronic bronchitis, lung cancer, foreign body, airway trauma	Carcinoid, endobronchial metastasis, Kaposi's sarcoma catamenial (endometriosis), broncholith
Parenchyma	Active tuberculosis, post-tubercular sequelae, pneumonia (viral, bacterial, fungal), aspergilloma, lung cancer, lung abscess, endobronchial biopsy, transbronchial biopsy), lung contusion, pneumoconiosis, inhalational injury (burns, cocaine), transthoracic lung biopsy)	Kaposi's sarcoma, catamenial (endometriosis), cavernolith, actinomycosis, cocardiosis, invasive fungal infections, parasitosis, non-tubercular *Mycobacteria*
Interstitium		Goodpasture's syndrome Idiopathic hemosiderosis Polyarteritis nodosa
Vascular	Pulmonary embolism Primary pulmonary hypertension	Tracheoinnominate fistula Aneurysm of aorta leading to fistulous communication with the airway
Systemic	Bleeding diathesis Leukemia Hemophilia	Wegener's granulomatosis Lupus pneumonitis, amyloidosis
Cardiac	Mitral stenosis with pulmonary hypertension Left ventricular failure Tricuspid valve endocarditis	VSD with pulmonary hypertension
Drugs	Warfarin, antiplatelet drugs, NSAIDs, thrombolytic agents	Bevacizumab, sildenafil, amiodarone
Cryptogenic	No known cause identified	

Pseudohemoptysis

This relates to the presence of red-colored sputum in the absence of red blood cells (RBCs). This is seen in *Serratia marcescens* infection and is due to the presence of a red-colored pigment known as prodigiosin, which is responsible for the color.

Clinical approach

A clinician's approach to a patient with hemoptysis should look into the localization of the source of bleeding, the cause of bleeding, and the management of hemoptysis.

Localization: Sometimes, the localization of the source of bleeding is easy as there is only one obvious source, for example, a cavity in the lung (Figure 4). In others, especially due to the bilateral bronchiectasis (Figure 5) or bilateral post-tubercular sequelae it may be difficult to know where the bleeding is coming from. In such situations, localization can be done either by bronchoscopy or by bronchial arteriography. Actual visualization during bronchoscopy can localize it to a particular segment or subsegment of the lung. One should be careful if those are the dependent regions of the lung, since blood from elsewhere can move into those segments due to gravitational aspiration. For an endobronchial lesion, bronchoscopy is ideal which in addition would help in the pathological diagnosis. In bilateral parenchymal lesions, bronchial arteriography is ideal to localize the bleeding. Some of the findings include a "flush" when the dye moves out of the arteries, hypertrophic and tortuous arteries, aneurysms, and anastomosis. There are instances when there is bleeding from more than one site (Figures 6 and 7). This subject had post-tubercular sequelae with partial destruction of the left upper lobe and very minimal bronchiectasis of the right lower lobe. On bronchial arteriography, there was evidence of bleeding from both the left upper lobe (not shown) and right lower lobe vessels.

Causes: To identify the cause of bleeding, a careful history, physical examination, and relevant investigations need to be undertaken (Table 4). HRCT

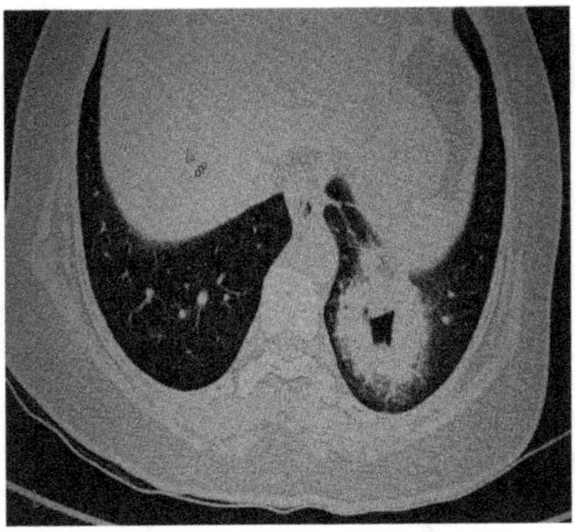

Figure 4: Cavity in left lower lobe causing hemoptysis.

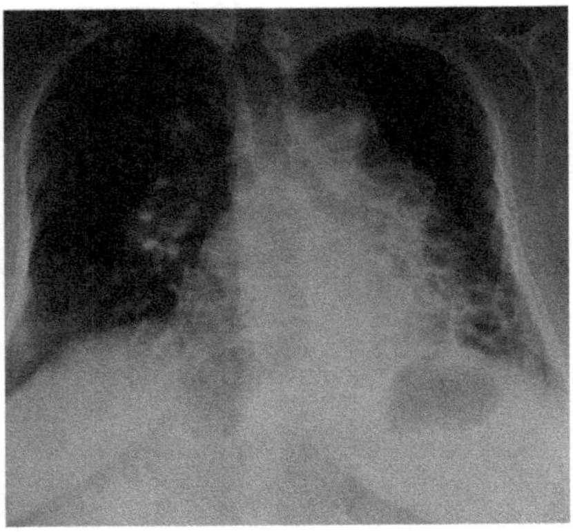

Figure 5: Bilateral bronchiectasis left more than right causing hemoptysis.

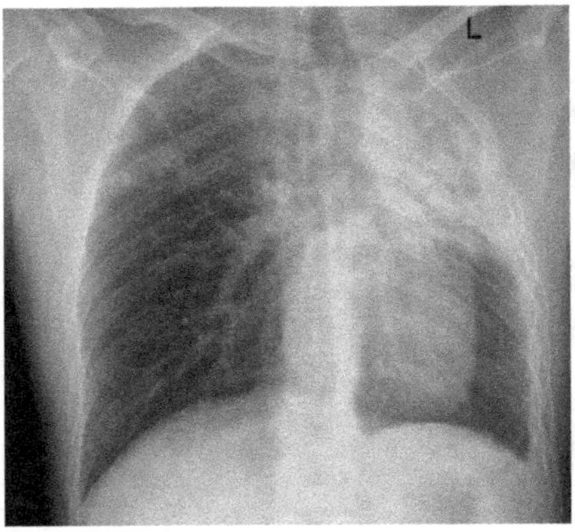

Figure 6: post tubercular sequlae the partial destruction on left upper lobe ad minimal bronchiectasis on right lower lobe.

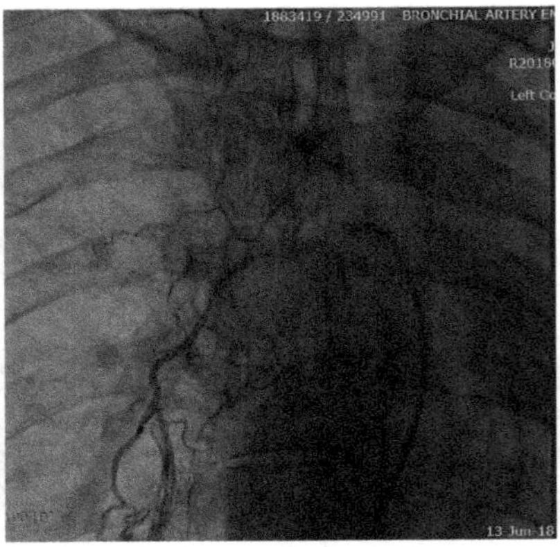

Figure 7: Bronchial arteriography, there was evidence of bleeding from both the left upper lobe (not shown) and right lower lobe vessels.

References — figure.

Source: By Hemoptysis.png: Original uploader was Garbass at en.wikipedia derivative work: Faigl.ladislav (talk) — Hemoptysis.png, Public Domain, https://commons.wikimedia.org/w/index.php?curid=8121077

is more sensitive than chest X-ray and is more important for parenchymal lesions as well as airway lesions such as bronchiectasis. Bronchoscopy is more useful for endobronchial lesions, especially mucosal abnormalities that cannot be visualized in an HRCT. The common causes are listed in

Table 4: Summary of clinical approach and important considerations in evaluating a patient with hemoptysis

Clinical approach	Important considerations
Demography	Variables such as age, gender, area of residence (endemic region for tuberculosis)
History	• Prior lung, cardiac, liver, or renal disease • Details of cigarette smoking and other recreational drugs such as marijuana and cocaine • Prior episodes of hemoptysis, quantity, duration, treatment taken, and other pulmonary symptoms including recent infections • Family history of hemoptysis or brain aneurysms (suggesting hereditary hemorrhagic telangiectasia) • History of skin rash • Travel history • Any asbestos exposure • Previous bleeding disorders or use of aspirin, non-steroidal anti-inflammatory drugs, or anticoagulants? • History of upper airway or upper gastrointestinal complaints or diseases
Clinical examination	• An erythematous skin rash which is non-blanching and having more pain than itching may be suggestive of vasculitis • Splinter hemorrhages suggest endocarditis or vasculitis • Clubbing may occur in many chronic diseases of the lungs, heart, and liver • Loss of lung volume may suggest fibrosis (usually post-tubercular) or collapse (malignancy in adults and foreign body in children) • Chronic thromboembolic pulmonary hypertension may be suggested by an augmented P2, murmurs of tricuspid regurgitation or pulmonic insufficiency, or a right ventricular lift • Cardiac murmurs also raise the question of congenital heart disease, endocarditis with septic emboli, or, when a diastolic rumble or opening snap is present, mitral stenosis

	• The lower limbs are examined for signs of deep venous thrombi • Bilateral pedal edema may suggest right ventricular failure • Presence of many telangiectasias suggests hereditary hemorrhagic telangiectasia
Laboratory investigations	• Chest X-ray for localization of lesion and cause • HRCT thorax for better localization of lesion and cause • Bronchoscopy for localization of lesion and cause • Bronchial arteriography for confirming bleeding vessels and plan intervention • Hematocrit, urinalysis, blood urea nitrogen, and plasma creatinine concentration, a coagulation profile • Sputum for cytologic and microbiologic studies, including Ziehl–Neelsen stain, fluorescence stain, or TB-PCR. • Serologic tests for Wegener's granulomatosis, systemic lupus erythematosus, or Goodpasture's syndrome • An echocardiogram may detect endocarditis, mitral stenosis, congenital heart disease, or pulmonary hypertension • A transesophageal echocardiogram may identify a thoracic aortic aneurysm as the cause of hemoptysis

Table 3, and the specific investigations for the diagnosis of each of those are enumerated in the respective chapters.

Acute management

Massive hemoptysis is one of the common and important medical emergencies, and the initial priorities include securing the airway for adequate airway protection, maintaining ventilation and cardiovascular function, and the control of bleeding. Life-threatening hemoptysis can lead to rapid exsanguination in a short time in some patients leading to hypotension and cardiovascular compromise. Bilateral extensive destroyed lung due to tuberculosis, aspergilloma with vasculitis, and Wegener's granulomatosis are some common causes of life-threatening hemoptysis. Even smaller hemoptysis that can clot in the trachea can be life-threatening. Patients with poor gas exchange (not maintaining saturation), rapid ongoing hemoptysis, hemodynamic instability, or severe shortness of breath should have their airways secured by a large bore endotracheal tube (size 8.0 or greater). Any coagulation disorders should be rapidly reversed. Once bleeding is controlled, then the subject should be investigated for the localization of the bleeding and the cause of bleeding.

Protection of the non-bleeding lung

In many cases, especially in those with unilateral disease, the side of bleeding is known and the bleeding lung should be in a dependent position. This will help to prevent blood spillage into the major airways or trachea and the non-bleeding lung. Alternatively, in an emergency, the placement of a typical, single-lumen endotracheal tube into the bronchus in the non-bleeding lung secures the airway from being flooded during massive hemoptysis. Where facilities are available, a double-lumen endotracheal tube specially designed for selective intubation of the right or left mainstem bronchi can be placed to secure the airway.

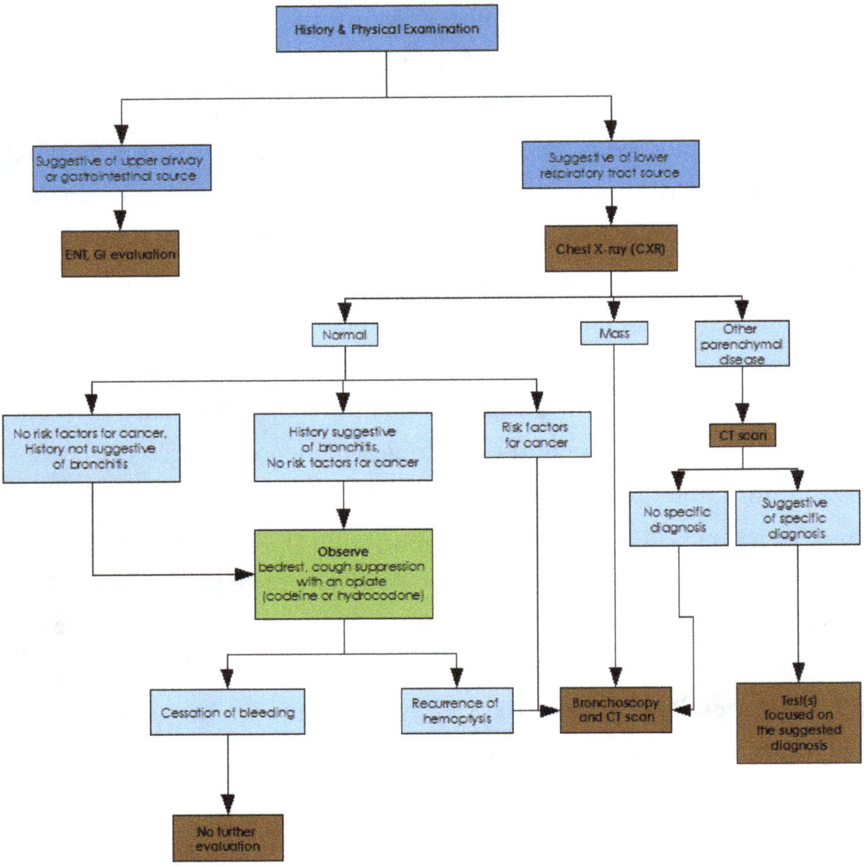

Algorithm for the investigational evaluation of a subject with hemoptysis
Source: By Hemoptysis.png: Original uploader was Garbass at en.wikipediaderivative work: Faigl.ladislav (talk) — Hemoptysis.png, Public Domain, https://commons.wikimedia.org/w/index.php?curid=8121077.

Use of bronchoscopy in the acute management

Initially performed with the rigid bronchoscopes only, now balloon tamponade is regularly performed with a flexible fiberoptic bronchoscope, which involves placing a Fogarty balloon catheter (number 4 French, 100 cm) in the subsegmental or segmental bronchus under vision to protect the contralateral aspiration of the blood into the non-bleeding lungs. The inflated balloon is left in situ for usually 24 hours, sometimes up to

48 hours. Then the balloon is deflated in situ, and the patient is observed for rebleeding for several hours. If there is no rebleeding the catheter is removed. This has been successfully used during the last few decades as an important life-saving tool in massive hemoptysis for causes ranging from tuberculosis, bronchiectasis, thoracic trauma, and iatrogenic complications such as rupture of the pulmonary artery during catheterization. There is a theoretical risk for ischemic mucosal injury at the site of inflation or atelectasis but have not been commonly reported.

Other bronchoscopic techniques that have not been tested in controlled trials but could be used in the management of hemoptysis are systematic lavage with iced saline, application of topical epinephrine (1:20,000), vasopressin, thrombin, or a fibrinogen–thrombin combination. If a localized mucosal lesion is identified, laser or electrocautery can be an option. Topical hemostatic tamponade therapy has been tried with good success. This uses a knitted fabric, oxidized regenerated cellulose that is placed at the site of bleeding. Many layers of cellulose (up to 10) can be used to tightly pack and close the bleeding airway. It can even be used on an endobronchial lung cancer. Once the cellulose is saturated with blood, it helps in clot formation due to its physical properties and helps to stop the bleeding.

Bronchial artery embolization

One of the key options for the evaluation and treatment of large or massive bleeding is bronchial artery embolization (BAE), which can be used as an emergency measure to control the bleeding as a "semidefinitive" measure or to stabilize the patient to prepare him for surgery. BAE is successful in stopping bleeding in more than 85% of the subjects. Over the next 6–12 months, up to 20% of the subjects may experience a recurrence of hemoptysis. The main reasons for late rebleeding are incomplete embolization, revascularization of the diseased lung, recanalization of the blocked artery, or the presence of non-bronchial systemic artery as the source of bleeding. It is the only treatment available for subjects who are not candidates for surgery due to poor lung reserve or bilateral lung disease.

Various materials are used to block the bronchial artery; some are permanent, others temporary. Permanent occlusive materials include polyvinyl alcohol (PVA), trisacryl gelatin microspheres, gelfoam, platinum microcoils, while the temporary materials include absorbable gelatin sponge and thrombin. Liquid embolic agents should always be avoided since they are known to cause tissue infarction.

The most important complication is transverse myelitis due to the occlusion of anterior spinal artery that may originate from the bronchial artery. The risks and benefits should be carefully evaluated in this situation, and BAE is done much more distally to avoid the possibility of the retrograde movement of embolizing material from the bronchial artery into the anterior spinal artery. Blocking of the anterior spinal artery leads to the disruption of the bilateral corticospinal tracts (motor deficit) and spinothalamic tract (sensory deficit). The most common complication is chest pain after the procedure. Another important complication is dysphagia due to the embolization of the esophageal branches. Equally serious but rare complications include aortic and bronchial necrosis, bronchoesophageal fistula, pulmonary infarction, and non-target organ embolization such as ischemic colitis.

Role of surgery in the management of hemoptysis

Surgical resection is an important consideration in subjects with localized disease with massive bleeding and should be assessed early in the course of disease. Surgery can be a definitive treatment for hemoptysis when the disease is not bilateral or progressive. For example, a post-tubercular cavity in the right upper lobe that is bleeding is a good candidate for surgery, whereas congenital bronchiectasis (e.g., ciliary dyskinesia such as Kartagener's syndrome) that is significant only in the left lower lobe at present and is minimal on the right lower lobe is not a good candidate for surgery due to the possibility of worsening in the right lung at a later date. Subjects have higher morbidity and mortality with emergency surgery for massive hemoptysis as compared to elective surgery after stabilizing the patient. Some contraindi-

cations for surgery include severe underlying bilateral pulmonary disease with poor lung reserve, active tuberculosis, or diffuse underlying lung disease (cystic fibrosis, multiple AVMs, multifocal bronchiectasis).

Dyspnea

Definition

- Dyspnea is defined as difficult or labored breathing or unpleasant awareness of one own breathing.
- American Thoracic Society defines dyspnea as a subjective experience of breathing discomfort that consists of qualitatively distinct sensations that vary in intensity.

Mechanism of dyspnea

- Respiratory consequences of interactions between the efferent sensations are the motor output from the brain to the ventilator muscles and the efferent, that is, sensory input from receptors throughout the body (feedback) which are integrated into the brain.

Peripheral chemoreceptors

- These are the carotid bodies and the aortic bodies, they sense the PCO_2 and pH of the blood.
- They are connected to the respiratory centers via the ninth (carotid bodies) and 10th (aortic bodies) nerves.
- When there is increased PCO_2, decreased PO_2, or decreased pH, they are stimulated and lead to the stimulation of respiration.

Central chemoreceptors

- The chemoreceptors present in the brain are called central chemoreceptors.
- Situation — they are situated in deeper parts of the medulla oblongata, close to the dorsal group of neurons. This area is a chemosensitive area, and neurons are called chemoreceptors.
- They are very sensitive to increase in hydrogen ion concentration.

- Hydrogen ion concentration cannot cross the blood–brain barrier (BBB) and blood–cerebrospinal fluid barrier.
- The hydrogen ion on crossing BBB stimulates the central chemoreceptors, which stimulates the dorsal group of the respiratory center (inspiratory group) and increases the rate and force of breathing.

Etiology of dyspnea

Causes of acute dyspnea

- Acute pulmonary edema
- Pneumothorax
- Acute pulmonary embolism
- Pneumonia
- Foreign body obstruction of the airway
- Myocardial infarction (MI)

Respiratory causes of dyspnea

- Diseases of airway — COPD, asthma, bronchiectasis, and bronchiolitis.
- Diseases of chest wall — kyphoscoliosis, weakness of respiratory muscles in diseases such as Gullian — Barre syndrome and myasthenia gravis.
- Diseases of lung parenchyma — destroyed lung, autoimmune disorders, infections, and occupational exposure.
- Diseases of interstitium — idiopathic pulmonary fibrosis, hypersensitivity pneumonitis, sarcoidosis, PCP, viral pneumonias, and atypical pneumonias.
- Diseases of pleura — massive pleural effusion, empyema, pneumothorax, hydropneumothorax and pyopneumothorax.
- Diseases of vessels — PTE, PAH and pulmonary vasculitis.

Cardiovascular causes

- Myocardial infarction
- Non-ischemic cardiomyopathy
- Constrictive pericarditis
- Cardiac tamponade

Miscellaneous causes

- Anemia
- Obstructive sleep apnea
- Anxiety disorder

Variants of dyspnea

- Hyperventilation.
- It is the state of breathing faster or deeper than normal.
- It can result from a psychological state such as panic attack or metabolic acidosis or can be brought about voluntarily.

It reduces the CO_2 concentration of the blood to below its normal level and thereby raising the blood pH (alkalosis) and causing muscle cramps and tetany.

- Orthopnea
  - It refers to dyspnea in a recumbent position relieved by sitting or standing.
  - Increased venous return increases in right ventricular pressure and pulmonary venous congestion.
  - In cor pulmonale, right-sided heart starts to fail because of high pulmonary artery pressure (pressure overload).

Causes:

- Left heart failure
- COPD
- Pericardial effusion (Figure 8)
- Constrictive pericarditis
- Massive ascites
- Right heart failure
- B/L diaphragmatic paralysis

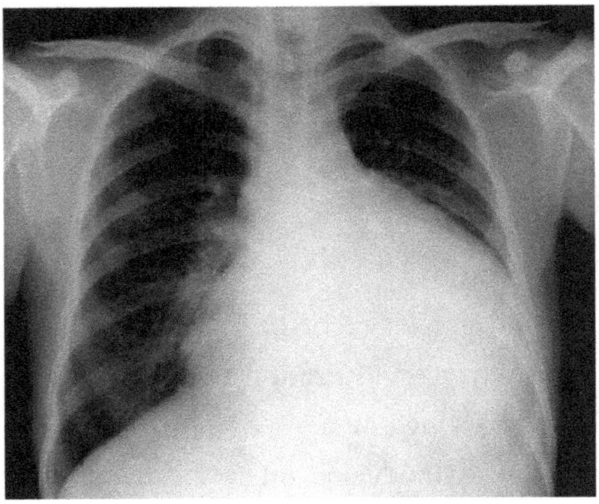

Figure 8: Pericardial effusion.

Paroxysmal nocturnal dyspnea

Dyspnea occurs at night that awakens the patient from sleep usually 1–3 hours after sleep. The patient may gasp and proceed to a window for fresh air. The dyspnea tends to resolve in 10–30 minutes. Paroxysmal nocturnal dyspnea (PND) almost always implies heart failure.

Conditions that mimic PND:

1. Nocturnal episodes of asthma
2. Sleep apnea with arousal
3. Cheyne stokes breathing
4. Postnasal drip (severe cough may end up with dyspnea)
5. Anxiety with hyperventilation
6. Nocturnal aspiration in GERD, especially when there is laryngospasm

- Trepopnea
  - Dyspnea occurring in lateral decubitus position.
  - It results from diseases of one lung, one major bronchus, or chronic congestive heart failure (CHF).

  - To maximize the function of the healthier lung, the best position for the patient is to lie on the side of the healthier lung, so that it maintains adequate perfusion.
- Platypnea
  - Dyspnea that worsens while standing or sitting and relieved in lying down position.
  - A related condition called orthodeoxia describes the clinical condition of low oxygen saturation in the upright position, which improves when lying down.
  - Platypnea and orthodeoxia often coexist, and this condition is named as orthodeoxia syndrome.
  - Causes: hepatopulmonary syndrome, right to left shunt.

Severity of dyspnea

Many scales are used for grading dyspnea. The most simple and important is the MMRC grading. The other scales are the Borg scale and the New York Heart Association classification.

MMRC grading for dyspnea

- Grade 0: breathlessness on exertion only
- Grade 1: breathlessness on hurrying on level ground or walking on uphill
- Grade 2: breathlessness while walking at same pace as a peer of your age or having to stop for breath when walking at my own pace on the level
- Grade 3: breathlessness on walking 100 m or for a few minutes on the level ground
- Grade 4: breathlessness on rest and not able to leave home

Borg scale

- 0: no breathlessness at all
- 0.5: very very slight (just noticeable)
- 1: very slight
- 2: slight breathlessness

- 3: moderate
- 4: somewhat severe
- 5: severe breathlessness
- 7: very severe breathlessness
- 9: very very severe (almost maximum)
- 10: maximum

Evaluation of patients with dyspnea

- Duration: depending on the duration of onset, dyspnea is classified into acute and chronic
- Acute onset: 24 to 48 hours
- Chronic: lasts more than 1 month
- Time of onset:

  Early morning — asthma

  Nocturnal — CHF

  COPD

  Asthma

  OSA

  Mitral valve disease — mitral stenosis
- Drugs causing dyspnea:
  - Beta-blockers (causes bronchospasm)
  - Nitrofurantoin and amiodarone (drug-induced lung diseases such as fibrosis)
  - Aspirin (hypersensitivity reactions causing bronchospasm)
  - Dapsone and sulfonamides — sulfhemoglobinemia
  - Nitrites and nitrates — methemoglobinemia
  - Quinidine and penicillin — hemolytic anemia
- Previous history:
  - Cardiac disease:
    - Enquire about cardiovascular risk factors (smoking, hypertension, diabetes, hypercholesterolemia).
    - If a risk factor is present, then enquire about previous MI, coronary angiography, or CABG surgery.

- Respiratory disease:
  - Enquire about the history of chronic lung diseases (asthma, COPD, bronchiectasis, ILD, sarcoidosis), thrombotic risk factors, and occupational history.
  - Thyroid disease
  - Renal disease
  - Deep vein thrombosis (DVT)
  - Breast cancer, bronchogenic cancer, and lymphoma
  - Previous thoracic radiation and chemotherapy with busulfan

Associated symptoms

- Chest pain suggest underlying cardiac ischemia but rarely may be a feature of asthma or COPD. Other causes are pulmonary embolism, pneumonia, pneumothorax, angina, and anxiety
- Wheezing (suggests airway narrowing which can occur both in lung and cardiac failure)
  - Asthma
  - CHF
  - COPD
  - Foreign bodies in the airway
- Syncope
  - Pulmonary hypertension
  - Pulmonary embolism
  - Aortic stenosis
  - Dysrhythmia
- Cough

Different types of cough receptors like RARs, SAR, C-fiber receptor, and J receptors are present in the airways and lung parenchyma. Stimulation of these receptors causes cough.

Dyspnea associated with cough is found in:

- ILD
- COPD

- CHF
- Asthma
- Pulmonary edema
- Pneumonia

➤ Dysphagia
  - Granulomatous laryngitis
  - Pneumomediastinum
  - Foreign body aspiration
  - Tetanus
  - Epiglottitis

➤ Hemoptysis
  - Lung neoplasm
  - Tuberculosis
  - Pneumonia,
  - Diffuse alveolar hemorrhage
  - Bronchiectasis
  - Mitral stenosis
  - AV malformation
  - COPD

General examination

- Nose and sinuses: Dyspnea may be due to nasal obstruction, allergic rhinitis, sinusitis, and asthma.
- Cyanosis: Cyanosis is an insensitive sign of hypoxemia except when it is extreme. Look for cyanosis and if present whether it is central or peripheral.
- Central cyanosis causes:
  - Respiratory: COPD, severe acute asthma, pulmonary embolism, ILD, severe pneumonia, and hypoventilation.
  - Cardiac: Congenital heart disease, heart failure, and MI.
  - Others: High altitude, congenital cyanosis, OSA, polycythemia, methemoglobinemia, and sulfhemoglobinemia.

- Peripheral cyanosis causes:
  - Raynaud's phenomenon, heart failure, DVT, cold exposure, and arterial obstruction.

Early clubbing is an easily overlooked sign of many processes notably cancer. Extent and symmetry of chest expansion may suggest a restrictive lung or musculoskeletal disease. Cough on deep inspiration and expiration may be an early sign of asthma or ILD. Forced expiratory maneuvers may elicit the wheeze of localized (eg, endobronchial tumor) or diffuse lung disease (asthma). Edema of lower extremities suggests congestive failure if symmetric and thromboembolic disease if asymmetrical. Other physical examinations include respiratory rate, body habitus (eg, cachexia, obesity), posture, use of pursed lips, and use of accessory muscle.

Laboratory evaluation

The most useful methods of evaluating dyspnea are ECG, chest X-ray, and routine blood examination. They can help to confirm or exclude many common diagnoses.

Routine blood examination

- Anemia: Severe anemia is unusual but important cause of chronic dyspnea.
- Leukocytosis: It accompanies dyspnea in any infectious process involving respiratory system as well as in sepsis, autoimmune disease, and leukemia.
- Eosinophilia: Parasitic diseases, vasculitides (eg, Churg–Strauss syndrome), asthma, and eosinophilic pneumonia.
- Thrombocytopenia: Viral infection including severe acute respiratory syndrome and Hantavirus pulmonary syndrome.
- Erythrocytosis: Secondary erythrocytosis may be present in patients with advanced COPD.

- Cardiac enzymes: Troponin I/T, myoglobin, and CK-MB elevated in acute MI, myocarditis, Takotsubo cardiomyopathy, and hypothyroidism.

Chest imaging

Cardiomegaly with pulmonary venous congestion (Figure 9) suggests CHF or valvular heart disease, a pericardial cyst, and cardiac tamponade. Dyspnea accompanied by parenchymal infiltrates may be present in infectious pneumonia, pulmonary edema, eosinophilic pneumonitis (Figure 10), radiation pneumonitis, ILDs, and pneumoconioses. Pleural effusion may accompany CHF, liver failure, uremia, nephrotic syndrome, malignancy, pneumonia, pulmonary embolism, or pleuritis. Lung hyperinflation may be present in COPD (Figure 11), exacerbation of asthma, or foreign body aspiration. Elevation of hemidiaphragm may indicate its paralysis due to phrenic nerve paralysis. Unilateral hyperlucent lung fields may indicate pneumothorax, large bulla, or a diaphragmatic hernia (Figure 12). Prominent hilar vessels may be apparent in pulmonary hypertension pleural calcification may indicate asbestosis (Figure 13).

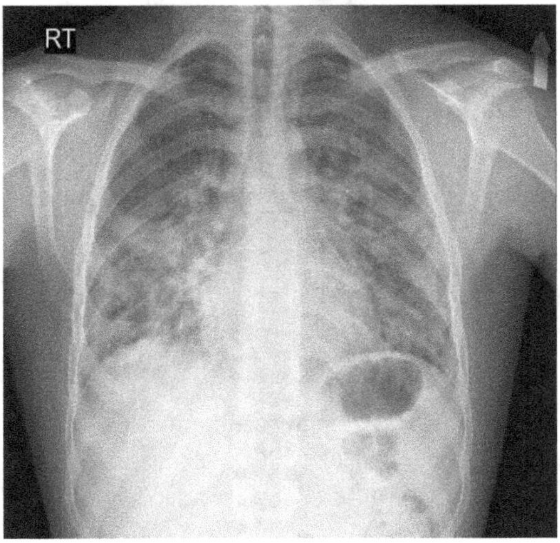

Figure 9: Venous congestion.

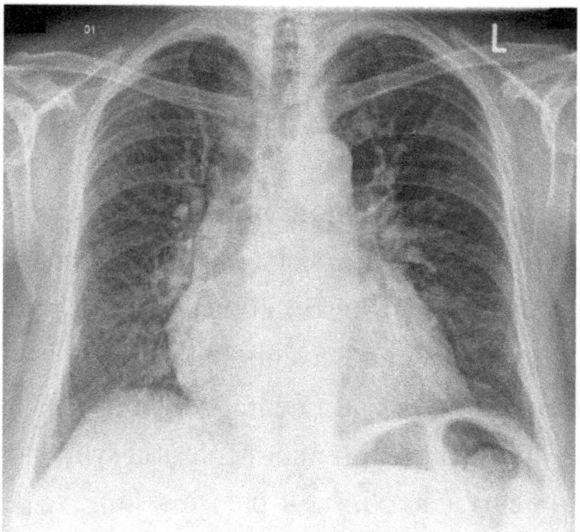

Figure 10: Eosinophilic pneumonitis.

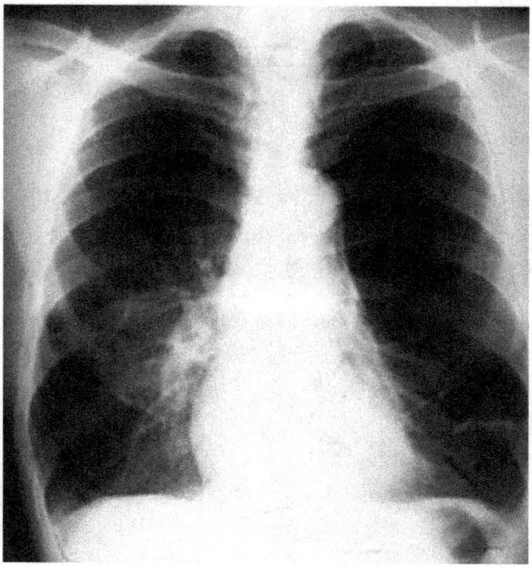

Figure 11: Gross hyperinflation–COPD.

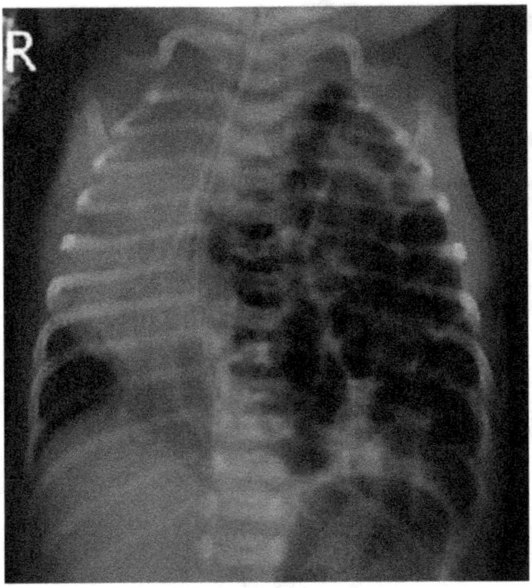

Figure 12: Diaphragmatic hernia.

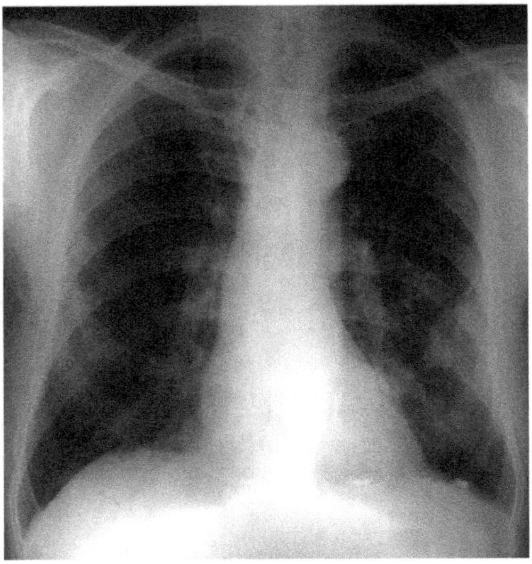

Figure 13: Pneumoconiosis-asbestosis.

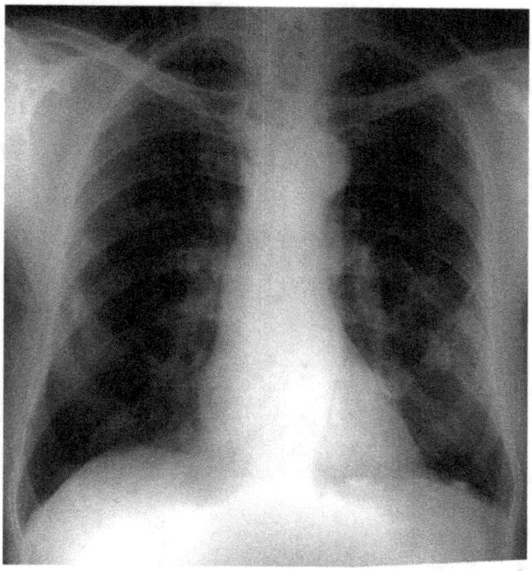

Figure 14: Pulmonary edema.

Electrocardiography

- The electrocardiogram can show abnormalities of the heart rate and rhythm or evidence of ischemia and injury of MI.
- Voltage abnormality suggests left or right ventricular hypertrophy if the voltage is excessive or pneumoconiosis-asbestosis (Figure 14) or obstructive lung disease with increased chest diameter if the voltage is diminished.
- In patients with dyspnea, ST-T segment changes in ECG are found in acute coronary syndromes, pericarditis, cardiac tamponade, and pulmonary embolism.
- Changes in the p-wave morphology help to diagnose right atrial enlargement (typical of a chronic pulmonary process) or left atrial enlargement (typical of valvular heart disease).
- Change in the QRS axis may indicate right (COPD, pulmonary hypertension) or left (hypertension, valvular heart disease) ventricular enlargement or hypertrophy.

Pulse oximetry

- It is a rapid, widely available, and non-invasive means of assessment and is accurate in most clinical situations.
- It uses an infrared light source to determine the hemoglobin oxygen saturation.
- A borderline normal oxygen saturation percentage may actually reflect an abnormally low PaO_2 in some cases.

Echocardiography

- It detects valvular abnormality in the heart and maybe diagnostically helpful in patients with cardiac murmurs with dyspnea.

A multigated cardiac acquisition scan or radionucleotide ventriculography can also be used to quantify the erection traction.

Spirometry

- It helps to differentiate obstructive lung disease and restrictive lung disease.
- COPD and asthma are the most common causes of obstructive spirometry pattern.
- Restrictive pattern can be caused by extrapulmonary factors such as:
- Obesity
- Skeletal abnormalities
- Neuromuscular disorders
- Systemic diseases such as rheumatoid arthritis, systemic lupus erythematosus, and sarcoidosis can cause ILD, which leads to restrictive pattern and spirometry.
- DLCO is used to indirectly measure the gas exchange of oxygen and carbon dioxide across the alveolar surface. It is often included in complete pulmonary function testing.

Arterial blood gas (ABG) analysis

- ABG helps to evaluate gas exchange abnormalities in conditions associated with hypoxemia.
- It provides information about altered pH, hypercapnia, hypocapnia, or hypoxemia.
- Hypercapnia: COPD exacerbation, neuromuscular disease, upper airway obstruction, and obesity hyperventilation syndrome.
- Hypocapnia: Anxiety states, hyperventilation, pulmonary embolism.
- Hypoxemia: Shunting (ARDS, pneumonia, pulmonary edema (Figure 15), cyanotic valvular diseases) V/Q mismatch (COPD, asthma, pulmonary embolism).
- Acidosis: Sepsis, pulmonary edema, exacerbation of COPD, renal failure, and cyanide toxicity.
- Alkalosis: Anxiety, panic attacks, dehydration, and pulmonary embolism.

Cardiopulmonary exercise testing

- This test quantifies cardiac function, pulmonary gas exchange, ventilation, and physical fitness.

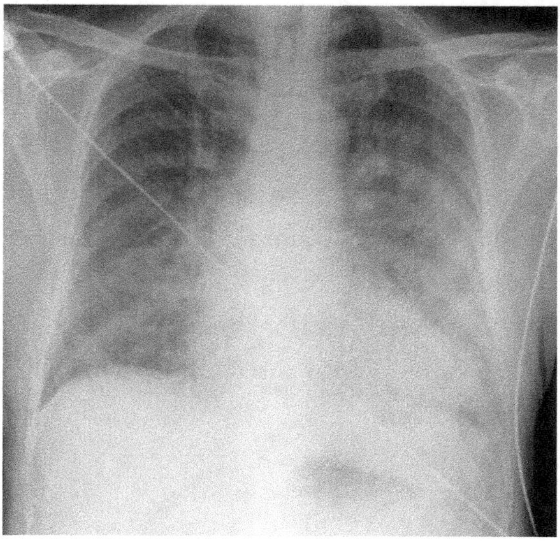

Figure 15: Pulmonary edema.

- This testing may be used in selected cases when the diagnosis is still unclear after the initial examination.
- Interpretation of the complete test requires analysis of oxygen consumption, carbon dioxide production, anaerobic threshold, heart rate and rhythm, blood pressure, minute ventilation, continuous exchange of gas, severity of perceived exertion, dyspnea, chest pain, and leg discomfort.
- This test helps to determine whether abnormality lies in pulmonary, cardiac, or skeletal muscle system.

Management of dyspnea

- Dyspnea is most effectively relieved by treatment of the underlying condition.
- Proper diagnosis as well as recognition of complications that may contribute to dyspnea will guide specific therapy.
- Until guidelines for specific therapy are established, one must take a generic approach to the treatment, with a focus of:
  - reducing the sense of effort in breathing.
  - decreasing the drive to breathe.
  - altering the way respiratory sensations are received or interpreted by the central nervous system.
  - exercise training.

Reducing sense of effort and improving respiratory muscle function

- Energy conservation techniques reduce physical effort so that less ventilatory effort is necessary.
- Breathing techniques (ie, pursed lip breathing and diaphragmatic breathing) reduce the sense of respiratory effort by slowing flow rates and improving arterial oxygen saturation.
- Other techniques include positioning (eg, leaning forward), correcting obesity or malnutrition, inspiratory muscle exercise, respiratory muscle rest (eg, cuirass, nasal ventilation, transtracheal oxygen), and medications (eg, theophylline).

Decreasing respiratory drive

- Oxygen: It reduces carotid body output and ventilatory response to exercise. Stimulation of nasal mucosa with oxygen cannula, facial stimulation with cold air, and chest vibration reduces dyspnea.
- Opiates and sedatives: It decrease the respiratory drive and thus reduces dyspnea.
- Surgical approaches may offer hope in extreme cases:
    - Vagal nerve block or actual nerve section has reduced breath-holding discomfort in healthy volunteers and dyspnea in pulmonary patients.
    - Bilateral carotid body resection has produced impressive long-term symptomatic relief of dyspnea without apparent serious side effects, but it is not an accepted approach.

Altering central perception

- When anxiety or depression contributes to dyspnea, as it often does in COPD, psychotherapy, counseling, progressive muscle relaxation, and even hypnosis may be useful adjuncts.
- Central-acting pharmacologic agents have a limited role in the treatment of dyspnea.
- The value of opiates is clearer for the palliation of dyspnea in a patient with terminal malignant disease, although the studies are still uncontrolled, and in this setting, the importance of relieving suffering at the risk of shortening life is more widely accepted.

Role of exercise training in relieving dyspnea

- The hope of most exercise and rehabilitation programs for patients with chronic lung disease is that improvement in one form of exercise (eg, treadmill walking or bicycle ergometry) will carry over into other activities of daily living and will be associated with improvement in dyspnea.
- Increases anaerobic threshold.
- Enhance self-esteem.

- Improve the efficiency of movement.
- Desensitization to dyspnea from repeated exercise.

References and suggested readings

1. Morice AH, Millqvist E, Bieksiene K, Birring SS, Dicpinigaitis P, Domingo Ribas C, Hilton Boon M, Kantar A, Lai K, McGarvey L, Rigau D, Satia I, Smith J, Song WJ, Tonia T, van den Berg JWK, van Manen MJG, Zacharasiewicz A. ERS guidelines on the diagnosis and treatment of chronic cough in adults and children. Eur Respir J. 2020 Jan 2;55(1):1901136. doi: 10.1183/13993003.01136-2019. Erratum in: Eur Respir J. 2020 Nov 19;56(5). PMID: 31515408; PMCID: PMC6942543.
2. Davis JA, Gudi K. Approach to the patient with cough. Med Clin North Am. 2021 Jan;105(1):31–38. doi: 10.1016/j.mcna.2020.08.013. PMID: 33246521.
3. McCallion P, De Soyza A. Cough and bronchiectasis. Pulm Pharmacol Ther. 2017 Dec;47:77–83. doi: 10.1016/j.pupt.2017.04.010. Epub 2017 Jun 7. PMID: 28602999.
4. Visca D, Beghè B, Fabbri LM, Papi A, Spanevello A. Management of chronic refractory cough in adults. Eur J Intern Med. 2020 Nov;81:15–21. doi: 10.1016/j.ejim.2020.09.008. Epub 2020 Sep 19. PMID: 32958373; PMCID: PMC7501523.
5. Weinberger M, Hurvitz M. Diagnosis and management of chronic cough: similarities and differences between children and adults. F1000Res. 2020 Jul 22;9:F1000 Faculty Rev-757. doi: 10.12688/f1000research.25468.1. PMID: 32765833; PMCID: PMC7385707.
6. Davidson K, Shojaee S. Managing massive hemoptysis. Chest. 2020 Jan;157(1):77–88. doi: 10.1016/j.chest.2019.07.012. Epub 2019 Jul 30. PMID: 31374211.
7. Deshwal H, Sinha A, Mehta AC. Life-threatening hemoptysis. Semin Respir Crit Care Med. 2021 Feb;42(1):145–159. doi: 10.1055/s-0040-1714386. Epub 2020 Aug 30. PMID: 32862418.
8. Marquis KM, Raptis CA, Rajput MZ, Steinbrecher KL, Henry TS, Rossi SE, Picus DD, Bhalla S. CT for evaluation of hemoptysis. Radiographics. 2021 May–Jun;41(3):742–761. doi: 10.1148/rg.2021200150. PMID: 33939537.
9. Atchinson PRA, Hatton CJ, Roginski MA, Backer ED, Long B, Lentz SA. The emergency department evaluation and management of massive hemoptysis.

Am J Emerg Med. 2021 Dec;50:148–155. doi: 10.1016/j.ajem.2021.07.041. Epub 2021 Jul 27. PMID: 34365064.

10. Reynolds C, Staples H. Hemoptysis in an adolescent with EVALI. Pediatr Pulmonol. 2022 Nov;57(11):2875–2876. doi: 10.1002/ppul.26090. Epub 2022 Aug 12. PMID: 35927938.
11. CerezoLajas A, Rodríguez Guzmán MDC, de Miguel Díez J. Hemoptysis associated with therapeutic doses of acenocoumarol. Arch Bronconeumol (Engl Ed). 2019 Jun;55(6):341–342. English, Spanish. doi: 10.1016/j.arbres.2018.10.019. Epub 2018 Dec 7. PMID: 30528810.
12. Budhwar N, Syed Z. Chronic dyspnea: diagnosis and evaluation. Am Fam Physician. 2020 May 1;101(9):542–548. PMID: 32352727.
13. Crombeen AM, Lilly EJ. Management of dyspnea in palliative care. Curr Oncol. 2020 Jun;27(3):142–145. doi: 10.3747/co.27.6413. Epub 2020 Jun 1. PMID: 32669923; PMCID: PMC7339837.
14. Binks AP. Dyspnea. Handb Clin Neurol. 2022;188:309–338. doi: 10.1016/B978-0-323-91534-2.00008-4. PMID: 35965030.
15. Hui D, Bohlke K, Bao T, Campbell TC, Coyne PJ, Currow DC, Gupta A, Leiser AL, Mori M, Nava S, Reinke LF, Roeland EJ, Seigel C, Walsh D, Campbell ML. Management of dyspnea in advanced cancer: ASCO guideline. J Clin Oncol. 2021 Apr 20;39(12):1389–1411. doi: 10.1200/JCO.20.03465. Epub 2021 Feb 22. PMID: 33617290.
16. Hanania NA, O'Donnell DE. Activity-related dyspnea in chronic obstructive pulmonary disease: physical and psychological consequences, unmet needs, and future directions. Int J Chron Obstruct Pulmon Dis. 2019 May 24;14:1127–1138. doi: 10.2147/COPD.S188141. PMID: 31213793; PMCID: PMC6538882.

https://doi.org/10.1142/9789811271410_0003

3 Clubbing

Introduction

Digital clubbing is an indicator of various internal disorders of different systems including cardiorespiratory systems. Digital clubbing is also called Hippocratic nails.

A number of subacute or chronic diseases affecting the respiratory, cardiovascular, hepatic, and alimentary systems may be seen in association with clubbing in more than three-fourths of cases. The condition can exist in an idiopathic or hereditary form. The latter condition develops during childhood without any associated disease state. In rare instances, clubbing may be limited to the toes only in association with patent ductus arteriosus with reversal of blood flow and in infected abdominal aortic prosthesis.

In the initial stages of clubbing, there is an increase in the thickness of the connective tissue in the nail bed (normal 2 mm–4 mm) due to an interstitial edema and cellular inflammation. This edema is replaced by collagen fibers later in the course of the disease when it becomes irreversible.

Definition

Clubbing refers to a bulbous enlargement of the terminal phalanges of the digits especially on the dorsal surface due to fibroelastic tissue overgrowth in the nail bed. Generally, it is bilateral. Occasionally it can be unilateral and even unidigital. Both fingers and toes are affected.

Diagnosis of clubbing

Usually, the index finger of the non-dominant hand is selected for examination. Applying gentle pressure to the proximal nail, just beyond the cuticle, helps to recognize minimal clubbing. It gives an impression of floating nail over a spongy pad (soft clubbing). There is disappearance of a diamond-shaped window which is normally seen if there is a mild enlargement of the soft tissue at the base of fingernails (Schamroth's sign).

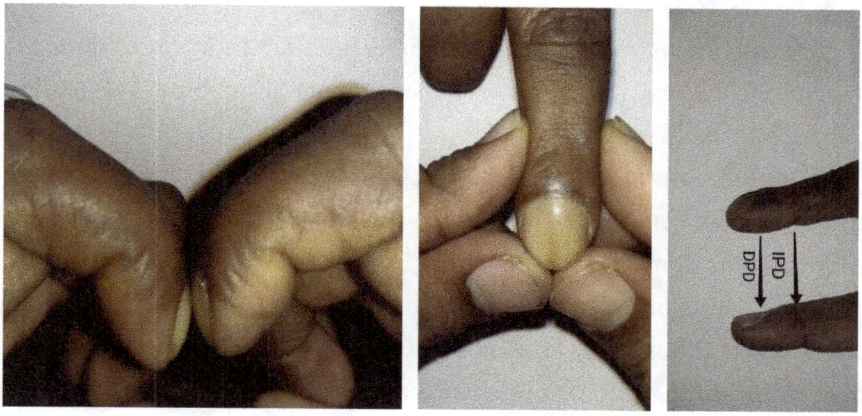

The connective tissue changes extend throughout the digits to give rise to prominent clubbing, which brings about change in the shape of the fingertips. The underlying bone remains normal. The enlargement is uniform with increased curvature of the nail in its longitudinal as well as transverse axes (hard clubbing, watch glass type). It may remain restricted to the proximal portion (Parrot's beak) or to the mid-portion (drum stick type) or the distal phalanx. These differences in the types of clubbing, however, have no clinical significance. The nails may look shiny. By viewing the index finger from the side the loss of the angle of the nail bed can be studied (Profile sign).

Objective assessment of clubbing is made either by measurement of the hyponychial angle between the nail and the proximal skin or the

interphalangeal depth ratio by viewing the index finger from the side against a dark background. The hyponychial angle is formed by joining a point of the distal finger crease and a point on the thickened skin underlying the free edge of the nail (hyponychia) to a point at the cuticle. Normally the angle is 180 degrees or less. It is increased in clubbing because the enlargement of the soft tissue at the base of the nail tends to lift the cuticle away from the underlying bone. This increases the angle and the depth of the fingertip (phalangeal depth ratio). The latter is assessed by measuring the depth of the distal phalanx (DPD) at the cuticle in relation to the depth at the distal interphalangeal joint (IPD) Normally the ratio of DPD to IPD is less than 1:0 and it is increased in clubbing. Digital clubbing is mostly bilateral. It can be unilateral or even unidigital.

Causes of clubbing

System	Causes
Respiratory	Lung abscess, bronchiectasis, empyema, lung cancer, mesothelioma of pleura, lung metastasis, idiopathic pulmonary fibrosis, asbestosis, berylliosis, some cases of fibrocaseous tuberculosis
Cardiovascular	Congential cyanotic heart diseases, Ebstein's anomaly, tetralogy of Fallot, transposition of aorta, subacute bacterial endocarditis, intrathoracic vascular anomalies
Gastrointestinal	Intestines: Crohn's disease (regional ileitis), ulcerative colitis, malabsorption syndrome, chronic diarrhea, carcinoma esophagus, carcinoma of the bowels Hepatic: liver cirrhosis, hepatocellular carcinoma, amoebic liver abscess

(*Continued*)

(*Continued*)

Unilateral clubbing	Hemiplegia Aneurysm of subclavian artery, brachiocephalic trunk, aortic arch, axillary artery Old dislocation of shoulder Carcinoma of right upper lobe bronchus Palmer arch aneurysm Traumatic obstruction of axillary vein Unilateral erythromelalgia and lymphangitis Causalgia Arteriovenous fistula used for hemodialysis Infected arterial graft Pulmonary hypertension with patent ductus arteriosus
Only upper limbs	Aneurysm of subclavian artery AV fistula used for dialysis Axillary vein thrombosis
Only lower limbs	patent ductus arteriosus associated with pulmonary artery hypertension and right to left shunt infected abdominal aortic aneurysm

Mechanism of clubbing

The specific pathophysiologic mechanism of digital clubbing remains unknown. Many theories have been proposed, yet none have received widespread acceptance as a comprehensive explanation for the phenomenon of digital clubbing.

Circulatory vasodilator

Variety of circulating vasodilators including ferritin, prostaglandins, bradykinin, adenine nucleotides, and 5-hydroxytryptamine that are released by normal tissue, which usually are inactivated as blood passes through the lungs, bypass the inactivation process in patients with right to left shunts patient with tof with substantial shunting high grade of clubbing after surgical correction diminishes the shunt, clubbing improves.

Neuronal mechanism

A neuronal mechanism has been proposed with particular consideration of the vagal stimulus. An increased incidence of digital clubbing has been associated with pathology and due to vagally innervated organs. Furthermore, regression of clubbing after vagotomy has been done. Although some factors related to vagus system is a possible contributor to the development of clubbing, especially clubbing occurring with hypertrophic osteoarthropathy, the hypothesis of neuronal mechanism has decreased in popularity due to the lack of evidence of clubbing in neurological disorders and the presence of clubbing in diseases of organs not innervated by systems.

Tissue hypoxia

Hypoxia has been proposed as an alternative explanation for clubbing in cyanotic diseases and pulmonary diseases. An increase in hypoxia may activate local vasodilators consequently increasing the blood flow to the distal portion of digits; however, in most cases, hypoxia in the presence of clubbing and many diseases with noted hypoxia are not associated with clubbing.

Genetic factors

Genetic inheritance and predisposition also may play a role in digital clubbing, hence clubbing is observed in two forms, including idiopathic hereditary clubbing and clubbing associated with pachydermoperiostosis. The two forms are believed to be separate entities. Both demonstrate autosomal dominant inheritance with incomplete penetrance.

Growth factors

More recently, platelet-derived growth factors released from the fragments of platelets or megakaryocytes have been proposed as the mechanism by which digital clubbing occurs; fragments are large enough to lodge in the vascular beds of the fingertips and subsequently release

platelet-derived growth factor. This factor has been shown to have general growth activity and causes increased capillary permeability and connective tissue hypertrophy.

Pseudoclubbing

Pseudoclubbing is an atypical presentation of clubbing, characterized clinically by asymmetrical involvement of the fingers and radiographically by resorption of the terminal tufts (acro-osteolysis). It has been described in chronic renal failure, subungual hemangioma, acrometastases, systemic sclerosis, etc. The exact mechanism is not known, but it could be the result of soft tissue collapse due to distal phalangeal osteolysis.

References and suggested readings

1. Romeo S, Neri B, Mossa M, Calabrese E, Lolli E, Sena G, Gesuale C, Chiaramonte C, Biancone L. Finger clubbing in inflammatory bowel disease: association with upper small bowel lesions and need of surgery in Crohn's disease. Eur J Gastroenterol Hepatol. 2021 Jun 1;33(6):844–851. doi: 10.1097/MEG.0000000000001966. PMID: 33136723.
2. Martínez-Lavín M. Hypertrophic osteoarthropathy. Best Pract Res Clin Rheumatol. 2020 Jun;34(3):101507. doi: 10.1016/j.berh.2020.101507. Epub 2020 Apr 11. PMID: 32291203.
3. Tyson N, Efthymiou C. Unilateral finger clubbing as an unusual manifestation of right atrial myxoma. Eur J Cardiothorac Surg. 2020 Sep 1;58(3):658. doi: 10.1093/ejcts/ezaa170. PMID: 32542368.
4. Gunasekera SN, Madurapperuma C, Weerasooriya N, Karunathilake H, Jayanaga A. A rare presentation of Takayasu's arteritis-unilateral finger clubbing — case report. BMC Rheumatol. 2020 Dec 10;4(1):66. doi: 10.1186/s41927-020-00166-z. PMID: 33298181; PMCID: PMC7727161.
5. Gunasekera SN, Madurapperuma C, Weerasooriya N, Karunathilake H, Jayanaga A. A rare presentation of Takayasu's arteritis-unilateral finger clubbing — case report. BMC Rheumatol. 2020 Dec 10;4(1):66. doi: 10.1186/s41927-020-00166-z. PMID: 33298181; PMCID: PMC7727161.

6. Ahmed AS, Divani GK, Arora GK. Differential clubbing with severe pulmonary hypertension. QJM. 2021 Nov 5;114(8):609–610. doi: 10.1093/qjmed/hcab128. PMID: 33956980.
7. Gunasekera SN, Madurapperuma C, Weerasooriya N, Karunathilake H, Jayanaga A. A rare presentation of Takayasu's arteritis-unilateral finger clubbing — case report. BMC Rheumatol. 2020 Dec 10;4(1):66. doi: 10.1186/s41927-020-00166-z. PMID: 33298181; PMCID: PMC7727161.
8. Shneerson J. Idiopathic digital clubbing. Br J Hosp Med (Lond). 2020 Dec 2;81(12):1. doi: 10.12968/hmed.2020.0687. Epub 2020 Dec 16. PMID: 33377843.
9. Crestani L, Fasciani IA, Kakizaki P, Valente NYS. Case for diagnosis. Single-digit clubbing. An Bras Dermatol. 2020 Jul–Aug;95(4):524–526. doi: 10.1016/j.abd.2020.01.006. Epub 2020 May 11. PMID: 32448714; PMCID: PMC7335881.
10. Fernandez-Quiroga C, Alfageme-Roldán F, Roustan-Gullón G. Digital clubbing: ultrasound findings. Actas Dermosifiliogr. 2022 May;113(5):522–523. English, Spanish. doi: 10.1016/j.ad.2020.05.018. Epub 2021 Sep 10. PMID: 35697412.

https://doi.org/10.1142/9789811271410_0004

4 Chest radiologic imaging

Chest X-ray is one of the most common investigations ordered by a chest physician for the diagnosis as well as follow-up assessments of impact of treatment. There is considerable improvement in the current chest X-rays, most being in the digital format unlike the previous conventional chest X-rays. The digital format is clearer and easier for storage and communications. The main drawback of the digital chest X-rays is that there are smaller in size and measurements cannot be taken unlike the conventional X-rays which were life sized. This chapter will deal with some of the basics of chest X-rays and its interpretation.

Chest X-ray positions

The commonest position used is the PA view. What is this view and why this view is preferred? Here the X-rays pass from the posterior chest to the anterior chest, which is touching the X-ray receptor. A close contact is necessary to obtain sharp images. The heart measurements in this view are a good reflection of the actual heart size and when greater than 50% of the thoracic diameter is indicative of cardiac enlargement. The AP view is mostly limited to bedside portable X-rays where the patient cannot stand and is taken in the ICU's and hospitalized patients. When the heart is away from the X-ray receptor as the rays pass from anterior chest to the posterior, the heart size appears enlarged, but it is a spurious enlargement. The structures seen in an AP view are not as sharp as seen in the routine PA view. There are several reasons why a PA upright chest X-ray is preferred over the AP supine bedside films. It is because there is less magnification in

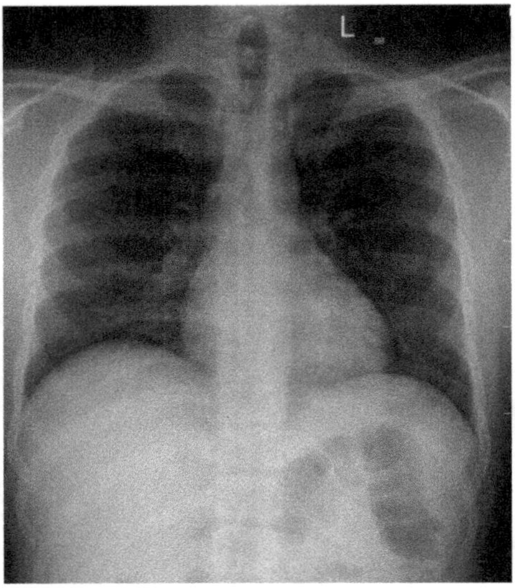

Figure 1: PA view.

a PA view and the image is sharper. Importantly, the erect patient breathes in more deeply, and this shows a greater portion of the lungs. The air in the pleura as well as the fluid shift with gravity more easily detected on the erect film as compared to the supine films.

With the advent of the CT scans, other views such as the lateral view, lateral decubitus view, and lordotic view are all less used these days. The lateral view can be either the right lateral view or the left lateral view. Along with the PA view, the additional lateral view helps to localize the lobe and the segment of the lung involved in the disease process. The lateral decubitus films were used to detect minimal pleural effusion and the lordotic view was used to detect upper lobe lesions that were masked by the ribs.

Indications of chest X-ray

1. Symptoms or signs of respiratory or cardiac disease
2. Preoperative evaluation of patients with known respiratory or cardiac disease or those patients with an indication for thoracic surgery
3. Tumor staging

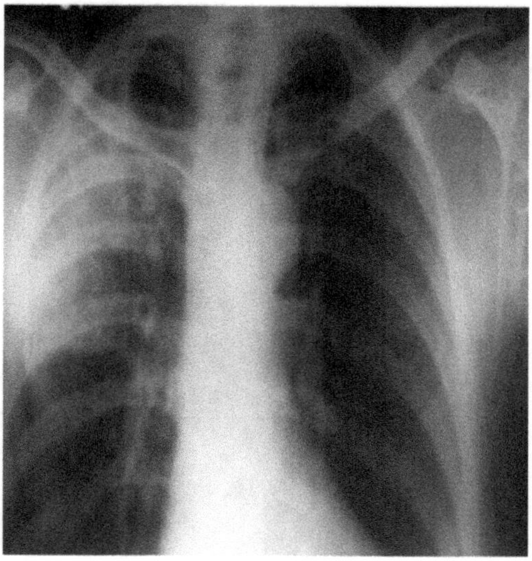

Figure 2: Early pneumonia.

4. Follow-up of a previous thoracic disease for resolution, persistence, or progression after treatment
5. Placement of chest tubes, endotracheal tubes, central venous catheters, and after interventions such as FNAC or tru-cut biopsy of the lung for development of pneumothorax
6. Follow-up of cases admitted to the ICU, especially on mechanical ventilation for development of complications related to barotrauma and ventilator-associated pneumonia

Tips to follow before reading a chest X-ray

1. Make sure you are reading the chest X-ray of the same patient, by checking the name, age, and ID number
2. If multiple chest X-rays are available, always start with the earliest chest X-ray
3. Useful to see the chest X-ray on the day you have examined the patient. The clinical picture may have changed if it is an old chest X-ray
4. It is always useful to have a good clinical correlation to be attempted with the findings on the chest X-ray

5. Understand that the chest X-ray is a two-dimensional image of many three-dimensional structures, the heart, lungs, mediastinum, and thoracic cage
6. Make sure you have access to a uniformly illuminated chest X-ray reading box with white light
7. Read the chest X-ray from a distance of 3–4 ft
8. Have a checklist and do not stop as soon as you find one abnormal finding as there may be more than one in a given patient

Checklist for reading a chest X-ray

It is very beneficial to train yourself to read the chest X-ray methodically from outside to inside or from inside to outside. All the structures listed below have to be given a close attention.

1. Heart and vasculature (pulmonary artery, aorta, and superior vena cava)
2. Lung fields
3. Major and minor fissures
4. Hilum
5. Mediastinum
6. Trachea and main bronchi
7. Domes of the diaphragm and infra-diaphragmatic areas, fundal gas shadow
8. Costophrenic and cardio phrenic angles
9. Skeleton — ribs, clavicle, scapulae, vertebrae, and costochondral junction
10. Soft tissue shadows including the breast shadows in women
11. Whether the inspiration is sufficient — if so, the anterior end of the 5th rib will be touching the diaphragm. If the inspiration is poor, it may give the findings of an interstitial lung disease
12. Whether exposure is correct — you should not be able to see the vertebral bodies below the tracheal bifurcation. If you can, it is an overexposed film and small radiologic abnormalities can be missed

13. Please see if there are any artifacts
14. Always check hidden areas, that are not visible at first look. A pneumonia behind the heart is usually missed. The clue is there is an increased density of the heart on that side. The apical areas of both lung fields need to be checked again. Small lesions can be missed due to the skeletal structure and after middle age, the cartilage starts getting calcified irregularly and can be mistaken for a pathology. The hilum is another area where pathologies are missed when they are small

Features of a normal chest X-ray

1. The cardiac shadow is normal in size and shape. It is less than 50% of the size of the transverse thoracic diameter. Two thirds of the heart are on the left side from the midline and one thirds is on the right
2. Both lung fields have equal blackness
3. Diaphragm is at the anterior end of the 5th rib on the right side and one space below on the left side
4. Tracheal air shadow is centrally located and right and left main bronchial air shadow are seen normally
5. No skeletal abnormalities. Anterior ribs are sloping downwards and posterior ribs are horizontal
6. Right hilum is usually one space below the left hilum
7. Cardiophrenic and costophrenic angles are sharp
8. Minor fissure when seen, is between the anterior end of 2nd to 4th ribs

Interpretation of chest X-rays and clinico-pathological correlations

For a clinician, it is useful to approach the chest X-ray similar to the clinical examination, wherein we collect information on the symptoms and signs to reach a diagnosis, which has three parts. We need to identify in order, the site of disease, the possible pathology and then infer the possible etiology. A similar model can be followed in reading the chest X-ray as well. The need for good clinical information before reading the chest X-ray cannot be over-emphasized.

Site of disease

There are classical signs in chest radiology that will offer adequate information to identify the site of disease. The sites of disease in the lungs are the airways, pulmonary parenchyma, pulmonary interstitium, pleural, and mediastinum. Airways are not clearly visible in the chest X-rays; however, there are indirect signs that point to the airway involvement. Generally the pulmonary parenchyma and pleural diseases are easily visualized except in the hidden areas which include areas behind the heart, in the posterior basal segments of the lower lobes behind the dome of the diaphragm (when a lateral view can clearly delineate the pathology), and sometimes small lesions behind the ribs are hidden from view.

Airway diseases

The most common diseases involving the airways are asthma, COPD, bronchiectasis, lung cancers, and small airway diseases. The signs of involvement are indirect and minimal airway obstruction may not lead to any radiologic abnormalities. When airway obstruction is significant as in severe asthma, especially during an attack, the signs of hyperinflated lung fields can be seen. Unlike asthma, COPD is a progressive disease and

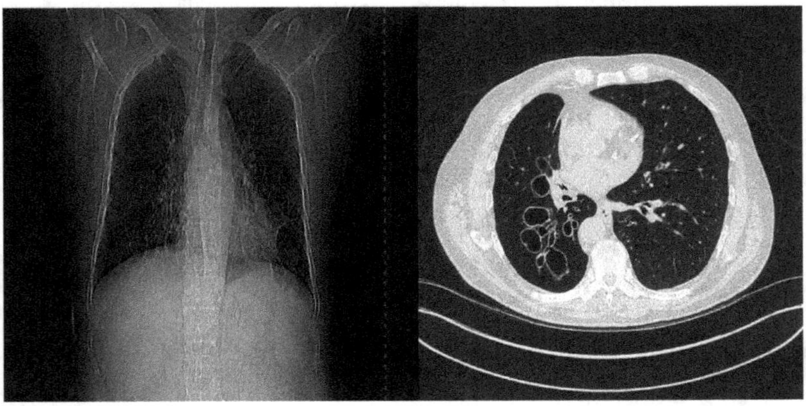

Figure 3: Cystic bronchiectasis — Chest X-ray and HRCT demonstrate thin-walled, cystic structures in lower lobe.

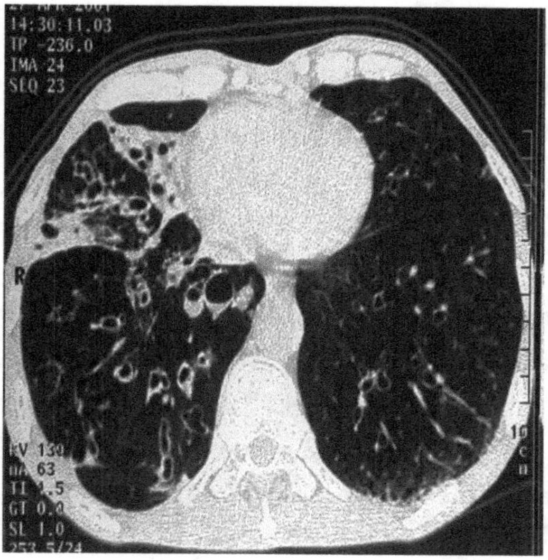

Figure 4: Middle lobe fibrosis and bronchiectasis, bilateral lower lobe bronchiectasis, and minimal lingular bronchiectasis.

usually presents late to seek medical attention. They usually present with features of fixed airway obstruction, which could include, hyperinflated lung fields (the level of the diaphragm is below the anterior end of the 6th rib and below the posterior end of the 10th rib). The heart size is smaller and is called a tubular heart when the size of the heart is below 11 cm. The ribs are usually horizontal when there is significant hyperinflation, and there are hyper-translucent lung fields. One needs to make sure that increased translucency is not due to greater exposure, which is easily identified if you can see the vertebral bodies behind the heart. Peripheral pruning of the pulmonary vasculature is another important sign to look for. It is usually seen in COPD and not in asthma. Normally, one can trace the pulmonary vessels up to two thirds of the lung fields from the mediastinum. If there is peripheral pruning, then we can trace the blood vessels for a much shorter distance.

Bronchiectasis is another common pulmonary disease and can occur due to a variety of causes. The main classification of bronchiectasis is

whether it is due to congenital causes or acquired causes. Usually, congenital bronchiectasis is more common in the left lower lobe, and acquired bronchiectasis is more common in the right lower lobe. The radiologic evidence of bronchiectasis includes the ring sign, which is due to dilated airway accompanied by the pulmonary vessel. On many occasions, there are multiple cavities if a large segment or lobe of the lung is involved. During active infection, one may see an air-fluid level within the cavities. In ABPA with proximal bronchiectasis, an inverted wine glass sign may be seen. Thickened bronchi are seen as "tram line" shadows in the X-ray.

Radiologic evidence when the lung cancer is only in the airways is very subtle. A mucosal lesion can be seen only on a bronchoscopy. If the tumor is large and infiltrating, a parenchymal lesion is usually seen. In some cases, a complete collapse of the lung can be due to a tumor obstructing the main bronchus and can be identified by a "bronchial cut-off sign." A tumor in the trachea or main bronchus can cause an abnormal indentation in the air shadow. A large lymph node in the sub-carinal region can cause widening of the sub-carinal angle. When there are associated hilar lymph nodes, the "hilum overlay sign" is positive.

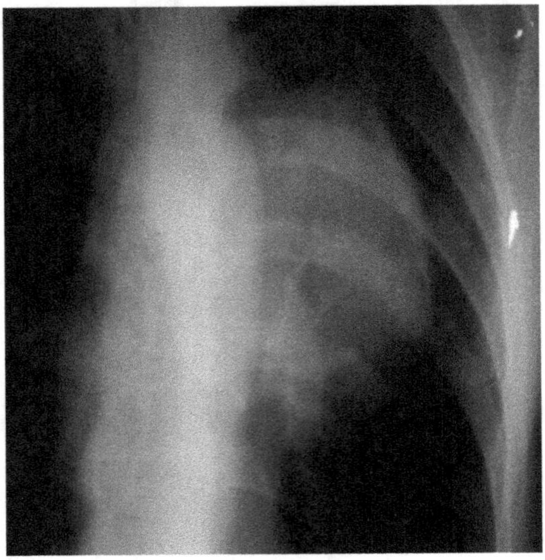

Figure 5: Hilum overlay sign.

Golden S sign

This sign is seen on chest radiology. The minor fissure is elevated with convexity upwards due to collapse of the right upper lobe fully or sometimes partially. There is a large central mass lesion near the hilum, both of which give the S-shaped curve as seen in the radiograph below.

Finger in glove

It is a sign seen either on a chest radiograph or an HRCT scan. It is typical of a bronchocele that is filled with impacted mucus. It starts from near the hilum and radiates to the periphery. It is classically described in ABPA.

Tree in bud

This is a sign seen in the HRCT and usually denotes an infectious etiology. Tuberculosis is a common cause, though there are several diseases including non-infectious diseases that can cause this sign. Mycobacterium other than tuberculosis (nontubercular mycobacteria), bacterial (Legionella,

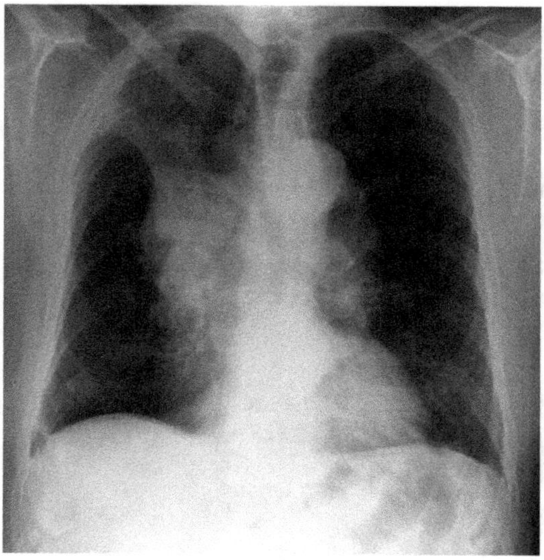

Figure 6: Golden S sign — Chest X-ray shows a right upper lobe collapse over a reverse S-shaped minor fissure and a prominent central mass lesion.

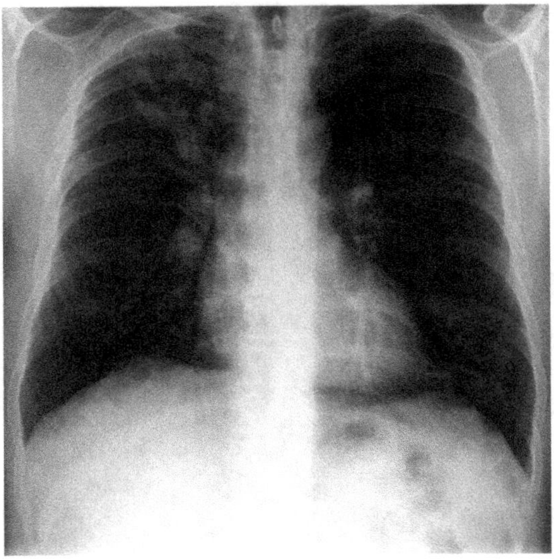

Figure 7: Finger in glove — Chest X-ray PA view shows finger-like opacities originating from the hilum and directed toward the periphery of the right upper lobe.

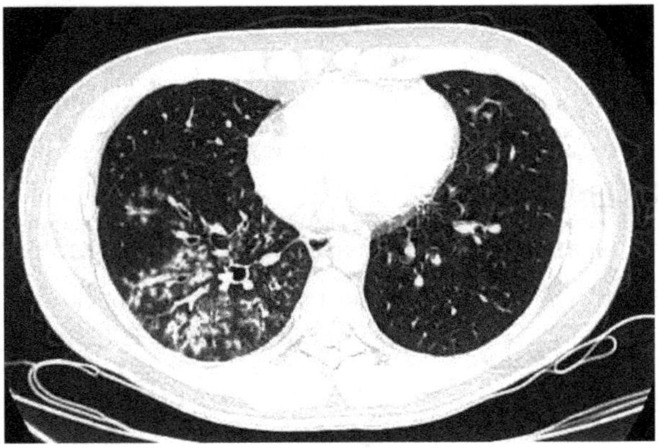

Figure 8: Tree in bud — CT Thorax shows multiple small centrilobular nodules of soft tissue attenuation connected to linear branching opacities in the right lung fields giving a tree-in-bud appearance. Associated bronchiectasis on the right lung is observed with the dilated bronchi larger than the accompanying blood vessel.

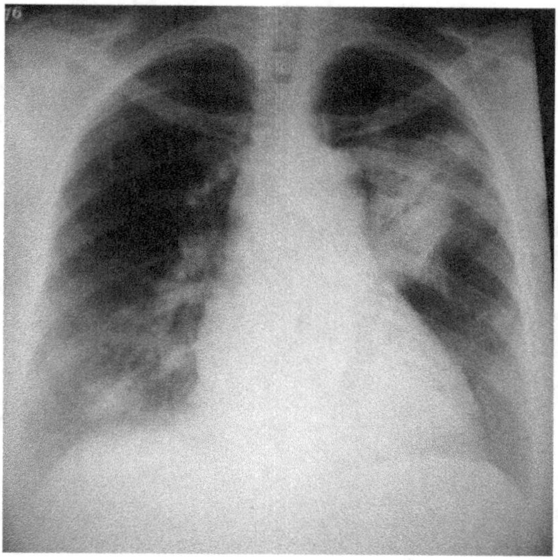

Figure 9: Airbronchogram — Tubular outline of the airway noted in the surrounding homogenous radio-opacity in the left upper zone indicative of airway disease.

Mycoplasma), fungal (Aspergillus, Pneumocystis), and viral diseases (Cytomegalovirus) are the infectious causes. Non-infectious causes include aspiration, intravenous injection of foreign substances, toxin inhalation, immunological diseases, inflammatory conditions, follicular bronchiolitis, pan bronchiolitis, and malignancies such as chronic lymphatic leukemia, intravenous tumor emboli can present with "tree-in-bud" sign. It has centrilobular nodules of soft attenuation with multiple linear structures from the same stalk.

Pulmonary parenchymal diseases

There are several features that suggest pulmonary parenchymal involvement, which may have a segmental, lobar, single lung, or bilateral lung distribution. The densities may be confluent or patchy and may involve more than one focal region. Presence of an air bronchogram or an air alveologram confirms lung involvement. The most common site of disease

that a parenchymal disease needs to be differentiated from is the pleural disease. When either air bronchogram or air alveologram is present, parenchyma disease is confirmed. But when they are absent, we cannot rule out parenchymal disease. The lobes are generally well demarcated by the major and minor fissure (right lung). Very few diseases cross the fissures and are an important clue to the etiology. The diseases that cross the fissures are tuberculosis, lung cancer, fungal infections, actinomycosis, and nocardiosis. Other bacterial infections are usually limited by the fissures and diseases such as a Klebsiella pneumonia are associated with a "bulging fissure sign" since they do not break through the fissures. It is possible to identify the exact bronchopulmonary segment involved when both the PA and lateral views are available, which gives an important clue to the etiology. The lesions involving the dependent areas of the lung indicate that the route of spread was an oropharyngeal microaspiration. A microaspiration involves inhaling minute quantities of the oro-pharyngeal secretions, which happens even in normal people. But usually, the flora is non-pathogenic in a healthy subject, and there is no disease. It is seen that subjects with poor oral hygiene and periodontitis are at risk for recurrent lung infections due to this microaspiration. When a large amount of oral secretions, food, or vomit reaches the lungs it is called as microaspiration. This is commonly seen during recovery from general anesthesia, altered consciousness, epileptic fit, and binge alcohol consumption when the consciousness and cough reflexes are impaired. The dependent areas of the lung are the posterior segment of the upper lobes, superior segment of the lower lobes, and the posterior basal segment (right is more involved than the left). When a non-dependent area of the lung is involved a specific pathology is likely. For example, when the anterior segment of the upper lobe is involved, specific diseases such as tuberculosis, lung cancer, and fungal infections need to be investigated. The only way a non-dependent area such as middle lobe is involved in if there is an aspiration when the subject is swimming or aspirates when the subject is leaning forward.

There are three classical signs that help to localize the pathology in the pulmonary parenchyma. The first is the location of the abnormal radiologic

shadow, second is the silhouette sign, and the third is the change in density of other normal structures such as the heart, mediastinal shadow, skeletal shadow, or the diaphragm.

Site of the shadow: One would need both PA and lateral view to be definite, but one could have a good idea even in a PA view. If the radiologic shadow is above the anterior end of the first rib, it is likely to be in the apical segment of the upper lobe. If it is between the first and second ribs, it is in the posterior segment of the upper lobe. If it is below the second rib until the minor fissure, it is in the anterior segment of the upper lobe. If it is in the paracardiac and parahilar region on either side of the heart, it is in the middle lobe (right) or lingula (left). The same region also represents the lower lobes which are posteriorly situated. This differentiation can be made out by identifying the silhouette sign discussed subsequently. If the shadows silhouette the right cardiac border, it is in the middle lobe, and if it silhouettes the left cardiac border, it is in the lingula. Posteriorly located shadows will not silhouette the heart borders, since heart is anteriorly situated. If the lesion is close to the hilum not silhouetting the cardiac borders and the shadow crosses the imaginary line drawn across the hilum it is most likely in the superior segment of the lower lobe. If the shadow

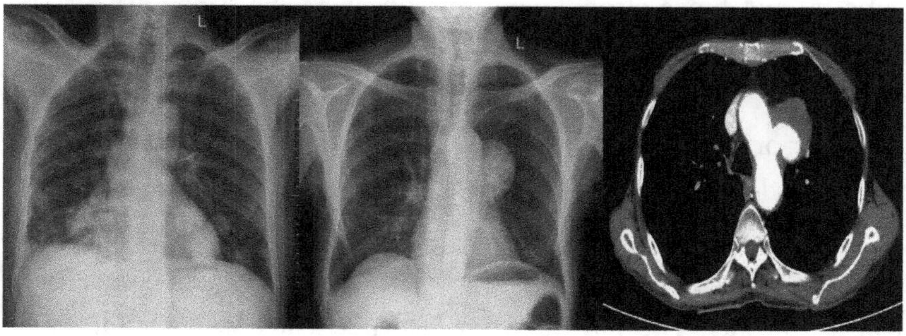

Figure 10: Silhouette sign — Chest X-ray PA view shows a large mass in the left upper lung field, that is "silhouetting" the left heart border which is no longer seen as a distinct edge. CT scan shows a partially thrombosed aortic aneurysm arising from the arch of aorta.

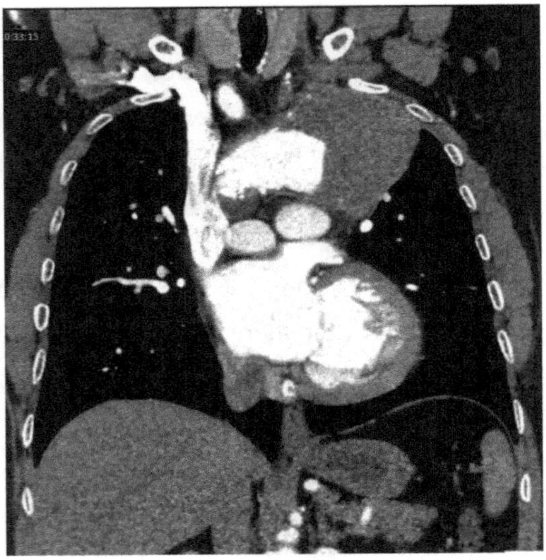

Figure 11: CT scan of thrombosed aortic aneurysm.

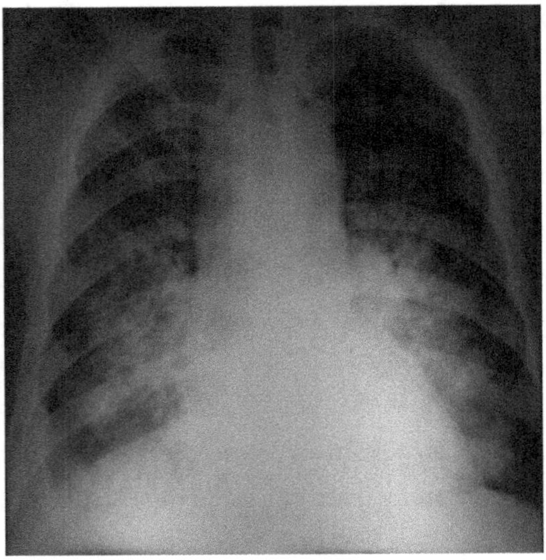

Figure 12: Pulmonary edema in a patient with hypertension, chronic renal failure, and congestive cardiac failure.

is present in the paracardiac region, but does not silhouette the heart, it is present in the medial basal (right) or posterior basal (right and left) segments of the lower lobe. If the shadow is present in the lower zones, but away from the cardiac shadow in the lateral half, the site of disease is in the anterior or lateral basal segments of the lower lobe.

Silhouette sign: This is one of the classical signs in chest radiology. Sometimes, it is the only sign that there is a pathology. The principle of the sign is that any shadow of any density will mask the clear border of the organ seen radiologically, if it abutting the organ. It gives an immediate clue as to the site of the disease. Examples have already been discussed in relation to the cardiac borders. It is also used in other sites. If the border of the ascending aorta is silhouetted, the lesion is in the anterior segment of the right upper lobe; if arch of aorta is silhouetted, the lesion is in the posterior segment of the left upper lobe; if the hemidiaphragms are silhouetted the lesion is in the lower lobes or pleura; and if the descending pulmonary artery is silhouetted it is in the lower lobe.

Change in density: This is another important sign that helps to identify pathologies that are sometimes missed. A denser right hilum as compared to the left hilum is indicative of a pathology in the right lung or pleura. An increased cardiac density is an indicator of a pathology in the lower lobes, mediastinum, or pleura. An increased density of the hemidiaphragm is indicative of a pathology, usually in the posterior basal segment of the lower lobe. In a lateral view, the density of the vertebral bodies generally reduces as one moves down from the upper thoracic vertebra. If there is a pathology, the density can increase and sometimes will be the only indication of a pathology.

Simon's foci and Assman's focus

This is a radiologic sign that is associated with tuberculosis. There is a progressive primary lesion or a hematogenous spread of tuberculosis to the upper lobe that heals by scarring and later by calcification which is seen on

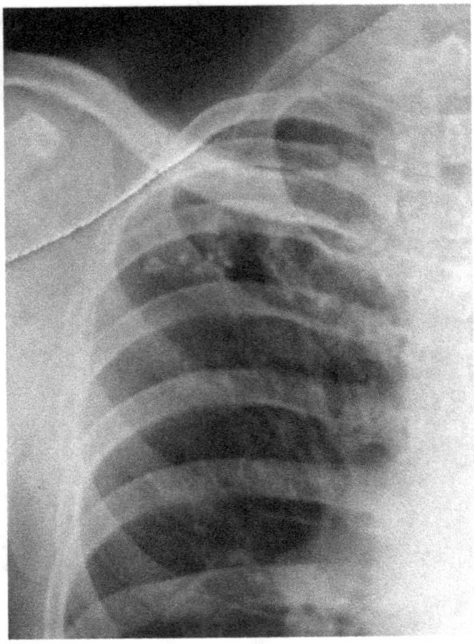

Figure 13: Calcified Simon's foci seen in the right upper lobe.

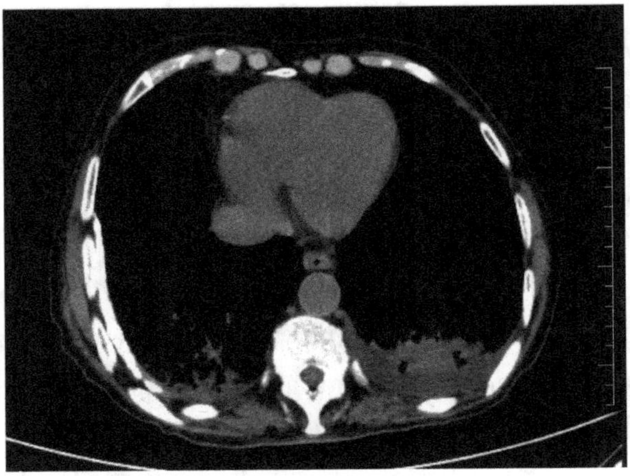

Figure 14: CT thorax, mediastinal window that shows extensive pleural calcification (same as bone density) in the right posterolateral pleura. There are pleural thickening and lung pathologies bilaterally.

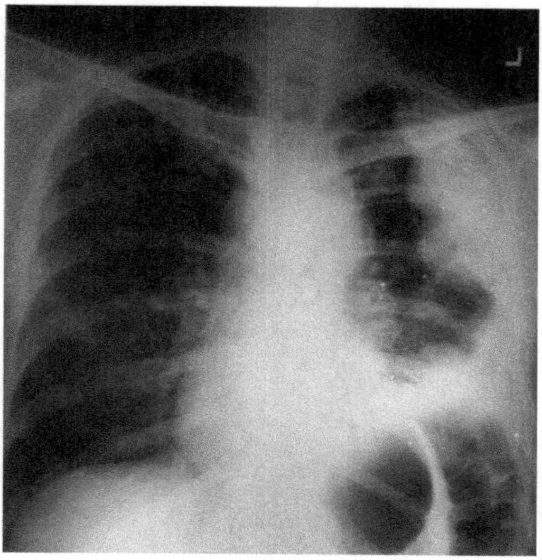

Figure 15: An irregular and nodular pleural mass. A case of Mesothelioma.

chest radiology. Simon's foci can be single or multiple, unilateral or bilateral. Sometimes the calcified nodules are extensive and are called as "the starry sky" appearance. Assman's focus is an infraclavicular calcified lesion which is usually single.

Pleural calcification

It is easy to diagnose pleural calcification in both chest X-ray and CT scan due to its high density which is similar to bone density. The most common reasons for pleural calcification are empyema and tuberculous pleural effusion. Other causes include hemothorax and occupational exposures such as asbestosis, which has a peculiar pattern of pleural calcification that spares the costophrenic angle. Asbestos exposure is risk factor for pleural mesothelioma. A talc pleurodesis can sometimes mimic a pleural calcification.

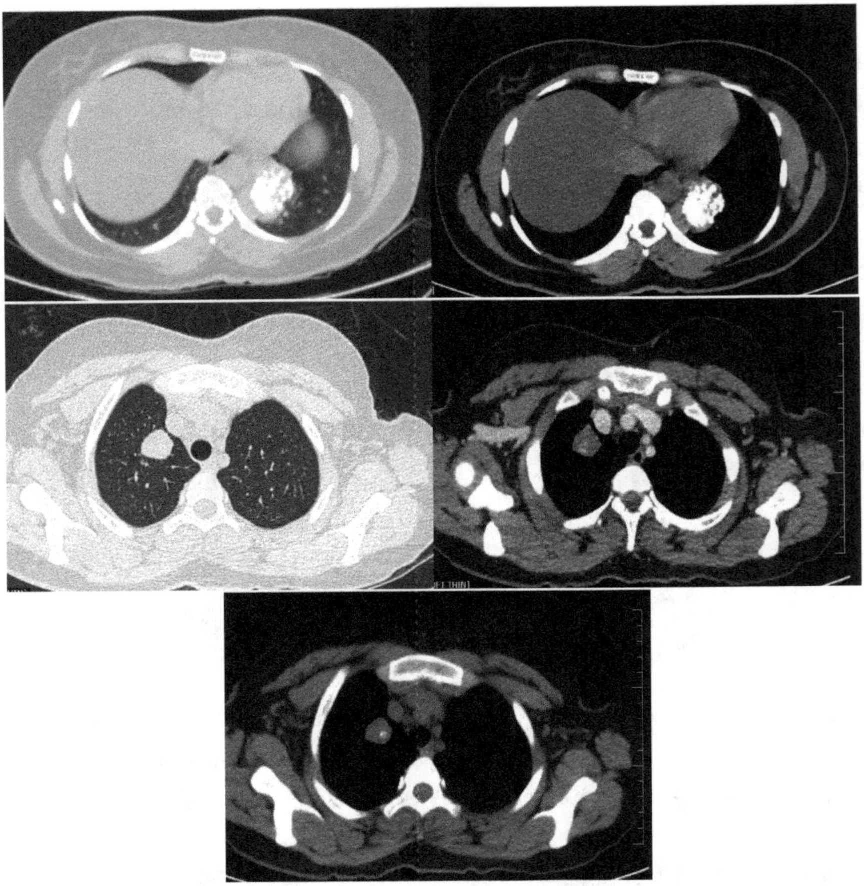

Figure 16: CT scans of two cases of Hamartoma-CT-lung window and mediastinal window of the first case shows typical popcorn calcification. CT-lung window and mediastinal window of the second case show very minimal calcification. While the first case can be diagnosed only by radiology, the second needed invasive tissue diagnosis to confirm that it is hamartoma and rule out malignancy.

Hamartoma

These are benign neoplasms comprising of bone, cartilage, connective tissue, muscle, and fat. Sometimes even epithelium is present. Usually, these are common to the lung, but their architecture is not preserved. The classical radiological sign of a hamartoma in chest C-ray and CT scan is called

the "popcorn" calcification. Hamartomas are usually well circumscribed as can be seen in any lobe. Size can vary, but are almost always single. They are situated in the periphery of the lung and very rarely are endobronchial. They are usually asymptomatic, unless they are endobronchial and detected incidentally. Endobronchial hamartomas can cause cough,

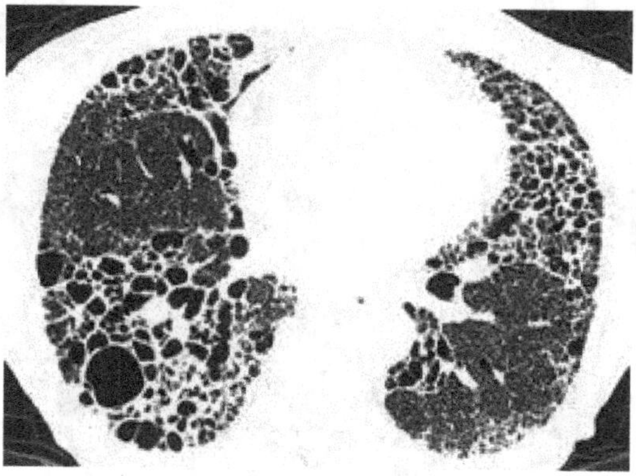

Figure 17: Honeycomb-HRCT thorax shows multiple small cystic spaces with thick dense fibrous tissue around it giving a honeycomb-like appearance — Typically indicative of Usual Interstitial Pneumonia.

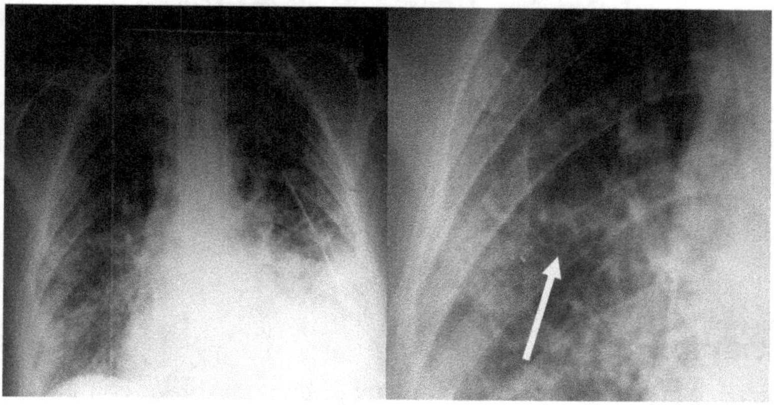

Figure 18: Lymphangitic carcinomatosis in a 58-year-old female. Here the tumor spreads through the lymphatics of the lung and a reticulo-nodular pattern is observed with thickening of the interlobular septa.

hemoptysis, or even collapse of the lung or lobe. The extent of calcium can vary from large to absent.

Interstitial diseases

The ideal tool to identify an early interstitial disease is an HRCT thorax and chest X-ray is not the ideal tool. In fact, an inching auscultation, especially of the lung bases to look for fine Velcro crepitations, is probably more sensitive than chest X-ray. One must make sure that the chest X-ray is not an expiratory film as the radiologic image will be similar to early ILD. The key indicator of interstitial involvement is reticulonodular opacities usually in the lower half of the lung fields. Reticulation can be defined as a mesh like a mosquito net and can be of variable size. In late ILD, the lung volume becomes smaller and the density of the mesh becomes thicker. Honeycombing can be observed in late-stage ILD's. Here, the lung parenchyma is replaced by small cysts which are separated by fibrous tissue. Interstitial diseases can be acute or chronic, infectious or non-infectious. The duration of clinical symptoms is a good marker to know whether we are dealing with an acute ILD or a chronic ILD. It is useful to review old films to understand the speed of progression of the disease.

Ground-glass opacity

This is the term used to describe an alveolitis wherein there is an increased haziness in the lung fields, best seen in an HRCT thorax, through which the shadows of the blood vessels and bronchial structures are preserved and can be visualized. It is a nonspecific sign and can be seen in both infectious and non-infectious causes. Early COVID-19 viral pneumonia typically presented with multiple patchy ground-glass opacities. Other viral pneumonias including H1N1 pneumonia can also present with ground-glass opacities. It can be either acute or chronic and any pathology causing alveolitis and interstitial involvement can give rise to this sign.

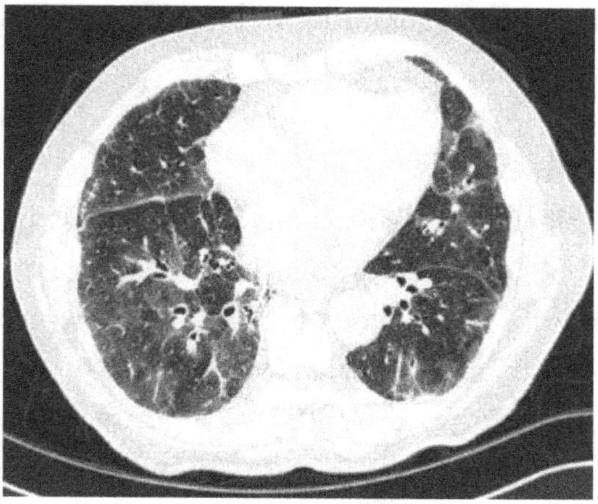

Figure 19: Ground-glass opacity — HRCT image at the level of cardia shows extensive ground-glass opacity across both lungs. There also is nonspecific interstitial thickening in lungs bilaterally.

Pleural diseases

Involvement of the pleura is a very common pulmonary problem along with pulmonary parenchymal diseases. Sometimes, it becomes difficult to differentiate between the two sites. Presence of an air bronchogram or an air alveologram makes it easy to confirm parenchymal disease, but the absence of these two signs makes it difficult to locate the disease as pleural or parenchymal in many situations. There are few signs that help to definitively conclude that the disease is pleural. First is a marker of pleural effusion and the most common sign; the blunting of the costophrenic and when pleural effusion is larger, blunting of the cardiophrenic angle as well. It is important to view earlier films is available to confirm that it is a recent finding. Old pleural diseases will lead to the same finding due to pleural thickening. It is sometimes difficult to see, when the costophrenic angle is behind the rib. Also, in an underexposed film, especially in an obese patient, it becomes difficult to interpret. Second, is the "pleural meniscus" sign. Here, the radiologic density is homogenous and the upper border is concave and is higher in the lateral half of the hemithorax. It is typical of

a pleural effusion and helps to distinguish it from a pneumonia. Third, the "extra pleural" sign. The margins of the opacity are clear cut, pencil sharp, and taper toward both ends. It is also called as the "D sign" when the opacity is abutting the chest wall. A mediastinal disease may also cause an extra pleural sign. Fourth, when the opacity is large one can observe that the pleural disease crosses the fissures. As discussed earlier, other than a few conditions, most parenchymal diseases are limited by the fissures. Pleural diseases easily cross the fissures. The margins of pleural diseases when it crosses the fissures are very sharp unlike the parenchymal diseases, when they cross the fissures, will be irregular. Fifth, movement of the fluid. When in doubt, it is useful to have a lateral decubitus view to confirm that the opacity is mobile. Pleural shadows invariably show movement unless they are encysted or organized. Sixth is the visualization of the underlying pulmonary vessels. While, in a pleural disease, the pulmonary vasculature is observed through the opacity, these are silhouetted if the

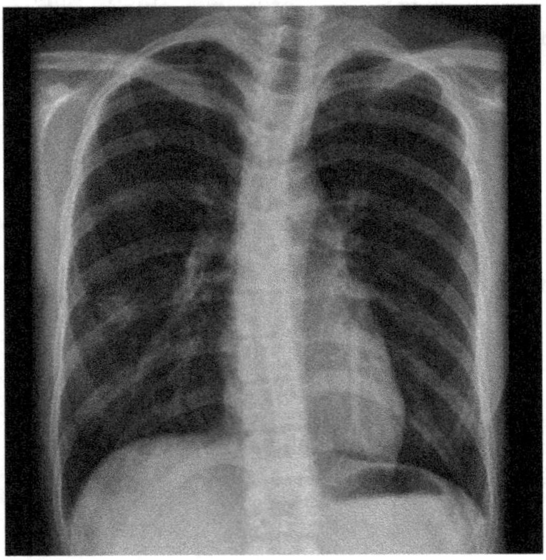

Figure 20: Air crescent sign — Chest radiograph shows a fungus ball (mycetoma or aspergilloma) in a pre-existing cavity. The characteristic crescent of air is seen over the superior margin of the fungus ball.

lesion is within the pulmonary parenchyma. Sometimes, there are fluid levels within the opacity and it is difficult to determine whether it is in the pleura (encysted hydropneumothorax or pyopneumothorax) or in the lung parenchyma (lung abscess). The seventh radiologic observation

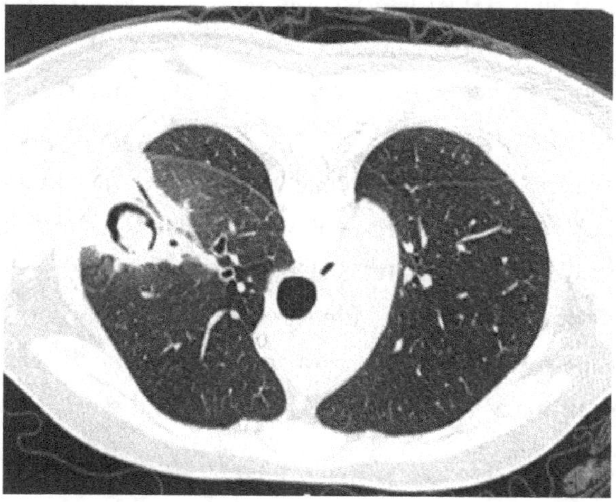

Figure 21: Air Crescent sign-CT Thorax in lung window done in prone position shows a fungal ball in the cavity with a rim of air around the lesion forming a crescent of air.

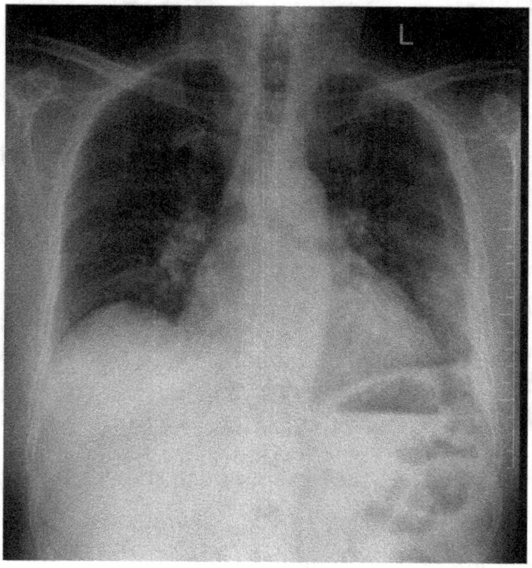

Figure 22: Blunting of the cardiophrenic angle.

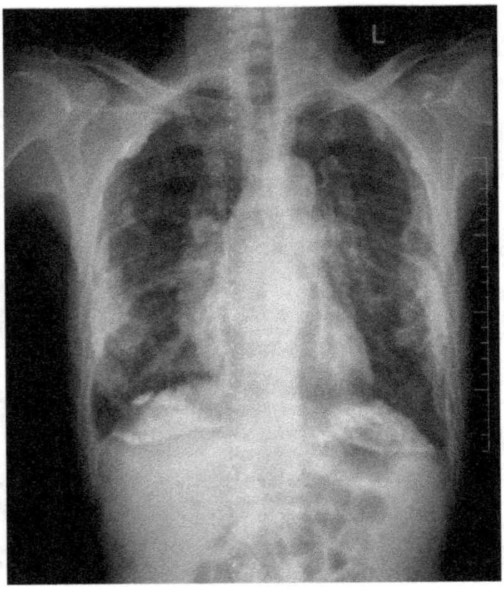

Figure 23: Extensive pleural plaques which are calcified.

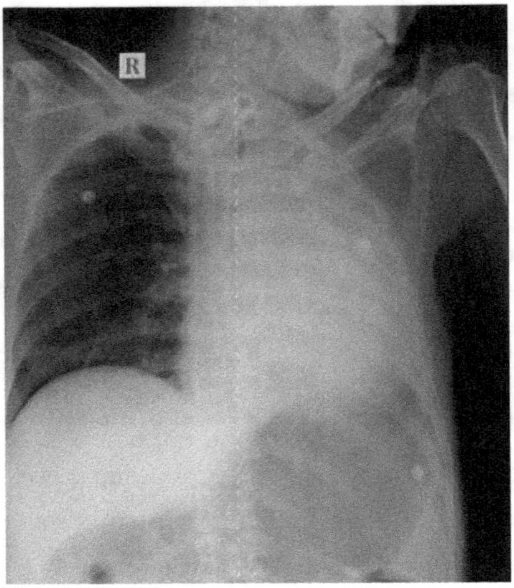

Figure 24: Collapse of left lung with minimal effusion.

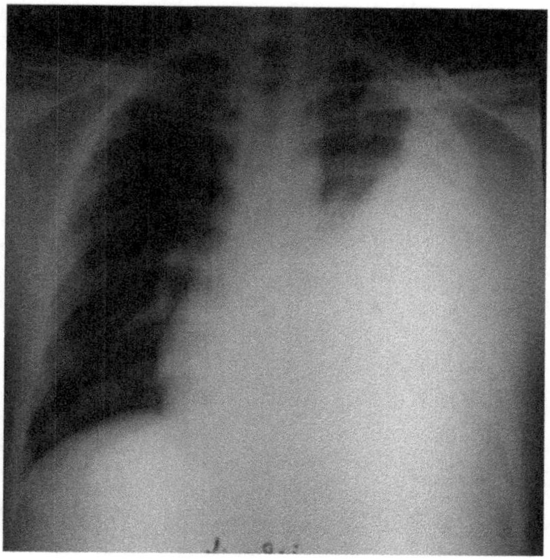

Figure 25: Massive effusion on left side. Ellis S-curve.

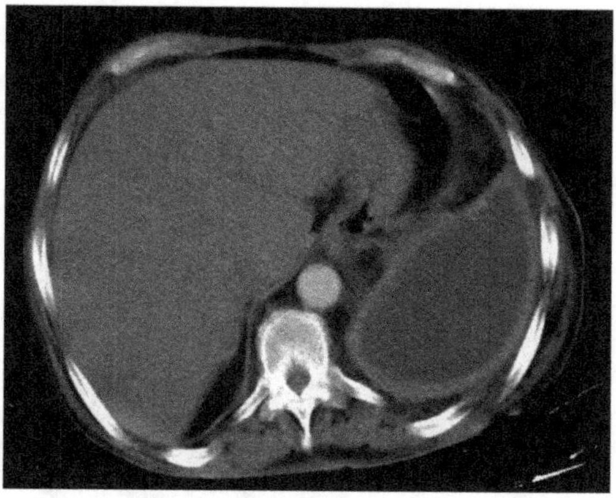

Figure 26: Split pleura sign-CECT thorax showing a well-defined loculated collection in the left pleural cavity along the posterolateral aspect showing the enhancing thickened split pleura sign suggestive of empyema.

would be to compare the diameter of the fluid in the PA and lateral films. If the opacity is within the lung parenchyma, the diameter will be the same in both views, while in a pleural lesion, the diameter would be different.

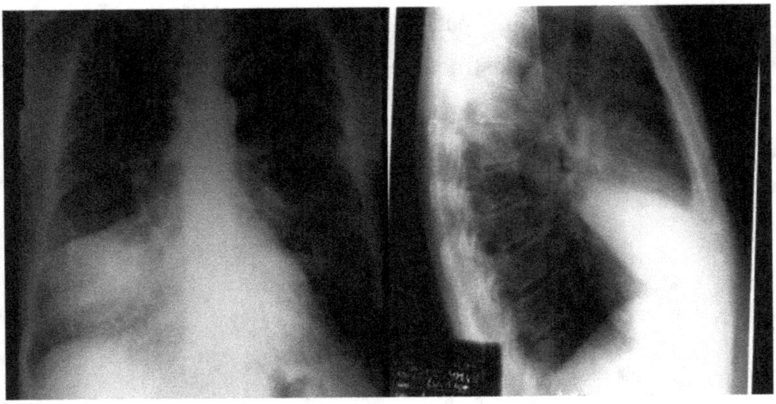

Figure 27: Chest X-ray PA and lateral view showing the loculated pleural effusion in the lower part of the oblique fissure and this is also called as phantom tumor, vanishing tumor, or pseudotumor.

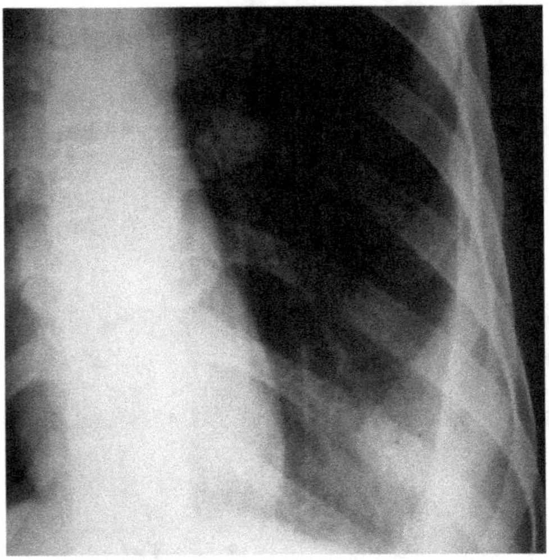

Figure 28: Left-sided pleural effusion encysted within the oblique fissure.

Mediastinum

The abnormal mediastinal shadows are cast due to a mediastinal mass, enlarged lymph nodes, aneurysmal dilation (Figures 16, 35, and 36) of

the large vessel (aorta), and dilation of the major pulmonary artery. The medial margin of the mediastinal opacity is generally not seen separately and merges with the mediastinum. The lateral wall is usually seen and has a clear cut, pencil sharp margins, the extra pleural sign is positive.

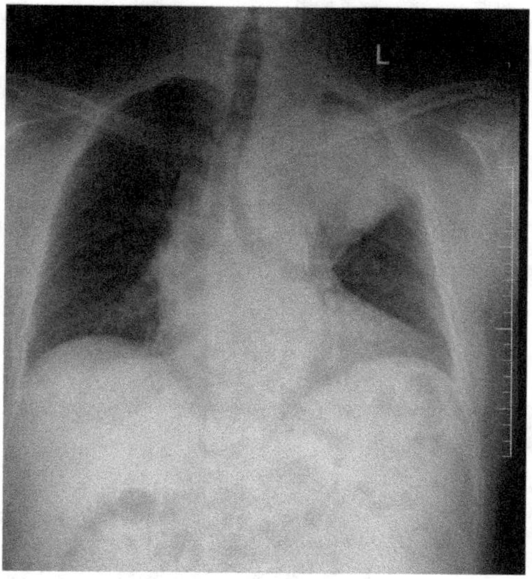

Figure 29: Aneurysmal dilation.

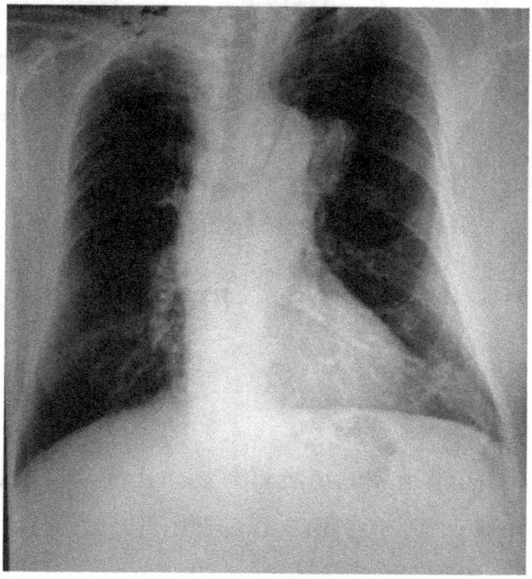

Figure 30: Aortic aneurysmal dilatation.

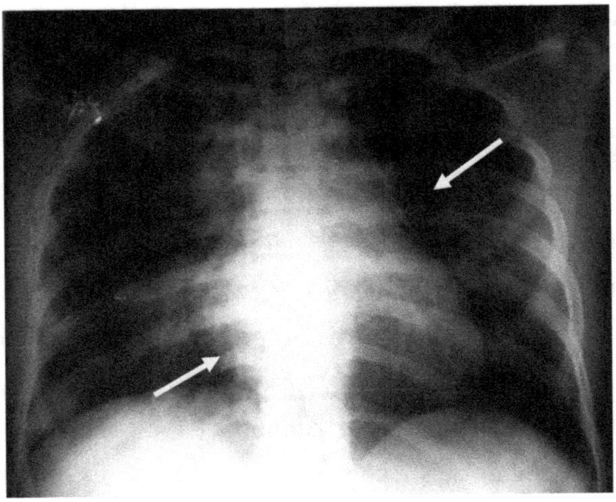

Figure 31: Pneumomediastinum (white arrows), there are bilateral lung infiltrates.

Difficulties can arise when an opacity, usually a benign lesion in the lung near the mediastinum is in contact with the mediastinal margin, and the lateral margin is clear cut and smooth. A malignant mediastinal lesion can infiltrate into the lung and then the lateral margin is irregular. Rarely, the mediastinal lesion is so large that the lateral margin is not seen at all.

Ring around the artery sign

This is a sign associated with pneumomediastinum. The air in the mediastinum is seen around the pulmonary artery in a lateral chest X-ray. It is usually a semi-circular radiolucent shadow around the main pulmonary artery. The other important signs of pneumo-mediastinum are the continuous diaphragm sign, Naclerio's V sign, Spinnaker's sail sign, and extrapleural air sign. Normally, the central part of the diaphragm is silhouetted due to the heart shadow, and in cases of pneumomediastinum, the whole diaphragm is clearly delineated in the continuous diaphragm sign. The Naclerio's V sign is seen usually in cases of pneumomediastinum due to an esophageal rupture and a V-shaped radiolucency is seen in the left cardiophrenic angle. The Spinnaker's sail sign is seen usually in neonates

and is due to the upward displacement of the thymus giving to the sail-shaped shadow.

Mediastinal tumors

Neurogenic tumors

These tumors are found in the posterior mediastinum, which is bordered anteriorly by the pericardium and posteriorly by the spine, and also for practical purposes include the paravertebral gutters. The common Neurogenic tumors are those of peripheral nerve origin such as neurofibromas and neurilemomas (schwannomas), those of sympathetic nerve origin such as ganglioneuromas which are usually benign and neuroblastomas and sympathicoblastomas which are usually malignant, and those of paraganglionic cells such as pheochromocytoma and chemodactomas (paragangliomas) which could be either benign or malignant. Around 30% of the posterior mediastinal tumors are usually malignant.

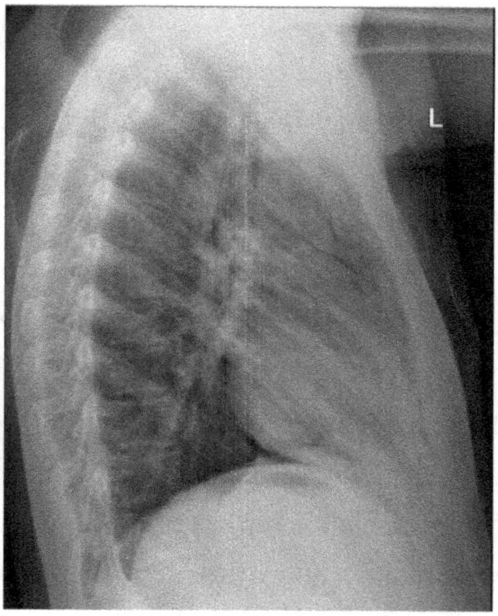

Figure 32: Ring around artery sign-Lateral X-ray of chest shows a rim of air around the pulmonary artery, and air in the anterior mediastinum, indicative of pneumomediastinum.

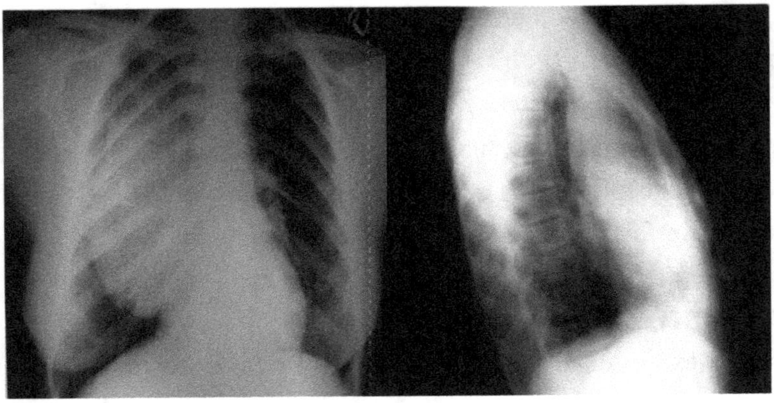

Figure 33: Chest X-ray PA view and lateral view showing an anterior mediastinal tumor.

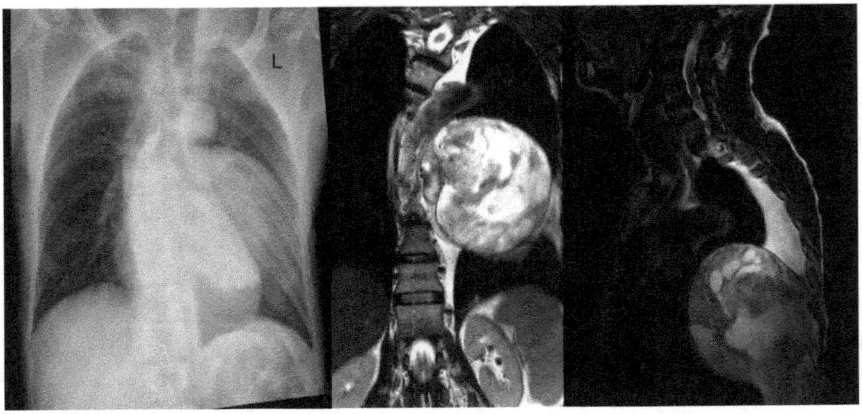

Figure 34: Neurogenic tumors.

Some of the common imaging features include erosion of ribs that may be seen in both benign and malignant tumors, scalloping of posterior vertebral bodies can be observed, both benign and malignant tumors may produce a scoliosis, both benign and malignant tumors may cause pleural effusion, and some of them may enlarge the neural foramina leading to a dumbbell tumor. A meningocele or a neuroenteric cyst also may be identified in the posterior mediastinum. The common differential diagnosis

includes lesions from other structures in and around the posterior mediastinum, cold abscess (Pott's spine), Lymphomas, Esophageal neoplasms, and esophageal duplication cysts, aortic aneurysm and aortic dissection, lipomas and liposarcomas, hiatus hernia and Bockdalek's hernia due to defects in the diaphragm, and extra-thoracic lesions extending to the thorax such as intra-thoracic goiter and pancreatic pseudocyst.

Teratoma

These are extra-gonadal germ cell tumors located usually in the anterior mediastinum in around 80%, posterior or middle mediastinum in 2%–8%. They usually present in the second to third decade and have no gender predilection. They contain a variety of tissues and therefore have different imaging features.

They are usually a well-demarcated mass lesions, displacing adjacent structures, are usually large sometimes as large as 25 cm, usually they are cystic which could be uni-loculated or multi-loculated, there is variable attenuation due to the multiple varieties of tissues in the mass, such as fat, water densities, calcification in a quarter of cases, and in some cases identifiable teeth or bone.

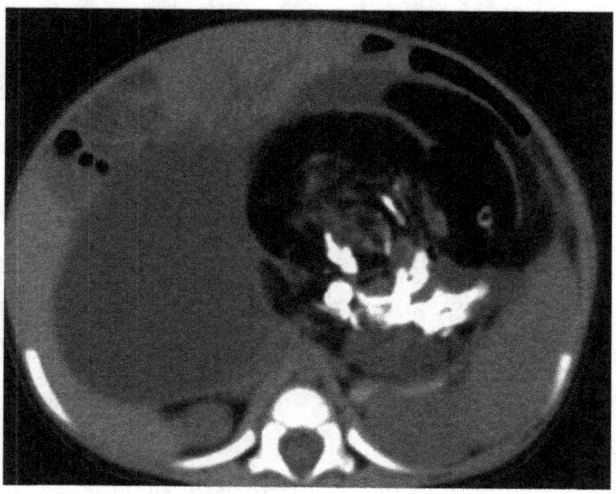

Figure 35: Teratoma.

Thymoma

Thymoma is an important cause of anterior mediastinal tumor which is round or ovoid, may or may not be lobulated, margins are smooth and well defined. This homogenous mass usually projects on the right side and rarely only on the left side or it can project on both sides of the mediastinum, when it is very large. Rarely, can show calcification. Usually benign but can be malignant. CT scans are the preferred modality for evaluation as compared to MRI scans for thymoma, which usually is seen as a sharply demarcated, can be round or oval-shaped soft tissue mass in the anterior mediastinum. When malignant, it can invade the fat or the mediastinal structures including the pericardium and have metastases including in the pleura.

Diaphragm diseases: Diaphragmatic palsy

There is elevation of the hemidiaphragm. Usually, the anterior end of the fifth rib touches the right hemidiaphragm in a chest X-ray PA. It can be elevated to reach the third or even second rib in some cases. On the left side, usually the left hemidiaphragm is one space below the right. If it is elevated 2 cm above the right hemidiaphragm then a diaphragmatic palsy should be suspected. A sniff test on fluoroscopy can help to confirm the diaphragmatic palsy. Alternatively, a real-time ultrasound can observe the

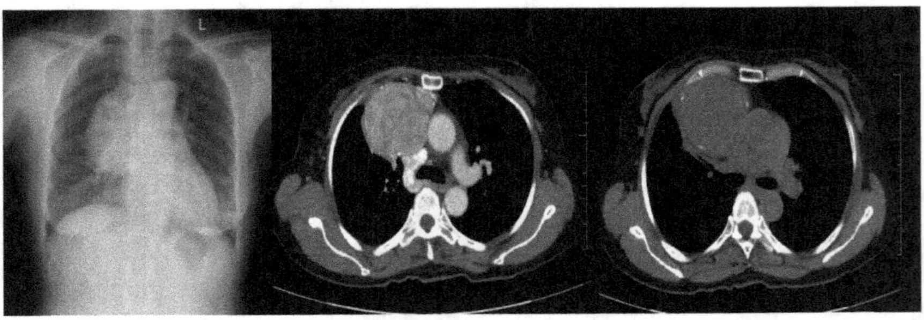

Figure 36: X-ray and CT scans of thymoma.

diaphragm movements and confirm that there is a palsy. The differential diagnosis includes eventration of the hemidiaphragm. The palsy is usually unilateral when it is usually asymptomatic. The cause is usually idiopathic, which is nearly three quarters of subjects, and the other important reason is phrenic nerve involvement due to malignancy such as lung cancer or injury during surgery. There are muscular disorders such as myasthenia gravis, polymyositis, and other muscular dystrophies that can cause diaphragm palsy.

Diaphragmatic hernia

There are several types of diaphragmatic hernia, which could be congenital or acquired which is traumatic. A chest X-ray is usually suggestive, though not always, and may need a CT thorax, barium swallow to have a confirmation. Typically, the chest X-ray will show the left hemithorax filled with cystlike structures which is due to the loops of bowels. The mediastinum is usually shifted to the right, and there will be less gas-filled structures in the abdomen.

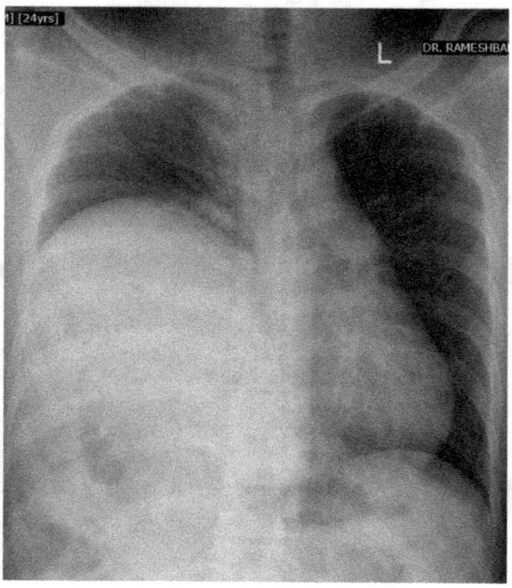

Figure 37: Diaphragmatic palsy showing a grossly elevated right hemidiaphragm.

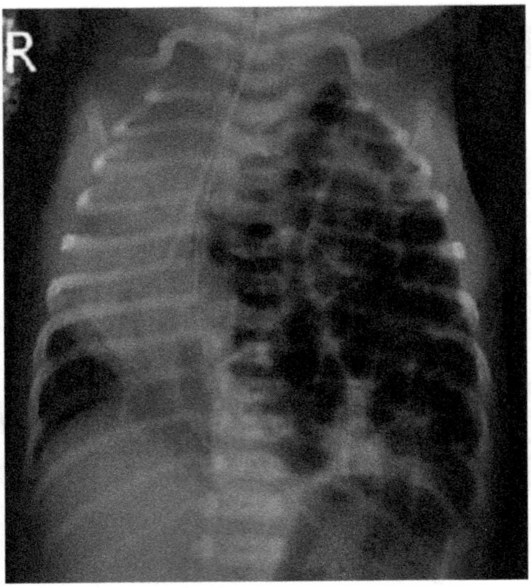

Figure 38: CXR of a child with diaphragmatic hernia of the intestines, with shift of the mediastinum.

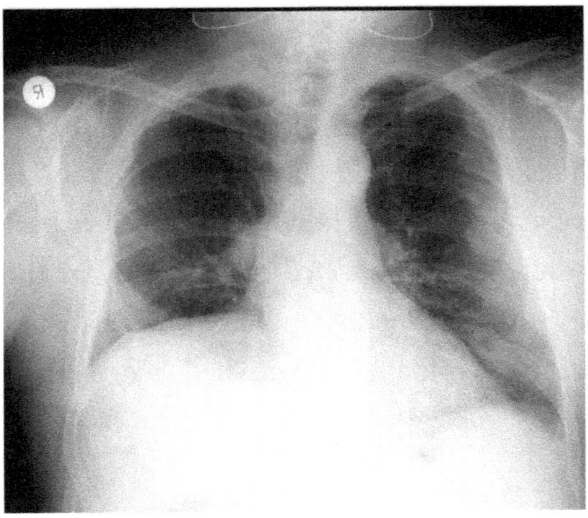

Figure 39: Elevated right hemidiaphragm due to complete eventration.

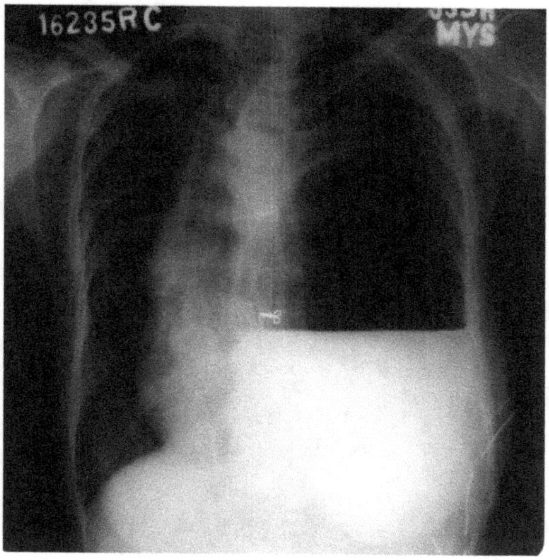

Figure 40: A 76-year-old female with diaphragmatic hernia of the stomach into the thorax shifting the mediastinum to the right side.

Chest wall

It is important to consider whether the lesion is outside the lungs or in the chest wall. A clinical examination before seeing the chest X-ray helps to identify any abnormalities in the chest wall. There have been instances of a CT scan being ordered for a suspected pathology in the thorax which was actually due to a radiologic shadow imparted by a hair tuft. One important clue would be to see if the radiologic shadow extends outside the lung fields.

Pathology

The second part of the diagnosis whether clinical or radiological is to identify the pathology. There are a large number of pathologies that can affect the lungs. As in clinical examination, they can be conveniently grouped under three categories: pathologies causing volume addition, pathologies causing volume loss, and pathologies retaining the same thoracic volume.

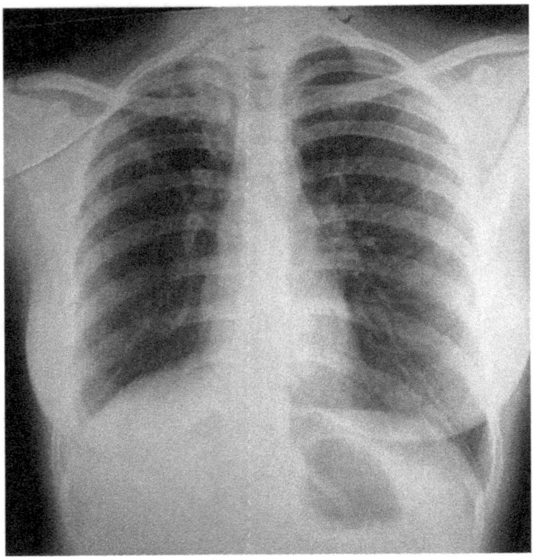

Figure 41: Chest X-ray of fibrosis or hair tuft density right upper lobe? It was a hair tuft!

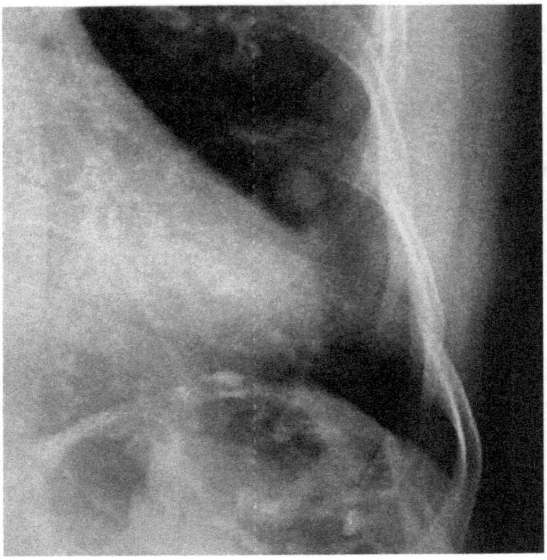

Figure 42: Nipple shadow A nodule seen on the left side.

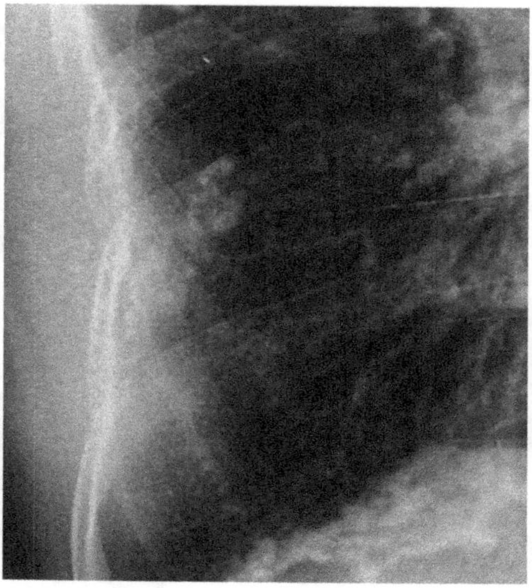

Figure 43: Nipple shadow right side.

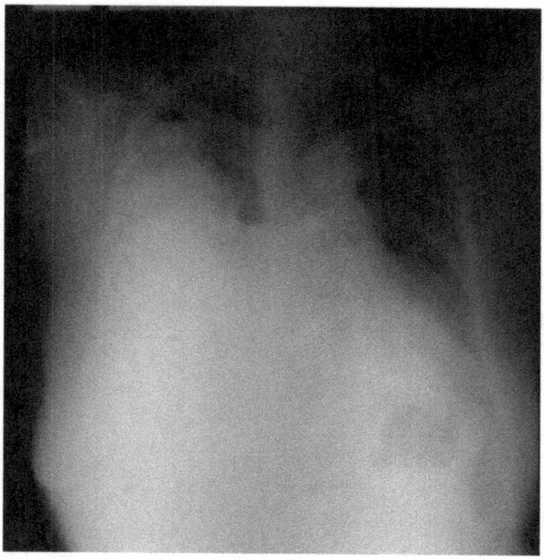

Figure 44: Right-sided massive empyema with shift of mediastinum to the left side.

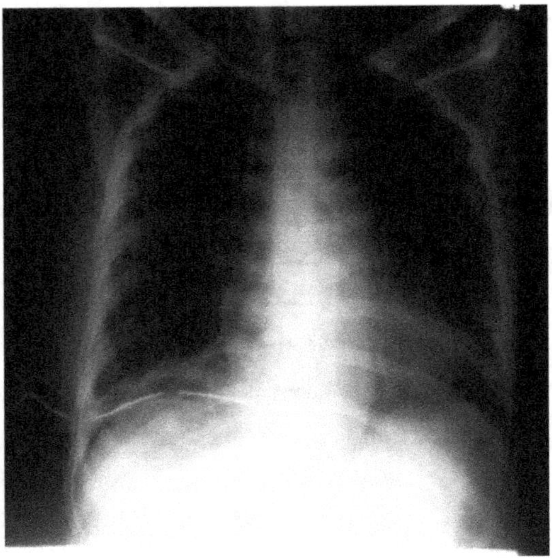

Figure 45: Same patient after drainage of the empyema.

These will be discussed briefly here and more detailed information will be available in the relevant chapters.

Pathologies causing volume addition

The most common of these pathologies causing volume addition to the hemithorax is due to pleural diseases. On clinical examination, one can observe the increased size of the hemithorax, which can be confirmed with a measuring tape. Radiologically, one can observe both in a chest X-ray as well as the CT scan, the increased volume of the involved hemithorax. Pleural diseases that lead to volume addition can be due to the presence of fluid, pus, blood, air, or any combination of the above. Rarely, volume addition can occur due to a pulmonary parenchymal abnormality such as a large bulla or a large mass lesion.

Pleural fluid

The pleural fluid can be either transudative or exudative and casts a shadow of an increased radiologic density. One cannot differentiate from

the radiologic opacity whether the pathology is transudative or exudative, which needs a biochemical examination of the fluid. A transudative effusion is commonly due to a cardiac failure, renal failure, liver failure, or hypoproteinemia. Cardiac failure is usually associated with an enlarged heart, while other conditions may have a normal cardiac size. Transudative effusions are generally mild to moderate and rarely massive. A pleural effusion is said to be mild if the upper border of the fluid is below the anterior end of the fourth rib. If it is above the anterior border of fourth rib and below the anterior border of the rib it is said to be moderate effusion and massive it the fluid levels extends above the anterior end of the second rib. Transudative effusions are also usually bilateral and symmetrical in size. If there is an asymmetry in size in a patient known to suffer from one or more of the conditions associated with transudative effusions, then it is an indication for thoracentesis and fluid examination, since these patients are also prone for respiratory infections and will need additional treatment. Exudative effusions cannot be radiologically differentiated from an empyema in a chest X-ray. Clinical examination, tenderness in the chest

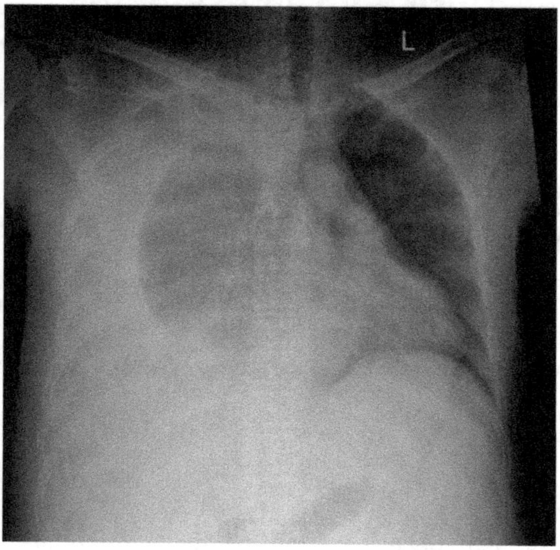

Figure 46: Pleural effusion with collapse.

wall, chest wall edema, and high-grade fever may point to an empyema. Hemothorax is usually associated with trauma and evidence of trauma may be observed in the form of rib fractures. Smaller pleural effusions, or encysted pleural effusions may not cause any volume addition. Fluid can also be collected between the lung and the visceral pleura which causes a thin peripheral opacity along the lungs and is called as a lamellar effusion.

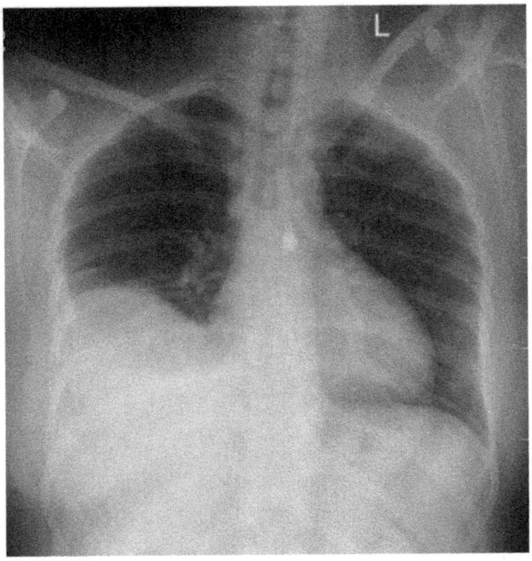

Figure 47: Subpulmonic effusion.

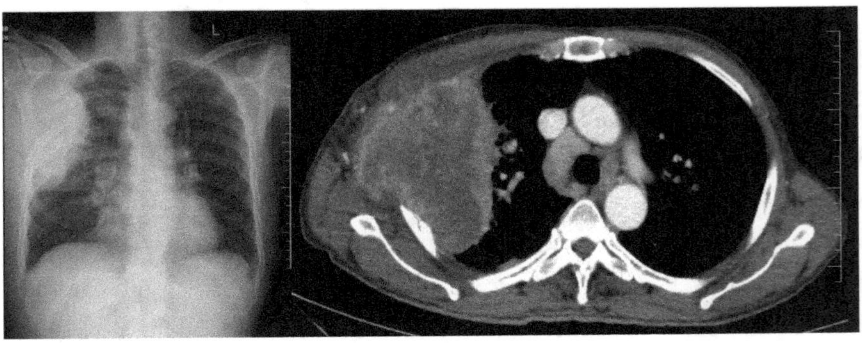

Figure 48: Is this an encysted pleural effusion? Please see the ribs carefully. X-ray and CT scan of Rib erosion due to malignancy.

Normally, in a pleural effusion, the fluid collects between the visceral and the parietal pleura. When fluid collects in the subpulmonic area, only an elevation of the hemidiaphragm is observed. The elevation is usually in the lateral part of the hemidiaphragm. The density of the diaphragm on that side may be greater than the density of the diaphragm on the opposite side. If it is on the left side an additional clue is the increased distance between the fundal gas shadow and the diaphragm. Sometimes, the pleural effusion is massive and is usually associated with a shift of the mediastinal structures such as the trachea and the heart to the opposite side. A massive effusion with the ipsilateral shift of the mediastinal structures usually indicates that there was a primary lesion of a lung collapse usually due to a malignancy, which later spread to the pleura causing a malignant pleural effusion. A chest X-ray is also taken after a pleural aspiration to assess the amount of remaining fluid, iatrogenic complications such as introduction of air into the pleural cavity as well as assessing the underlying lung for a pneumonia or a tumor.

Pneumothorax

Another common cause of increased volume of the hemithorax is the collection of air in the pleural cavity, a pneumothorax, which causes increased radiologic translucency or reduced radiologic density. It is fairly easy to diagnose a pneumothorax when it is moderate or large, but can be difficult if it is small or in the ICU when most chest X-rays are AP views. A small pneumothorax is best seen in the expiratory films. Another method not commonly used now due to the easy availability of CT scans is the contralateral decubitus view, the side in which the pneumothorax is suspected is above. In the ICU, the deep sulcus sign is an important clue for a pneumothorax. Sometimes, when the film is overexposed, there may be difficulties as well to identify a small pneumothorax. One should carefully look for the collapsed lung margin and the absence of any lung vascular markings from that lung margin to the chest wall confirms a pneumothorax. An encysted pneumothorax can be difficult to differentiate from

a bulla, especially when present close to the chest wall. Some of the points of differentiation include a concave medial border in a bulla while it will be convex in an encysted pneumothorax. An encysted pneumothorax may cross the fissures, while a bulla usually does not, though it may push the fissures. A tension pneumothorax is identified by the shift of the mediastinal structures including the trachea and the heart to the opposite side, low flattened or rarely inverted diaphragm, and a complete collapse of the affected lung. It is a medical emergency and can be life threatening if not managed immediately. A chest X-ray needs to be taken after the intercostal tube drainage to observe the tube placement as well as the lung expansion and any underlying cause for the pneumothorax. A line on the chest X-ray which may mimic a collapsed lung margin can be seen due to the pectoral fold. Two clues help to differentiate; the first is the presence of lung markings between the line and chest wall and the second is that the line can be traced outside the lung fields. Another finding is that the collapsed lung margin is usually convex, while here the line may be straight. This is termed as a pseudo-pneumothorax.

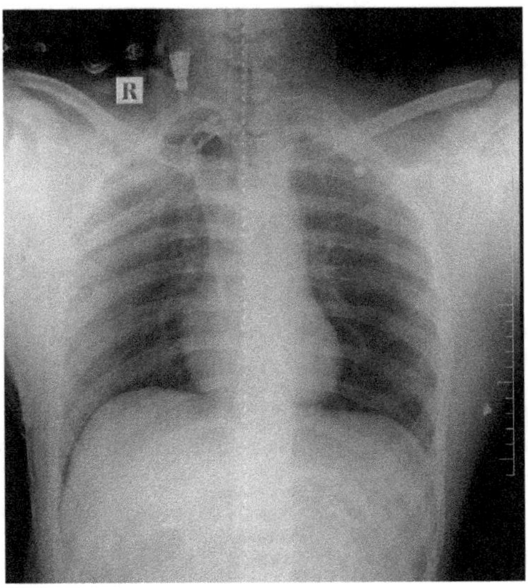

Figure 49: Right deep sulcussign.

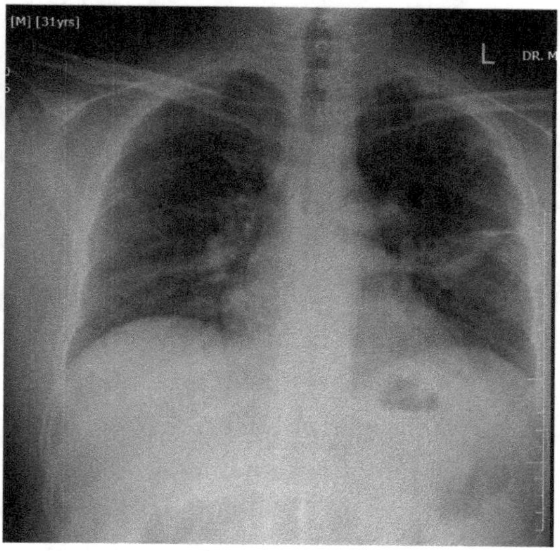

Figure 50: X-ray showing fluid in the left fissure.

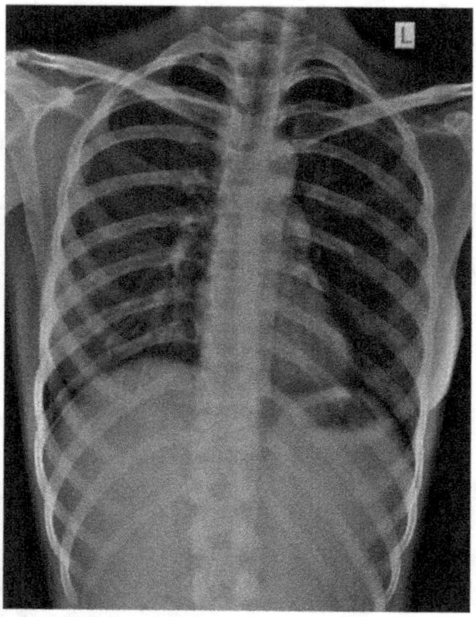

Figure 51: Overexposed film pseudo-pneumothorax.

Hydropneumothorax

It is usually easy to diagnose a combination of air and fluid in the pleural cavity. Difficulties arise when there is an encysted hydropneumothorax and needs to be differentiated from a lung abscess close to the chest

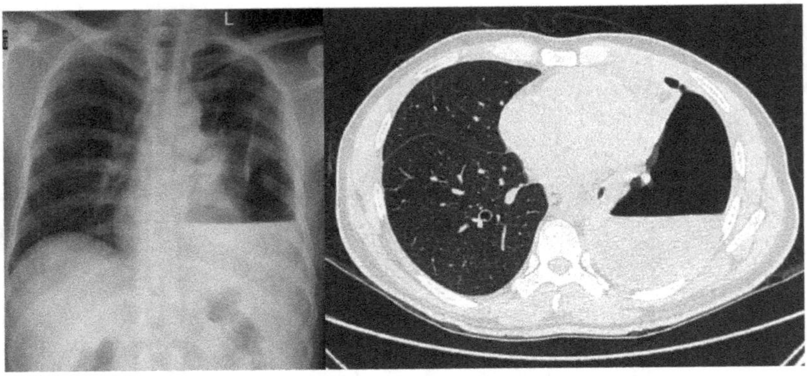

Figure 52: Hydropneumothorax on the left side with air-fluid level and collapsed lung. It is encysted and there is no shift of the mediastinum.

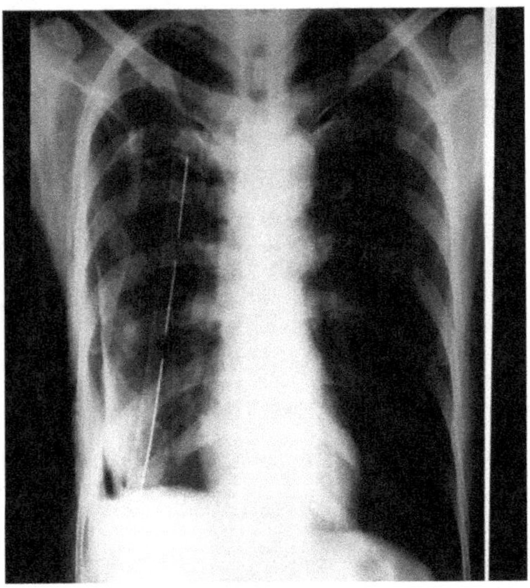

Figure 53: Right-sided hydropneumothorax with intercostal chest tube in-situ.

wall, which will also have an air-fluid level. One of the ways to differentiate it in chest X-rays is to study both the PA and the lateral views. In the lung abscess, which is usually spherical and the diameter of the fluid level will be the same in both the PA and lateral views. In contrast, the diameter of the fluid level will be different in the PA and lateral views

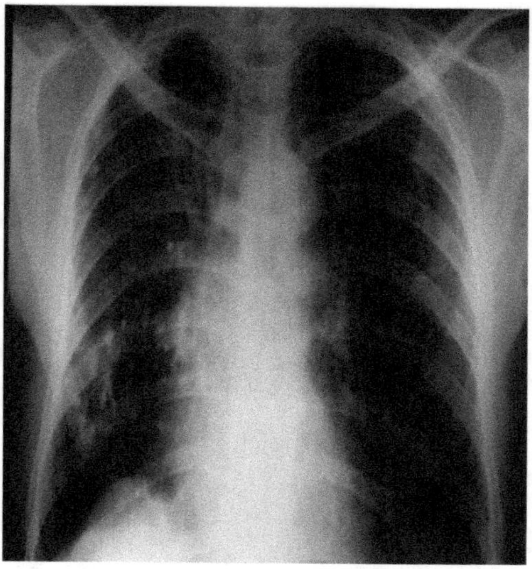

Figure 54: Post TB sequelae with fibrosis and calcification.

in a pleural lesion. The most common cause of hydropneumothorax is tuberculosis. Unless a needle is inserted one cannot be sure whether it is a hydropneumothorax or a pyopneumothorax, which has a combination of pus and air.

Pathologies causing volume loss

This can be due to pathologies in several parts of the thorax including the airways, lung parenchyma, interstitium, pleural, chest wall, and the diaphragm. The common airway diseases causing loss of lung volume are due to collapse which could be due to an intraluminal obstruction (foreign body, mucus plug), intramural obstruction (benign and malignant tumors or bronchial stenosis due to endobronchial lesions such as tuberculosis), and extraluminal obstruction due to a mass or enlarged lymph nodes. Once there is complete obstruction to the main, lobar, or segmental bronchus, the air in the lung gets absorbed into the bloodstream within 24 hours usually leading to a collapse. The other pathology causing volume loss is due to fibrosis.

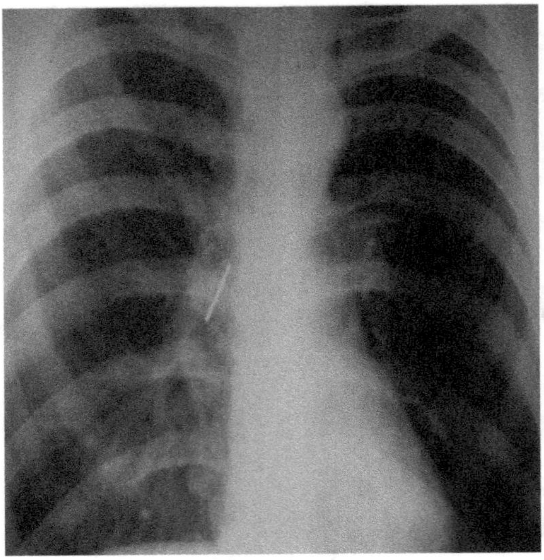

Figure 55: A 48-year-old male with a foreign body in the right main bronchus.

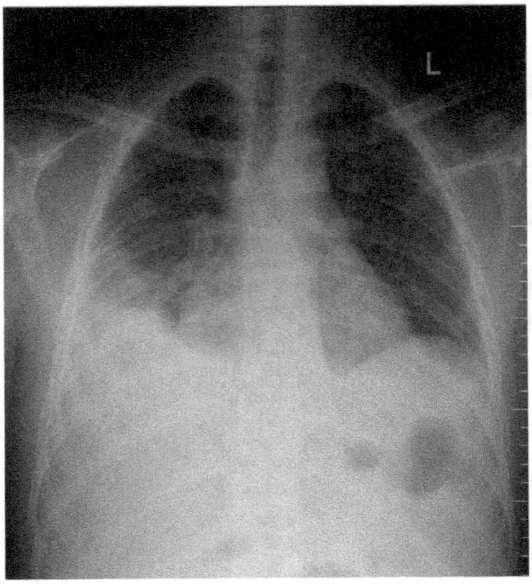

Figure 56: Collapse of a segment of the lower lobe.

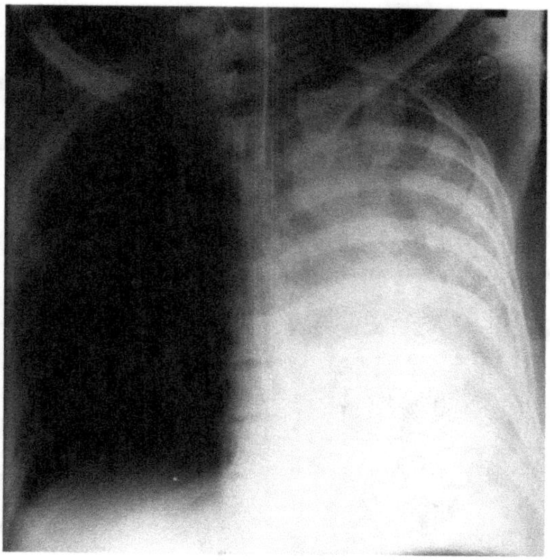

Figure 57: Patient on ventilator. Complete collapse of left lung.

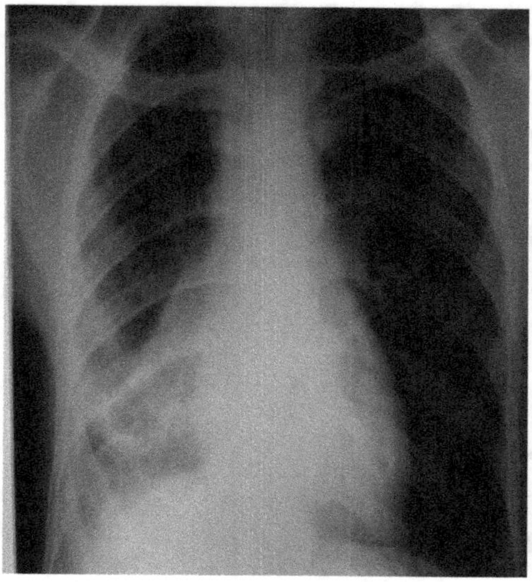

Figure 58: Right lower lobe collapse.

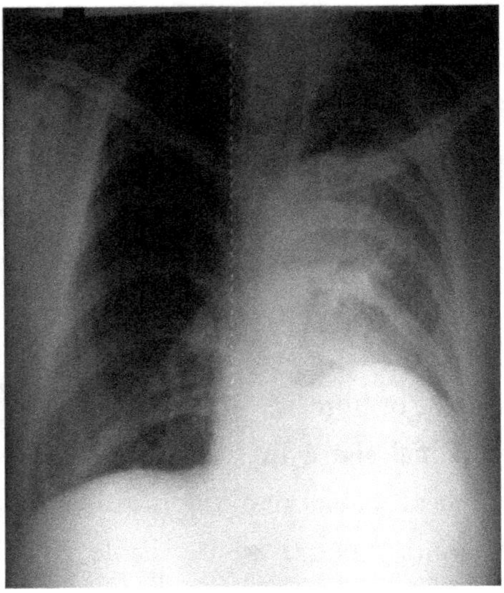

Figure 59: Left lower lobe collapse.

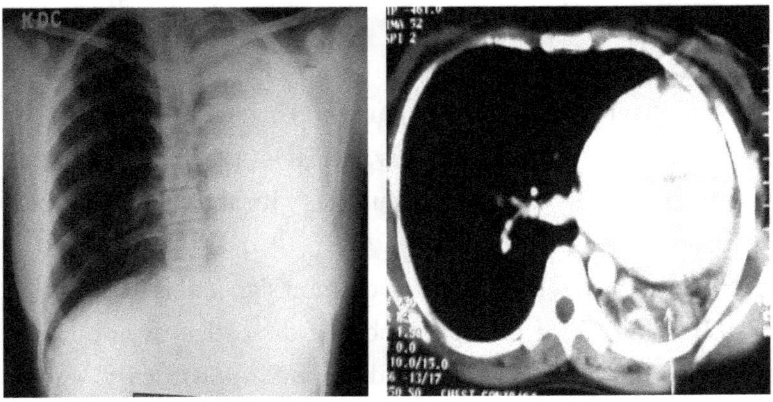

Figure 60: Complete collapse of the left lung.

The radiological evidence of collapse and fibrosis is quite similar. The similarities and the differences in signs are discussed below. Felson has classified these radiological signs into two categories as direct and indirect.

Direct signs:

1. Displaced septa: Septa includes the major or minor fissures. This is one of the most reliable signs of lobar collapse. The extent of displacement depends on the severity of collapse. The decreased volume of the lung becomes easily discernible if we can visualize these septa.
2. Loss of aeration: When there is a collapse, there is loss of aeration, leading to opacity in the affected lobe. It is important to look for other signs that suggest collapse. Presence of silhouette sign is helpful in determining the site of collapse or fibrosis.
3. Vascular and bronchial signs: In the collapsed lobe, sometimes, the vascular marking or bronchial marking is visible for example, if there is an air bronchogram. When these are visible, if there is crowding of the bronchial and vascular markings, it suggests that there is a loss of volume such as collapse or fibrosis. CT scan is ideal to investigate for collapse.

Indirect signs:

1. Unilateral elevation of diaphragm: Both collapse or fibrosis of the lower lobes leads to elevation of the diaphragm. This sign is uncommon when lower lobe is not involved. But this sign is not specific and can be seen as a normal variation as well as in subjects with abdominal disease, such as hepatomegaly or splenomegaly.
2. Deviation of the trachea: This is a common sign and is usually noted in collapse or fibrosis of the upper lobes. If the patient is not positioned properly, it may lead to "spurious deviation of the trachea" and therefore each chest X-ray has to be carefully taken. In a properly positioned chest X-ray, the medial end of the clavicles will be equidistant from the spinous process. It is easy to differentiate between collapse and fibrosis by looking carefully at the tracheal shadow. When due to collapse, tracheal borders will be straight, called as a "pendulum shift." When due to fibrosis, the trachea shadow will appear distorted and irregular, called as "kinking of the trachea." This is an important sign that helps differentiate collapse from fibrosis as a cause for the loss of volume.

3. Displacement of the heart: displacement of the cardiac opacity toward the collapsed or fibrosed hemithorax may occur when the loss of volume is significant due to the size of the heart and is usually seen in lower lobe collapse or fibrosis. The collapsed of the upper and middle lobes generally, does not cause any shift of the heart, as they cannot generate sufficient negative pressure to move the heart.
4. Decrease in the size of the hemithorax: it occurs in the hemithorax where there is a collapsed or fibrosed lung, but needs to be substantial in size to cause a decrease in hemithorax volume. There will be crowding of the rib spaces as compared to the contralateral rib spaces. In subjects with congenital agenesis of a lobe or lung, generally, there is no or very minimal decrease in the size of the hemithorax.
5. Hilar displacement: Shift of the hilum is one the key indirect evidence of loss of lung volume. In the usual normal chest X-ray, the right hilum is lower than the left and in more the 80% of the cases it is about one rib space. In <5% of the normal population both the right and left hila are in the same level. Elevation of the hilum is usually seen in upper lobe collapse or fibrosis. The hilum is likely to be displaced downwards in a lower lobe collapse.
6. Compensatory over aeration: Whenever, there is a collapse or fibrosis of a lobe or lung, the adjacent lobes or the lung, if they are normal and have good elasticity can stretch to fill the space left behind, and the normal lung becomes hyperlucent (more black) and the vascular marking may appear to be spread out as compared to a normal lung and may appear to have oligemia as compared to the other lung. Compensatory over aeration needs to be differentiated from other forms of pulmonary hyperlucency such as Macleod syndrome. Easy differentiation is on fluoroscopy, when the lung with compensatory over aeration cloud-up on expiration. Clinical examination of the patient is easily accessible and very important. Compensatory hyperinflation has key criteria for clinical diagnosis; normal movement of the affected hemithorax, percussion is hyper-resonant, intensity of breath sounds is normal and there are no adventitious sounds.

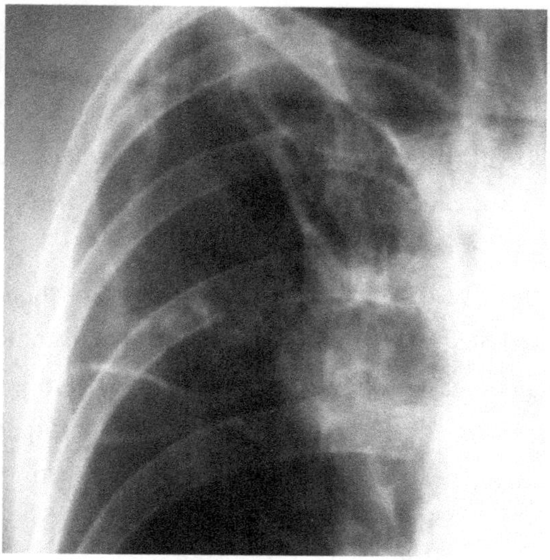

Figure 61: Indirect sign: elevated minor fissure on right side.

Fibrosis:

Another key feature differentiating fibrosis and collapse is fibrotic strands. The smooth counter of the shadows in the thorax such as diaphragm and the cardiac borders will be quite irregular due to the pull from the fibrosis. Unlike in collapse, in fibrosis, the loss of aeration in the involved lung fields is not uniform and is irregular. In the upper lobes, kinking of the trachea due to irregular pull of fibrotic strands helps to differentiate between fibrosis and collapse wherein a pendular shift of the trachea is noted. Fibrosis can be noted in various diseases in the lung; airways as in bronchiectasis, parenchyma as in tuberculosis, interstitium as in interstitial pulmonary fibrosis due to idiopathic pulmonary fibrosis, rheumatoid lung, scleroderma, and other connective tissue diseases, pleura as in organized empyema, or tuberculous effusion, asbestos-related pleural effusion, which can become calcified. It is not possible from clinical examination to comment that there is bilateral fibrosis, as we always comment on the loss of volume by comparing with the contralateral hemithorax. In imaging, it is possible to diagnose bilateral fibrosis. Radiologically, many signs can be applied individually to the hemithorax.

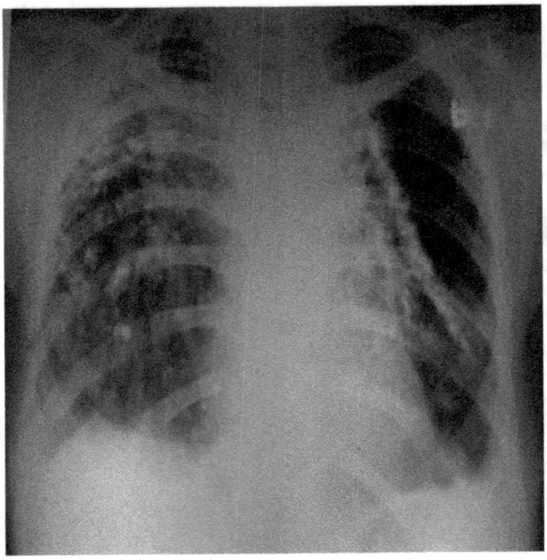

Figure 62: Bilateral extensive pleuropulmonary calcification, elevated hilum is noted on the right lung leading to the waterfall sign of the descending pulmonary artery.

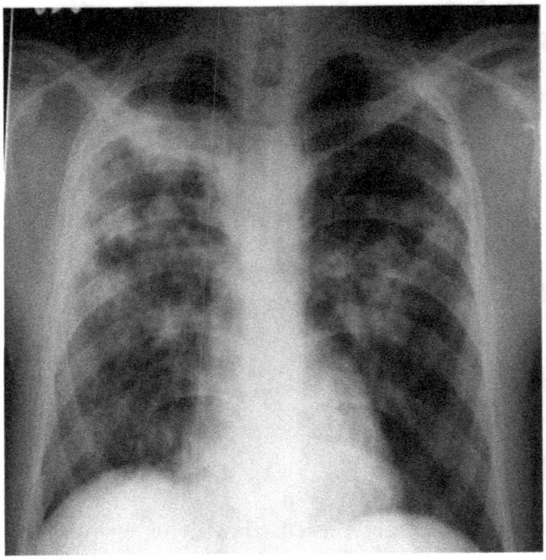

Figure 63: Bilateral pulmonary infiltrates predominately in the upper and mid zones. A case of sputum-positive pulmonary TB.

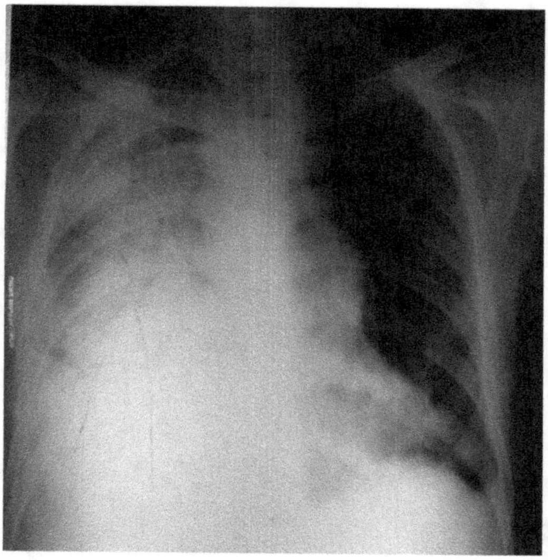

Figure 64: Massive consolidation with air bronchogram and pleural effusion.

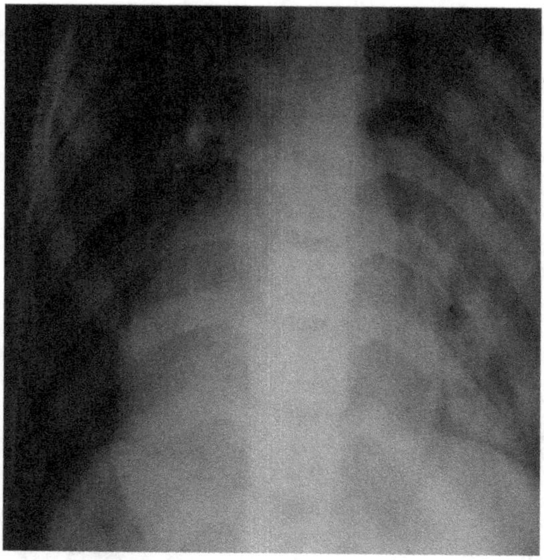

Figure 65: A 16-year-old male presented with extensive infiltrate in the left lung with severe anemia and shortness of breath. A case of idiopathic pulmonary hemosiderosis.

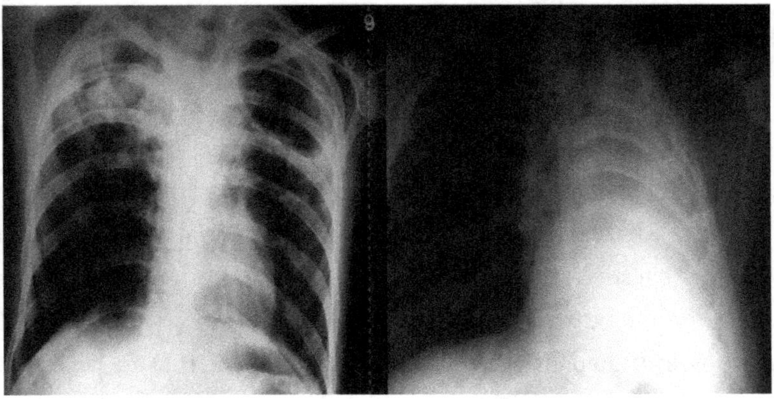

Figure 66: Left lung collapse with pendular shift of the trachea, shift of the mediastinum, silhouette sign, left cardiac border, and left hemidiaphragm.

Volume loss related to parenchymal disease is seen after lobectomy or pneumonectomy, after surgical resection. The key differential diagnosis is a collapse, which it can mimic radiologically. Clinical history and review of the old records and images are the most important and confirmatory. If old records or history is not forthcoming, the total isolation of the bronchus and rib resection in a radiograph should suggest previous thoracotomy and resection. A rib resection is different (smooth margins) from rib destruction in malignancy (irregular margins). The aplasia of the lung has similar radiological features. In aplasia, there is complete suppression of key lung structures such as bronchial, parenchymal, and vascular tissues and only a small bud may be visualized.

Diseases of the interstitium

Loss of volume due to interstitial diseases is a late feature and is generally bilateral, though likely asymmetrical. The volume of both lungs is reduced. The level of both the right and the left hemidiaphragms is elevated. In a chest X-ray, it is commonly mistaken as an "expiratory film," which has the similar findings. Easy to differentiate when a good clinical history and examination are performed. In a patient with interstitial lung disease breathlessness, initially on exertion such as climbing stairs, then progresses to dyspnea at rest is pathognomonic. Additionally, dry cough, tachypnea, and bibasilar crepitations are common. Other differential diagnosis that causes elevation of both the hemidiaphragm is a tense ascites.

A reticular, short linear pattern is typical of interstitial disease. There are situations where the patient has extensive interstitial disease, but a normal-looking chest X-ray, since the individual nodules are very small and therefore cannot be visualized by conventional radiography. An HRCT therefore is indicated in every patient suspected of ILD to have a clear picture. Patients with diffuse interstitial diseases such as IPF and other late-stage ILD's diseases show honeycombing, identified as small air cysts. These cysts, 1–10 mm in diameter, are actually, dilated terminal and respiratory bronchioles.

Disease of the pleura

Usually, pleural disease causes an increase in the hemithorax volume due to addition of fluid, pus, air, and blood, either alone or in combinations of air and other fluids leading to hydropneumothorax, pyopneumothorax, and hemopneumothorax. In certain conditions such as empyema, or high protein pleural exudates, late in the course of the disease, after the "stage of organization," contraction of the lung fields can occur. The diagnosis can be made by adequate history-talking and examining earlier chest X-rays. The loss of the volume is usually associated with pleural thickening, and after a minimum of 2 years, pleural calcification may set in. Any calcification in the lung or pleura confirms that the age of the lesion is more than 2 years.

Pleural thickening usually follows inflammation of the pleura secondary to exudative pleural effusion with high proteinaceous content or empyema. One of the most common causes of pleural thickening and calcificatios. Tuberculosis. The other reasons are empyema and hemothorax, and occupational exposure such as asbestosis. In asbestos exposure, the pleural thickening and calcification is usually bilateral with a predilection

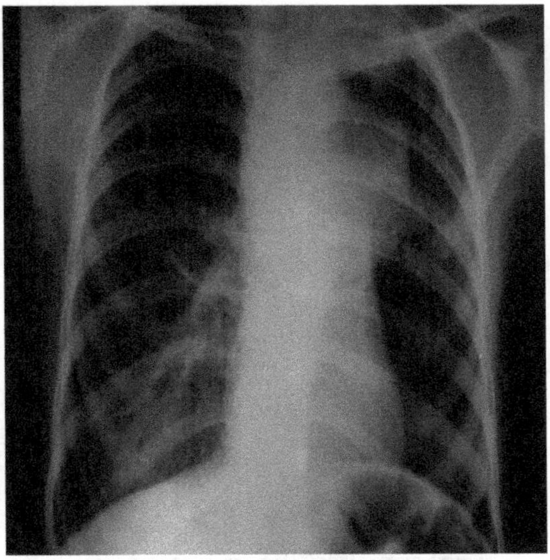

Figure 67: Bronchiectasis.

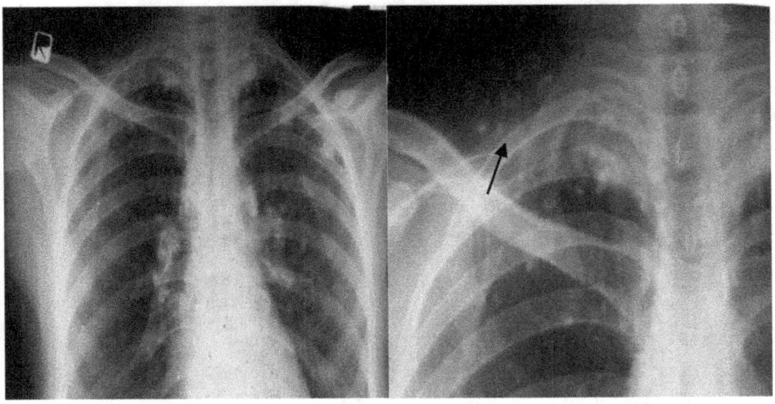

Figure 68: Intra-pulmonary, lymph node (both hilar and paratracheal), and extra-thoracic calcification.

for lower zones and diaphragmatic pleura. Calcium deposits are found in the visceral and parietal pleura due to faulty wound healing. The thickening varies in size; when a significant portion of the pleural is involved, it can lead to impairment of respiratory movements. When causing distress,

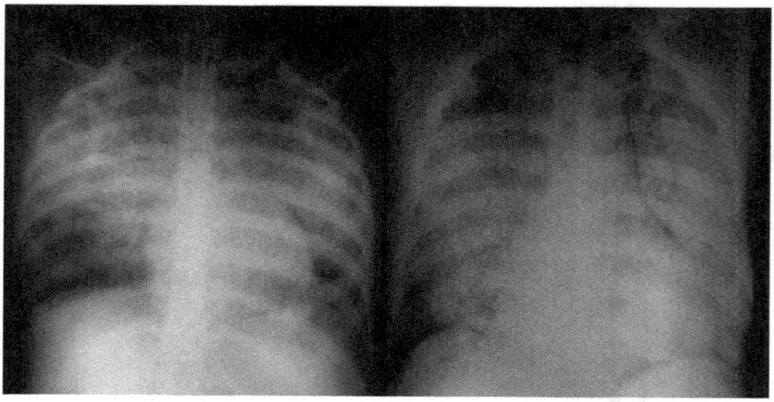

Figure 69: Chest X-ray showing ARDS.

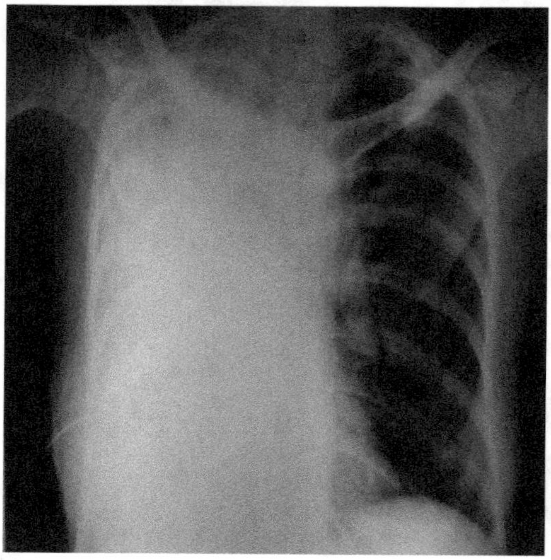

Figure 70: Right-sided empyema with shift of mediastinum to the same side.

it needs to be surgically resected to release the underlying lung. Pleura thickening at the apex of the lung, is termed as pleural cap, and the most common reason is due to tuberculosis.

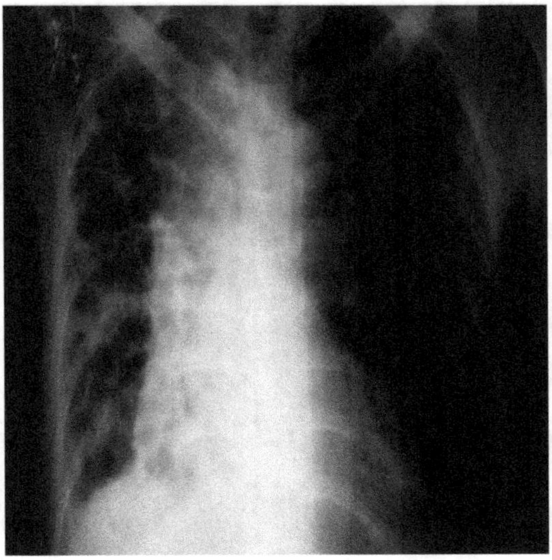

Figure 71: Empyema was secondary to bronchiectasis which was visible after drainage of the empyema and lung fibrosis secondary to bronchiectasis led to volume loss.

Diseases of the diaphragm

Volume loss of the lung is commonly accompanied by an elevated ipsilateral hemidiaphragm especially, when the lower lobes or the entire lung is involved. A disease limited to the upper lobe does not cause an elevation of the hemidiaphragm. Whenever there is a raised hemidiaphragm consider the following possibilities

1. Supradiaphragmatic disease: these groups of conditions include diseases between the undersurfaces of the lungs and pleura. Here, the contour of the diaphragm is retained. Classical example is the "subpulmonic" pleural effusion. The entire hemidiaphragm may appear to be elevated. Diagnosis of the site of the disease can be ideally confirmed by ultrasound. In centers, where ultrasound is not easily available, then

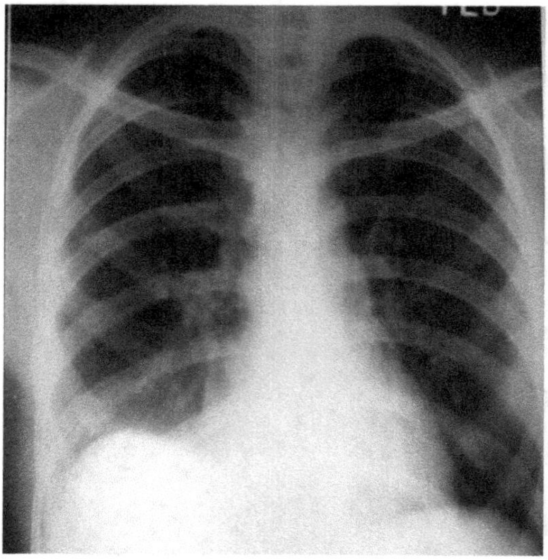

Figure 72: Right-sided subpulmonic.

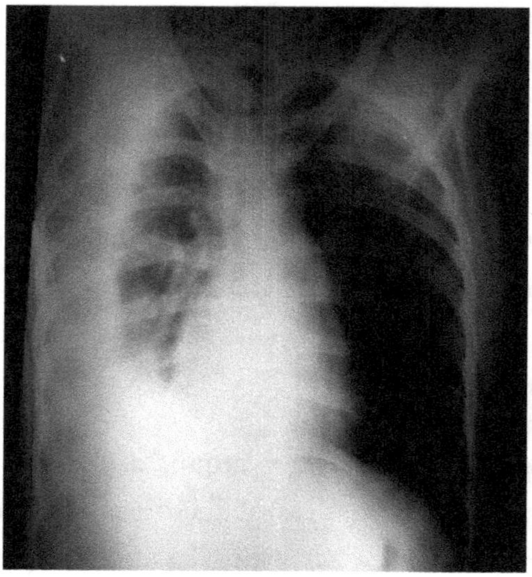

Figure 73: Lateral decubitus view showing effusion shifting of the fluid from the sub-pulmonic area.

the presence of fluid can be confirmed in cases where the fluid is not encysted by a lateral decubitus film, where, the fluid will gravitate out of the subpulmonic region and is easily detected. In subpulmonic effusion, only the lateral part of the hemidiaphragm can be elevated. A similar elevation of the medial part of the hemidiaphragm is usually due to a diaphragmatic hump which is a natural variation or due to irregular contraction of the diaphragm.

2. Diaphragmatic diseases: Unilateral diaphragmatic paralysis affecting one of the hemidiaphragms can be seen in several conditions; ipsilateral phrenic nerve infiltration due to tumor, phrenic nerve damage due to trauma, surgery, or radiation. A congenital condition leading to elevation of the hemidiaphragm mimicking diaphragmatic paralysis is seen in complete eventration of the diaphragm. This condition commonly affects the left hemidiaphragm and can show marked elevation and is rarely seen on the right side. It is due to the complete absence or reduced number of muscle fibers in the affected hemidiaphragm. In partial eventration of the hemidiaphragm only a part is elevated. Eventration can be differentiated from the paralysis of the diaphragm by the "sniff test" during fluoroscopy. When the subject takes a rapid sniff, there is a paradoxical movement of the affected hemidiaphragm in subjects with a paralysis of the diaphragm compared to the contralateral side. Earlier a fluoroscopy was used, now an ultrasound gives the same information. The hemidiaphragm moves by 1–3 cm in quite breathing and 3–9 cm in deep breathing, higher in athletes compared to average subjects.
3. Infra-diaphragmatic diseases: There are conditions of the abdomen which cause an elevation of one or both the hemidiaphragm. Large ascites is a common condition which can be due to several diseases and is associated with elevation of both the hemidiaphragms. In addition, this leads to a reduction of lung volume. Enlargement of the liver, spleen, kidney, and subphrenic abscess are some of the causes, for elevation of one of the hemidiaphragm. In a chest X-ray, it is easily diagnosed

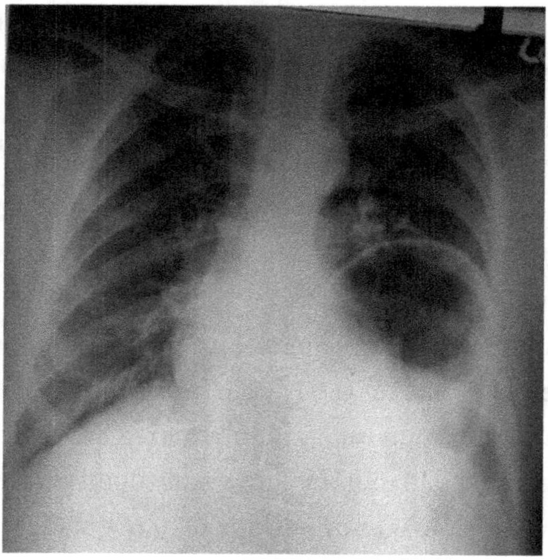

Figure 74: Eventration.

on the left side by looking at the distance between the contour of the diaphragm and the fundal gas shadow. In normal subjects it is about 1 cm. An ultrasound examination can confirm it easily. Other than fluids, air under the diaphragm also can lead to similar findings and a common cause is intestinal perforation leading to gas collection under the diaphragm which leads to elevation of both the hemidiaphragms and reduce the lung volumes.

Diseases of the chest wall and spine

Diseases of the chest wall, muscles, and spine are also associated with loss of lung volume. Congenital kyphoscoliosis, causes in many cases large loss of lung volume due to inadequate lung development. Acquired conditions such as thoracoplasty and lung surgeries that led to collapse of the involved lung to treat complication of tuberculosis, the classical example being massive hemoptysis. Spinal injuries especially in younger ages led to loss of lung volume due to poor lung development.

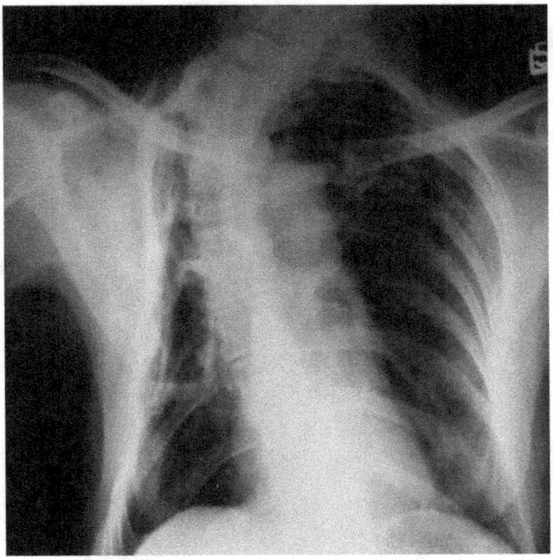

Figure 75: Thoracoplasty.

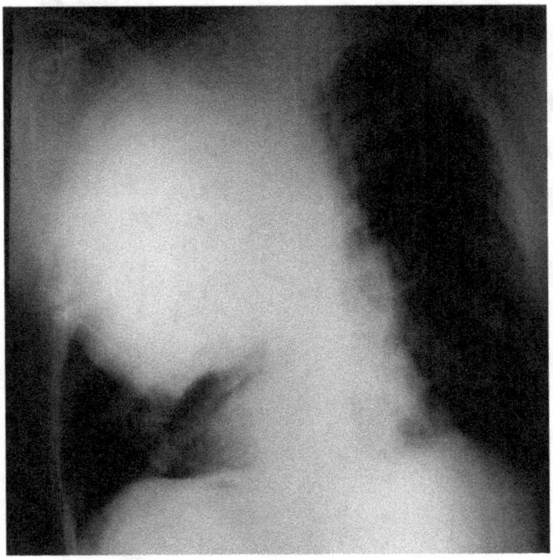

Figure 76: Large tumor in the right lung in case of squamous cell carcinoma.

Pathologies causing volume replacement

Some diseases cause volume replacement, in which the air that is normally present in the lungs is replaced by either fluid, pus, inflammatory cells, tumor cells, or calcium. On both clinical and imaging evaluation,

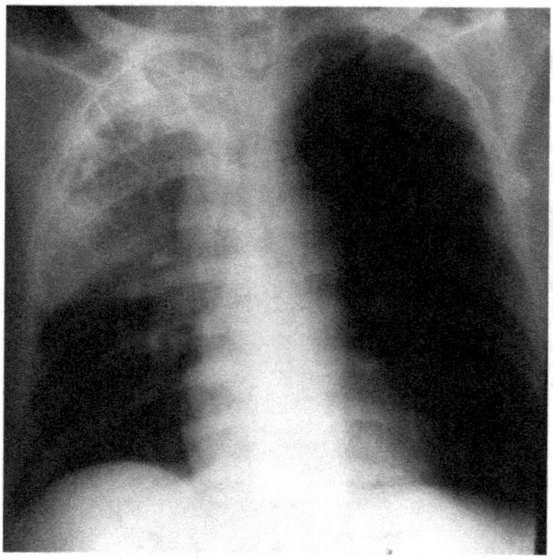

Figure 77: Right upper lobe pneumonia and the lower end are limited by the minor fissure.

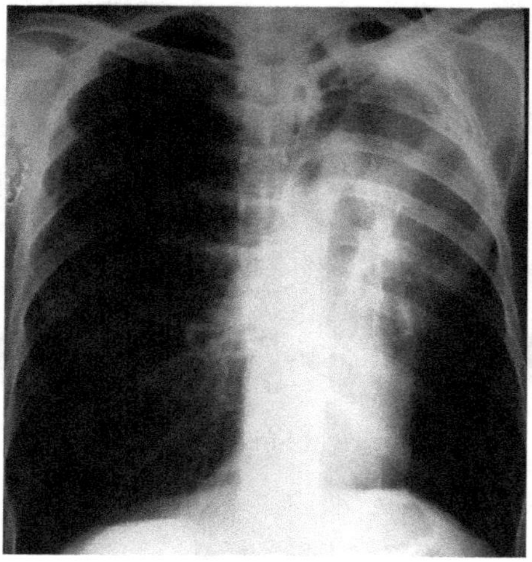

Figure 78: Post-obstructive pneumonia presented with rapid onset breathlessness. Chest trauma few months ago and patient.

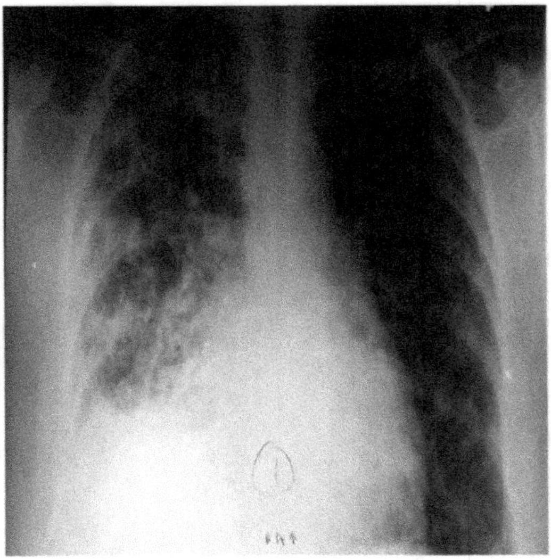

Figure 79: A 48-year-old female patient presented with bilateral infiltrates more the right lower and mid zones. She was treated with antitubercular drug for 5 months and was referred for the evaluation of nonresponsiveness and possible drug-resistant TB. She was never sputum positive. Bronchoscopy confirmed adenocarcinoma. This was a case of bronchioloalveolar carcinoma which commonly presents as a non-resolving pneumonia.

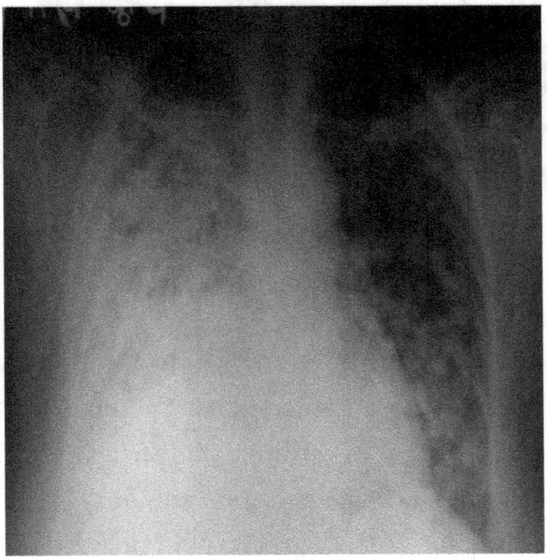

Figure 80: A 35-year-old female patient for evaluation of non-resolving pneumonia. A case of bronchioloalveolar carcinoma.

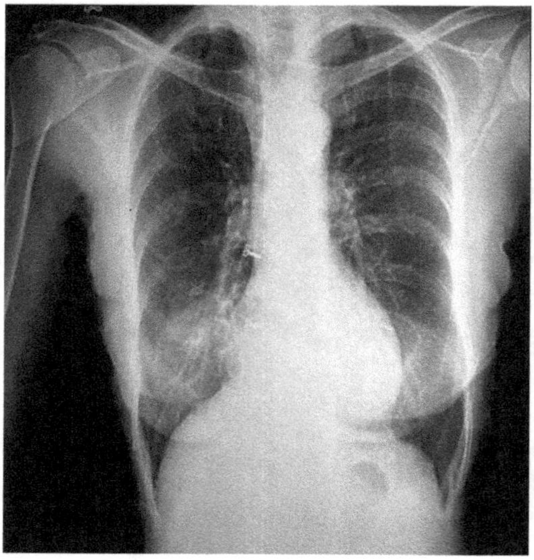

Figure 81: Increased density right lower zone, early pneumonia.

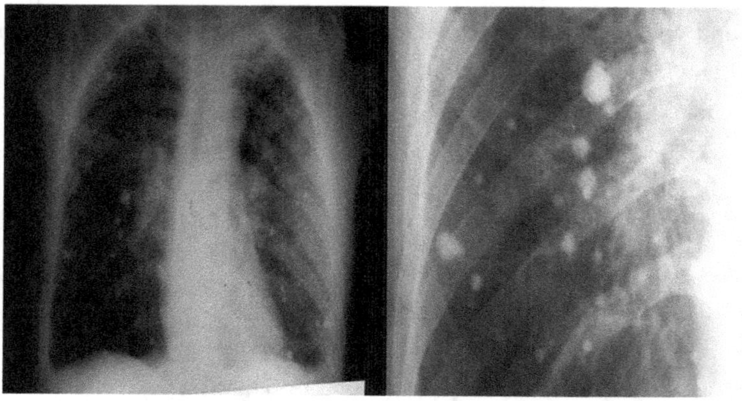

Figure 82: Bilateral pulmonary calcification due to post tubercular sequelae (Simons foci, starry sky appearance).

the volume of the affected hemithorax looks identical to the contralateral hemithorax. Clinically, one can observe that the movement of the hemithorax is reduced. The diseases causing volume replacement, commonly are various pneumonias which in some cases may be associated with parenchymal destruction, including TB, pulmonary nodules and mass lesions, cysts and cavities, and pulmonary calcification.

Pneumonias

Pneumonias are fairly common in routine clinical practice and may involve any part of the lung and can be sub-segmental, segmental, or lobar or involve the whole lung. It can also involve different areas of both the lungs. It could be due to infective or non-infective causes.

Infective

a) Pyogenic: gram-positive, gram-negative, and anaerobic organisms are common. Examples include *Streptococcus*, *Pneumococcus*, *Klebsiella*, *Pseudomonas*, *Acinetobacter*, *Escherichia coli*, and *Staphylococcus*.
b) Tubercular — Both mycobacterium tuberculosis and mycobacterium other than tuberculosis (MOTT) or nontubercular mycobacteria (NTM).
c) Fungal
d) Various opportunistic infections in immunocompromised patients

Pneumonia with destruction

It is common for pneumonias to be associated with parenchymal destruction, which is seen in pyogenic necrotizing pneumonias, lung abscesses, and tuberculosis. They are initially seen in imaging evaluation as breaking down lesions and progress to a cavity with or without fluid levels. The cavity can vary in size and usually has satellite lesions. The wall of the cavity is usually less than 1.5 mm in a benign lesion. A cavity with a fluid level is called a lung abscess, which can be easily made out in a chest X-ray. There are pyogenic organisms which commonly cause destruction such as Staphylococcus and Klebsiella. Both of these infections can lead to air-filled cavities, and these are called pneumatoceles, where the air is under tension with a high risk for rupture leading to a pneumothorax or a pyopneumothorax with or without tension and are life threatening. Paradoxically, they occur during treatment and the mechanism is due to the ball valve effect due to the granulation tissue that develops during healing, in the

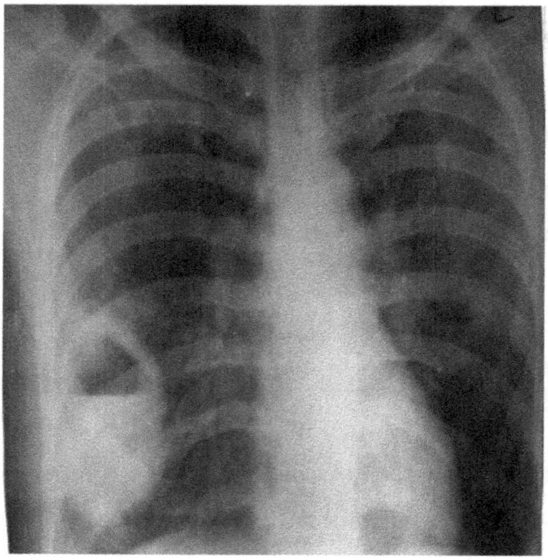

Figure 83: Lung abscess.

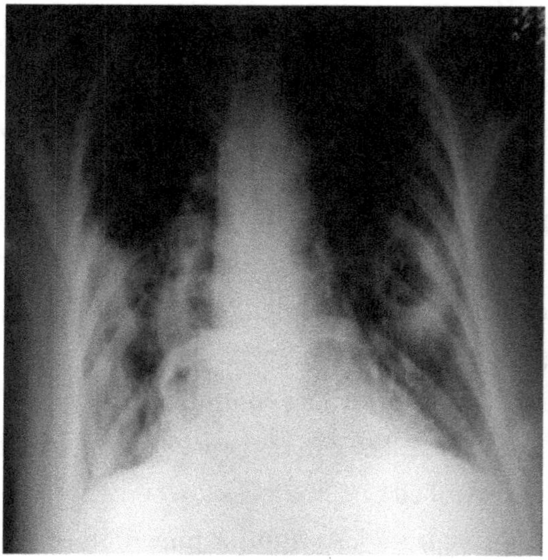

Figure 84: Lung abscess in TB (Sputum +).

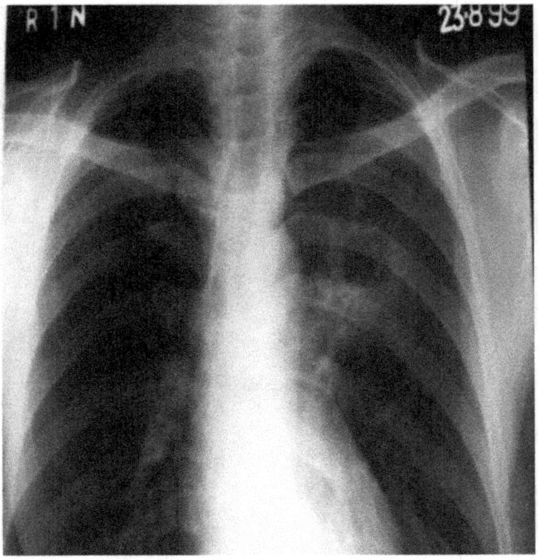

Figure 85: Left upper lobe cavity with air fluid level (lung abscess).

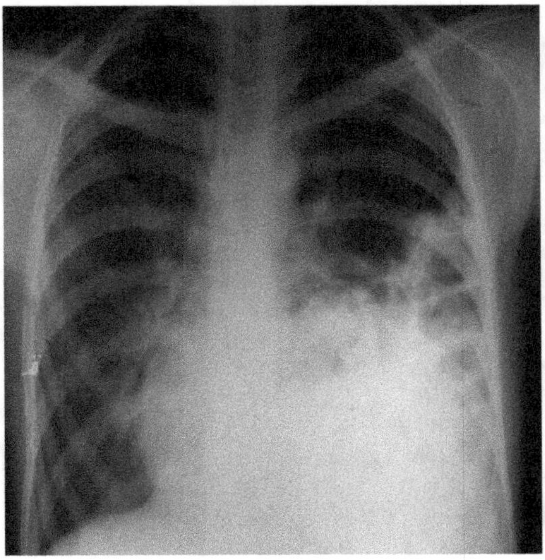

Figure 86: Left-sided diaphragmatic hernia showing intestine within the thoracic cavity.

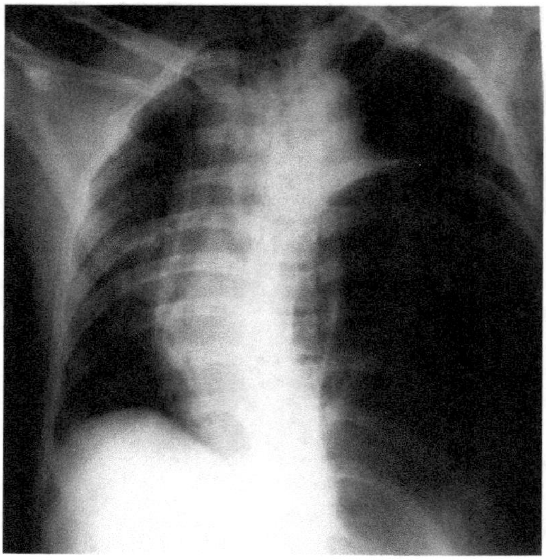

Figure 87: Traumatic diaphragmatic hernia.

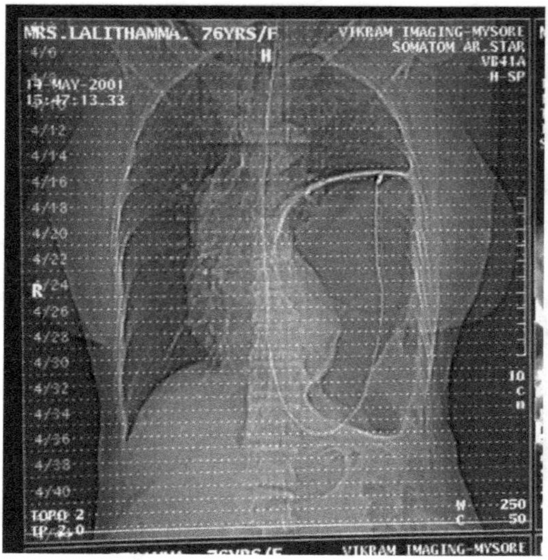

Figure 88: A CT scanogram of the same patient showing ryle's tube within the stomach and in the thorax.

small airways leading to air trapping and development of tension air-filled cavities.

Nodules and mass lesions

Pulmonary nodule

Many diseases present as nodules in the lungs which can be solitary or multiple. A nodule is clearly circumscribed and is usually surrounded by air-containing lung. A nodule has a clear sharp outline and can be of different size. A large nodule of greater than 3 cm is called a mass lesion. A nodule may be solid or can be filled with fluid.

1. Presence of calcification is seen in a benign lesion. Rarely, calcification is seen in malignant lesions.
2. The borders of a benign nodule or mass lesion are smooth and sharp, while shaggy and irregular borders are seen in malignancy

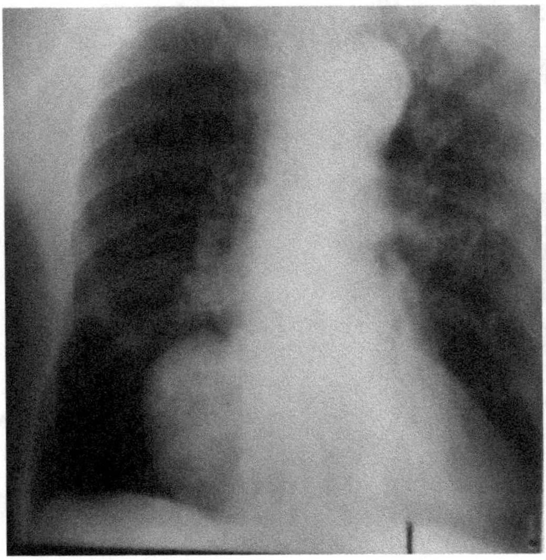

Figure 89: Patient with COPD suffering for 2 years present with mass lesion with right paracardiac region. A case of lung cancer. Sometimes in cancer the borders can be smooth as well.

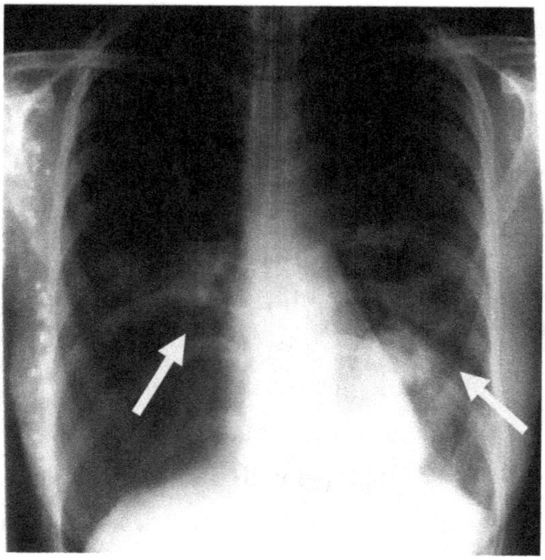

Figure 90: Multiple nodules in both lung fields due to TB.

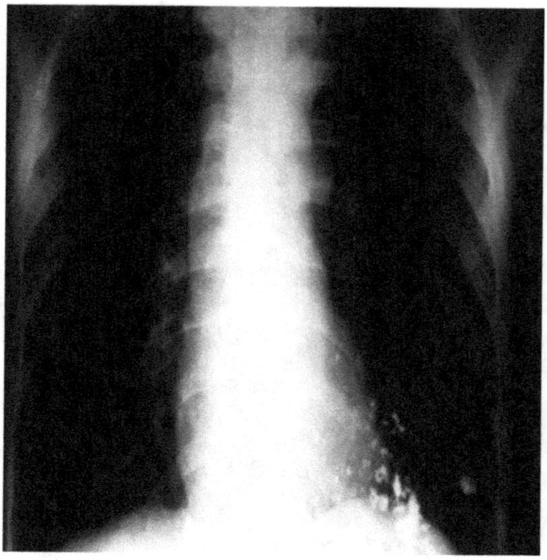

Figure 91: A case of carcinoma esophagus which has infiltrated into the airways. A barium swallow has entered the lungs through the esophago-bronchial fistula.

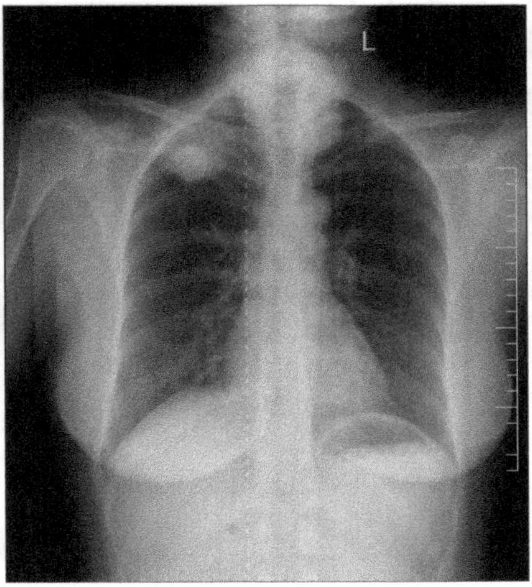

Figure 92: Hair artifact. A repeat chest X-ray revealed normal lung fields when the artifact was removed.

Table 1:

Solitary		Multiple	
Benign	**Malignant**	**Benign**	**Malignant**
Granulomas Lung abscess Encysted pleura fluid Hydatid disease Hamartoma Benign tumors: lipoma, fibroma, Neurofibroma, bronchial adenoma	Lung cancer Solitary metastasis	Granuloma Lung abscess. Hydatid disease Encapsulated pleural fluid Wegener's granulomatosis	Lung cancer Metastatic cancer

3. Rate of growth: This is measured by the doubling time and that is the time taken for the volume of the mass to double and not the diameter. The volume has doubled if there is an increase in the diameter by a factor of 1.25. For example, if the diameter of a lesion is 3 cm, then for the

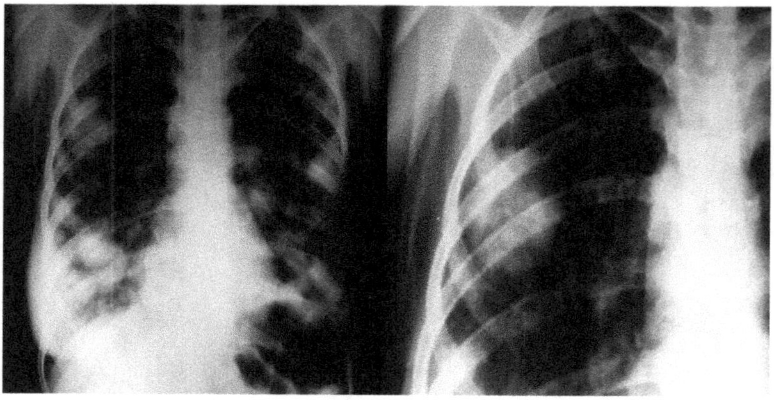

Figure 93: A case of 26-year-old female with choriocarcinoma and lung metastasis (cannon ball metastases).

volume to have doubled it should reach a diameter of 3.75 cm. When the lesions are benign they grow very fast (classic example is inflammatory lesions) or very slowly (classic example are benign tumors)

4. The diagnosis of these mass lesions has to be confirmed with histopathology. Serial X-ray are very useful. If there is no change in the radiologic opacity for over 2 years, the lesion is most likely benign. However, in the early course of the disease, where previous chest X-ray are not available, invasive investigations are necessary to confirm the diagnosis.

Pulmonary mass

A mass lesion is a solitary radiologic opacity, usually homogenous, and is more than 3 cm in its maximum diameter, with a high possibility of being cancerous. In a malignant mass, the margins are usually shaggy, but is smooth in metastatic lesions like a single cannon ball metastasis. Cavitation can be seen in malignant lesions and hilar and mediastinal lymphadenopathy can be observed. Pressure effects such as those on the phrenic nerve causing ipsilateral diaphragmatic paralysis or on the left vocal cord, leading to hoarseness of voice due to left vocal card palsy. Bronchioloalveolar carcinoma usually presents as unresolved pneumonia with presence of air bronchograms.

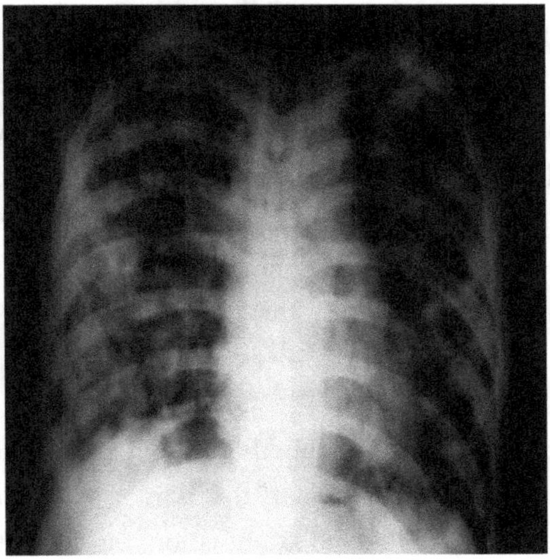

Figure 94: Metastatic cancer.

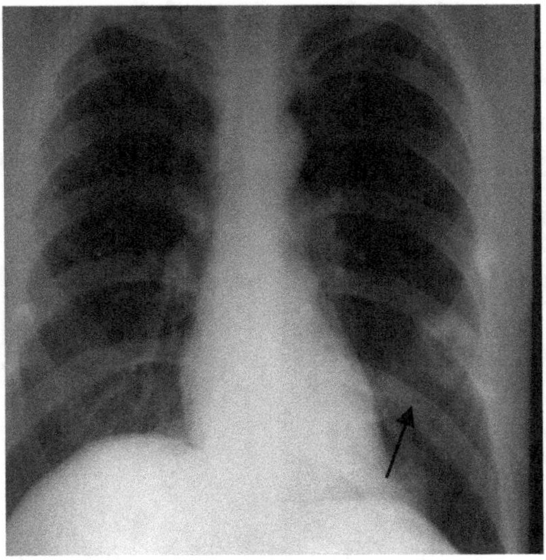

Figure 95: Adenocarcinoma left lung.

Pulmonary interstitial nodules

These nodules are present in the interstitium and can accumulate due to hematogenous dissemination, classically seen in miliary tuberculosis, or due to inhalation of inorganic dusts causing pneumoconiosis or due to unknown reasons as in sarcoidosis. Various sizes have been described and have been categorized as micronodular (<1 mm), small (1–3 mm), medium (3–5 mm), and large (>5 mm) nodules.

Cysts and cavities

A cavity is air-containing space within the lung surrounded by a wall that is more than 1 mm thick. A cyst is a cavity that is lined by epithelium and this cannot be made out by radiologic examination, but by histopathological examination. Cysts and cavities may be solitary or multiple and benign or malignant. Fraser has presented important information on wall thickness that is measured in the thickest part of the cavity, and this information is useful in differentiating a benign and malignant lesion.

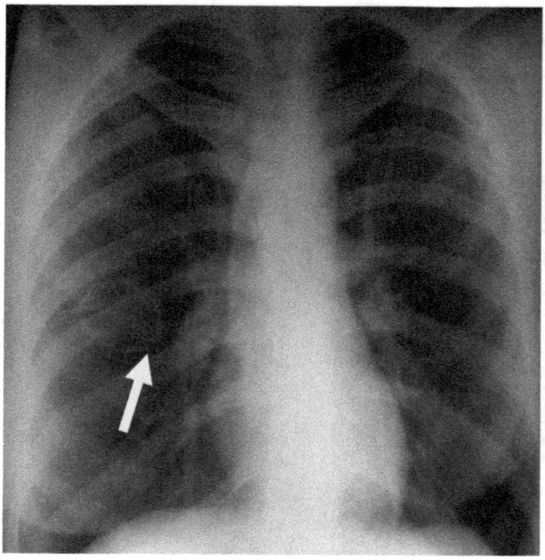

Figure 96: Small cavity in the right mid zone.

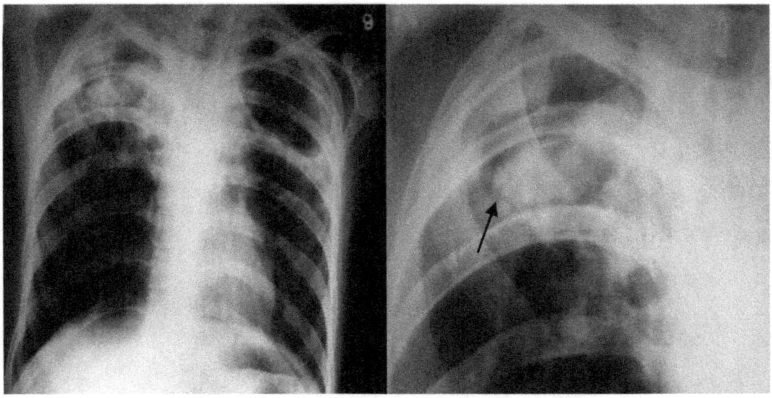

Figure 97: A cavity in the left upper lobe under tension. A fungal ball is seen in the right upper lobe.

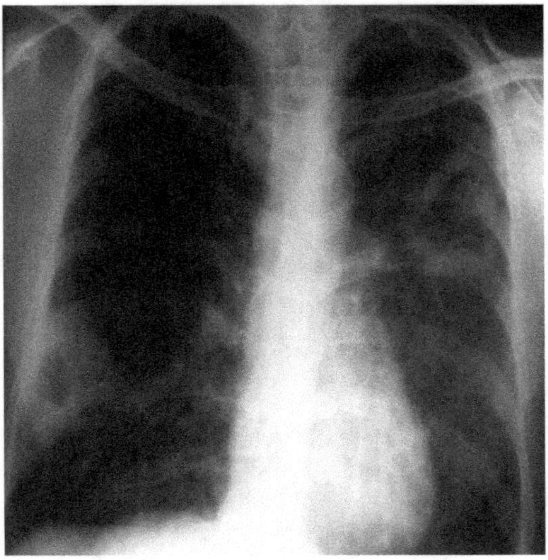

Figure 98: Bilateral cavity in the left upper zone and right upper zone of infective etiology.

Table 2:

Cavity wall thickness	Possibility of benign lesion or malignancy
1 mm	Benign–almost 100%
1–4 mm	Benign (92% chance)
5–15 mm	Malignant (50% chance)
More than 15 mm	Malignant (92% chance)

A cyst that is filled with fluid but not communicating with the bronchus can appear as solid nodule, which is usually benign. One of the features of a malignant cavity is nodular inner or outer wall. Hydatid cysts are common in the lower half of the lung fields, but can be seen in other lung zones. They are unusual in that they mold themselves to the contours of the surrounding mediastinal structures. Some of the common causes of the cysts are listed below:

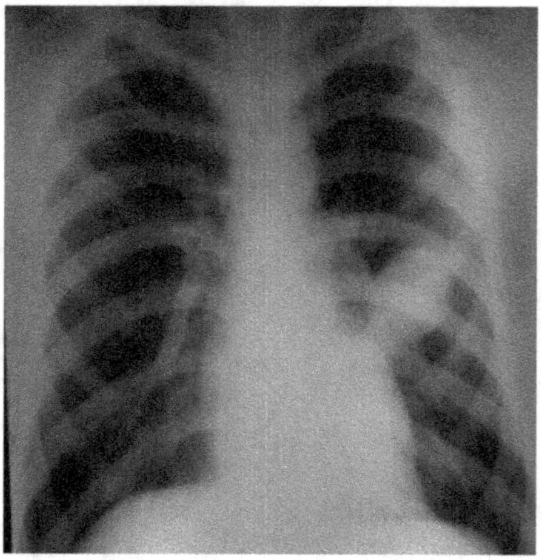

Figure 99: Hydatid cyst.

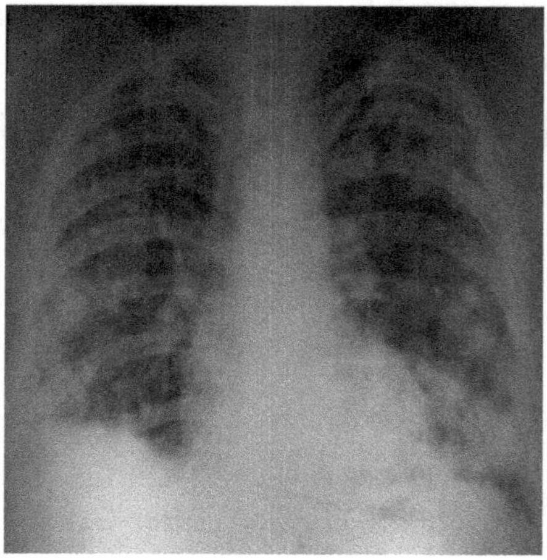

Figure 100: Malignant metastases.

Table 3:

Solitary cysts		Multiple cysts	
Benign	**Malignant**	**Benign**	**Malignant**
Lung abscess	Cavitating lung cancer	Lung abscess	Cavitating metastasis
Infected bulla		Bronchiectasis	
Wegener's granulomatosis		Infected bulla	
Hydatid cyst		Hydatid cyst	

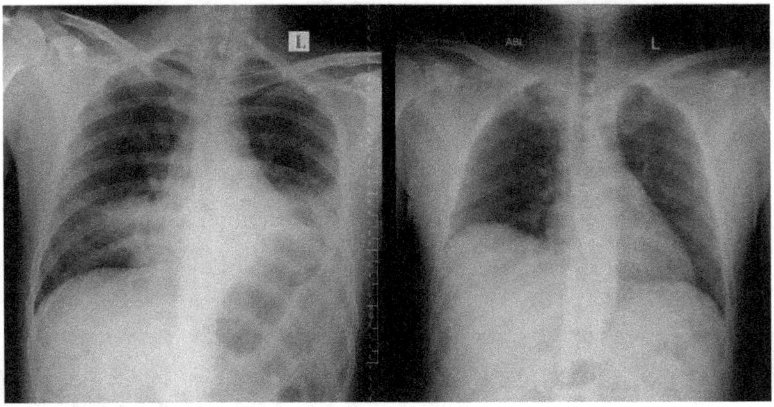

(a) (b)

Figure 101: Complete eventration of diaphragm (a): left hemidiaphragm (b): right hemidiaphragm.

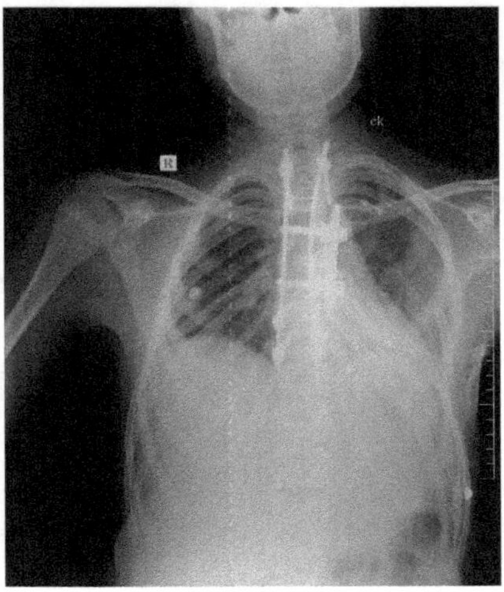

Figure 102: Spinal fixation.

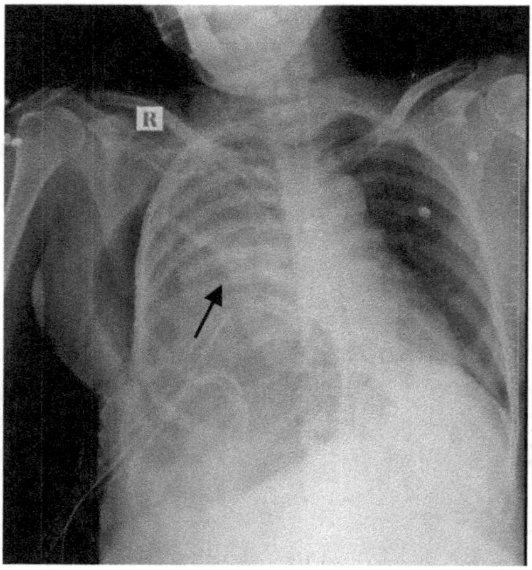

Figure 103: Thoracotomy. Rib resection is seen.

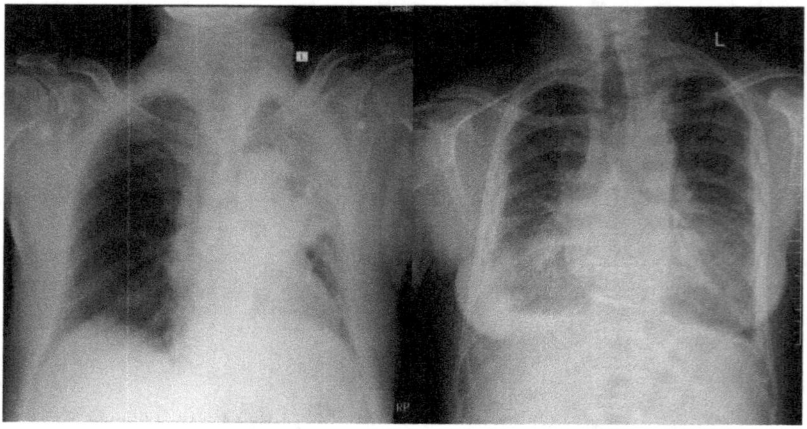

Figure 104: Pleural thickening causing loss of lung volume.

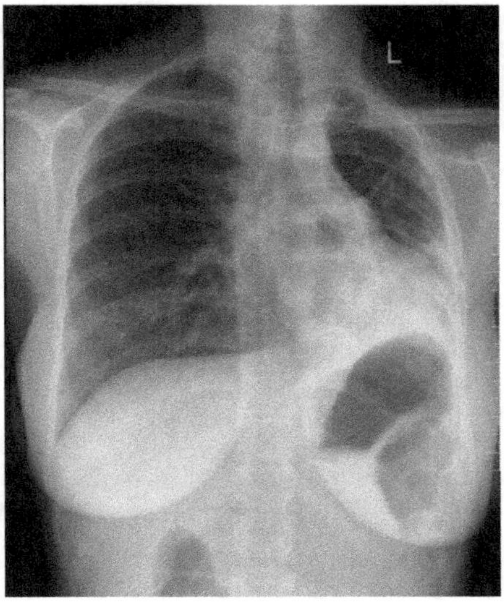

Figure 105: Collapse — Left lower lobe.

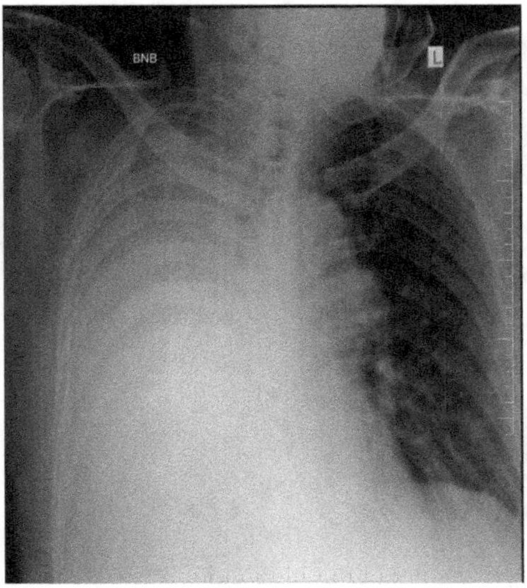

Figure 106: Collapse — Right lung.

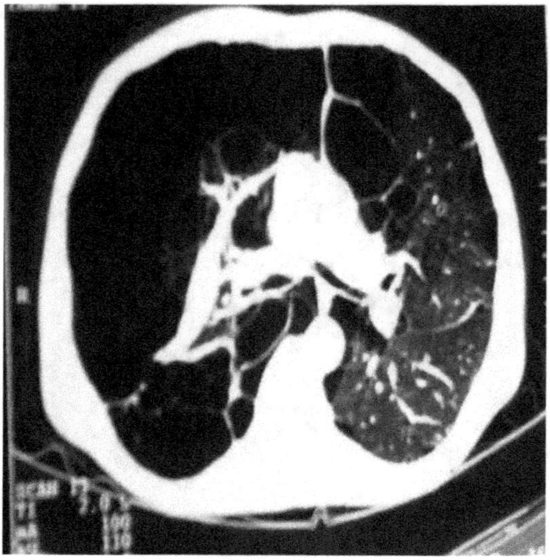

Figure 107: Gross emphysema with near destruction of the right lung and multiple bulla in the left lung.

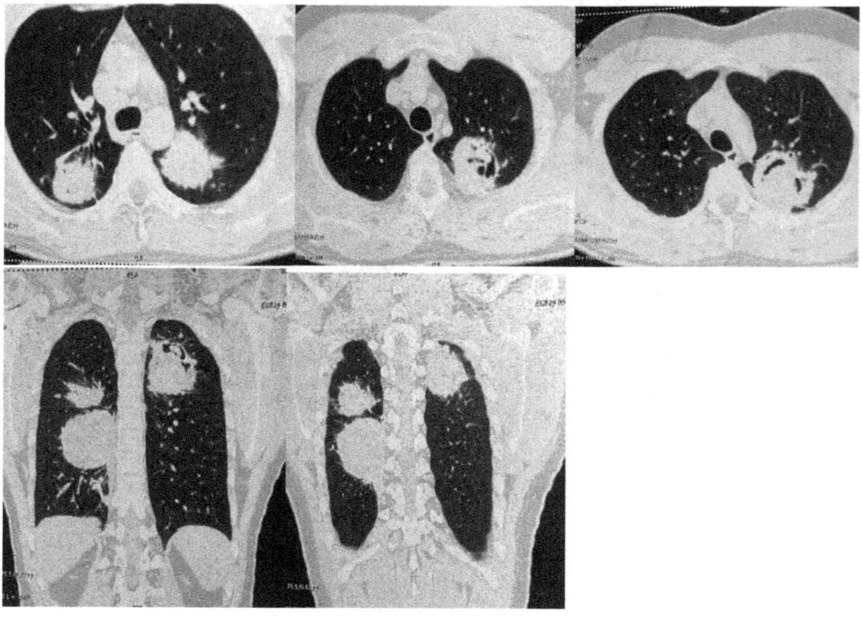

Figure 108: Series of CT scans of 18-year-old patient with Wegener's granulomatosis with multiple nodules.

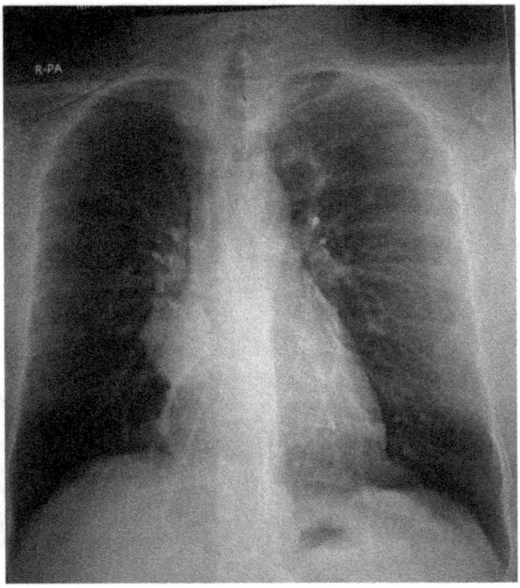

Figure 109: Chest X-ray of the same patient after treatment with Rituximab.

References and suggested readings

1. Ye Z, Zhang Y, Wang Y, Huang Z, Song B. Chest CT manifestations of new coronavirus disease 2019 (COVID-19): a pictorial review. Eur Radiol. 2020 Aug;30(8):4381–4389. doi: 10.1007/s00330-020-06801-0. Epub 2020 Mar 19. PMID: 32193638; PMCID: PMC7088323.
2. Bansal T, Beese R. Interpreting a chest X-ray. Br J Hosp Med (Lond). 2019 May 2;80(5):C75–C79. doi: 10.12968/hmed.2019.80.5.C75. PMID: 31059330.
3. Chassagnon G, Vakalopoulou M, Paragios N, Revel MP. Artificial intelligence applications for thoracic imaging. Eur J Radiol. 2020 Feb;123:108774. doi: 10.1016/j.ejrad.2019.108774. Epub 2019 Dec 11. PMID: 31841881.
4. Garg M, Prabhakar N, Bhalla AS, Irodi A, Sehgal I, Debi U, Suri V, Agarwal R, Yaddanapudi LN, Puri GD, Sandhu MS. Computed tomography chest in COVID-19: when & why? Indian J Med Res. 2021 Jan & Feb;153(1 & 2):86–92. doi: 10.4103/ijmr.IJMR_3669_20. PMID: 33402610; PMCID: PMC8184074.
5. Oterino Serrano C, Alonso E, Andrés M, Buitrago NM, Pérez Vigara A, ParrónPajares M, Cuesta López E, Garzón Moll G, Martin Espin I, Bueno Barriocanal M, De Ceano-Vivas la Calle M, Calvo Rey C, Bret-Zurita M. Pediatric chest x-ray in covid-19 infection. Eur J Radiol. 2020 Oct;131:109236.

doi: 10.1016/j.ejrad.2020.109236. Epub 2020 Aug 26. PMID: 32932176; PMCID: PMC7448740.

6. Benveniste MF, Cuellar SLB, Szarf G, Benveniste APA, Ahuja J, Marom EM. Imaging of the chest after radiotherapy and potential pitfalls. Semin Ultrasound CT MR. 2021 Dec;42(6):574–587. doi: 10.1053/j.sult.2021.04.012. Epub 2021 May 8. PMID: 34895613.
7. Walkoff L, Hobbs S. Chest imaging in the diagnosis of occupational lung diseases. Clin Chest Med. 2020 Dec;41(4):581–603. doi: 10.1016/j.ccm.2020.08.007. PMID: 33153681.
8. Li K, Wu J, Wu F, Guo D, Chen L, Fang Z, Li C. The clinical and chest CT features associated with severe and critical COVID-19 pneumonia. Invest Radiol. 2020 Jun;55(6):327–331. doi: 10.1097/RLI.0000000000000672. PMID: 32118615; PMCID: PMC7147273.
9. Vulasala SSR, Wynn GC, Hernandez M, Kadambi I, Gopireddy DR, Bhosale P, Virarkar MK. Dual-energy imaging of the chest. Semin Ultrasound CT MR. 2022 Aug;43(4):311–319. doi: 10.1053/j.sult.2022.03.007. Epub 2022 Mar 26. PMID: 35738816.
10. Lau KK, Troupis JM, Parsons D. Transformative radiology: chest imaging is being re-defined. Respirology. 2022 Oct;27(10):815–817. doi: 10.1111/resp.14358. Epub 2022 Sep 7. PMID: 36070934.
11. Yun G, Kazerooni EA, Lee EM, Shah PN, Deeb M, Agarwal PP. Retained surgical items at chest imaging. Radiographics. 2021 Mar–Apr;41(2):E10–E11. doi: 10.1148/rg.2021200128. PMID: 33646907.
12. De Smet K, De Smet D, Ryckaert T, Laridon E, Heremans B, Vandenbulcke R, Demedts I, Bouckaert B, Gryspeerdt S, Martens GA. Diagnostic performance of chest CT for SARS-CoV-2 infection in individuals with or without COVID-19 symptoms. Radiology. 2021 Jan;298(1):E30–E37. doi: 10.1148/radiol.2020202708. Epub 2020 Aug 10. PMID: 32776832; PMCID: PMC7418927.
13. Machnicki S, Patel D, Singh A, Talwar A, Mina B, Oks M, Makkar P, Naidich D, Mehta A, Hill NS, Brown KK, Raoof S. The usefulness of chest CT imaging in patients with suspected or diagnosed COVID-19: a review of literature. Chest. 2021 Aug;160(2):652–670. doi: 10.1016/j.chest.2021.04.004. Epub 2021 Apr 20. PMID: 33861993; PMCID: PMC8056836.

14. Adams HJA, Kwee TC, Yakar D, Hope MD, Kwee RM. Chest CT imaging signature of Coronavirus disease 2019 infection: in pursuit of the scientific evidence. Chest. 2020 Nov;158(5):1885–1895. doi: 10.1016/j.chest.2020.06.025. Epub 2020 Jun 25. PMID: 32592709; PMCID: PMC7314684.
15. Willer K, Fingerle AA, Noichl W, De Marco F, Frank M, Urban T, Schick R, Gustschin A, Gleich B, Herzen J, Koehler T, Yaroshenko A, Pralow T, Zimmermann GS, Renger B, Sauter AP, Pfeiffer D, Makowski MR, Rummeny EJ, Grenier PA, Pfeiffer F. X-ray dark-field chest imaging for detection and quantification of emphysema in patients with chronic obstructive pulmonary disease: a diagnostic accuracy study. Lancet Digit Health. 2021 Nov;3(11):e733–e744. doi: 10.1016/S2589-7500(21)00146-1. PMID: 34711378; PMCID: PMC8565798.

https://doi.org/10.1142/9789811271410_0005

5 Ultrasonography in chest disorders

Background: Transthoracic ultrasonography (USG) is a useful diagnostic tool for respiratory physicians,[1] which can be utilized for respiratory monitoring as well. It is a bedside investigative tool for the diagnosis of pleural effusion, pneumonia, pneumothorax, tumor, atelectasis, and chest wall contusion. It can also be utilized for the evaluation of pleural fibrosis.[2] In critical illness,[3] USG is being used as a bedside tool for predicting pulmonary artery occlusion pressure,[4] lung consolidation, and ateilectasis.[8] Following cardiac surgery, postoperative pleural effusion volume and alib be assessed by ultrasound.[6] Consensus conference of lung ultrasound provides evidence-based unified approach and language for terminology, technology, technique, clinical outcome, cost-effectiveness, and future research.[7] It is being increasingly used in respiratory emergencies for being safe and simple in the procedure. Chest computed tomography (CT) is useful for diagnosing missed lung lesions, but USG is better than chest radiography (chest X-ray) for its safety and simplicity as a bedside diagnosing tool,[8] and many times may obviate CT thorax.[9] Endoscopic ultrasound has been used for TBNA as a bedside investigative tool. EBUS is useful in accessing mediastinal adenopathy,[9] whereas EBUS–TBNA helps in differentiating tuberculosis and sarcoidosis as well as benign hyperplasia, anthracosis, and malignancy.

Introduction: The use of ultrasound in the chest was first applied in 1964 in a patient with pleural effusion. Later on, the application was well established in chest opacities. Ultrasound is a reliable, efficient, and revealing imaging technique in evaluating various clinical problems as well as in guiding a variety of interventional procedures in the chest.[11] The ribs, spine, and air-filled lung usually act as a barrier to ultrasound visualization of some intrathoracic lesions; however, tumor, consolidation, or atelectasis in the lung can very well be evaluated sonographically. Endoscopic ultrasound-guided fine-needle aspiration (FNA) for diagnosing and staging mediastinal masses is quite useful. Safety and simplicity of the procedure and the advantage of repeatability make it an excellent diagnostic tool as a bedside investigation, even in pulmonary emergencies such as acute pulmonary embolism, tension pneumothorax, pneumonia, and pleural effusion. Convex probe — endobronchial ultrasound is the best investigative tool of recent times being used for pulmonary embolism,[12] pulmonary artery sarcoma,[13] bronchogenic cysts,[14] puncturing of tumor embolism,[15] and transvascular TBNA.[16] It is useful in a patient with excessive cough or poor lung function. Cytologists, however, must be informed about the esophageal route as squamous lining cells may lead to confusion.

Summary of the utility of ultrasonography

Sonography can differentiate pleural from parenchymal lesions. It can detect diseases of parenchyma hidden by pleural effusion. It can differentiate which pleural effusions can be aspirated and which cannot. It can differentiate solid from cystic lesions. Apart from the clear demarcation of the diaphragm, ultrasound can differentiate subpulmonary effusions from the subphrenic abscess. Being portable, ultrasound can easily be used as a bedside investigation in a critically ill patient, as it causes minimal discomfort.[18] Transthoracic ultrasound can be used in chest wall soft tissue and bony lesions. In subcutaneous emphysema, the presence of characteristic E-lines poses limitations to lung ultrasound. In COPD, asthma, and pulmonary embolism, subpleural aeration is not affected. However, lung sliding is reduced by hyperinflation. BLUE protocol is used for pulmonary embolism, and a search for venous thrombosis is suggested if 'A' profile is present.

Ultrasonographic signs of pneumothorax include an absence of lung sliding (Figure 1), B-lines and lung pulse, and the presence of lung point

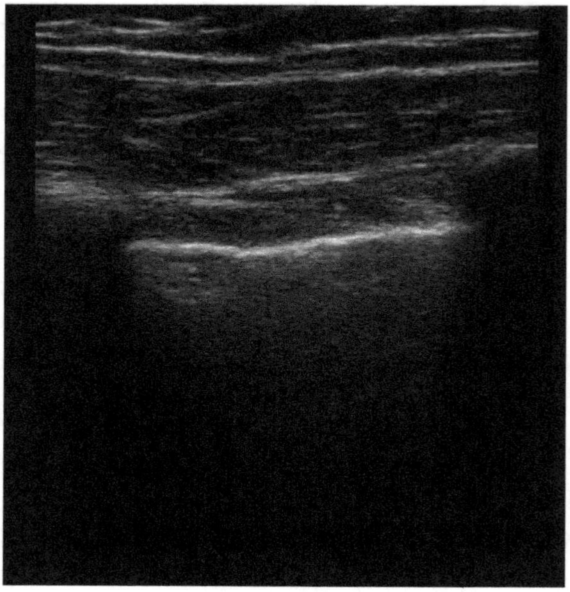

Figure 1: Lung sliding — normal.

(Figure 2). Lung ultrasound is as good as CT and superior to a plain X-ray chest in diagnosing pleural effusion (Figure 3). The nature of ultrasound images depends on the appearance of effusion between parietal and visceral pleura. Hydropneumothorax is identified by dynamic air field margin with features of pneumothorax above air–fluid levels.

Regularly spaced B-lines suggest septal or interstitial edema, and crowded or coalescent B-lines suggest alveolar edema. Non-homogeneous B-line positive areas in both lungs with reduced/absent lung sliding are features in acute lung injury (ALI)/acute respiratory distress syndrome (ARDS). Bilateral interstitial syndrome with non-homogeneous B-line positive areas, along with pleural line thickening, irregularities, fragmentation, and subpleural echo-poor areas are suggestive of pulmonary fibrosis.

Dynamic air and fluid bronchogram along with shred lines are lung ultrasound features of lung consolidation. In lung atelectasis, abolished lung sliding with lung pulse and stand-still cupola are early signs and residual trapped air with static air bronchogram is a late sign.

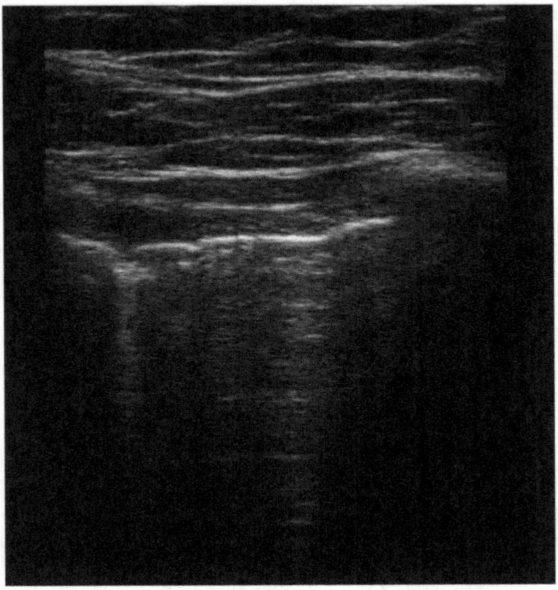

Figure 2: Lung point.

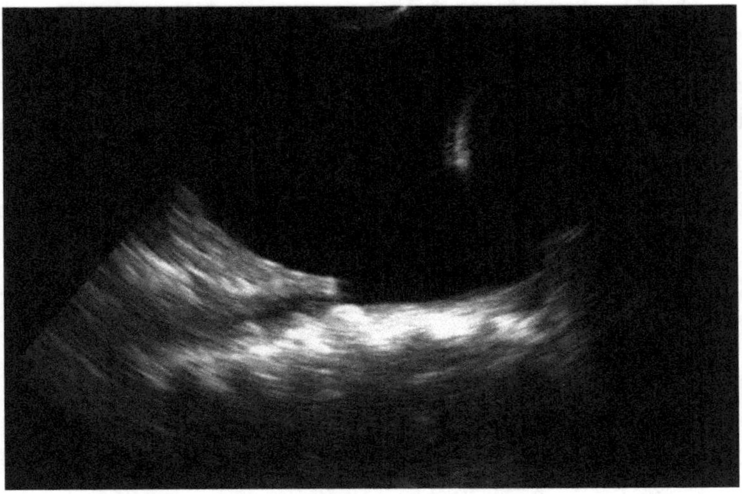

Figure 3: Pleural effusion.

Pleura

Pleural space can be examined ultrasonographically, utilizing either a direct or an abdominal approach. A high frequency (5 MHz) linear transducer applied directly to the chest provides a broad near field, thus allowing an excellent view of the pleural space. The lower areas of the pleural space can be examined via an abdominal approach by using a lower frequency (3.5 MHz) sector transducer directly superiorly from the abdomen. The liver and spleen provide sonography windows to the thorax. Thorax can be examined deep through the fluid in the pleural space, without any hindrance.

Pleural fluid can be detected even in small amounts by using a high-resolution linear assay transducer. Mostly pleural fluid is relatively anechoic and is easily recognized as an area of echolucency separating the parietal and visceral pleura (Figure 3). Sonography is helpful when conventional radiology fails in making a confident diagnosis in the event of a whole hemithorax looking opaque or the fluid is encysted. The diagnostic sensitivity for pleural effusion has been reported from 93% to 96.90%.[11] At the same time, the ultrasonic intensity used is entirely harmless.[18]

Pleural effusions may be detected during the routine ultrasonographic abdominal examination as a hypoechoic fluid above the diaphragm, along with the visualization of the interior of the thorax through fluid collection. Ultrasound may also be used to evaluate pleural abnormalities seen on chest X-ray. Focal pleural lesions may be loculated pleural effusions or solid pleural tumors. Pleural masses are usually well-circumscribed and hypoechoic or of mixed echogenicity. The lesion is considered solid if the internal echoes which do not move with respiration are detected.

Empyema: The findings are similar to a pleural effusion with greater echogenic debris within a pleural effusion. An echogenic swirling fluid within a pleural effusion is characteristic. Multiple thick septations are usual (Figure 4). The debris is highly echogenic and coarse. Other causes of

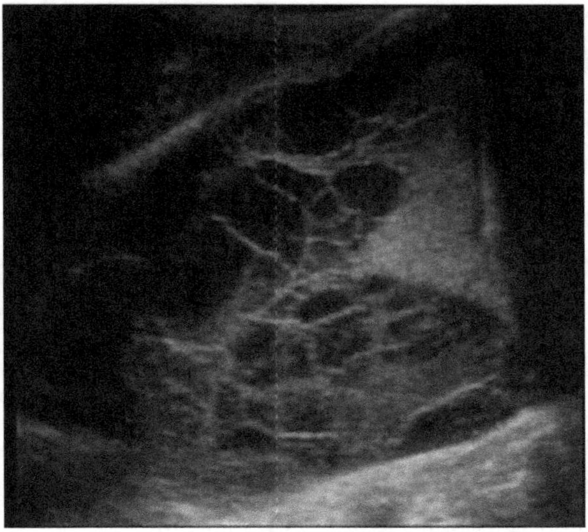

Figure 4: Empyema.

echogenic debris within a pleural effusion are hemothorax, chylothorax, and highly proteinaceous exudate such as tuberculosis or malignancy.

Pneumothorax: Pneumothorax can be detected by ultrasound by using the three important signs: lung sliding, lung point, and A-lines. The pleural line is the clear line seen on USG at the interface of the visceral pleura and the lung. The respiration alters the pleural line and this movement is called lung sliding. The presence of lung sliding excludes pneumothorax with a negative predictive value of 100%. When lung sliding is not visualized, there are other differential diagnoses along with pneumothorax such as pleural adhesions, collapse, lung contusion, or ARDS. Lung point is the point where the visceral and the parietal pleural leaves separate. Lung point will be identified as the point where there is an intermittent visualization of lung sliding when during breathing, intermittently, the collapsed lung slides into the pneumothorax area. This sign confirms pneumothorax. The more inferior and lateral the lung point, the larger is the pneumothorax. The absence of a lung point suggests a very large pneumothorax. Several lines run parallel to the pleural line called as A-lines. The A-lines are classically seen in a pneumothorax but can also be seen in a well-aired lung. A normal lung and a pneumothorax can only be differentiated with the presence of lung sliding, which excludes pneumothorax. The absence of lung sliding with A-lines is a strong pointer for pneumothorax.

Diagnostic thoracentesis: Ultrasonographic guidance of diagnostic thoracentesis can be done whenever clinical thoracentesis is likely to fail or be difficult. It is especially useful when the interpretation of chest X-ray is difficult to differentiate between subpulmonic or subphrenic collection. Sonography can identify the largest and most accessible pocket of pleural fluid. The location and depth of the fluid are determined, and vital structures such as the heart and aorta are identified. A safe site for thoracentesis can be selected based on ultrasound examination.

Lung parenchyma

Ultrasound evaluation of the lung parenchyma is inhibited by the air in the periphery of the lung. However, when the airspaces are collapsed or filled with fluid, an ultrasound evaluation is possible and can help to determine the nature of the lesion.

Consolidation: The lung airspaces are filled with fluid and inflammatory cells in consolidation (Figure 5) and hence the aerated lung is converted into a firm dense mass with good sound transmission. The consolidated lung is hypoechoic as compared with a highly reflective aerated normal lung and is usually hypoechoic as compared with liver and spleen because of its high fluid content. The consolidated lung is poorly defined and is wedge-shaped. The air within the bronchi surrounded by a consolidated lung produces highly reflective linear bronchial echoes that can be recognized as sonographic air bronchogram.[20]

Lung abscess: Lung abscess is a localized suppurative process characterized by the necrosis of lung tissue. Lung abscesses have thick irregular walls with echogenic debris and air is present within the internal fluid. A lung

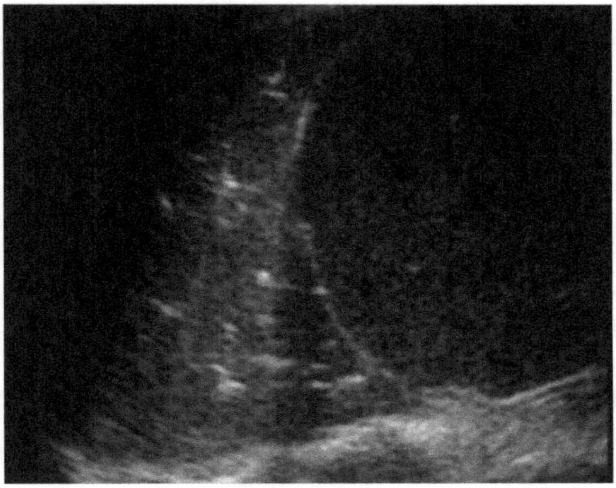

Figure 5: Pneumonia with airspace consolidation.

abscess, on sonography, will demonstrate the expansion of its circumference with inspiration.

Lung tumor: Lung tumors pushing the pleural surface can be visualized sonographically as masses partially surrounded by aerated lungs with well-defined margins.[20]

ALI/ARDS: USG is useful in ALI/ARDS to rule out other etiologies of an alveolar interstitial syndrome involving both lungs.

Lung contusion: Chest USG is useful in diagnosing lung conditions following blunt trauma. Nevertheless, CT chest remains the gold standard in investigation.

Atelectasis lung: Lung ultrasound is a complementary investigative tool in diagnosing atelectasis especially due to the increasing pleural effusion. It also helps in differentiating from pneumonia.

Pulmonary fibrosis: Lung ultrasound is a complementary investigative tool in pulmonary fibrosis in diagnosing and assessing the severity and management of this disease of diverse etiology.

Subcutaneous emphysema: USG is useful in diagnosing subcutaneous emphysema but with certain limitations due to the hindrance in imaging caused by subcutaneous air.

Airway obstructive disease: In chronic obstructive airway disease, bronchial asthma, and pulmonary embolism, subpleural aeration is not affected, and USG is usually present with a similar picture of the aerated lung. In the presence of venous thrombosis, diagnosis of pulmonary embolism is considered in patients with acute respiratory failure.

Lung biopsy: Percutaneous transthoracic biopsy using fluoroscopic guidance is a standard invasive method of obtaining tissue diagnosis of pulmonary parenchymal masses.[21] However fluoroscopic visualization of lung nodules may become difficult or impossible when the nodules are located at:

1. Pleural base
2. On the lung apex
3. In the axilla
4. Near the diaphragm
5. Near mediastinum

In such situations, the masses are easy and best visualized by USG.

Ultrasound-guided biopsy is quick, convenient, and safe because USG can visualize aerated lung adjacent to pleural-based nodules better than fluoroscopy, and the aerated lung can be avoided more easily.[22] Complication such as pneumothorax following biopsy of pleural-based nodules is 2% with ultrasound guidance as compared to 11% with fluoroscopic guidance.[23] Both procedures, however, have similar (90%) sensitivity for the diagnosis of lung cancer. Looking at the chest X-ray as a first requisite is essential in planning the approach to ultrasound-guided biopsy. Most lung lesions may be visualized and biopsied through the intercostal space. Lesions at the lung apex may be approached from either above or below the clavicle. Lesions on the diaphragm may be visualized and biopsied using an upward angle through the liver. Once the lesion is visualized, a safe course for the needle is determined. The needle pass into the lesions may be performed either freehand or by the use of a needle guide attached to the transducer. The patient is asked to suspend respiration while the needle is being advanced into the lesion. The patient may then resume shallow respiration while the needle is allowed to swing freely. The patient is again asked to stop breathing while the biopsy is being taken. The specimens are immediately sent for cytopathological examination. Comparison of non-invasive conventional and minimal invasive endobronchial ultrasound-guided procedure of transbronchial aspiration has been documented.[24,25] Endoscopic ultrasound-guided FNA for diagnosing and staging mediastinal mass as well as diagnosis of sarcoidosis has been utilized.[26]

FNA biopsy guided by real-time USG was studied in 25 patients with peripheral lung lesions, and the lesions were visualized in 88% of patients and aspiration was diagnostic in 85% of patients (FNA biopsy under USG guidance is a safe, simple, and economical method with high diagnostic yield in the evaluation of pleural and peripheral lung lesions). The examination is non-invasive and more comfortable as a bedside investigation for a sick patient. The intensity of ultrasonics used for a diagnostic purpose is generally accepted to be safe for the patient.

Besides ultrasound is helpful in diagnosing pulmonary emergencies, such as acute pulmonary embolism, tension pneumothorax, pneumonia, and pleural effusion.[27,26] Its use and extended focused utility can be encased in assessment with sonography in chest trauma, directly at the bedside to identify hemothorax, pericardial/pleural fluid, and solid organ injury. It is superior to chest X-ray in diagnosing pneumothorax/hemothorax.

Endobroncial ultrasound is the recent advancement in pulmonary medicine in nodal staging in lung malignancy, almost replacing mediastinoscopy. However, it stands inferior to mediastinoscopy in lymphoma as architectural pattern of nodes would be reguired.[36] EBUS is contraindicated in bleeding disorders, anticoagulant therapy, recent myocardial infarction, severe hypoxemia, and lymphoma. Complications of EBUS include hemorrhage 1.23%, infection 0.19%, and rarely pneumothorax and mediastinal abscess.[31]

References and suggested readings

1. Koegelengerg CR, et al. Transthoracic ultrasonography for respiratory physicians. Respiration. 2012;84:337–350.
2. Sperendeo M, et al. Transthoracic ultrasound in the evaluation of pulmonary fibrosis — our experience. Ultrasound Med Biol. 2009;35:723–729.
3. Lichtenstein DA. Lung ultrasound in the critically ill. Ann Intensive Care. 2014;4:1.
4. Lichtenstein DA, et al. Lung ultrasound as a bedside tool for predicting pulmonary artery occlusion in the critically ill. Chest. 2009;136:1014–1020.
5. Wang XT, et al. The value of bedside ultrasound in emergency — plus protocol for the assessment of lung consolidation and atelactasis in critical patients. Zhoughua Nei Ke Za Zhi. 2012;51:948–951.
6. Usta E, et al. Ultrasound estimation of volume of post-operative pleural effusion in cardiac surgery patients. Inter Cardiovascular Thoracic Surg. 2010;10:204–207.
7. Saraogi A. Lung ultrasound — present and future. Lung India. 2015;32:250–257.
8. Ghosh UC, et al. Chest radiography. Med Update API. 2016;26:472–478.
9. Prasad BNBM, et al. USG in chest diseases. Med Update API. 2016;26:1939–1943.
10. Dhamija A, et al. Mediastinal adenopathy in India through FRU&JAPI. 2015;63:15–IR.
11. Sohan S, et al. Role of sonography in diagnosis of pleural and lung disease. Lung India. 2005;22:97–98.
12. Aumiller J, et al. Endobronchial ultrasound for detecting central pulmonary emboli — a pilot study. Respiration. 2009;77:298–302.
13. Shingyoji M, et al. Pulmonary artery sarcoma diagnosed by endobronchial ultrasound guided transbronchial needle aspiration. Ann Thorac Surg. 2013;96:33–35.
14. Twebues A, Islam S. Cystic lesions of the thoeax — role of endobronchial ultrasound guided transbronchial needle aspiration. J Bronchol Intery Pulmonol. 2011;18:65–66.
15. Chamorro N, et al. The expanding horizons of endobronchial ultrasound: Diagnosis of a tumor embolism. Chest. 2012;142:1134–3.

16. Francho J, Monclou E. Transesophageal endobronchial ultrasound guided fine needle aspiration. Arch Bronchoneumol. 2011;47:418–1.
17. Vallandramam PRR, et al. EUSB-FNA — pulmonologist's viewpoint whose tube is it anyway? Lung India. 2015;32:285–286.
18. Yu CJ, et al. Diagnostic and therapeutic use of chest sonography — value in critically ill patients. AJR. 1992;159:695–701.
19. Narang P, Bharagava SK. Ultrasonic features of tuberculous pleural effusion. Ind J Radio Imag. 1993;2:217–220.
20. Weinberg B, et al. The air bronchogram sonographic demonstration. AJR. 1986;147:593–595.
21. Westcott JL. Percutaneous transthoracic needle biopsy. Radiology. 1988;169: 593–601.
22. Ciniti D, Hawkins HB. Aspiration biopsy of peripheral pulmonary mass using real-time sonography guidance. AJR. 1984;142:1115–1116.
23. Khan GO, et al. Fine needle aspiration biopsy of peripheral pulmonary lesions under real-time sonographic guidance. Abstract. JIMA. 1995;2–135.
24. Herth FJ, et al. Trans-bronchial and transesophageal ultrasound guided aspiration of enlarged mediastinal lymphnodes. Amer J Resp Grit Care Med. 2005;171:1164–1167.
25. Rintoul RC, et al. Endobronchial and endoscopic ultrasound guided realtime FNA for mediastinal staging. Eur Resp J. 2005;25:416–421.
26. Annema JT, et al. Ultrasonic ultrasound guided FNA for diagnosis of sarcoidosis. Eur Resp J. 2005;25:405–409.
27. Khan GQ, Basher I. Ultrasonography in chest medicine. IN: RS Bhatia, ed. Pulmonary Med. New Delhi: Pee Pee Publ. 2007;2:06–1.
28. Mishra R. Role of ultrasound in managing life threatening emergencies. IN: SR Joshi, ed. Med Update; API. 2014;24:580–587.
29. Shankar PS. Imaging in pulmonary thrombolism. API. 2001;11:59–64.
30. Pattabhi Raman VR. Overview of endobronchial ultrasound (EBUS) — the route to enter mediastinum. IN: R Upadhyay, ed. 2015;25:473–474.
31. Vora A. Endoscopic ultrasound – Indian prospective. JAPI. 2015;63:11–13.

https://doi.org/10.1142/9789811271410_0006

6 Spirometry

Background

Spirometry is one of the most commonly performed dynamic pulmonary function tests worldwide. It was invented by John Hutchinson in 1846 (1). It is compact, portable, inexpensive, and sensitive, making it the gold standard in diagnosing several diseases. It has, over time, demonstrated its excellent effectiveness in the detection and prognosis of obstructive lung diseases like asthma and COPD; however, it is not effective in identifying the site of pathology in restrictive lung diseases, which could be in the lung parenchyma, pleura, chest wall or due to neuromuscular abnormalities. Spirometry measurements reflect the ability of the lungs to blow out air and consequently the patient's ability to breathe. This chapter deals with the performance of spirometry in the clinical setting and various measurements that can be made with a spirometer along with their interpretations and their clinical significance. It is assumed, in this chapter, that the reader is well acquainted with the basic parts of a modern spirometer.

Indications and relative contraindications for spirometry

Spirometry is indicated in diagnosis, evaluation, monitoring, epidemiology, and many other conditions (table 1). The list recommended by the ATS-ERS guidelines 2019 has been given below. There are several contraindications to spirometry as well. An easy way to remember them is to realize that spirometry routinely has either forced expiratory maneuvers or bronchoprovocative challenge tests (such as the methacholine challenge).

Therefore, any condition that gets worse by an increase in intrathoracic, intracranial, or intra-abdominal pressure is contraindicated. The pressure increase is also transmitted to the sinuses and middle ear through the nose, which must also be noted. Challenge tests should be performed with utmost care and with emergency kits close by. The list of relative contraindications as recommended by the ATS-ERS guidelines 2019 has also been given in the table below.

Purpose	Indications
Diagnosis	Evaluation of clinical manifestations or laboratory results
	Measurement of physiological effects of a particular disease
	Screening high-risk population
	Preoperative risk assessment
	Prognosis assessment
Monitoring	Assessment of response to therapy
	Monitoring of exacerbations and recovery from exacerbations
	Adverse reaction monitoring: adverse reactions to drugs with known pulmonary toxicity and/or reactions to inhaled agents (eg, chemicals)
Disability/impairment evaluation	Assessment of patients who are part of rehabilitation programs
	Evaluation for insurance/legal reasons
Miscellaneous	Research, clinical trials, and/or epidemiology
	Derivation of reference equations
	General health monitoring including preoccupational for all high-risk occupations
	Health assessment before at-risk physical activities

Table 1: Indications of spirometry as recommended by ATS-ERS guidelines (2019) (2)

Conditions	Contraindications (duration of contraindication)
Surgery	Abdominal surgery (4 weeks)
	Thoracic surgery (4 weeks)
	Brain surgery (4 weeks)
	Eye surgery (1 week)
	Sinus surgery/middle ear surgery/infection (1 week)
Cardiovascular diseases	Myocardial infarction (1 week)
	Systemic hypotension or severe hypertension
	Uncompensated cardiac failure
	Arrhythmias (sinus or ventricular)
	Uncontrolled pulmonary hypertension
	Acute cor pulmonale
	History of syncope related to cough/forced expiration
Increase in intracranial pressure	Aneurysms
	Concussions (recent with continuing symptoms)
Increases in intrathoracic or intra-abdominal pressures	Pneumothorax
	Late-term pregnancy
Infection	Acute or transmissible respiratory infection including tuberculosis
	Signs/physical conditions predisposing to infections like hemoptysis or increased secretions

Lung volumes and capacities

One of the most basic, yet major topics that are talked about while discussing pulmonary physiology is different lung volumes and capacities. It is so because, they are the most intuitive, non-invasive, and hassle-free methods to measure objectively the functional state of the lung. While a traditional vitalograph could only measure lung volumes, modern-day spirometers can measure airflow as well. This has led to the classification of lung volume measurements into two types:

1. Static lung volumes
2. Dynamic lung volumes

Static lung volumes are those which emphasize more on the volume of air inspired or expired by the patient. These include tidal volume (TV), inspiratory reserve volume (IRV), expiratory reserve volume (ERV), and residual volume. Dynamic lung volumes, on the other hand, emphasize not only the volume of air being moved but also the time taken to move that volume of air into and out of the lungs. These include, but are not limited to, forced expiratory volume in 1 s, forced vital capacity, and mid-expiratory flow. These will be dealt later in the chapter.

Static lung volumes

Tidal volume

TV is defined as the volume of air inhaled or exhaled during normal, unforced breathing, with normal inspiratory effort from the resting position of the chest and the lung. In a normal person, it is roughly 500 mL. TV is subject to normal variation between breaths or variation due to the patient knowing that they are being examined.

Inspiratory reserve volume

It is the volume of air that can be forcefully inspired after the inspiration of the TV.

Expiratory reserve volume

It is the volume of air that can be expired in addition to the air expired by the normal expiratory effort. In other words, the voluntary effort of expiration begins at the resting position of the lung and chest and continues till maximal expiration. The volume of air that is exhaled during this process is the ERV.

Residual volume

This refers to the volume of air that is left behind in the lungs even after maximal expiration. This volume of air cannot be expelled. Therefore, it is not possible to measure the residual volume in a given individual using spirometry.

Lung capacities

Lung volumes can be thought of as measurements that cannot be sensibly divided further. Lung capacities, however, are composed of at least two volumes. We can define four lung capacities:

Total lung capacity
It is the sum of all the lung volumes discussed above.

$TLC = V_T + IRV + ERV + RV$

Inspiratory capacity
It is defined as the maximum volume of air that can be inhaled after a tidal expiration. This, therefore, includes IRV and V_T.

$IC = IRV + V_T$

Functional residual capacity (FRC)
It is the volume of air that remains in the lung after a tidal expiration. In other words, it is the volume of air that remains in the lung after it reaches the resting position. Therefore,

$FRC = ERV + RV$

Vital capacity (VC)
It is defined as the maximum volume of air that can be exhaled after a maximal inspiration. Therefore,

$VC = IRV + ERV + V_T$ or $IC + ERV$

Note that VC does not contain RV and TLC does include RV.

Impulse oscillometry

Introduction

Definition

Impulse oscillometry (IOS) is a **sensitive, non-invasive** method of measuring the **mechanical properties of the lungs** using **sound waves** towards that end.

Principle of IOS

- IOS is based on the principle of **Forced Oscillation Technique (FOT)**.
- The sound waves that are generated using a loudspeaker are transmitted into the lungs of the subject.
- **Sound waves** can be imagined as changes in air pressure traveling at a particular frequency and velocity, that is, **pressure waves.**
- These **pressure waves**, when transmitted through the airway, cause **changes in the pressure**, which in turn produces **changes in the airflow.**
- These **pressure and flow changes** can be **measured** and used to derive the **mechanical properties of the lung.**

The mechanical properties of the lung as a whole have limited usefulness. It was found, during a series of experiments, that **sound waves of different frequencies travel different distances before reflecting back towards the mouthpiece**. Therefore, to solve the problem of measuring mechanical properties at different locations in the lungs, sound waves of different frequencies are used.

- Sound waves of **lower frequencies** travel **further into the lungs** and **reach the alveoli** before reflecting back to the mouthpiece.
- Sound waves of **higher frequencies** are reflected back from **higher points in the airway**.

- Frequencies ranging from **5 Hz to 30 Hz** are used in routine clinical practice as frequencies **above 30 Hz** not only have **limited usefulness** but also **cause discomfort to the subject.**

In **FOT**, the **sound waves** of different frequencies are **transmitted sequentially**. This is **a time-intensive** process. Therefore, **each of these waves** having different frequencies is **combined mathematically** into a "summated" wave, which is then transmitted into the lungs in the form of **impulses**. This technique is called **impulse oscillometry**. The **resulting wave** that is reflected back from the airways **can be mathematically decomposed** into the parent waves and properties at those frequencies can be measured all at once. This greatly **reduces the time of testing.**

Proper technique for performing IOS

IOS is a highly sensitive test. Therefore, it is of utmost importance to follow proper techniques, standardized for all patients to ensure not only accurate measurements but also both intra- and intersubject repeatability of those measurements. This technique is given below in a simple, easy-to-follow manner:

1. Subject should be seated on a stool or a chair with back support in a relaxed, yet erect position.
2. Head of the subject should be in neutral or slightly extended position.
3. A disposable mouthpiece may be used. If not, the mouthpiece should be cleaned and sanitized thoroughly as per the manufacturer's guidelines, both inside and out, to prevent transmission of infection.
4. The level of the mouthpiece should be adjusted such that the subject is not hyperextending their neck.
5. The subject should put their lips around the mouthpiece such that they form a tight seal with the mouthpiece. Teeth should not be used to hold the mouthpiece in the mouth.
6. A nose clip should be placed to prevent leakage of air from the nose.

7. The cheeks of the subject should be firmly supported either by a technician or by the subject themselves.
8. It must be ensured that the tongue of the subject lies below the mouthpiece within the mouth and does not block, even partially the opening in the mouthpiece.
9. Sound is transmitted using a loudspeaker and the recording is started.
10. The subject is asked to relax and breathe tidally during the whole procedure.

Some need-to-know terminologies to interpret an IOS report:

1. **Impedance**: When an impulse is transmitted into the airway, the mechanical properties of the lung and the airways oppose that impulse. The sum of all the forces that oppose the impulse is called Respiratory Impedance (Z). This impedance is frequency dependent, that is, it varies with the frequency of the impulse used to measure it. Since different frequencies of sound travel different distances in the airway, the frequency dependence of impedance can be used to our advantage. Impedance measured at a given frequency is the ratio of change in pressure to change in flow at that frequency. We can measure impedance at different points in the airway using different frequencies of the input sound. Obviously, these measurements would be different from each other in the same person. For instance, the total impedance of the airways can be measured using the pressure difference between the mouth and the alveoli. This uses low-frequency sounds (5 Hz). Similarly, one can define the impedance of the respiratory system (Zrs) by simply measuring the difference between pressures in the mouth and pleural pressures.
2. **Resistance (R)**: Since IOS can only measure impedance directly, resistance is therefore derived from the measured impedance. This derived resistance includes resistance from central airways, peripheral airways as well as a negligible contribution from the chest wall and lung tissue. The

contribution of central and peripheral airways is highly age dependent. The physiology and age dependence are discussed elsewhere in the chapter. In an average healthy individual, resistance is frequency independent. In other words, the resistance measured at each of the frequencies from 5 to 30 Hz has roughly the same value. However, interestingly, in central airway obstruction resistance is increased at all frequencies, while in peripheral airway obstruction, only lower frequencies are affected. The reason for this is given in the aforementioned content and should serve as an exercise for the reader.

3. **Reactance (X)**: It reflects the elastic properties of the lungs. It consists of two components: capacitance and inertance. At lower frequencies, in a normal individual, the reactance is negative, while at higher frequencies the reactance is positive. Therefore, reactance is said to be frequency dependent. Reactance values become more negative in peripheral airway disease irrespective of whether it is an obstructive or restrictive disease.
4. **Resonant frequency (Fres)**: It is the frequency at which the total reactance is zero. It is mainly used to separate low frequencies from high frequencies. In other words, frequencies above the resonant frequency can be thought of as higher frequencies reflecting larger airways while those below are lower frequencies that reflect smaller airways. In disease states of the lung, it was found that the resonant frequency is higher than normal as the reactance becomes more negative. It is also the case in children as reactance is higher than normal adults even in normal children.
5. **Area under the curve**: This includes the area under the reactance curve from the lowest frequency to Fres. This parameter also behaves like Fres and X, in that it increases in any peripheral lung disease and is normally higher in children.
6. **Coherence**: It is a parameter that indicates the reproducibility of the results of impedance measurements. It is a value between 0 and 1. In adults, a coherence value >0.8 at 5 Hz and >0.9 at 20 Hz is ideal. Coherence can reduce because of improper technique, swallowing, or glottis closure.

References and suggested readings

1. Langan RC, Goodbred AJ. Office spirometry: indications and interpretation. Am Fam Physician. 2020 Mar 15;101(6):362–368. PMID: 32163256.
2. Rivero-Yeverino D. Espirometría: conceptosbásicos [Spirometry: basic concepts]. Rev Alerg Mex. 2019 Jan–Mar;66(1):76–84. Spanish. doi: 10.29262/ram.v66i1.536. PMID: 31013409.
3. Lopes AJ. Advances in spirometry testing for lung function analysis. Expert Rev Respir Med. 2019 Jun;13(6):559–569. doi: 10.1080/17476348.2019.1607301. Epub 2019 Apr 23. PMID: 30977428.
4. Agusti A, Fabbri LM, Baraldi E, Celli B, Corradi M, Faner R, Martinez FD, Melén E, Papi A. Spirometry: a practical lifespan predictor of global health and chronic respiratory and non-respiratory diseases. Eur J Intern Med. 2021 Jul;89:3–9. doi: 10.1016/j.ejim.2021.04.027. Epub 2021 May 18. PMID: 34016514.
5. Sullivan KA, Churchill IF, Hylton DA, Hanna WC. Use of incentive spirometry in adults following cardiac, thoracic, and upper abdominal surgery to prevent post-operative pulmonary complications: a systematic review and meta-analysis. Respiration. 2021;100(11):1114–1127. doi: 10.1159/000517012. Epub 2021 Jul 16. PMID: 34274935.
6. Morais-Almeida M, Barbosa MT, Sousa CS, Almeida I, Pimenta L, Aguiar R. Spirometry outside the hospital. Arch Bronconeumol (Engl Ed). 2021 Mar;57(3):236. doi: 10.1016/j.arbres.2020.10.011. Epub 2020 Oct 28. PMID: 33309419; PMCID: PMC7832428.
7. Seyller H, Gottlieb M, Colla J. The role of incentive spirometry for patients with COVID-19. Am J Emerg Med. 2021 Sep;47:292–293. doi: 10.1016/j.ajem.2021.05.034. Epub 2021 May 15. PMID: 34020843; PMCID: PMC8123532.
8. Noth I, Cottin V, Chaudhuri N, Corte TJ, Johannson KA, Wijsenbeek M, Jouneau S, Michael A, Quaresma M, Rohr KB, Russell AM, Stowasser S, Maher TM; INMARK trial investigators. Home spirometry in patients with idiopathic pulmonary fibrosis: data from the INMARK trial. Eur Respir J. 2021 Jul 8;58(1):2001518. doi: 10.1183/13993003.01518-2020. PMID: 33419890; PMCID: PMC8264778.

9. Morais-Almeida M, Barbosa MT, Sousa CS, Almeida I, Pimenta L, Aguiar R. Spirometry outside the hospital. Arch Bronconeumol (Engl Ed). 2021 Mar;57(3):236. doi: 10.1016/j.arbr.2020.10.011. Epub 2021 Mar 10. PMID: 33994647; PMCID: PMC7945879.
10. Gupta A, Mishra P, Gupta B, Kakkar K. A kid-friendly approach to *Incentive Spirometry*. Ann Card Anaesth. 2021 Apr–Jun;24(2):238–240. doi: 10.4103/aca.ACA_188_19. PMID: 33884984; PMCID: PMC8253039.
11. Lone HU, Al-Ishaq F, Carr CS. Patient adaptation for effective incentive spirometry. Asian Cardiovasc Thorac Ann. 2021 Mar;29(3):227. doi: 10.1177/0218492320986278. Epub 2021 Jan 5. PMID: 33401922; PMCID: PMC7941497.
12. Aaron SD, Boulet LP, Reddel HK, Gershon AS. Underdiagnosis and overdiagnosis of asthma. Am J Respir Crit Care Med. 2018 Oct 15;198(8):1012–1020. doi: 10.1164/rccm.201804-0682CI. PMID: 29756989.
13. Halpin DMG, Criner GJ, Papi A, Singh D, Anzueto A, Martinez FJ, Agusti AA, Vogelmeier CF. Global initiative for the diagnosis, management, and prevention of chronic obstructive lung disease. The 2020 GOLD Science Committee Report on COVID-19 and Chronic Obstructive Pulmonary Disease. Am J Respir Crit Care Med. 2021 Jan 1;203(1):24–36. doi: 10.1164/rccm.202009-3533SO. PMID: 33146552; PMCID: PMC7781116.

https://doi.org/10.1142/9789811271410_0007

7 Arterial blood gases

Introduction

The analysis of arterial blood gases (ABGs) plays an important role in making correct diagnoses in critically ill patients. It provides valuable information about the biochemical status of a patient and clues about the underlying pathophysiology of a patients' disease process. ABG analysis is used to measure the partial pressures of oxygen and carbon dioxide and the pH in arterial blood. The ABG provides information on the following three important physiological processes that maintain the normal homeostasis of the body: alveolar ventilation (VA), oxygenation and acid–base balance. However, the investigation does not give a diagnosis and the results should be considered in the context of the patient's symptoms and disease process.

Alveolar ventilation

Lungs play a major part in the excretion of CO_2 which results in excreting of over 10,000 mEq of carbonic acid every day. As the majority of the carbon dioxide excretion is by the lungs, VA (which determines CO_2 elimination) has the greatest impact over acid–base balance. The maintenance of CO_2 level is reflected by the quantity of CO_2 produced in the body and its excretion through VA. It is given by the equation **$PaCO_2$=CO_2 production/VA** (when CO_2 production is constant), where $PaCO_2$ is the partial pressure of arterial carbon dioxide. VA is best represented by $PaCO_2$. A $PaCO_2 > 45$ mm Hg is suggestive of alveolar hypoventilation, whereas $PaCO_2 < 35$ mm Hg suggests alveolar hyperventilation.

Oxygenation

The ultimate aim of oxygenation is to provide adequate delivery of oxygen to tissues. The oxygen that reaches alveoli is best described by the partial pressure of alveolar oxygen (P_AO_2), which is given by the alveolar gas equation:

$$P_AO_2 = (FiO_2 \times (P_{atmosphere} - P_{H20})) - (PaCO_2 / \text{Resp Q})$$

P_AO_2 → Partial pressure of alveolar oxygen
FiO_2 → Fraction of inspired oxygen, 0.21 in room air
$P_{atmosphere}$ → Atmospheric pressure: 760 mmHg at sea level
P_{H20} → H20 vapor pressure in the alveolus
$PaCO_2$ → From the ABG
Resp Q → Respiratory quotient, which is 0.8

and substituting the values in the equation gives a P_AO_2 of approximately 100 mm Hg. Ideally, the arterial side should also have the same partial pressures as that of the alveoli, but due to the presence of physiological ventilation and perfusion mismatch, there exists an alveoli–arterial difference in partial pressures of oxygen. This is termed as A-a gradient. A-a gradient varies with age and helps in determining the cause of hypoxemia.

Once oxygen reaches blood, only 1.5% of total oxygen is transported as dissolved content in plasma. It is mainly transported as oxyhemoglobin binding to four globin chains of hemoglobin molecule. Each globin chain carries one oxygen molecule and the binding of one molecule increases the affinity of the globin chains for binding to the next oxygen molecule. This is known as cooperative binding which also explains the sigmoid shape of oxygen dissociation curve. Thus, the total oxygen transported by plasma is the sum of oxygen transported via hemoglobin and dissolved oxygen. Thus, the oxygen content in the blood is given by the formula.

$$C_aO_2 = \text{Hb} - \text{bound}\,O_2 + \text{dissolved}\,O_2$$

$$C_aO_2 = (O_2 \text{ carrying capacity} \times S_aO_2) + (P_aO_2 \times 0.0031)$$

$$C_aO_2 = (1.34 \times [\text{Hb}] \times S_aO_2) + (P_aO_2 \times 0.0031)$$

Hemoglobin-bound oxygen

The amount of oxygen carried by hemoglobin is the product of a person's hemoglobin levels, the amount of hemoglobin saturated with oxygen (given by the saturation of arterial oxygen — SaO_2), and the Huffner's constant-1.34 (the amount of oxygen in milliliters carried by each hemoglobin molecule).

Dissolved oxygen

According to Dalton's law of partial pressures, the amount of oxygen dissolved in the plasma is directly proportional to the partial pressure exerted by oxygen. Hence the total amount of dissolved oxygen is the product of PaO_2 (partial pressure of arterial oxygen) and the constant 0.003. (It is the amount of dissolved oxygen carried by 100 mL of blood at 1 atmospheric pressure.)

To summarize, normal tissue oxygenation requires perfusion by blood adequate in oxygen content, which is dependent on the factors described above. The PaO_2 provides an important contribution as it exerts a partial pressure sufficient to saturate hemoglobin molecules.

Acid–base physiology

An acid is a substance that dissociates, giving H+ ions whereas a base is a substance that accepts H+ ions, and an alkali is a substance that dissociates, giving OH− ions that react with H+ ions.

Acid production: Every 24 hours, approximately 60 mmol/L of H+ ions are produced. Inorganic acids such as hydrochloric acid (HCl), sulfuric acid (H_2SO_4), and phosphoric acid (H_3PO_4) and organic acids like amino acids, lactic acid form the end product of metabolism which carry these H+ ions. The organic acids are converted into carbon dioxide and water, which is excreted by the body in the following forms: bicarbonate dissolved in plasma (60%), bicarbonate within the erythrocytes (29%), and hemoglobin carbamate (Hb–NH.COO–) in the erythrocytes, CO_2 dissolved in plasma. The inorganic acids are excreted by the kidneys as their respective anions (NH_4–, HSO_4–, and H_2PO_4–).

Input of alkali: This occurs primarily when fruit and vegetables are ingested because they contain the K+ salts of organic acids that are metabolized to yield HCO_3– anions.

Elimination of alkali is achieved in a two-step process: the alkali load stimulates the production of H+ ions via the production of endogenous organic acids (eg, citric acid), which eliminate HCO_3– anions, and the kidneys excrete these organic anions (eg, citrate anions) with K+ ions in the urine. Thus, acids, bases, and alkali together determine the H+ ion concentration in blood. The process is summarized in Figure 1.

pH is the negative logarithm to base 10 of the concentration of hydrogen ions in solution, where "p" denotes power and "H" denotes hydrogen

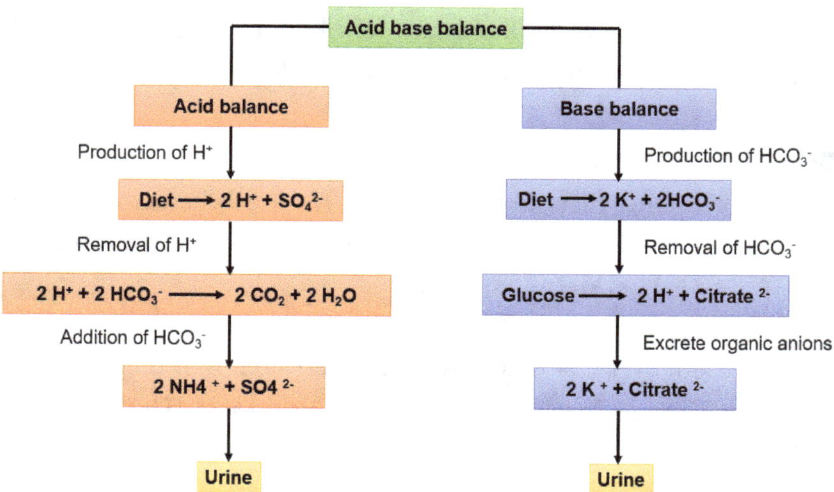

Figure 1: Acid–base load in diet and its handling by the body.

and the measure of the activity of dissolved hydrogen (H+) ions in a solution. Maintaining a normal pH is important as abnormal acid–base balance can lead to protein denaturation and enzyme inactivation.

$$pH = -\log_{10}(H+)$$

The acid–base homeostasis is maintained by the interaction of blood buffers, kidneys, and lungs. These are the three main lines of defense against changes in the pH of body fluid: the buffers system acts in a few seconds, whereas the respiratory system acts in a few minutes by bringing changes in $PaCO_2$, and the kidney acts in hours to days by regulating bicarbonate concentration to bring back the pH to normal.

Buffer system: It is a solution with two or more chemical compounds, which combine with strong acid or base to form weak acid or base. The effectiveness of a buffer depends on the quantity available and its pKa (defined as the logarithm to base 10 of the acid dissociation constant, Ka). It is the pH at which 50% of the buffer is in ionized form. The closer the pKa of the buffer is to the pH of the solution, the more effective it is.

$$\boldsymbol{pH = pKa + log10\ [A\text{-}]/[HA]}$$

- **The relationship between pH, pKa, and the concentrations of ionized [A–] and unionized [HA] acid.**
- **When [A–] = [HA], log10[A–]/[HA] = 0; thus pH = pKa.**

There are two types of buffer systems in the body: bicarbonate buffer system and non-bicarbonate buffer system.

Bicarbonate buffer system: In blood, bicarbonate is the most significant buffer despite low pKa (6.1) compared to blood pH due to the large quantity available. Also, since it is an open-ended buffer system [an open buffer system can have the amount of chemical at one (or both) end removed by physiological means], it can alter pH either via lungs or kidneys by affecting CO_2 and HCO_3- levels.

$$H_2O + CO_2 \leftrightarrow H_2CO_3 \leftrightarrow H+ + HCO_3-$$

Applying values for pKa and substituting the values in the Henderson–Hasselbalch equation pH = pKa + log (base/acid), we get pH = pKa + log (HCO_3-/H_2CO_3). Since carbonic acid (H_2CO_3) production and elimination are directly proportional to partial pressure carbon dioxide, we get

$$pH = pKa + \log (HCO_3-/PaCO_2)$$

removing logarithm, H+ = Ka * $PaCO_2/HCO_3-$
substituting Ka = 24, H+ = 24 * $PaCO_2/HCO_3-$

Bicarbonate is not actually measured in ABG machine but instead is calculated using the above formula. Hence, this equation is used to check the validity of ABG.

Non-bicarbonate buffers: In intracellular fluid, proteins and phosphate are the main buffers. Hemoglobin is the predominant buffer. Phosphate buffer is more effective as their pKa matches the pH of the plasma. However, the quantity of phosphate buffer is less. All non-bicarbonate buffers are closed systems as the end products remain in the system after buffering. Nevertheless, non-bicarbonate buffers are important as they buffer both carbonic and non-carbonic acids.

Pulmonary compensation

These changes are important in the immediate defense against marked changes in pH during metabolic disturbances. In metabolic acidosis, the decreased pH causes a rise in cerebrospinal fluid $PaCO_2$, leading to the stimulation of medullary respiratory centers, which causes hyperventilation and washout of carbon dioxide. The reverse is true in metabolic alkalosis leading to the retention of CO_2 in the blood. However, the magnitude of compensation is lesser than that of metabolic acidosis.

Renal compensation

The kidney's abilities to control the amount of HCO_3 reabsorbed, to form new HCO_3, and to eliminate the H^+ in the form of titrable acids and NH_4

ions allow them to exert a major influence on patients during acid–base disturbances. In respiratory acidosis, there is an increased reabsorption of filtered HCO_3-, increased excretion of titrable acids, and increased ammonia production. In acute respiratory acidosis, renal compensation begins after 6–12 hours and takes several days to complete. Kidneys can filter and excrete tremendous amounts of HCO_3 as a compensation for metabolic alkalosis.

Interpretation of ABG

There are three main methods of evaluating acid–base status of the patient: the Fencl–Stewart method, the Boston method (bicarbonate-centered approach), and the Copenhagen method. The most robust approach is the Fencl–Stewart approach. However, the most commonly used is the Boston method, which will be discussed in this section.

It is important to confirm whether the sample is indeed an arterial sample. Many times, venous samples are drawn by inexperienced personnel which can lead to unnecessary confusion. When drawing the sample, the technician needs to observe the flash of blood which is due to the high pressure in the arteries. Earlier, glass syringes were used and the blood would fill very easily when the needle was in the artery. The other clues are incompatibility of values with clinical conditions, low PO_2, and high PCO_2, and the oxygen saturation by pulse oximeter is greater than the oxygen saturation in the ABG report.

Boston approach/physiological approach

This is based on the assumption that components of the HCO_3–CO_2 are in equilibrium with non-bicarbonate buffers (albumin, phosphate, and hemoglobin). Also, bicarbonate buffer is the main buffering system of extracellular fluid. Hence, bicarbonate-centered approach better reflects the acid–base status of the patient. It was developed at Tufts University, Boston. Investigators Schwartz and Relman conducted a series of experiments on healthy volunteers, pregnant women, smokers, and sick patients with metabolic acid–base disorders and categorized acid–base disorders into six primary disorders and developed six equations to calculate expected compensation in these disorders. This is given in Table 1.

Table 1: Compensatory response in a primary acid–base disorder.

Primary disorder	Expected compensation
Acute respiratory acidosis	• Expected 1 mmol/L increase in HCO_3 per 10 mm Hg rise in $PaCO_2$
Chronic respiratory acidosis	• Steady within 24 – 36 hours • Expected 3 – 5 mmol/L increase in HCO_3 per 10 mm Hg rise in $PaCO_2$
Acute respiratory alkalosis	• Expected 1-2 mmol/L fall in HCO_3 per 10 mm Hg fall in $PaCO_2$
Chronic respiratory alkalosis	• Expected 4-5 mmol/L fall in HCO_3 per 10 mm Hg fall in $PaCO_2$
Metabolic acidosis	• Steady within 12 – 24 hours • Expected $PaCO_2$ = 1.5 [measured HCO_3] + 8 ± 2 mm Hg (Winter's formula)
Metabolic alkalosis	• Most variable • Expected 0.5 mm Hg increase in $PaCO_2$ per 1 mmol/L increase in HCO_3 • Expected $PaCO_2$ = 0.7 [measured HCO_3 24] = 40 ± 2 mm Hg

Step-by-step analysis of ABGs

The normal values obtained in an ABG test are given in Table 2. The following steps must be followed while analyzing ABG by the Boston approach.

Step 1: Checking the validity and patient details.
Step 2: Checking oxygenation status.

Table 2: Normal values of variables commonly displayed in an ABG.

Parameters	Arterial	Venous
pH	7.35–7.45	7.31–7.41
$PaCO_2$	35–45 mm Hg	41–51 mm Hg
HCO_3	24 ± 4 mmol/L	22–29 mmol/L
PaO_2	85–100 mm Hg	30–40 mm Hg
O_2 saturation	96%–100%	60%–85%
BE	0 ± 2 mmol/L	0 ± 4 mmol/L

Step 3: Checking ventilation status.
Step 4: Determine the primary disorder from blood, pH, HCO_3, and PCO_2 values. Calculate the compensatory response. Calculate the anion gap (AG). Calculate the delta ratio/corrected HCO_3.
Step 5: Examine the patient to determine whether the clinical signs are compatible with the acid–base analysis thus obtained.

Step 1: Checking the validity of ABG

Due to errors in sampling like the presence of air bubbles, excessively cooled sample, clotting of the sample or excess heparin, or uncalibrated ABG machine, the values obtained in ABG may be invalid. Hence, ABG has to be checked for validity using the equation:

$H+ = 24*PaCO_2/HCO_3-$.

Corresponding values of H+ ion concentration for a pH are shown in Figure 2.

Step 2: Check oxygenation status

Using the alveolar gas equation (described in page 3), calculate the P_AO_2. Then obtain the A-a gradient by the difference between P_AO_2 and PaO_2

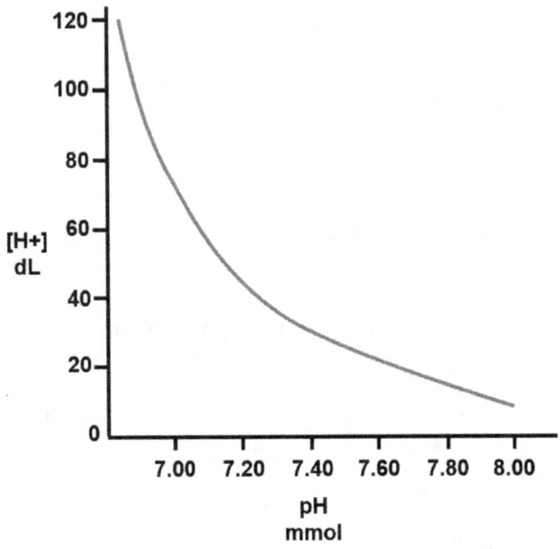

pH	Log10 [H+]
7.50	32
7.42	38
7.40	40
7.38	42
7.30	50
7.20	64
7.10	80
7.00	100
6.90	125

Figure 2: Concentration of H+ ions for various values of pH.

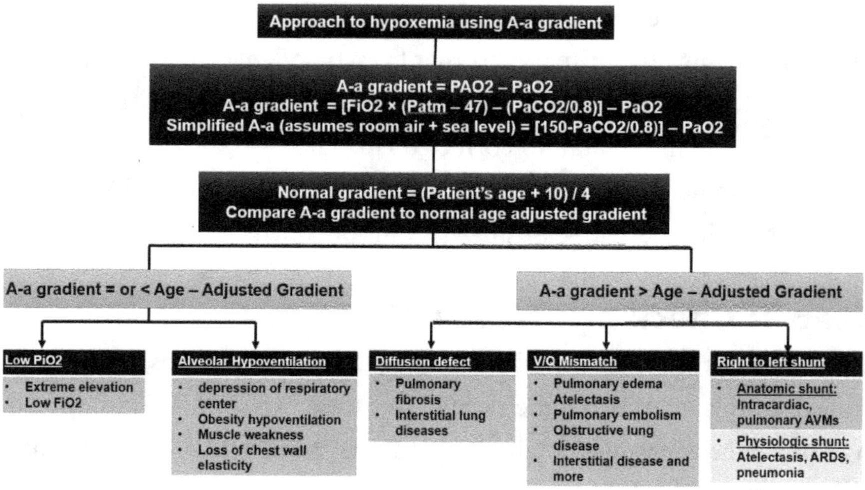

Figure 3: Approach to determine the cause for hypoxemia using A-a gradient.

(A — alveolar, a — arterial). The approach to causes of hypoxemia using A-a gradient is given by Figure 3.

Step 3: Check ventilation status

A $PaCO_2 > 45$ mm Hg is suggestive of alveolar hypoventilation leading to respiratory acidosis, whereas $PaCO_2 < 35$ mm Hg suggests alveolar hyperventilation causing respiratory alkalosis. The causes for respiratory acidosis and respiratory alkalosis are given in Table 3.

Step 4:

a. **Determine the primary disorder from blood, pH, HCO_3, and $PaCO_2$ values.**

Approach to determine the primary disturbance using pH, bicarbonate, and $PaCO_2$ is shown in Figure 4.

In mixed disorders, calculating the percentage change in baseline $PaCO_2$ and HCO_3- helps in diagnosing the dominant acid–base disturbance. For example, in an ABG with pH 7.55 HCO_3 30 mmol/L and PCO_2 35 mm Hg, there are both metabolic alkalosis and respiratory alkalosis.

Table 3: Depicting causes for acute and chronic hypercarbia

Causes	Acute hypercapnia	Chronic hypercapnia
Central depression of respiratory drive	Sedatives Opiates Anesthetic agents CNS lesions or trauma Stoke Encephalitis	Primary alveolar hypoventilation
Neuromuscular	Spinal cord lesions or trauma High central neural blockade Tetanus Poliomyelitis Amyotrophic lateral sclerosis Myasthenia gravis Organophosphate poisoning Muscular relaxants Dyselectrolytemia	Chronic neuro – myopathies Poliomyelitis Dyselectrolytemia Malnutrition
Chest wall	Flail chest Diaphragmatic dysfunction	Kyphoscoliosis Obesity Thoracoplasty
Pleura	Pneumothorax	Chronic large effusions
Lung parenchyma	Cardiogenic pulmonary edema ARDS Pneumonia	Longstanding and severe ILD
Airways	Upper airway obstruction Aspiration Asthma or COPD	Persistent asthma Severe COPD Bronchiectasis
Other	Circulatory shock Sepsis Malignant hyperthermia CO_2 insufflation into the body	

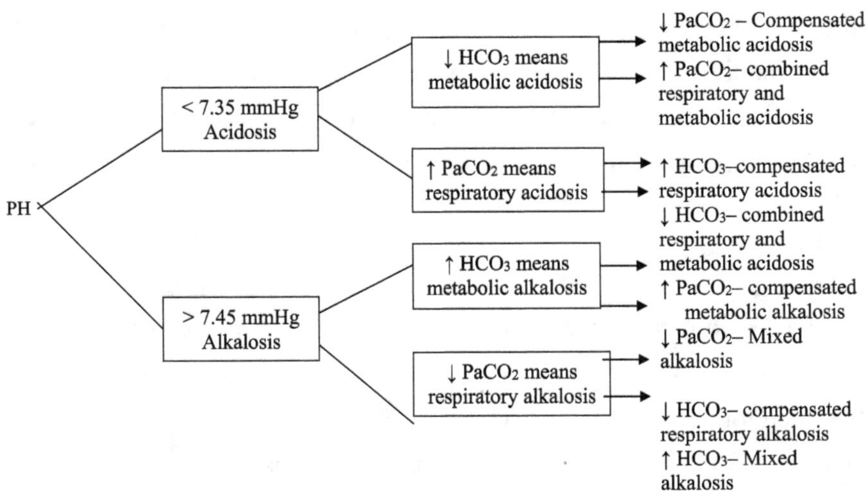

Figure 4: Approach to diagnose primary acid–base disorder and its compensation.

By calculating the percentage change in $PaCO_2$ and HCO_3-, the dominant disturbance can be diagnosed.

The percentage change in HCO_3- = 6/24*100 = 25%
The percentage change in $PaCO_2$ = 5/40*100 = 12.5%
So, the metabolic component is dominant.

b. **Calculate the compensatory response.**

Compensatory response depends on the proper functioning of organ system and severity of acid–base disturbances. Refer to Table 1 for calculating the compensation for a primary acid/base disturbance. The general rules of compensation include the following:

- Acute compensation occurs within 6–24 hours.
- Chronic compensation occurs within 1–4 days.
- Respiratory response occurs faster than metabolic component.
- Suspect mixed disorder if compensation does not occur.

c. **Calculate the anion gap.**

This is an extension to the Boston's approach. All body fluids are electrically neutral. The number of anions is equal to number of cations in plasma. The anions in extracellular fluid (ECF) include bicarbonate, chloride, phosphates, proteins, and inorganic anions and cations in ECF include sodium, potassium, calcium, and magnesium. AG represents the difference between measured anion and cation. It is routine to measure sodium, potassium, chloride, and bicarbonate ions as these are the important ions in terms of concentration in the plasma.

In plasma,

$$\text{Na} + \text{unmeasured cation} = \text{Cl} + HCO_3 + \text{unmeasured anion}$$

Therefore, AG = Na − (HCO_3 + Cl). Normal AG is 12 ± 4 mEq/L. Calculating AG helps in classifying metabolic acidosis into two types: high anion gap metabolic acidosis (HAGMA) and normal anion gap metabolic

Table 4: Causes for normal and high anion gap metabolic acidosis.

High anion gap	Normal anion gap
Renal failure	Gastrointestinal losses of bicarbonate
Ketoacidosis	Renal tubular acidosis
Lactic Acidosis	Treatment with carbonic anhydrase inhibitors
Salicylate poisoning	Urinary diversion procedure
Glycol ingestion (ethylene glycol, propylene glycol) Methanol ingestion	Excessive administration of 0.9 % saline

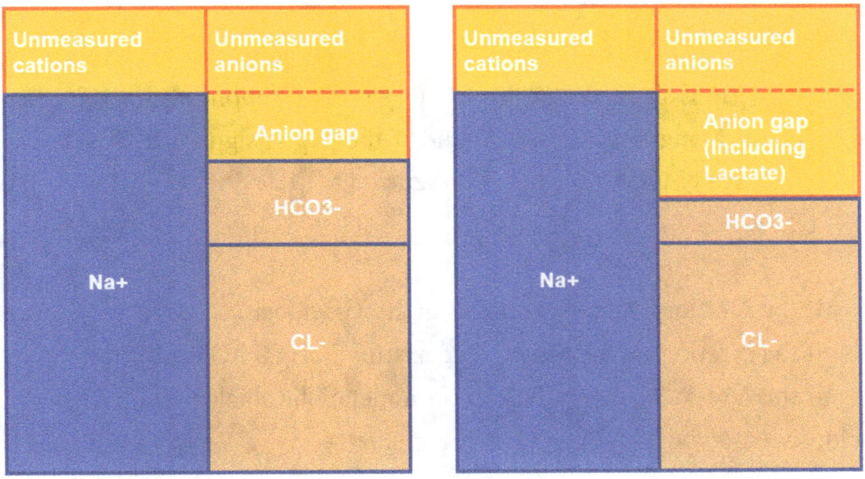

The anion gap contains unmeasured anions [Na+] – [Cl] + [HCO3] = Anion gap.

In HAGMA, e.g. lactic acidosis, the anion gap will increase following addition of "new" anions (lactate) with a corresponding fall in bicarbonate as it buffer the additional acid.

Figure 5: Gamblegram depicting increased anions in high anion gap metabolic acidosis.

acidosis (NAGMA). The causes for HAGMA and NAGMA are given in Table 4. Thus, AG helps in determining the etiology of metabolic acidosis. However, in mixed acid–base disorders, calculating the change in AG with respect to the change in bicarbonate (termed as delta–delta ratio) is necessary to arrive at the diagnosis.

d. **Calculate the delta gap/delta ratio**

In HAGMA, for every 1 mmol/L increase in the AG, there should be associated decrease of 1 mmol/L in the bicarbonate (HCO_3-) concentration. Any noteworthy change from this suggests the presence of a mixed acid–base disorder. Thus, delta gap is calculated as follows: Δ gap = Δ AG – Δ HCO_3-.

The Δ AG and Δ HCO_3- are calculated by the formulas

Δ AG = observed AG – 12
Δ HCO_3- = 24 – observed bicarbonate

If this gap is significantly positive (> +6), a metabolic alkalosis is usually present along with HAGMA, and if the gap is significantly negative (< –6), then a NAGMA is usually present.

Similarly, calculating the Δ ratio $= \frac{\Delta AG}{\Delta HCO_3}$

If the Δ ratio = 1, then it implies high AG acidosis.

If the Δ ratio < 1, then there is coexisting normal AG acidosis.

If the Δ ratio > 1, then there exists a metabolic alkalosis with high AG acidosis.

Step 5: Examine the patient to determine whether the clinical signs are compatible with the acid–base analysis thus obtained.

This is the most important step as correct interpretation leads to successful outcomes. This will be explained in examples section.

Urinary AG

Evaluating urinary AG (calculated by urine sodium + urine potassium – urine chloride) helps in identifying the cause for normal AG acidosis by differentiating between gastrointestinal or renal cause. This is usually positive and is a measure of urinary excretion of H+ ions in the form of ammonium ions. Usually, NAGMA is caused by the loss of bases by gut (diarrheal illness) or loss of bases by kidney (renal tubular acidosis). In cases of loss of bicarbonate by gastrointestinal system, kidney compensate by increasing excretion of ammonium ions (in the form of ammonium chloride). This leads to the decrease in urinary AG. If the loss of bases is of renal origin, then urinary AG is unchanged.

Summary

ABG status provides a window to ventilation, oxygenation, and acid–base pathophysiology of the patient. Correct interpretation of complex acid–base disorders is vital for initiating appropriate management of the deranged physiology.

Case studies

1. A 60-year-old man was admitted with gluteal abscess. He is also known diabetic who was on oral hypoglycemic agents. His oral intake has reduced for 2 days and complains of breathing difficulty today. His blood pressure was low and was resuscitated with intravenous fluids after which it normalized. He was started on 6 L of oxygen via face mask. ABG done in ward shows this. What is the cause for his breathing difficulty? What is the acid–base disturbance?

- **ABG**
- **pH** 7.30 **Na** 138 **lactate** 4.2
- **PCO_2** 18 **K** 4.1 **AG** 17
- **HCO_3** 9 **CI** 113 **PaO_2** 56

Answer

Check the validity of ABG

$H+ = 24 * PaCO_2/HCO_3-$

$= 24 * 18/9 = 48.$

Referring to Figure 2, the corresponding expected pH is 7.3, which shows that the ABG is valid. If the pH was not the same obtained in ABG, then it is considered an invalid ABG. The sample should to be redrawn and processed again.

To evaluate oxygenation status, first calculate the P_AO_2 (partial pressure of alveolar oxygen) using alveolar gas equation. FiO_2 for 6 L of supplemental oxygen is 44% or 0.44 (FiO_2 = 20% + 4 * liters of oxygen). Therefore, substituting the values in this equation

$$P_AO_2 = FiO_2\,(Pb - PH_2O) - PaCO_2/R, \text{ where } PH_2O \text{ is 44 mm Hg and } R=0.8.$$
$$= 0.44\,(760 - 44) - 44/0.8$$
$$= 258 \text{ mm Hg}$$

Now calculate A-a gradient = $P_AO_2 - PaO_2$ = 258 − 56 = 202 mm Hg. Expected normal age-adjusted A-a gradient = (age + 10)/4 = 70/4 = 17.5 mm Hg.

Referring Figure 3, since A-a gradient is increased, there is additional shunt or ventilation perfusion mismatch causing hypoxemia and breathing difficulty. The clinician must now rule out pneumonia, pulmonary embolism, and other causes as given in Figure 3.

Now evaluate the acid–base status

Since pH is less than 7.4, there is acidosis and primary disorder is metabolic because of low HCO_3. The expected compensation in $PaCO_2$ is given by Winter's formula:

$$PaCO_2 = 1.5 \times HCO_3 + 8 \pm 2$$
$$PaCO_2 = 1.5 \times 9 + 8 = 21.5 \text{ mm Hg.}$$

The actual $PaCO_2$ is less than expected $PaCO_2$, hence there is additional respiratory alkalosis.

The diagnosis in this patient is metabolic acidosis with additional respiratory alkalosis. Since AG is 17, this is HAGMA.

Check delta – delta gap to rule out additional NAGMA.

Delta AG = 17 − 12 = 5

Delta HCO_3- = 24 − 9 = 15

Delta – delta gap = Δ AG – Δ HCO_3– = 5 – 15 = –10
Any delta – delta gap more negative than –6 is suggestive of additional NAGMA.

Putting it all together

Patient has hypoxemia with respiratory alkalosis. The clinician must now rule out pneumonia, pulmonary embolism, and other causes for elevated A-a gradient as given in Figure 3. Patient has HAGMA. Since lactate is only mildly elevated, the clinical suspicion should be of diabetic ketoacidosis. Urine ketone bodies will confirm the diagnosis. The additional NAGMA is due to the excessive normal saline resuscitation as evidenced by high chloride levels. Thus, patient has mixed triple disorders: HAGMA, respiratory alkalosis, and NAGMA.

2. A 50-year-old man with chronic renal failure on maintenance hemodialysis has missed his last dialysis session now comes with complains of breathing difficulty. He is also case of chronic obstructive pulmonary disease (COPD) on inhalers and gives history of increased cough with pink sputum. His saturation in room air is 70% ABG done in emergency is

• **ABG**				
• **pH**	7.1	**Na**	140	**lactate** 4.2
• **PCO_2**	50	**K**	5	**AG** 20
• **HCO_3**	15	**CI**	105	**PaO_2** 40

What is the acid–base disturbance? What is the clinical diagnosis?

Answer

Check the validity of ABG

$$H+ = 24 * PaCO_2/HCO_3$$
$$= 24 * 50/15$$
$$= 80$$

Referring to Figure 2, the corresponding expected pH is 7.1, which matches with pH on ABG. Hence, the ABG is valid.

Evaluate oxygenation status

Here FiO_2 is 0.21, substituting the values in the equation $PaO_2 = FiO_2$ (Pb – PH_2O) – $PaCO_2$/R where PH_2O is 44 mm Hg and R=0.8,

$$PaO_2 = 0.21 * 713 - 50/0.8$$
$$= 149 - 62 = 87 \text{ mm Hg}$$

Calculate A-a gradient = $P_AO_2 - PaO_2 = 87 - 40 = 47$ mm Hg.

Expected normal age – adjusted A-a gradient = (age + 10)/4 = 60/4 = 15 mm Hg

Since A-a gradient is increased, there is additional mechanism of ventilation perfusion mismatch or shunt along with hypoventilation (elevated $PaCO_2$).

Evaluate the acid–base status

It is acidosis because pH < 7.4.

The diagnosis is both metabolic acidosis with respiratory acidosis as bicarbonate is low and there is elevated $PaCO_2$. To calculate the primary disorder, check the percentage change, that is, the percentage change in HCO_3- = 9/24 * 100 = 37.5%.

The percentage change in $PaCO_2$ = 10/40 * 100 = 25%.

Hence the dominant primary disturbance is metabolic acidosis.

Since the AG is elevated, it is HAGMA.

Check delta – delta gap to rule out additional NAGMA.

Delta AG = 20 – 12 = 8
Delta HCO_3- = 24 – 15 = 9
Delta – delta gap = Δ AG – Δ HCO_3- = 8 – 9 = –1

There is no additional acid–base disorder.

Correlating the ABG findings to the patient's clinical status, the clinical diagnosis is chronic renal failure and COPD causing HAGMA and respiratory acidosis. The cause of hypoxemia might be due to pulmonary edema due to missed dialysis (as there is complaints of pink sputum) or ventilation perfusion mismatch seen in COPD patients.

3. A 73-year-old woman with rheumatoid arthritis on home oxygen increased her dose of salicylates because of a flare-up. She then developed epigastric pain and vomited frequently for 2 days. She went to the local hospital, where the following blood results were obtained. Her saturation is low but reaches 92% with 15 L of oxygen.

   - **pH** 7.70
   - **PaCo$_2$** 25 mm Hg
   - **Anion gap** 17 mEq/L
   - **PaO$_2$** 60 mm of Hg
   - **Lactate** 6 mmol/dL
   - **HCO$_3$−** 30 mEq/L

   Evaluate her ABG and give clinical diagnosis.

Answer

Check the validity of ABG

$$\begin{aligned} H+ &= 24 * PaCO_2/HCO_3- \\ &= 24 * 25/30 \\ &= 20 \end{aligned}$$

Referring to Figure 2, the corresponding expected pH is 7.7, which matches with pH on ABG. Hence, the ABG is valid.

To evaluate oxygenation status, first calculate the P_AO_2 (partial pressure of alveolar oxygen) using alveolar gas equation. FiO_2 for 10 L of supplemental oxygen is 60% or 0.6 (FiO_2 = 20% + 4 * liters of oxygen). Therefore, substituting the values in this equation

$$\begin{aligned} P_AO_2 &= FiO_2\,(Pb - PH_2O) - PaCO_2/R, \text{ where } PH_2O \text{ is 44 mm Hg and } R=0.8 \\ &= 0.6\,(760 - 44) - 25/0.8 \\ &= 401 \text{ mm Hg} \end{aligned}$$

Now calculate A-a gradient = P_AO_2 − PaO_2 = 401 − 60 = 341 mm Hg. Expected normal age adjusted A-a gradient = (age+10)/4 = 83/4 = 20.75 mm Hg.

Referring to Figure 3, since A-a gradient is increased, there is additional shunt or ventilation perfusion mismatch causing hypoxemia. Causes as given in Figure 3 in this patient are interstitial lung disease (ILD) secondary to rheumatoid arthritis (suggested by use of home oxygen) or aspiration pneumonia during repeated vomiting.

Evaluating the acid–base status

She has metabolic alkalosis (low [H+] and elevated plasma [HCO_3]). However, her $PaCO_2$ is low (the expected response during metabolic alkalosis is hypoventilation to return the (H+) in cells towards normal), and she is hyperventilating; therefore, she has a second primary acid–base disorder respiratory alkalosis secondary to salicylate intoxication. In addition, the small rise in her plasma AG raises the possibility of a third acid–base disorder, HAGMA, resulting from added acids (salicylic acid and lactate, most likely).

The clinical diagnosis is salicylate poisoning causing metabolic alkalosis, respiratory alkalosis, and HAGMA with hypoxemia secondary to suspected aspiration pneumonia and ILD.

4. Consider the following values in a patient who complains of diarrhea and vomiting.

Na+	140 mmol/L	**pH**	7.4
K+	2.3 mmol/L	**$PaCO_2$**	40 mm Hg
Cl	103 mmol/L	**Anion gap**	12 mEq/L
HCO_3	25 mmol/L		

What is the acid–base disorder?

Answer

On the surface, most of the laboratory data do not suggest an acid–base disturbance, but the hypokalemia must be explained. It is most likely that the patient has a mixed metabolic acidosis (HCO_3 loss due to diarrhea) and metabolic alkalosis (HCO_3 gain due to vomiting) with the hypokalemia associated with excessive renal loss of K+. The acid–base status, which results from the combination of these two disorders, is normal when judged solely by the four parameters in plasma (pH, $PaCO_2$, HCO_3-, and AG). The physical examination test results were not normal: The ECF volume was contracted. In therapy containing K+ (40–60 mmol/L), half-normal saline plus KCI is a good initial solution.

5. A 38-year-old woman who is known asthmatic had preoperative check ABG done on room air before undergoing cholecystectomy.

   ABG measurements are the following:

   pH 7.31, $PaCO_2$ 60, HCO_3 23, PaO_2 95

   Comment on her ABG.

Answer

Acute hypercapnia is incompatible with the history of stable asthma. PaO_2 should proportionately decline in response to rise in $PaCO_2$ on room air. The sum of PaO_2 and $PaCO_2$ is 155. On room air, the sum of PaO_2 and $PaCO_2$ should be less than 140. Also checking the validity of ABG,

$$\begin{aligned} H+ &= 24 * PaCO_2/HCO_3- \\ &= 24 * 60/23 \\ &= 62 \end{aligned}$$

Referring to Figure 2, the corresponding expected pH is 7.2 that does not match with pH on ABG. Hence, the ABG is invalid. The sample should to be redrawn and processed again.

6. A 60-year-old admitted with gluteal abscess, known diabetic.

• **ABG**				
• **pH**	7.18	**Na**	138	
• **PCO_2**	18	**K**	4.1	AG 23.1
• **HCO_3**	9	**CI**	110	

What is the acid–base disturbance?

pH < 7.4 — acidosis

Metabolic or respiratory?

Metabolic — because of low HCO_3 and low PCO_2

Whether compensated?

Expected PCO_2

$= 1.5 \times HCO_3 + 8$

$= 1.5 \times 9 + 8 = 21.5$

When actual PCO_2 is less than expected PCO_2 — respiratory alkalosis.
When actual PCO_2 is greater than expected PCO_2 — respiratory acidosis.

The diagnosis in this patient is:

Metabolic acidosis with partially compensated respiratory alkalosis.

How much is AG?

$(Na+ + K+) - (HCO_3 + CI) = \text{normal} - 16 + -4$

In known case, it is 23. It is increased AG metabolic acidosis.

The clinical diagnosis is:

Diabetic ketoacidosis with sepsis.

Management

How to calculate the dose of sodium bicarbonate?

BE: Normal ± 2

$$= \frac{BE \times 0.3 \times \text{Body weight (kg)}}{2}$$

Half correction is done within ½ hour, and rest is given as slow infusion over 4 hours and ABG is repeated.

7. A 50-year-old with chronic renal failure, smoker.

• **ABG**				
• **pH**	7.1	**Na**	140	
• **PCO_2**	50	**K**	5	AG 23
• **HCO_3**	15	**CI**	105	

What is the acid–base disturbance?
It is acidosis because pH < 7.4.

Is it metabolic or respiratory?
Metabolic acidosis because of low HCO_3.

Expected $PCO_2 = 105 \times 15 + 8 = 30.5$
Now, actual PCO_2 > expected PCO_2
Then there is added respiratory acidosis.

The diagnosis of the metabolic acidosis with respiratory acidosis. The clinical diagnosis is chronic renal failure with COPD and increased AG metabolic acidosis.

Management: Soda bicarbonate administration? and elective mechanical ventilation weaning with permissible hypercapnia.

8. A 35-year-old, collapsed on physical exertion was brought to hospital.

• **ABG**			
• **pH**	6.99	**Na**	141
• **PCO_2**	34	**K**	6.0
• **HCO_3**	8	**CI**	105

What is the acid–base disturbance?
Acidosis because pH < 7.4.

It is metabolic because of low bicarbonate.
Expected PCO_2 is $1.5 \times 8 + 8 = 20$.
Actual PCO_2 > expected PCO_2 = Respiratory acidosis.
AG is 28. It is increased AG metabolic acidosis.

Hyperkalemia with metabolic and respiratory acidosis.
Clinical diagnosis is cardiorespiratory arrest.

Management
Cardiopulmonary resuscitation.
Mechanical ventilation.
Correction of hyperkalemia and metabolic acidosis.

9. A 70-kg healthy man had acute airway obstruction during induction of anesthesia.

- **pH** 7.1
- **PCO_2** 70
- **HCO_3** 21

pH < 7.4, it is acidosis.
PCO_2 > 40, it is respiratory.

Is there a component of metabolic acidosis ?

Rule of thumb
Acute hypercapnia: HCO_3 increases 1 mmol for every increase in 10 mm Hg of PCO_2 above 40.

Then HCO_3 should be 3 mmol above 24, if PCO_2 only is changed. Predicted HCO_3 is 27.

But actual is 21, a deficit of 6 mmol/L. Hence it is combined respiratory and metabolic acidosis.

10. A 56-year-old male patient, with COPD having resting PCO_2 of 70 sustains perioperative myocardial infarction, blood pressure is 80/60 mm Hg, is sweating, cool, and clammy.

    - **pH** 7.1
    - **PCO_2** 70
    - **HCO_3** 21

    pH < 7.4, it is acidosis.
    PCO_2 > 40, it is respiratory.

    Rule of thumb

    Chronic hypercapnia: HCO_3 increases by 4 mmol/L for every 10 mm Hg increase of PCO_2 above 40 mm Hg.

    Predicted HCO_3 is 36 mmol/L, whereas actual is 21, deficit is 15 mmol/L.

    Metabolic component is much greater despite the same value as in the above case.

11. A 23-year-old woman with rheumatoid arthritis increased her dose of salicylates because of a flare-up. She then developed epigastric pain and vomited frequently for 2 days. She went to the local hospital, where the following blood results were obtained.

    - **pH** 7.70
    - **H+** 20 nmol/L
    - **$PaCO_2$** 25 mm Hg
    - **Anion gap** 17 mEq/L

    What is her acid–base disorder (s)?
    The pH of her blood is very alkalemic ([H+] = 20 nmol/L, pH = 7 – 70). Her [HCO_3] can be calculated from the Henderson equation:

    $[HCO_3] = 24 \times PaCO_2/[H+] = 30$ mmol/L

Thus, she has metabolic alkalosis (low [H+] and elevated plasma [HCO_3]). However, her $PaCO_2$ is low (the expected response during metabolic alkalosis is hypoventilation to return the (H+) in cells towards normal), and she is hyperventilating; therefore, she has a second primary acid–base disorder, and respiratory alkalosis was secondary to vomiting and HCI loss. Her respiratory alkalosis was secondary to salicylate intoxication. In addition, the small rise in her plasma AG raises the possibility of a third acid–base disorder, metabolic acidosis, resulting from added acids (salicylic acid and the more negative valence of albumin, most likely).

12. Consider the following values in a patient who complains of diarrhea and vomiting.

Na+	140 mmol/L	**H+**	40 nmol/L
K+	2.3 mmol/L	**$PaCO_2$**	40 mm Hg
Cl	103 mmol/L	**Anion gap**	12 mEq/L
HCO_3	25 mmol/L		

What are the acid–base disorders?

On the surface, most of the laboratory data do not suggest an acid–base disturbance, but the hypokalemia must be explained. It is most likely that the patient has a mixed metabolic acidosis (HCO_3 loss due to diarrhea) and metabolic alkalosis (HCO_3 gain due to vomiting) with the hypokalemia associated with excessive renal loss of K+. The acid–base status, which results from the combination of these two disorders, is normal when judged solely by the four parameters in plasma (pH, $PaCO_2$, (HCO_3), and AG). The physical examination test results were not normal: The ECF volume was contracted. In therapy containing K+ (40 – 60 mmol/L), half-normal saline plus KCI is a good initial solution.

13. A 38-year-old woman who is known asthmatic had preoperative check ABG done on room air before undergoing cholecystectomy.

ABG measurements are the following:
pH 7.3, $PaCO_2$ 60, HCO_3 23, PaO_2 95.

Acute hypercapina is incompatible with the history of stable asthma. PaO_2 should proportionately decline in response to rise in $PaCO_2$ on room air. Sum of PaO_2 + $PaCO_2$ is 155. On room air, the sum of PaO_2 and $PaCO_2$ should be less than 140.

14. A 50-year-old asthmatic woman presented with progressive SOB in emergency.

    ABG was done on room air:
    pH 7.68, $PaCO_2$ 20, HCO_3 22, PaO_2 115.

    Though it is non-compensated not only in acute respiratory alkalosis but even in acute asthma, $PaCO_2$ falling to 20 mm Hg is rare. Excepted PaO_2 is either in normal range or hypoxemia to varying degree. Here PaO_2 is 115, which is even more than P_AO_2 (PO_2 in alveolar air).

    Normal P_AO_2 is 100 – 105 mm Hg on room air in normal lungs. Here because of V/Q mismatch expected is lower than normal. Possibly atmosphere air was mixed with arterial blood in syringe while sampling, giving falsely high PaO_2 and low $PaCO_2$.

    PaO_2 can never be higher than expected P_AO_2.

15. An insulin-dependent diabetic patient with several days of vomiting developed diabetic ketoacidosis. His ABG was the following:
    pH 7.18, $PaCO_2$ 38, PaO_2 70, HCO_3 15
    Na+ 140, K+ 5, CI 190
    Identify the acid–base disturbance.

    Metabolic acidosis is present because pH < 7.4 and $HCO_3 < 24$
    Actual $PaCO_2$ (38) is greater than expected (30) compensatory $PaCO_2$ ($1.5 \times 15 + 8 = 30$), hence respiratory acidosis is present.

    AG is raised: (140 [Na] – 90 [CI] 15 (HCO_3) = 35
    Normal AG is 12 ± 2 [HCO_3] + – in AG > 24 (note: A change in AG above 12).

    that is, ($15 + 23 = 38 > 24$).
    Hence superimposed metabolic alkalosis present.

Measurement of AG is very important in metabolic acidosis to assess for associated another metabolic disorder and also to explain the cause of metabolic acidosis.

16. A 17-year-old 48-kg woman with known insulin-dependent diabetes mellitus entered the emergency department with Kussmaul breathing and an irregular pulse. Room air arterial blood gas values were the following:

- **pH** 7.05
- **PCO_2** 12 mm Hg
- **PO_2** 108 mm Hg
- **HCO_3** 5 mmol/L
- **BE** −30 mmol/L

Interpretation

This is a mixed acid–base abnormality, severe partly compensated metabolic acidosis, and respiratory alkalosis without hypoxemia.

Intravenous glucose and insulin were immediately administered. A judgment was made that the severe acidemia was adversely affecting cardiovascular function, and it was elected to restore the pH to the vicinity of 7.20. Calculate the amount of sodium bicarbonate you would administer.

HCO_3 deficit = body weight/2 (target − actual HCO_3) $48/2 \times 24 - 5 = 456$ mL.

Because the goal was to partly correct the acidemia, approximately one-half of the calculated deficit was intravenously administered over a 15-minute time interval. Room air arterial blood gas values were the following:

- **pH** 7.27
- **PCO_2** 25 mm Hg
- **PO_2** 92 mm Hg
- **HCO_3** 11 mmol/L
- **BE** −14 mmol/L

17. A 66-year-old woman with a history of COPD entered the emergency department in respiratory distress with bilateral rales. A presumptive diagnosis of cardiogenic pulmonary edema was made. Room air arterial blood gas values were the following:

- **pH** 7.10
- **PCO_2** 25 mm Hg
- **PO_2** 40 mm Hg
- **HCO_3** 8 mmol/L
- **BE** −20 mmol/L

Interpretation

Partly compensated metabolic acidosis with severe hypoxemia. Tissue hypoxia must be assumed when acidemia and hypoxemia coexist. The patient was mechanically ventilated. 100% oxygen was administered and treated with inotropes, furosemide, and morphine. On FiO_2 of 1.0, arterial blood gas values were the following:

- **pH** 7.38
- **PCO_2** 25 mm Hg
- **PO_2** 110 mm Hg
- **HCO_3** 16 mmol/L
- **BE** −7 mmol/L

The acidemia was revered, most probably because aerobic metabolism was restored by improving both cardiac output and arterial oxygen content.

Significant pulmonary disease is reflected in the PaO_2 of 110 mm Hg despite an FiO_2 of 1.0.

18. A 17-year-old girl with severe kyphoscoliosis entered the hospital with pneumonia.

- **pH** 7.37
- **PCO_2** 25 mm Hg
- **PO_2** 70 mm Hg
- **HCO_3** 14 mmol/L
- **BE** −7 mmol/L

Interpretation

Chronic alveolar hyperventilation (respiratory alkalosis) with uncorrected hypoxemia. The patient was treated with appropriate antibiotics. Intravenous fluids consisted of 5% dextrose/0.45 NaCl, but she refused to eat. On the third day, despite the resolution of the pneumonia, she began to complain of weakness and difficulty in breathing. Room air arterial blood gas values are the following:

- **pH** 7.53
- **PCO_2** 38 mm Hg
- **PO_2** 62 mm Hg
- **HCO_3** 32 mmol/L
- **BE** +7 mmol/L

Interpretation

Uncompensated metabolic alkalosis with mild hypoxemia. Serum electrolyte studies revealed a low potassium level (2.6 mmol/L). After appropriate potassium chloride (KCl) replacement, the complaints of dyspnea and weakness disappeared. Room air arterial blood gas values were the following:

- **pH** 7.41
- **PCO_2** 24 mm Hg
- **PO_2** 68 mm Hg
- **HCO_3** 16 mmol/L
- **BE** −6 mmol/L

Interpretation

Chronic alveolar hyperventilation (compensated respiratory alkalosis) with mild hypoxemia. This most likely represents her baseline state.

Her chronic restrictive pulmonary disease is responsible for the baseline state of chronic alveolar hyperventilation and renal compensation hypokalemia resulted in a metabolic alkalosis, some respiratory compensation, and the feeling of muscular weakness.

References and suggested readings

1. Claassen JAHR, Thijssen DHJ, Panerai RB, Faraci FM. Regulation of cerebral blood flow in humans: physiology and clinical implications of autoregulation. Physiol Rev. 2021 Oct 1;101(4):1487–1559. doi: 10.1152/physrev.00022.2020. Epub 2021 Mar 26. PMID: 33769101; PMCID: PMC8576366.
2. Doaei S, Gholami S, Rastgoo S, Gholamalizadeh M, Bourbour F, Bagheri SE, Samipoor F, Akbari ME, Shadnoush M, Ghorat F, Mosavi Jarrahi SA, Ashouri Mirsadeghi N, Hajipour A, Joola P, Moslem A, Goodarzi MO. The effect of omega-3 fatty acid supplementation on clinical and biochemical parameters of critically ill patients with COVID-19: a randomized clinical trial. J Transl Med. 2021 Mar 29;19(1):128. doi: 10.1186/s12967-021-02795-5. PMID: 33781275; PMCID: PMC8006115.
3. Adly AS, Adly MS, Adly AS. Telemanagement of home-isolated COVID-19 patients using oxygen therapy with noninvasive positive pressure ventilation and physical therapy techniques: randomized clinical trial. J Med Internet Res. 2021 Apr 28;23(4):e23446. doi: 10.2196/23446. PMID: 33819166; PMCID: PMC8080964.
4. Valizad Hassanloei M, Mahoori A, Karami N, Sina V. The relationship between arterial and central venous blood gases values in patients undergoing mechanical ventilation after cardiac surgery. Anesth Pain Med. 2018 Jun 23;8(3):e74243. doi: 10.5812/aapm.74243. PMID: 30214888; PMCID: PMC6119237.
5. Salvarani C, Dolci G, Massari M, Merlo DF, Cavuto S, Savoldi L, Bruzzi P, Boni F, Braglia L, Turrà C, Ballerini PF, Sciascia R, Zammarchi L, Para O, Scotton PG, Inojosa WO, Ravagnani V, Salerno ND, Sainaghi PP, Brignone A, Codeluppi M, Teopompi E, Milesi M, Bertomoro P, Claudio N, Salio M, Falcone M,

Cenderello G, Donghi L, Del Bono V, Colombelli PL, Angheben A, Passaro A, Secondo G, Pascale R, Piazza I, Facciolongo N, Costantini M; RCT-TCZ-COVID-19 Study Group. Effect of Tocilizumab vs standard care on clinical worsening in patients hospitalized with COVID-19 pneumonia: a randomized clinical trial. JAMA Intern Med. 2021 Jan 1;181(1):24–31. doi: 10.1001/jamainternmed.2020.6615. PMID: 33080005; PMCID: PMC7577199.

6. Scott T, van Waart H, Vrijdag XCE, Mullins D, Mesley P, Mitchell SJ. Arterial blood gas measurements during deep open-water breath-hold dives. J Appl Physiol (1985). 2021 May 1;130(5):1490–1495. doi: 10.1152/japplphysiol.00111.2021. Epub 2021 Apr 8. PMID: 33830815; PMCID: PMC8354821.
7. Lambert LL, Baldwin MB, Gonzalez CV, Lowe GR, Willis JR. Accuracy of Transcutaneous CO_2 values compared with arterial and capillary blood gases. Respir Care. 2018 Jul;63(7):907–912. doi: 10.4187/respcare.05936. Epub 2018 May 8. PMID: 29739856.
8. Storgaard LH, Hockey HU, Laursen BS, Weinreich UM. Long-term effects of oxygen-enriched high-flow nasal cannula treatment in COPD patients with chronic hypoxemic respiratory failure. Int J Chron Obstruct Pulmon Dis. 2018 Apr 16;13:1195–1205. doi: 10.2147/COPD.S159666. PMID: 29713153; PMCID: PMC5909797.
9. Adamidi ES, Mitsis K, Nikita KS. Artificial intelligence in clinical care amidst COVID-19 pandemic: a systematic review. Comput Struct Biotechnol J. 2021;19:2833–2850. doi: 10.1016/j.csbj.2021.05.010. Epub 2021 May 7. PMID: 34025952; PMCID: PMC8123783.
10. Beyer AM, Norwood Toro LE, Hughes WE, Young M, Clough AV, Gao F, Medhora M, Audi SH, Jacobs ER. Autophagy, TERT, and mitochondrial dysfunction in hyperoxia. Am J Physiol Heart Circ Physiol. 2021 Nov 1;321(5):H985–H1003. doi: 10.1152/ajpheart.00166.2021. Epub 2021 Sep 24. PMID: 34559580; PMCID: PMC8616608.
11. Longhini F, Bruni A, Garofalo E, Ronco C, Gusmano A, Cammarota G, Pasin L, Frigerio P, Chiumello D, Navalesi P. Chest physiotherapy improves lung aeration in hypersecretive critically ill patients: a pilot randomized physiological study. Crit Care. 2020 Aug 3;24(1):479. doi: 10.1186/s13054-020-03198-6. PMID: 32746877; PMCID: PMC7396943.

12. Shaw K, Butcher S, Ko J, Zello GA, Chilibeck PD. Wearing of cloth or disposable surgical face masks has no effect on vigorous exercise performance in healthy individuals. Int J Environ Res Public Health. 2020 Nov 3;17(21):8110. doi: 10.3390/ijerph17218110. PMID: 33153145; PMCID: PMC7662944.
13. Bergamaschi G, Borrelli de Andreis F, Aronico N, Lenti MV, Barteselli C, Merli S, Pellegrino I, Coppola L, Cremonte EM, Croce G, Mordà F, Lapia F, Ferrari S, Ballesio A, Parodi A, Calabretta F, Ferrari MG, Fumoso F, Gentile A, Melazzini F, Di Sabatino A; Internal Medicine Covid-19 Collaborators. Anemia in patients with Covid-19: pathogenesis and clinical significance. Clin Exp Med. 2021 May;21(2):239–246. doi: 10.1007/s10238-020-00679-4. Epub 2021 Jan 8. Erratum in: Clin Exp Med. 2021 Mar 17. PMID: 33417082; PMCID: PMC7790728.
14. Aslanidis T, Grosomanidis V, Karakoulas K, Chatzisotiriou A. Electrodermal activity during blood pooling for arterial blood gases analysis in sedated adult intensive care unit patients. Med Sci (Basel). 2018 Mar 6;6(1):20. doi: 10.3390/medsci6010020. PMID: 29509711; PMCID: PMC5872177.
15. Deng T, Liu M, Pan L, Jiang K, Li Y. A comparison of arterial blood glucose and peripheral blood glucose levels in critically ill patients: measurements using the arterial blood gas analyzer and the rapid glucose meter. Ann Palliat Med. 2021 Mar;10(3):3179–3184. doi: 10.21037/apm-21-354. PMID: 33849103.
16. Zwisler ST, Zincuk Y, Bering CB, Zincuk A, Nybo M, Mikkelsen S. Diagnostic value of prehospital arterial blood gas measurements — a randomised controlled trial. Scand J Trauma Resusc Emerg Med. 2019 Mar 18;27(1):32. doi: 10.1186/s13049-019-0612-8. PMID: 30885262; PMCID: PMC6421666.

https://doi.org/10.1142/9789811271410_0008

8 Bronchoscopy

Introduction

Bronchoscopy is a procedure that allows a bronchoscopist (usually a pulmonologist or a thoracic surgeon) to visualize and examine the patient's airways and lungs, including larynx, vocal cord, trachea, and many branches of bronchi. It allows direct view of the tissue and permits to take samples of biopsied lung tissue through the bronchoscope for histological studies in the laboratory.

Two types of bronchoscopes are available: a flexible fiberoptic bronchoscope (FOB) and another rigid bronchoscope. For the last four decades, flexible bronchoscopy has taken away almost all the preferential indications from rigid bronchoscopy, because of convenience and patients not requiring general anesthesia.

However, the indication favoring use of rigid bronchoscope in case of massive bleeding as it offers better optics for view at a large or in failure of flexible bronchoscopy are still being kept reserved with rigid bronchoscopy.

Types: A rigid bronchoscopy is a straight, hollow metal tube that is used:

- When a large tissue sample is to be removed.
- When flexible bronchoscope's view is blocked due to massive bleeding.
- When a foreign body (FB) such as a piece of food particle that cannot be removed by flexible bronchoscopy.
- When a special procedure such as widening (dilating) the airways or debulking or destroying of tumor is to be done using a laser.

For laser bronchoscopy stent placement and removal. It is contraindicated in the unstable cervical spine, non-obstructive hypoxemia, unstable cardiovascular status, and importantly in the hands of an inadequately trained person.

A flexible bronchoscopy is a long, thin tube that contains many small, clear fibers or a small camera that can transmit light images as it bends. It is a safe procedure in expert hands and does not require general anesthesia.

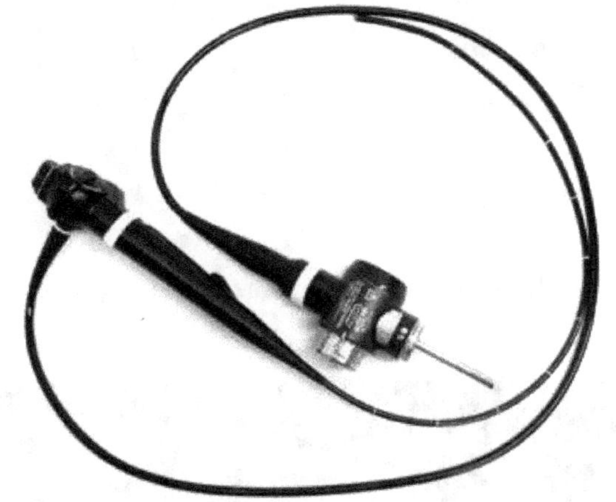

Image 1: Flexible bronchoscopy.

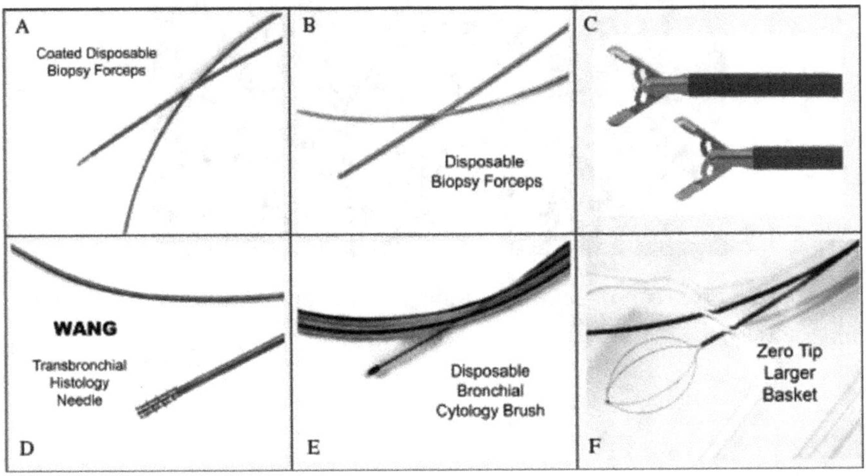

Image 2: Various accessories for flexible bronchoscopy.

Radiological findings

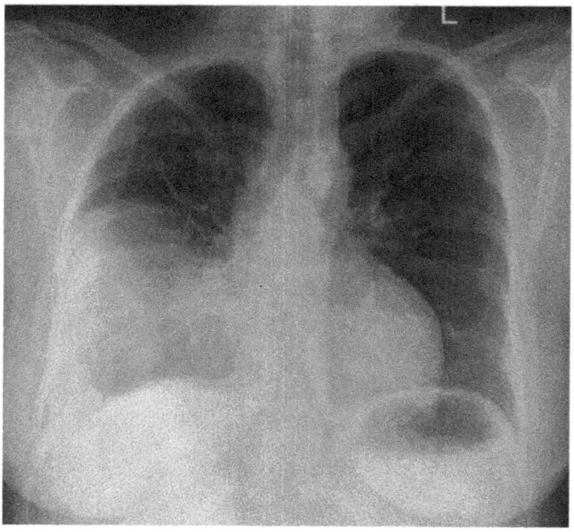

Chest X-ray: Right middle and lower zone non-homogeneous opacity.

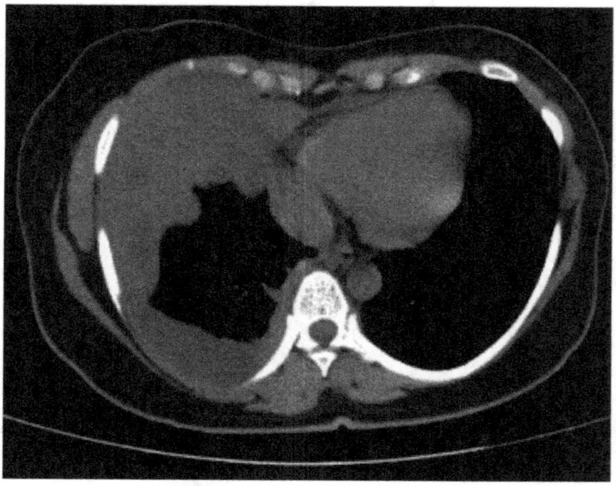

CT thorax: Lobar consolidation of right middle lobe with air bronchogram/ mucus plugging.

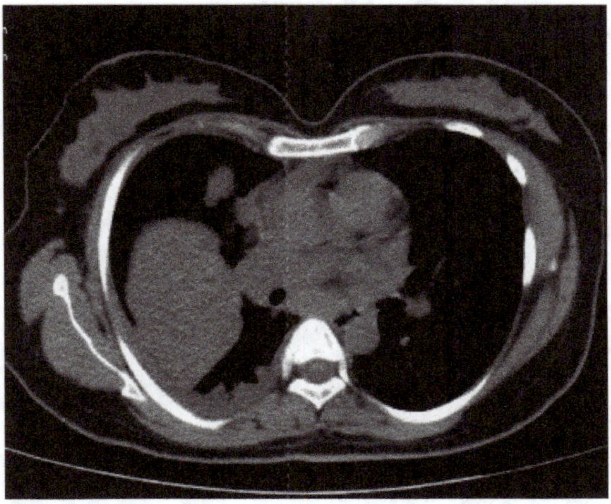

Computed tomography (CT)-guided biopsy was done and sent for histopathological examination (HPe). The specimen consisted of multiple grayish-white tissue fragments of HPe, which showed fibrocollagenous and fibromuscular tissues.

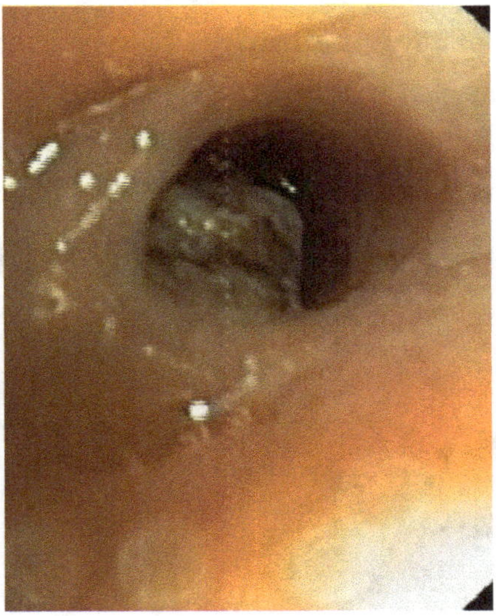

Flexible bronchoscopy showed a right middle bronchus lesion causing partial obstruction to the right middle lobe.

Indications

Bronchoscopy is done to identify the cause of inflammation and bleeding. It may be indicated to collect secretions from the airways for identifying certain specific abnormalities or infections.

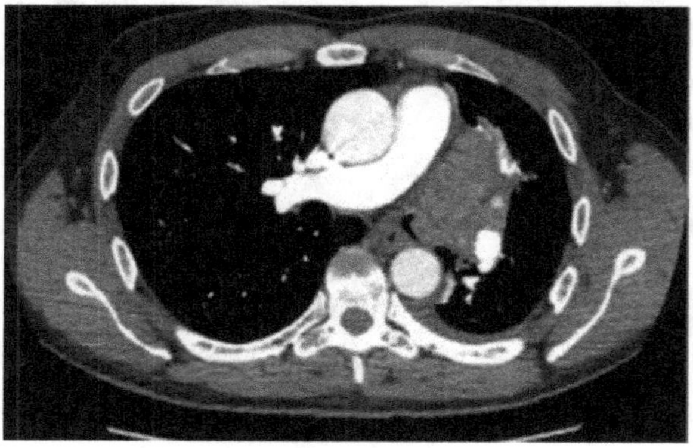

It can be performed for magnified diagnostic viewing or for collecting samples of biopsied lung tissue to be differentiated histologically for diagnosis in the laboratory, or it may be used to diagnose and determine the extension of lung cancer. It can be used to find the cause of wheezing or difficulty in breathing and also to evaluate previously diagnosed lung cancer and following chest trauma.

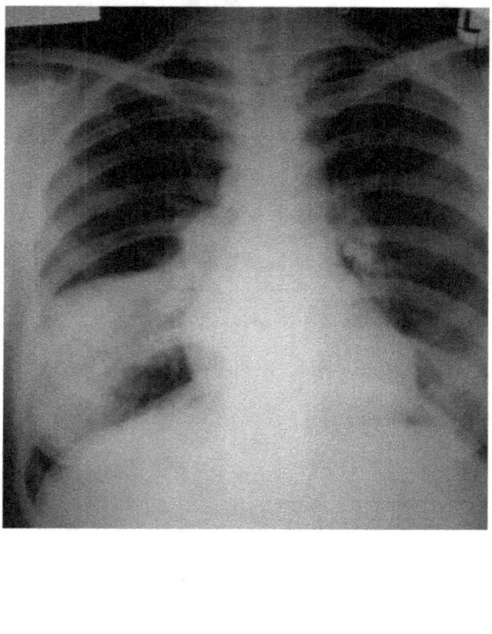

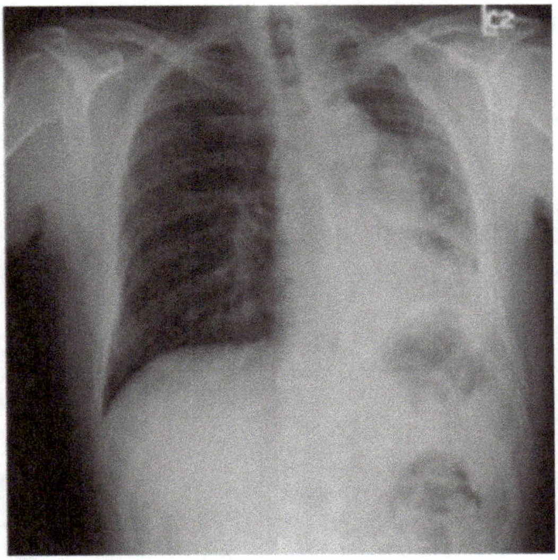

It may be used to control bleeding, to remove an FB or thick mucus to clear the blocking airways, to debulk or destroy the intraluminal growth in the airways, and to determine the degree and extent of airway obstruction for the placement of a stent. It can be therapeutically used to deliver laser treatment, radiation therapy (brachytherapy), or cautery (burning) of the

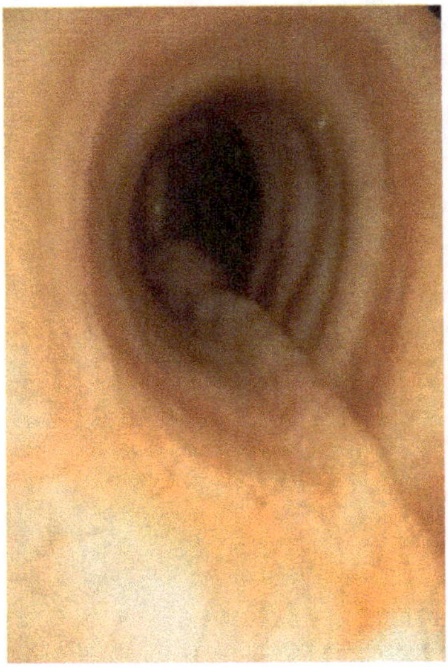

Figure 1: Trachea in expiration — normal anatomy.

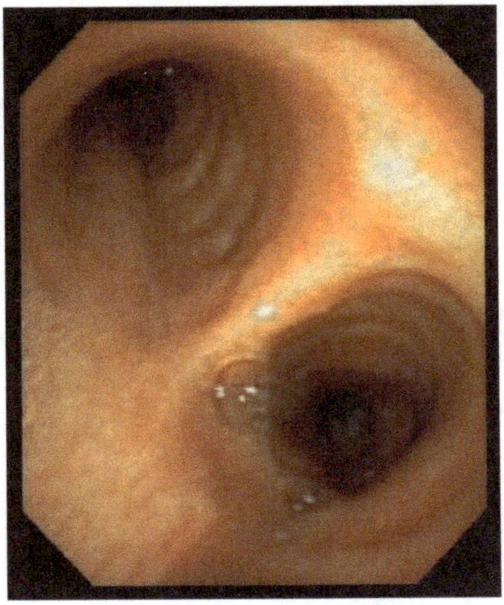

Figure 2: Carina — normal anatomy.

lesion in the airway. Various indications and therapeutic utility have been listed in Tables 1 and 2.

Normal bronchial anatomy (bronchoscopy images)

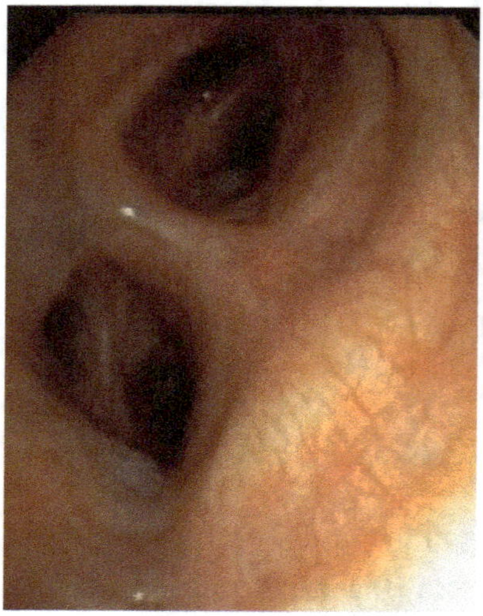

Figure 3: Right middle lobe bronchus (left) and right lower lobe bronchus (right).

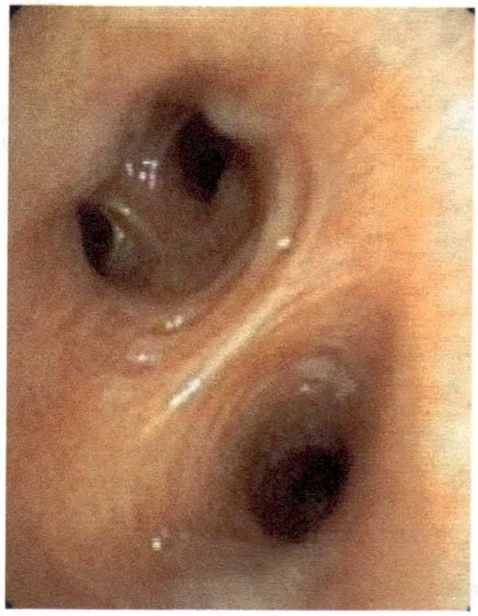

Figure 4: Right upper lobe bronchus and bronchus intermedius.

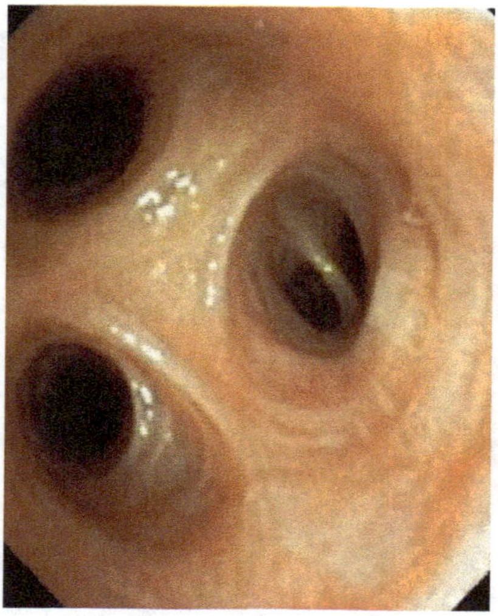

Figure 5: Right upper lobe bronchus with segmental bronchus to right apical, right anterior, and right posterior segments.

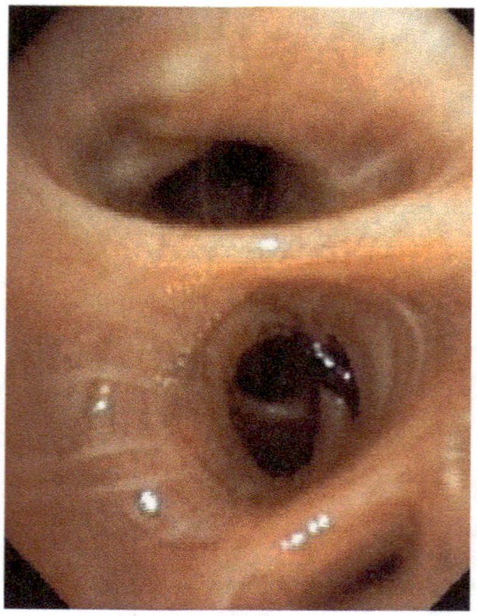

Figure 6: Blood clot in the lateral segment of the right lower lobe.

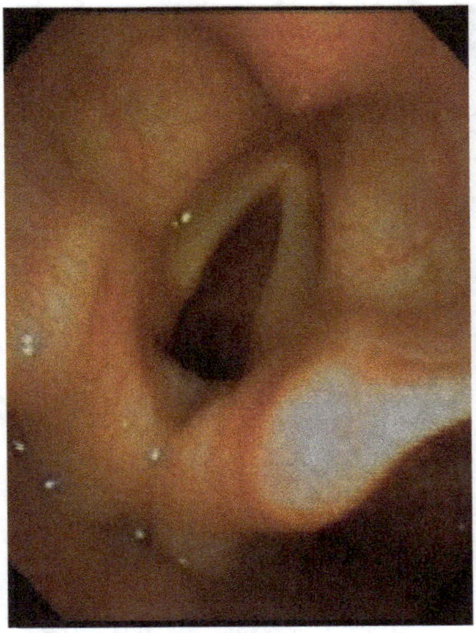

Figure 7: Vocal cords with cartilages.

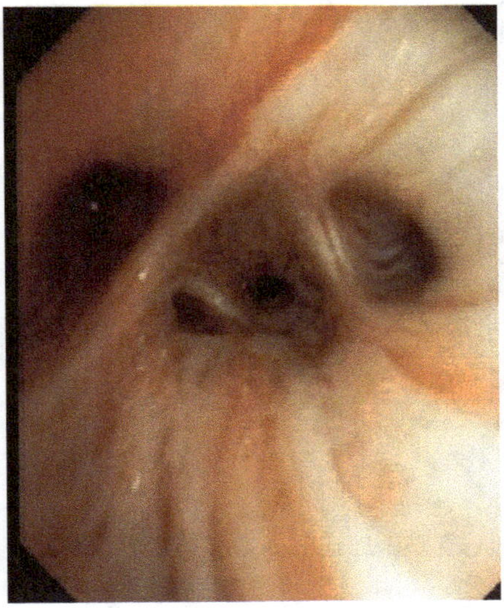

Figure 8: Partial narrowing of middle lobe subsegments and mucosal irregularity.

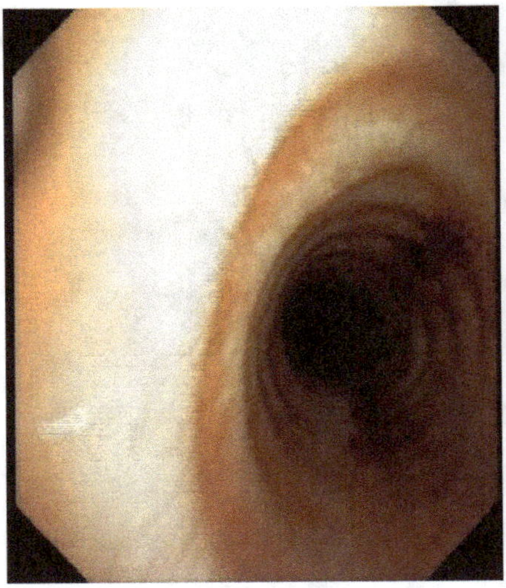

Figure 9: Submucosal hemorrhage — case of hemoptysis.

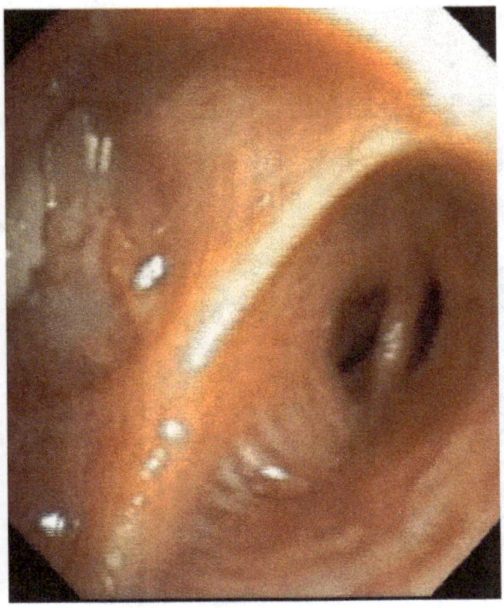

Figure 10: Growth in the right upper lobe posterior segmental bronchus with complete occlusion.

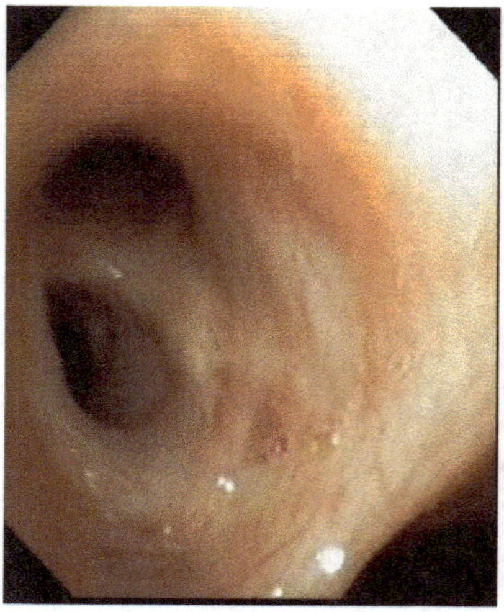

Figure 11: Lingular bronchus.

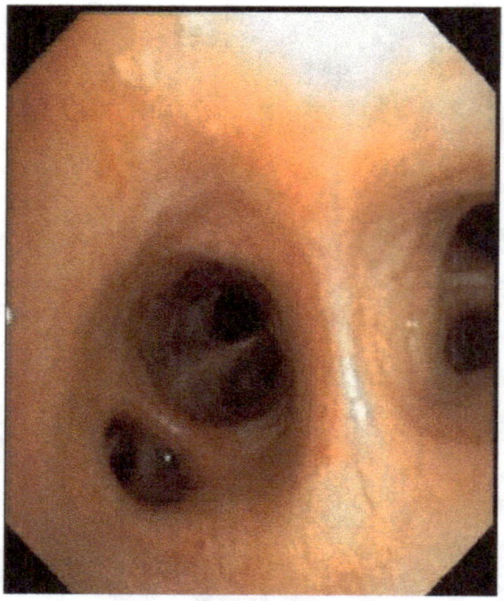

Figure 12: Right lower lobe (left) and middle lobe bronchus (right).

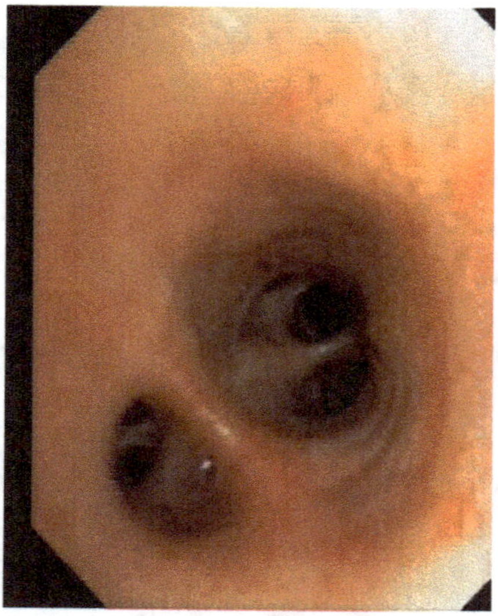

Figure 13: Right lower lobe.

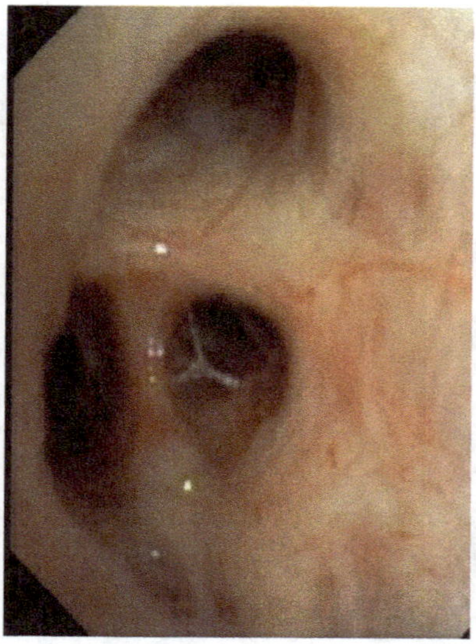

Figure 14: Right upper lobe bronchus.

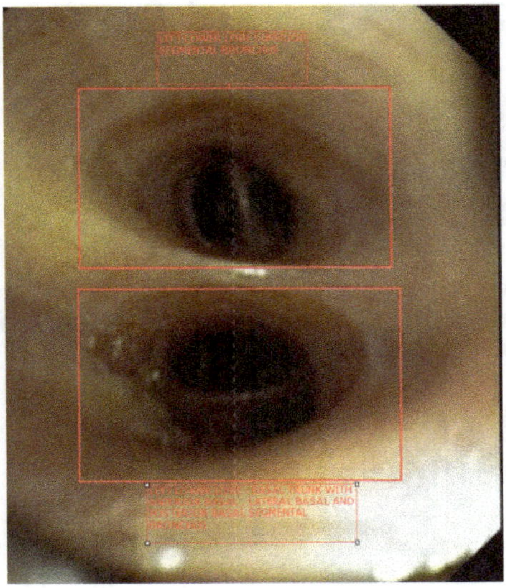

Figure 15: Left lower lobe bronchus with superior and basal segmental bronchus.

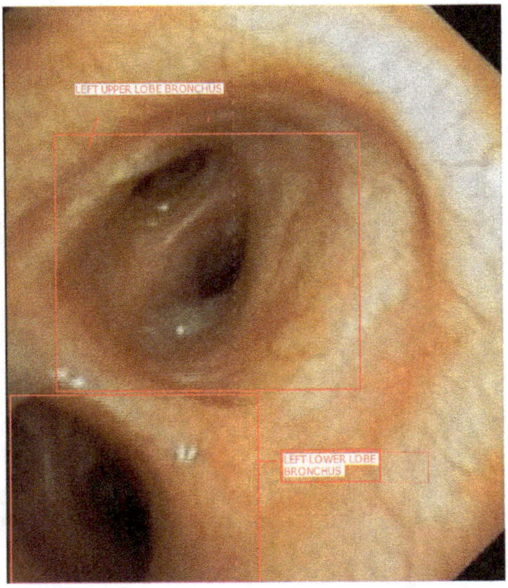

Figure 16: Left main bronchus — short bronchus showing division into upper and lower lobe bronchus (magnified view).

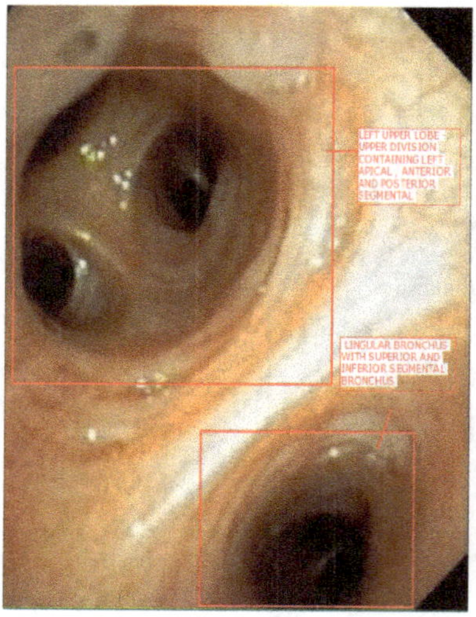

Figure 17: Left upper lobe — upper division with segmental bronchi.

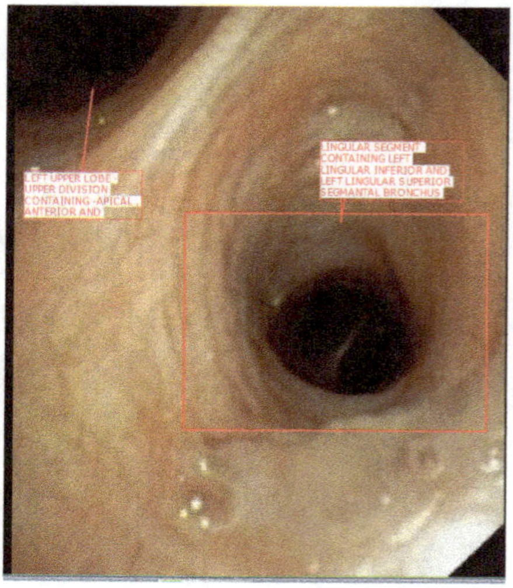

Figure 18: Left upper lobe with lingular bronchus.

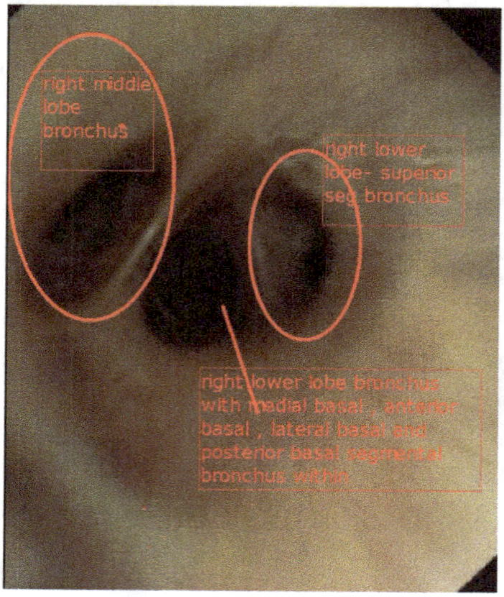

Figure 19: Bronchus intermedius.

Preparation of patient

Patients' preparation includes taking the history of any drug intake especially aspirin, history of diabetes, or bleeding diathesis, history of being pregnant (in females) and history of drug allergy to any medication including anesthetics. Patients are advised and thoroughly explained about the procedure. Routine investigations including chest X-ray are ordered, and a consent form is signed. An overnight fast is important and all accompaniments such as contact lenses, dentures, jewelry, and wigs are removed. Urinary bladder is emptied and the patient is given the hospital gown to wear. Premedication to help relax the patient and dry up the secretion of the mouth and respiratory tract is given.

Procedure

The patient lies on his or her back on the table; sometimes, the procedure is done in a sitting position. Dim light in the bronchoscopic suite allows to observe a better image on the video monitor. Intravenous sedative allows the patient to feel relaxed but awake during the procedure. A local spray of local anesthesia is made into the nose and mouth, which numbs the throat and reduces the tendency to gag during the bronchoscopic insertion. An anesthetic ointment is applied, and slowly the bronchoscope is inserted and advanced to near the vocal cord, where another spray of anesthesia is sprinkled and further advanced, with the help of the patient who is asked to make a high-pitch sound, to easily pass the scope through vocal cord. An X-ray machine (fluoroscope) is rightly placed above the patient to transmit the pictures to the video monitor. The bronchoscope is then slowly passed down to larger bronchi.

The air passages are viewed and secretion samples or tissue samples may be collected by inserting brush or tiny forceps through the scope. Figures 20–24 depict the normal trachea, carina, and the view at the entry to the right middle lobe, right upper lobe, and right lower lobe. Bronchoalveolar lavage (BAL) with a saline wash may be collected along with a tissue biopsy to be sent to the laboratory for analysis. In case a transbronchial lung biopsy is required, a small biopsy needle may be used to penetrate the lung through the bronchial tube to obtain the sample of the lung tissue from the appropriate site.

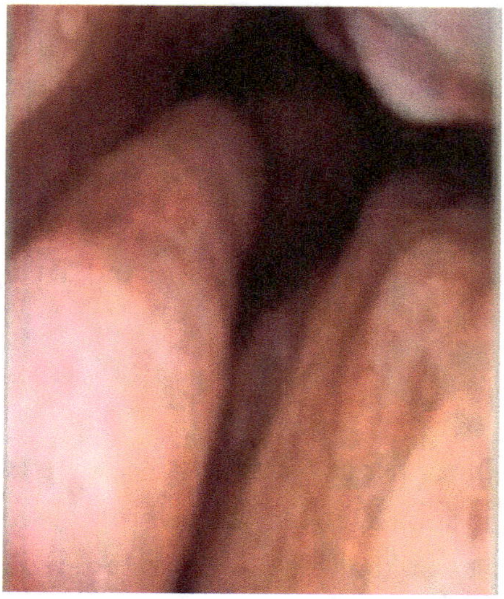

Figure 20: The upper airway.

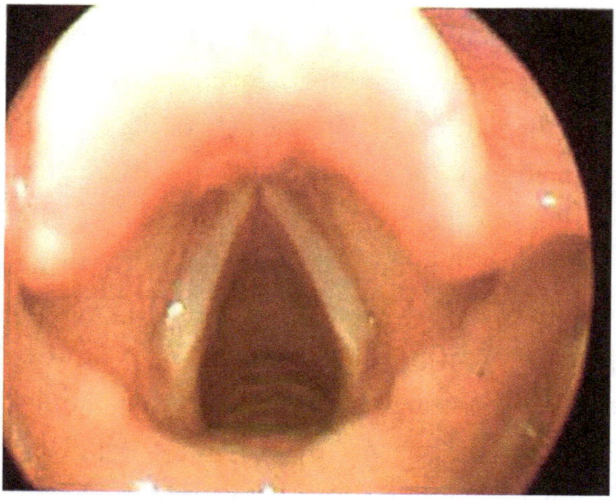

Figure 21: Laryngopharynx.

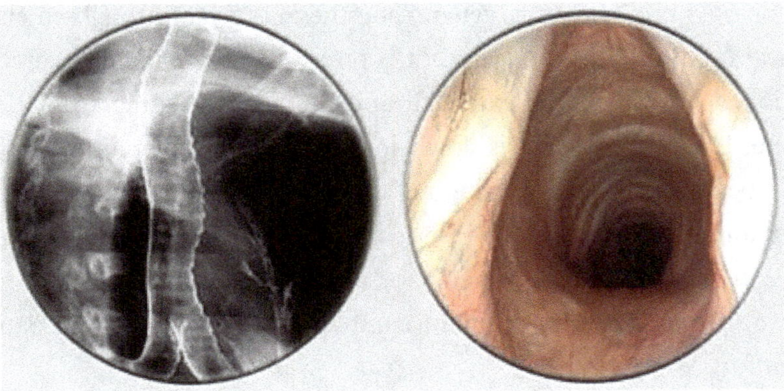

Figure 22: Trachea.

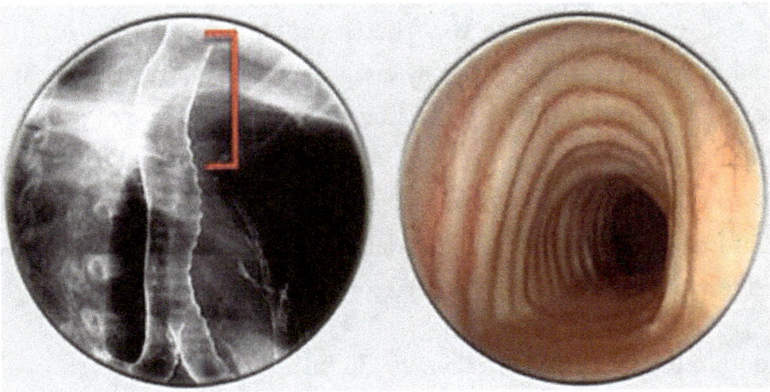

Figure 23: Cervical trachea.

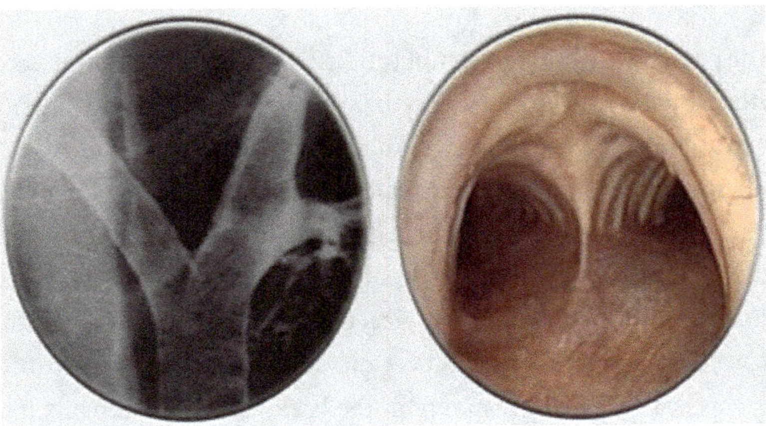

Figure 24: Carina.

For rigid bronchoscopy, general anesthesia is given through an endotracheal tube (ET). Muscle relaxant is given, and the patient is carefully positioned with the neck extended and on the ventilating machine to breathe. The bronchoscope is slowly inserted through the mouth into the windpipe by adjusting the position of the head as and when required. Tiny brush, forceps, or laser can be inserted through the scope. Usually, it may take ½ to 1 hour, but the time factor is not important; important is to achieve the target, with minimum complications and minimum patient discomfort.

Follow-up with the patient is important. Post procedure, nil orally is to be strictly observed for at least 2 hours. Spit-out salivary secretion is ordered to avoid choking. Avoid harsh coughing for several hours if a biopsy has been taken. Patient may cough and gag and complain of discomfort in the chest along with a feeling of tiredness. In case of use of local anesthesia, it may cause bitter taste, dryness of mouth, and difficulty in swallowing. Sore throat and hoarseness of voice may be observed. Blood of 10–20 mL in the sputum is noted. Patient is advised accordingly and always looked for (postprocedure), if there is any:

- Blood in the sputum more than 20–30 mL.
- Rise in temperature lasting more than 24 hours.
- Difficulty in breathing.

The procedure is safe but complications such as bronchospasm, cardiac arrhythmias, and infection may occur, and requires immediate attention. Complications following biopsy such as bleeding and infections including tuberculosis and pneumothorax have been reported. The inference of bronchoscopy removed can be normal or an FB can be shown, or sample of secretions or lung tissue biopsy has to be sent to the laboratory for culture for bacteriological and histological decisions. Nil orally till anesthetic effect waves off; a little water intake may cause choking. Return of gag reflex, checked by placing a spoon on the back part of the tongue, means anesthetic effect is gone.

The procedure as such is a three-hand procedure, where a failure can be faced in the form of difficulty in extending the neck or a nasal bridge fracture; a failure can be faced when the laboratory report is unable to convey a definite diagnosis because of inadequate sample; or a failure can also be faced when a diagnosis is missed since needle biopsy had been taken from an inappropriate area.

The physician pulmonologist has to face the horrible situation when he is unable to give a final diagnosis after bronchoscopy or a solution to the problem of the patient and the attempts to request for a repeat bronchoscopy. It is always better to enrich your skill with a battery of investigations with plain X-ray and computed tomography (CT) scan (must), using an electromagnetic navigator to guide to the area of biopsy, to take an adequate sample of lung biopsy, to practice several times on model sample before actually performing on the patient and to target to achieve the 100% success and 0% complication rate, using endotracheal ultrasound and virtual CT scan and leaving no chance to say or hear "inconclusive" at the end.

Lung biopsy through bronchoscope is a procedure that is indicated most often in diffuse infiltrative lung disease, tumors, rejection of transplanted lung, and in cases where open lung biopsy cannot be performed. It is always kept in mind that the bronchoscopy procedure must be performed with concentration on ensuring 100% outcome in an atmosphere conducive to patients' comfort and with negligible complications. The satisfaction and success that a bronchoscopist achieves and the relief and comfort provided to the patient do help in contributing life to extending the role of diagnosis and therapeutic bronchoscopy.

Pediatric bronchoscopy is indicated in stridor, persistent wheeze, chronic cough, atelectasis, and infection/pneumonia. It is used in airway management in the operating room, difficult intubation in the intensive care unit (ICU), routine inspection of the respiratory tract, and stent placement in selected patients.

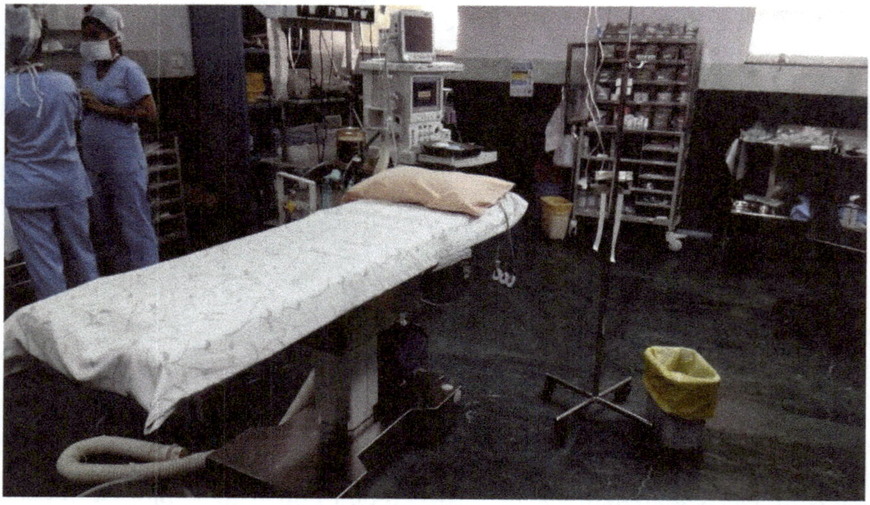

Figure 25: Operation table.

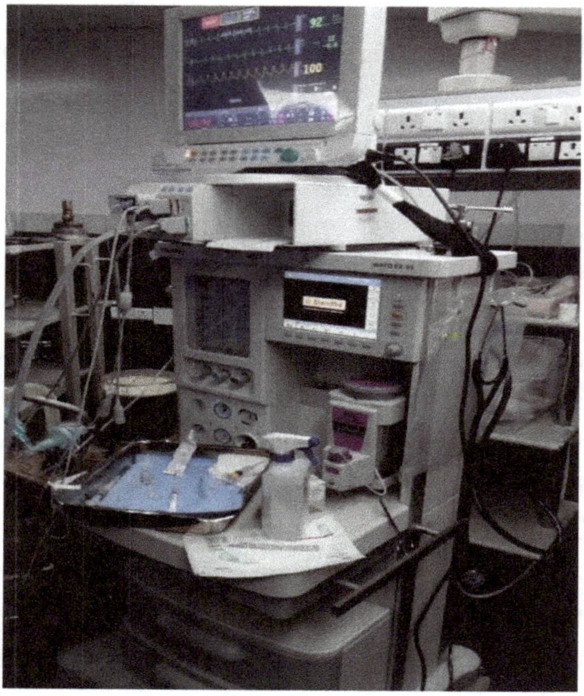

Figure 26: Cardiorespiratory monitors.

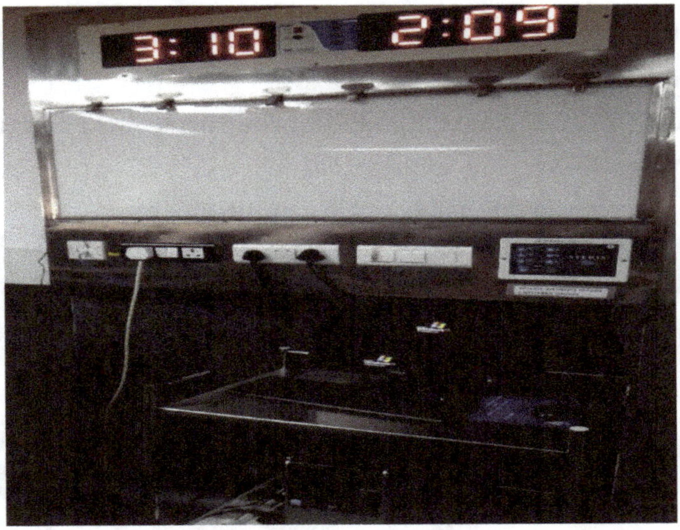

Figure 27: Radiographs display.

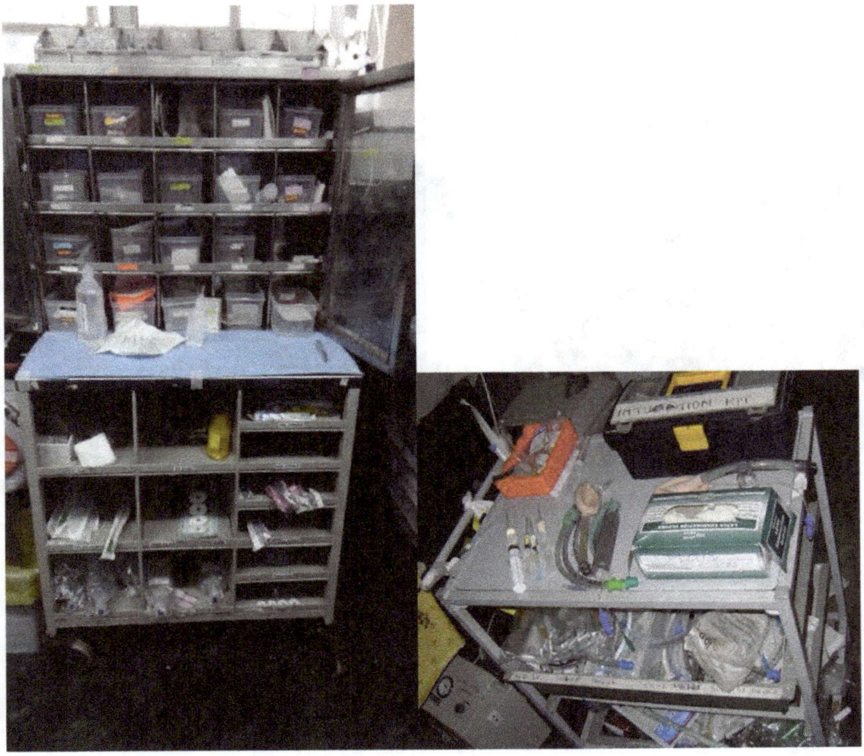

Figure 28: Full resuscitation facilities.

Specimen collection — bronchoscopy-extended indications

The specimens are obtained from the lung segment with a new infiltrate based on chest X-ray or the segment that on inspection has purulent secretion. In patients without radiographic densities, the right middle lobe or the lingula is to be chosen as the sampling area. Usually, a combination of specimens is required to increase the yield.

Some of the findings on abnormal bronchoscopic images are described in the following.

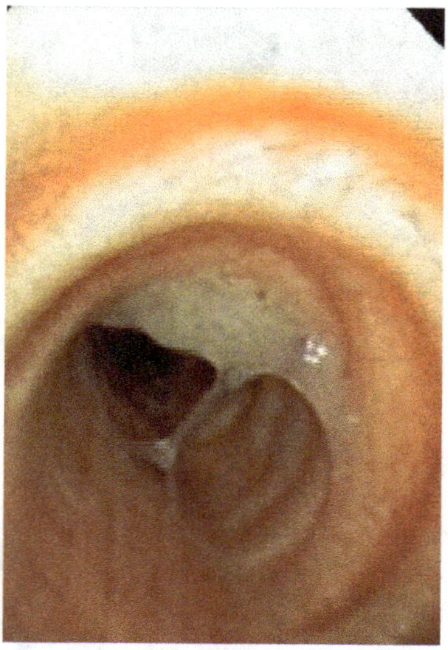

Figure 29: Thick secretions in the left main bronchus.

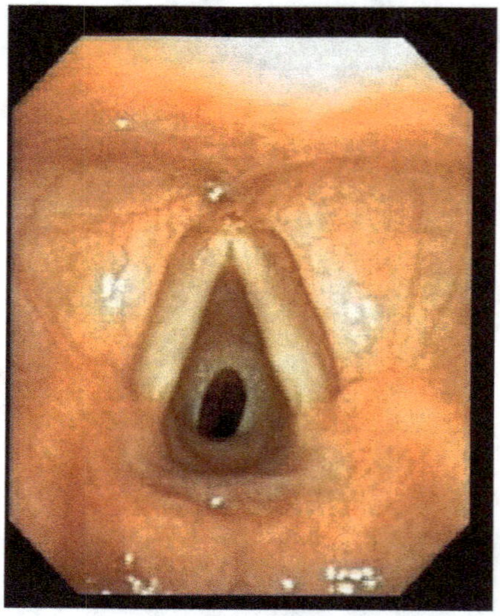

Figure 30: Membranous subglottic stenosis.

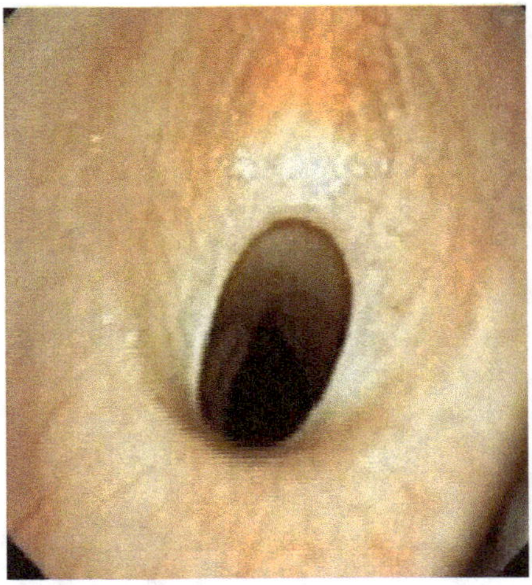

Figure 31: Magnified and closer view of membranous subglottic stenosis.

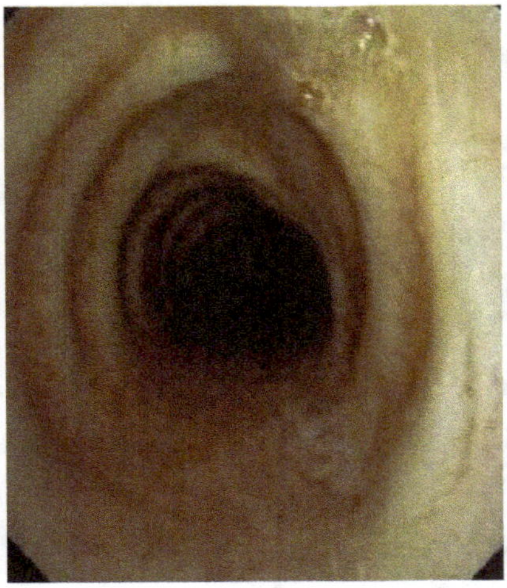

Figure 32: A case of hemoptysis with tracheal blood-tinged secretions — nocardiosis.

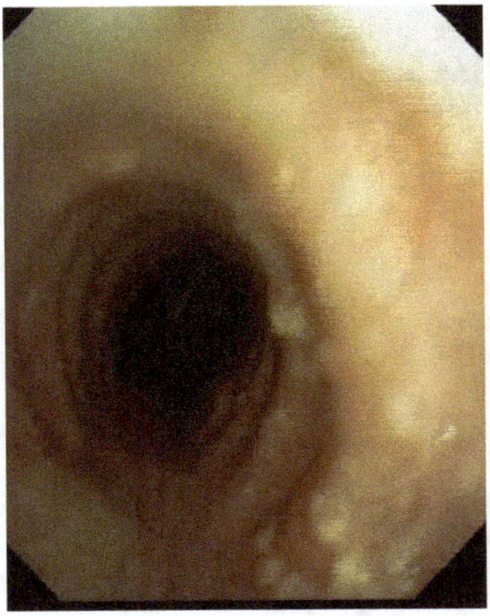

Figure 33: Mucosal nodular lesions — a case of bronchoalveolar lavage (BAL) proven with pulmonary tuberculosis.

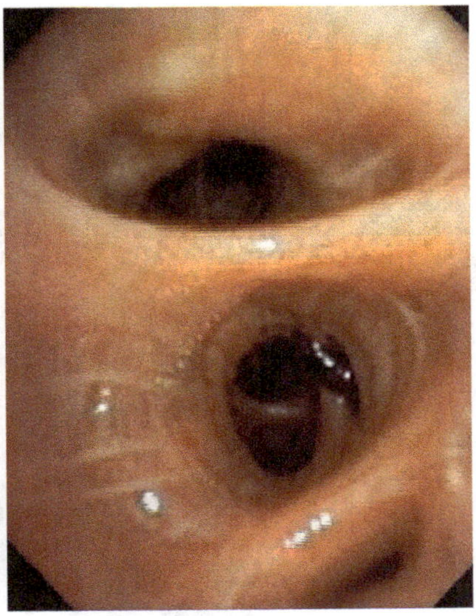

Figure 34: Blood clot in the lateral segment of the right lower lobe.

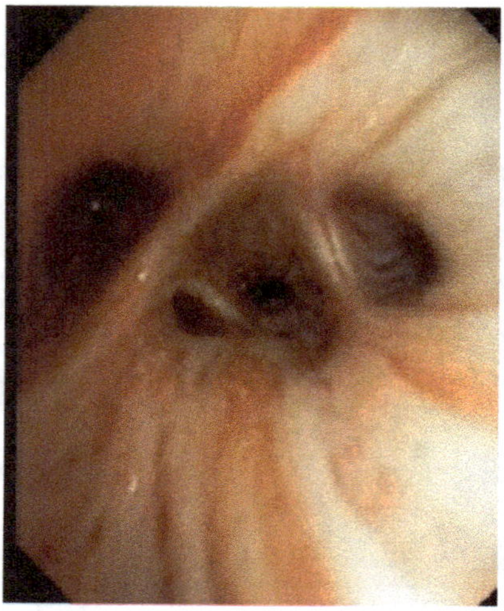

Figure 35: Partial narrowing of middle lobe subsegments and mucosal irregularity.

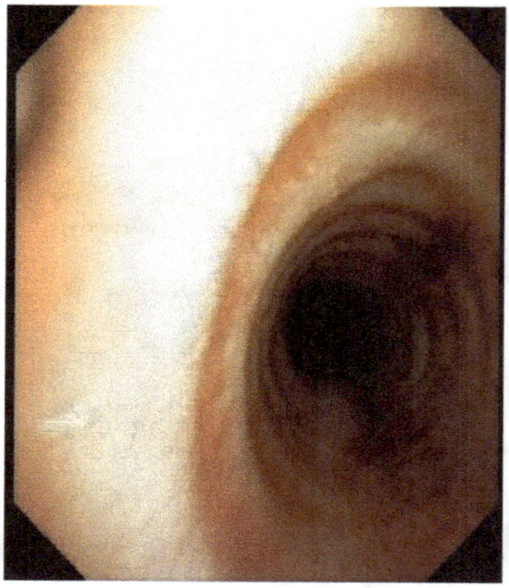

Figure 36: Submucosal hemorrhage — a case of hemoptysis.

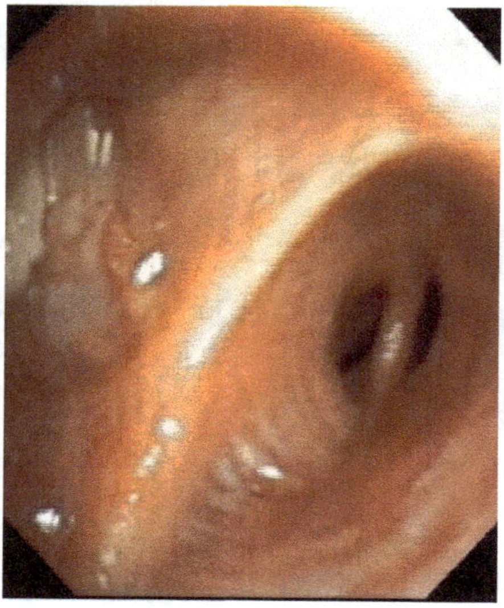

Figure 37: Growth in the right upper lobe posterior segmental bronchus with complete occlusion.

1. **Brush biopsy and protected specimen brushing:** Only those types of cytology brushes, which have a protective sheath, should be used. The ordinary single-sheathed brush is inadequate for taking specimens for bacteriological examination other than *Mycobacterium tuberculosis* because contamination by nasopharyngeal commensal organisms occurs too frequently. For optimal results, topical analgesia should be applied without injecting into the bronchoscopic channel, that is, aerosol or nebulized lignocaine may be preferred. No suction should be applied before taking specimens. After obtaining the specimen, smear should be prepared on a glass slide immediately to avoid drying and should be stained for various bacteria, fungi, and cytology (neoplastic cells, inclusion bodies). The brush can also be agitated in 1 mL of sterile Ringer's lactate solution, and this fluid is used for direct plating onto several media, for example, blood agar, Sabouraud agar (fungi). MacConkey's agar (intestinal organism), Lowenstein–Jensen medium (*M. tuberculosis*), slopes, and tissue cultures (for viruses).
2. **Bronchial washing:** Usually 5–10 mL of 0.9% saline is instilled with each wash and about 25%–50% of this can be aspirated into the trap. A yield of 5–10 mL of aspirate is usually sufficient. Culturing the trapped specimen of bacteria other than *Mycobacteria* is not helpful because contamination with nasopharyngeal secretions occurs in the majority of cases.
3. **BAL:** BAL should be performed in an affected segment preferably other than that from which selective culture and brush biopsy have been taken. Sterile buffer saline is infused in 50 mL aliquots to a cumulative amount of 200–300 mL. The fluid is aspirated with a low-pressure suction of 150–100 mm after each aliquot of fluid is inserted. They can be kept at room temperature instead of in ice if transported to the laboratory within an hour with no loss of viability in the cells or overgrowth from contaminating bacteria. BAL fluid is examined for total and differential cell count, protein estimation, enzyme estimation, cytological examination, and quantitative culture.

4. **Protected BAL:** For this, a protected transbronchoscopic balloon-tipped catheter should be used. It has two lumens, the larger one for irrigation and aspiration and the smaller one communicates with the latex balloon at the distal end of the catheter and allows optimal occlusion at the level of the third-generation bronchi. Protective specimen brushing and protected BAL are the effective ways for collecting uncontaminated specimens from lower airways with the specificity of 92% for protected specimen brushing and 97% for protected BAL.

Biopsy: Endobronchial biopsy is an effective way to obtain a specimen from directly visualized lesion and a histopathological diagnosis can be made immediately. When the lesion is in a segmental or subsegmental bronchus or distal to a bronchial stenosis, it can be biopsied with a curette. A clotting screen must be performed before it. Platelet count should be more than 1 lakh/microliter, and bleeding time, clotting time, prothrombin time, and prothrombin concentration should be normal. Ideally, transbronchial biopsy (**TBB**) should be performed with fluoroscopic control and should always be confined to one lung because of the risk of inducing bilateral pneumothorax. When the disease is unilateral, on X-ray, the segment with the highest density of shadowing is chosen for me site of biopsy with the bilateral extensive disease the lateral segment of the right lower lobe is selected. Usually, — four to six specimens are taken. Specimen obtained should be fixed in a 10% formaline solution, and it should be 2 mm in diameter and float in the fixative indicating that they include alveolar tissue. Occasionally consolidated lung will sink. A chest X-ray should be done routinely after TBB to rule out pneumothorax. In diagnosing infectious agents, bronchoscopy protected brush specimen should be taken before protected BAL. Finally biopsy specimen should be obtained if indicated. P carinii pneumonia in particular is amenable to diagnosis by this investigation, and other opportunistic infections with Cryptococcus, Aspergillus, Phycomycetes, Candida, Histoplasma, Coccidioides, Blastomyces, Penicillium, Nocardia, viruses, mycobacteria, protozoa, and helminths have all been identified.

Transbronchial needle aspiration can also be done to sample mediastinal lymph nodes in tuberculosis and fungal diseases.

Bronchoscope — cleansing, sterilization, and precautions

The standard of cleanliness used for FOB has changed with time.

It is very essential to follow strict cleansing. Sterilization and universal precaution prevent cross infection to other patients and healthcare personnels.

1. Cleansing: It should be done using a detergent antiseptic solution, clean water, and 50%–70% alcohol as usual.
   A. Sterilization: All bronchoscopes, biopsy forceps, and other instruments should be totally immersible and following routine cleansing, they should be sterilized by 30-min immersion in 2% glutaraldehyde. A syringe is used to suck the solution into the aspirating channel and is left attached to ensure continued contact with the solution during the period of immersion. The instrument subsequently must be washed and irrigated in sterile water before use.
   B. Precaution during procedure: All patients must be assumed to be potential infectious cases and hence the following precautions must be taken routinely in all bronchoscopies to limit possible infection to staff and subsequent patients.

1. The bronchoscopist and assistant should wear disposable or washable gowns, disposable gloves, and eye protection in the form of close-fitting spectacles or goggles. Operator must wear a surgical mask to prevent contamination by droplet infection.
2. All detritus collected during bronchoscopy should be disposed of properly considering potential infection.
3. All contaminated surfaces should be cleaned with a 10% solution of household bleach (sodium hypochlorite).
4. Specimens obtained at bronchoscopy should be packed carefully and labeled. Thigh risk of Adequate care should be taken if a procedure is done in immunocompromised host.

5. Lignocaine should not be injected into the area, which is to be sampled as it may inhibit the growth of some bacteria but probably not *M. tuberculosis.*
6. It is optimal to use the totally immersible newer generation instruments for proper sterilization.

Bronchoscopy is the visual examination of the airways. Since its first reported use in children 30 years ago. In the years since, the technique has improved and continued to develop. In addition to direct visualization of the upper and lower airways, bronchoscopes also provide an effective means to obtain specimens from the lungs and airways. Tissue samples may be obtained by biopsy forceps, secretion may be aspirated from the airways, and BAL yields samples of the fluid resident on the surfaces of the alveoli and distal airways. Recent advances in endoscopic technique and instrumentation have greatly enhanced the improvement in diagnosis and treatment. While most bronchoscopic procedures are performed for diagnostic purposes, bronchoscopes are also useful for certain therapeutic maneuvers. Extraction of foreign bodies from the airways, removal of masses or other forms of airway obstruction such as mucus plugs, and therapeutic BAL are primary examples.

Bronchoscopy may be performed with either rigid or flexible FOBs, depending on the particular needs of the patient and the skills and instrumentation of the bronchoscopist. The most important step in pediatric bronchoscopy is to decide what outcome needs to be procured during the procedure. This will determine what type of bronchoscope is used and how the child should be sedated and anesthetized. However, there are some specific situations in which an FOB instrument has special advantages. These include examination of lower airways in a patient who is intubated with an ET or tracheostomy tube (TT) and a patient in whom there is an unstable cervical fracture or mandibular hypoplasia. A flexible bronchoscope has a much smaller diameter than a rigid instrument and can be passed further into the distal airways. Because it is flexible it can be passed further and also reach the upper lobes more easily than a rigid bronchoscope.

Rigid bronchoscope is preferred for the extraction of tracheal or bronchial foreign bodies, evaluation of patients with suspected H-type tracheaesophageal fistula, laryngoesophagus, and bilateral abductor paralysis of vocal cords. It provides a better view of the posterior aspect of the larynx and trachea as compared to flexible instrument, giving a better view of the anterior part of the larynx and upper trachea. It allows the patient to breathe through its lumen (either spontaneously or by positive pressure), and the flexible bronchoscopes force the patient to breathe around the instrument, thus former method affords better control of the airways as compared to the latter. Flexible bronchoscopes have very small operating channels, and thus have limited ability to accommodate instruments through them. Flexible bronchoscopy as compared to rigid does not require general anesthesia and can be done under local anesthesia with or without sedation. Overall, rigid and flexible bronchoscopies complement each other rather than compete.

Advances in instrumentation allow FOB to be safely performed in even very small, sick infants, provided proper precautions are taken but inexperienced bronchoscopist can readily get into trouble.

FOB in pediatric population

Diagnostic indications	Therapeutic/procedural indications
Early or persistent stridor Persistent wheezing • Atelectasis • Localized hyperinflation • Compression of the trachea of major bronchi Recurrent and persistent pneumonia Pneumonia in the immunocompromised host Suspected case of FB aspiration Hemoptysis Vocal cord paralysis Tracheostomy evaluation	Removal of mucus plug Removal of FB Resection of upper from endobronchial lesions Therapeutic lavage Difficult or complicated intubation Removal of bronchial cast

Diagnostic indications

(a) Stridor: Ideally, the patient should be examined during a time when the stridor is audible, and the vibrating structures, for example, in nasopharynx, larynx, or trachea that cause stridor will then be visible. Flexible laryngobronchoscopy is a better method because it permits visualization of the laryngeal apparatus while the patient is breathing spontaneously without any loss of muscle tone due to deep sedation or anesthesia. It should be performed in any child with severe or persistent symptoms, if associated with hoarseness of voice or if it leads to hypoxia or apnea. Similarly, any infant who has stridor from a very early age, before 4 weeks of age, needs evaluation as the causes other than laryngomalacia are present early.

(b) Localized hyperinflation: This may occur due to localized partial obstruction due to mucous plug, FB aspiration, extrinsic bronchial compression, severe localized bronchomalacia, or intrinsic airway masses. Mucous plug in the main or segmental bronchi can cause air trapping or collapse depending on the type of obstruction.

(c) Atelectasis: Patients with persistent atelectasis, or in whom the atelectasis is massive or of functional consequence, may benefit from bronchoscopy. Unsuspected FB aspiration, anatomic abnormalities, mucous plug, and other causes of atelectasis are commonly found. Valuable information was obtained from the microscopic and microbiologic evaluation of BAL specimens.

(d) Persistent wheezing: Often the persisting wheezers who do not respond to bronchodilator and anti-inflammatory therapy may have an organic obstruction. FOB is useful in such cases.

(e) Compression of the trachea or major bronchi: It can be confirmed by endoscopy and will help to define the functional consequences of the compression. Common causes of airway compression include vascular structures (e.g., vascular rings), enlarged lymph nodes, tumors, and congenital abnormalities such as bronchogenic cysts.

(f) Recurrent and persistent pneumonia: Recurrent pneumonia is a productive indication for diagnostic bronchoscopy. In addition to visual inspection of the airways, GAL may give definitive information with which to guide therapy. The absence of any findings on bronchoscopy is equally important as it conclusively excludes surgical causes like anatomic lesions or occult FBs.

(g) Pneumonia in the immunocompromised host: Immunocompromised host can get pneumonia due to the usual as well as the unusual organisms. Isolating the organisms from the GAL may be useful.

(h) Suspected case of FR aspiration: All patients presenting with a history of choking and respiratory symptoms should undergo diagnostic bronchoscopy. The yield of bronchoscopy is very high. Most centers prefer rigid bronchoscopy as the FB can be removed after confirmation in the same sitting. The flexible instrument is preferred for the initial evaluation. If the evidence of FB aspiration or equal.

Therapeutic indications

They include primarily the restoration of airway potency. Even though the rigid bronchoscope has been preferred due to its ability for better airway control, yet considerable therapeutic benefits can be achieved with a flexible instrument as well.

The surgeons primarily operate with the rigid bronchoscope, whereas the pediatricians or chest physicians primarily operate with the flexible bronchoscope.

(a) Removal of the FB: Although flexible bronchoscopy has been found useful for FB removal in adults and adolescents, open tube extraction remains the procedure of choice in children with a definite history of FB aspiration.

If rigid bronchoscopy did not reveal an FB but there was still a high suspicion of its presence, flexible endoscopy could be performed to locate an FB in distal airways.

If there is a definite history of FB inhalation in a child with a choking episode or when he presents with asphyxial features, he should be taken up straight for rigid therapeutic bronchoscopy. However, if history is not forthcoming or when other methods have yielded equivocal results, then doing a diagnostic FOB can be rewarding. FOB for all cases with FB aspiration, a very high success rate can only be achieved in expert hands.

(b) Mass lesions: Most common causes of mass lesions in pediatric airways are granulation tissue due to tuberculosis or as a reaction to FB. Less common tumor masses may be found.

(c) Mucous plug: Most mucous plugs or blood clots in airways can be removed by suction through a flexible bronchoscope. Local lavage with saline or a mucolytic agent can also be helpful to dislodge a mucous plug.

The future is likely to increase the intervention potential as stents for the narrowed airways, lasers, and other instruments appropriate for use with pediatric flexible bronchoscope become available.

Another aspect of bronchoscopy is the information provided by the BAL. It provides useful information regarding the offending organism or type of inflammation

Pediatric bronchoscopy

When all aspects of the study such as observation, cytology, and bacteriology are considered, the overall incidence of a clinically meaningful bronchoscopy was 90.5% of all bronchoscopies. The yield from the inspection was low in recurrent pneumonia and immunocompromised groups, but can be improved by adding BAL and microbiological studies.

Relative contraindications (some of which may in themselves be indications) include massive hemoptysis, severe airway obstruction, severe hypoxemia, and severe bronchospasm needing diathesis. All these conditions require additional care with sedation and anesthesia instrumentation, airway management, preparation of the patient, and monitoring before, during, and after the procedure. None, however, is an absolute contraindication to bronchoscopy if the potential benefit of the procedure exceeds the potential risks.

Complications of pediatric FOB

The complications of bronchoscopy depend on the technique and instruments used. The underlying risks for the patient include the skill, experience, and diligence of the bronchoscopy team, and of course, luck. Most of the life-threatening adverse events involve drug overdose, inadequate monitoring, or inappropriate sedation. Upper airway pathology, persistent radiographic change, % oxygen dependency, and a weight <10 kg are major risk factors associated with adverse events. The commonest problems encountered are transient hypoxia, minor bleeds, and postprocedural pyrexia. In skilled hands. the procedure is quite safe and useful.

Transbronchial needle aspiration

Introduction

Transbronchial needle aspiration (TBNA) is mainly used as a diagnostic procedure to take samples from peribronchial or submucosal lesions,[1] using a needle attached to a catheter which is introduced through a rigid or flexible bronchoscope. It is a safe, efficacious, and cost-effective method to diagnose and stage lung cancer as well as to diagnose granulomatous lesions such as sarcoidosis and tuberculous lymphadenitis. The method has not gained its popularity with as much pace as it could have been since its introduction six decades back; the higher cost and slower pace in imparting training might have played some role. More than 50% of TBNAs are performed in the United States, the real cause of its being underused more so in Asia lies in cost factor, undertraining, lack of experience, poor safety profile, and concerns expressed about poor diagnostic yields.[2,3]

Diagnostic indications

A. Main diagnostic indications of TBNA
   1. Diagnosis and staging of lung cancer
   2. Identifying inoperable cancers
   3. Diagnosis of peripheral nodule and mass

B. Relative indications included diffuse infiltrative lung disease, tumors, rejection of transplanted lung, and severe illness that does not allow open lung biopsy.

The sensitivity, specificity, and accuracy of TBNA in lung cancer[4] are variable from 60% to 90%, 98% to 100%, 60% to 90%, respectively, depending on technique, method, patient selection, and mediastinal metastatic involvement. These indicators in comparison with granulomatous lung disorders[5–9] are shown in Table 1.

Diagnostic yield of TBNA can be as low as 0%–20% in the hands of experienced bronchoscopists with a complication rate of 0.26%.[10] It is always better to update theoretically, practice on lung models, review the CT scans before undertaking TBNA, and develop expertise with trained staff to work in a bronchoscopy suite. Important points during the procedure include placement of the needle at an angle of 45 degrees to the airways, ensuring the penetration of the needle up to the hub, supporting the TBNA catheter by channel of the scope, and stopping the aspiration before putting the needle into the airways. Two adequate specimen smears in alcohol and two samples along with all flush solutions are to be sent to cytopathologists. Following these guidelines has improved the diagnostic yield from 21% to 48% and from 33% to 81%. Rapid on-site evaluation

Table 1: Comparison of TBNA utility

Disorder	Sensitivity	Specificity	Accuracy
Lung cancer	60%–90%	98%–100%	60%–90%
Sarcoidosis	53%–66%	100%	54%–65%
Tuberculosis	45%–83%	100%	50%–85%

Table 2: Abnormal yield of TBNA

1. Bronchial or endobronchial tumors
2. Infections
   - — Aspergillosis
   - — Coccidioidomycosis
   - — Actinomycosis
   - — Tuberculosis
   - — Cytomegalovirus
   - — PCP
   - — Anaerobic bacterial infection
3. Hypersensitivity pneumonitis
4. Rheumatoid lung disease
5. Systemic vasculitis
6. Alveolar proteinosis
7. Granulomas
   a. Non-necrotizing granulomatous inflammation
   b. Necrotizing granuloma
   c. Caseating granuloma
   d. Sarcoidisis
   e. Peribronchial granuloma

improves lamostic accuracy[11] and obviates the need for invasive and costly investigations. Abnormal yield of TBNA has been given in Table 2.

To improve diagnostic yield by TBNA, various adjuvants have been used as shown in Table 3.

Risks and complications of bronchoscopy have been listed in Table 4.

Local anesthesia is sprayed topically before flexible bronchoscopy is done. This will initiate coughing but this will settle as the anesthesia begins to work. A feeling of thickness conveys sufficient numbness. If there is cough during the procedure, it means more anesthesia is required. Premedication with a sedative does help in allowing relaxation during the procedure.

Conventional fluoroscopy is being used to guide TBNA in peripheral pulmonary lesions of more than 2 cm diameter.[12] CT is used to pinpoint

Table 3: Adjuvant methods of TBNA (to improve diagnosis yield)

1. Fluoroscopy
2. CT/CT fluoroscopy
3. Virtual bronchoscopy
4. Tip position technology
5. Endobronchial ultrasound (EBUS)
6. Position emission tomography (PET)
7. Combined PET and CT
8. Electromagnetic navigation

Table 4: Risks and complications'

Major:

- Pneumothorax
- Hemorrhage
  - Radiation exposure

Minor:

- Cardiac arrhythmias
- Cardiac ischemia
- Hypoxemia

In case of general anesthesia:

- Nausea/vomiting
- Sore throat
- Difficulty breathing
- Muscle pains
- Bradycardia
- Altered blood pressure
- Kidney damage
- Choking (If water is ingested by mistake before anesthesia, *effect* goes off.)

puncture sites with a sensitivity of not more than 57% and specificity of not more than 74% as it has limitations in lesions that lack good contrast with surrounding tissues.[13] Sensitivity TBNA can be improved by 83%–87% by using a spiral CT scanner (CT fluoroscopy), but it requires more time and thus excessive unnecessary radiation exposure occurs both to the patient and the assisting staff.[14] Virtual bronchoscopy using spiral CT for TBNA has been used with success, but does not provide final needle placement to the point. Three-dimensional (3-D) data have been used in real-time bronchoscopy tip position technology for TBNA, especially in non-visible extrabronchial lesions.

Ultrasound used endobronchially has increased the yield of conventional TBNA from 58% to 76%–86% in mediastinal lymph node lesions.[15] The EBUS guided transbronchial yield of 85% and transesophageal yield of 78%, and if combined, provide results, comparable to mediastinoscopy results of 94% in mediastinal staging of lung cancer.[16,17] Similarly, a diagnostic yield of 82% by EBUS-guided TBNA has been recorded in stage I and II sarcoidosis.[18]

A metabolic imaging technique based on the biological activity of a neoplastic cell, thus using tissue function rather than its anatomy is PET, where PET camera identifies the neoplastic or inflammatory cells having increased cellular uptake of glucose and higher rate of glycolysis. PET serves as a guide to TNBA in evaluating lymphadenopathy in lung cancer as it has higher accuracy and sensitivity than TBNA alone (88% compared to 67%) in differentiating benign and malignant mediastinal lymphadenopathy.[19] Combined EBUS in PET gives 94% accuracy in mediastinal lesions with TBNA.[20] Integrated PET and CT can also provide successful results.[21]

Electromagnetic navigator using virtual bronchoscopy and 3-D CT images in combination with a steerable prove that peripheral lung lesions can be successfully sampled (69%–88%) by TBNA along with transbronchial lung biopsy, brushing, and curettage.[22,23] Initiated by Shieppati in 1949[24] as rigid TBNA and performed over flexible bronchoscope in 1983 by Wang and Terry present time TBNA — an invasive bronchoscopic technique, needs to be more utilized as a routine bronchoscopic procedure. Young bronchoscopists need to develop skills and expertise and strictly follow *guidelines. Cutting* down the cost of the needle for TBNA shall improve the diagnostic yield as well as optimally utilize this presently underused technique, especially in developing countries like India. This would broaden the spectrum of diagnostic bronchoscopy as well as bring forth newer diagnostic yields in respiratory medicine.

Bronchoalveolar lavage

Introduction

BAL today is a useful and safe method of sampling cellular and biochemical components from the lung. BAL performance and BAL fluid processing have recently been standardized from technical angles to improve diagnostic yield and diagnostic accuracy.

Technique

BAL technique involves the introduction of sterile saline into the lung through FOB to obtain secretions, cells, and proteins from the lower respiratory tract. This has been in used for many years in treating cystic fibrosis and severe asthma and to remove mucous plugging in patients not responding to other treatments. It remains the only effective treatment for alveolar proteinosis. Meticulous technique and expertise are essential for successful studies.

Indication

BAL can be used to confirm asbestos exposure identification of reactivated tuberculosis and cytological diagnosis of tumors beyond the visual range of FOB. Diagnosis of centrally situated lung tumor is easy with FOB, but diagnostic accuracy in peripheral lung lesions which is poor with FOB has improved with BAL. A success rate of 65% diagnosis has been obtained in an Indian study. CBAL cellular analysis may help in identifying interstitial lung disease. The normal range of BAL cytology is provided in the Table.

Raised lymphocytes in BAL fluid are found in sarcoidosis and extrinsic alveolitis.[1] An increase in mast cells in sarcoidosis could represent the initiation of fibrosis. Raised neutrophils, macrophages, and eosinophils are found in cryptogenic fibrosing alveolitis. Similar changes are seen in collagen vascular disorder. However, mast cells in extrinsic alveolitis and lymphocytes in cryptogenic fibrosing alveolitis have also been reported. The alteration in cell count may provide a clue to the activity of the disease in sarcoidosis and may guide the treatment in cryptogenic fibrosing alveolitis. The lymphocytosis seen in some early cases of idiopathic pulmonary fibrosis may represent a subgroup that improves with steroids.

Table 5: Cellular components of BAL fluid in normal

Total cell count	$10–15 \times 10^6$/dL
Macrophages	84 ± 1%
Lymphocytes	11 ± 1%
T cells	62 ± 2%
Helper T (CD4) cells	46 ± 3%
Suppressor T (CD8) cells	25 ± 2%

Table 6: Indications for BAL

Diagnostic indications
— Pulmonary infections
— Pulmonary malignancy
— ARF
— Diffuse pulmonary disease
— Occupational lung disease
— Monitoring lung allograft
— Following transplantation
Therapeutic
Total lung lavage for pulmonary alveolar proteinosis

Table 7: Useful evaluation clues of BAL

A. Polymorphs — bacterial infections
B. Lymphocytes — tuberculosis, sarcoidosis, radiation pneumonitis
C. Eosinophils — eosinophilia, pneumonia, fungi, drugs, PCP, systemic vasculitis
D. Hemosiderin-laden macrophages — alveolar hemorrhage

It can be used to understand the pathogenesis of diseases like drug hypersensitivity, emphysema, occupational diseases, adult respiratory distress syndrome, and bronchial asthma. Carrying out BAL in various stages of the disease/disorder could illustrate the varying cytological and biochemical responses found in these disorders with time. BAL technique has also been used with good tolerability in establishing the diagnosis of pneumocystis carinii and cytomegalovirus, legionella pneumonia, fungi, and mycobacterial lung infections. Sputum induction with nebulized saline may be used to replace BAL in a small number of patients. In patients with human immunodeficiency syndrome infections, BAL is a much preferred investigative tool over invasive procedures like transthoracic needle biopsy and exploratory thoracotomy.

Table 8: Utility of BAL as a diagnostic tool

1. Agents which causes Infectious diseases
Pneumocystis carinii
Legionella pneumonia
Mycobacterium tuberculosis
Hemophilus influenza
Mycoplasma pneumonia
Histoplasma capsulatum
Toxoplasma gondii
Strongyloides stercoralis
Respiratory syncytial virus
2. Non-infectious diseases
Alveolar proteinosis
Histiocytosis X
Pulmonary malignancies
Possibly helpful
Pulmonary hemorrhages
Eosinophilic lung disease
Asbestosis
Hypersensitivity pneumonitis
Idiopathic pulmonary fibrosis
Sarcoidosis

Adverse effects

Minor side effects after the procedure include fever, chills, and transient alveolar opacities seen radiologically. More serious complications include delayed recovery from the procedure, nosocomial infection (including mycobacteriosis), and pulmonary hemorrhage. Following guidelines improves yield and cuts down complications.

The removal of tenacious mucous plugs in severe unremitting asthma and exacerbations of severe infection in cystic fibrosis may be life-saving, but lavage risks in silicosis and alveolar microlithiasis have not been a proven success. As of now, BAL remained an investigative technique and a research tool. It has attained the status of an important diagnostic tool over these years.

Bronchoscopic removal of FB in airways: procedure and precautions

The technique of bronchoscopically removing an airway FB is a state of the art, best conducted successfully by an adept bronchoscopist, who has excellent support of an experienced and a trained team around. For excellent results, selection of the patient for appropriate indication is of utmost importance that yields successful outcomes with minimum complications. The procedure to success depends on the preparation of the patient for the procedure, the assistance of a trained technician to insert and manipulate the grasping instruments, with the bronchoscopist's primary concern to maneuver the bronchoscope to the target position to achieve. Even *the* expert bronchoscopist must have multiple practice sessions in the lung model prior to the actual performance to realize using the appropriate instrument if and when required, depending on the radiology film, and identifying the desired position. Thus, all the baskets and grasping instruments are needed to be actually tested before putting to use in the bronchoscopic procedure.

The infrastructure and the assisting team are assigned specific work for each member for the uneventful procedure. A team member looks after sedation and monitors the vital signs, while a bronchoscopic assistant who is adept in the removal of an instrument helps the bronchoscopist in doing so during the procedure. The backup support of anesthesiologist and thoracic surgeon should always be ready to meet any untoward complications during the procedure. These precautions are always rewarding when an unwanted complication is faced unexpectedly.

The running time is not always short in the case of a non-asphyxiating FB in an adult but the caring time and commitment of the attending bronchoscopist are always rewarding. The presence of erythema, edema, infection, and granulation is always faced as long as the FB remains in the airway, and usually, an inflammatory reaction develops within 24 hours of FB aspiration in most cases. And if acute respiratory distress is not warranting, a well-planned procedure can be undertaken, where rushing for the procedure has no value and is replaced with a commitment to remove the FB, after properly studying the place, shape, size, and structure of FB, in relation to the surrounding areas before a successful attempt is made. Radiological view during the procedure is very essential. Early management helps in reducing both morbidity and mortality. Presence of bleeding and granulation tissue often adds to the agony, and many workers do use a short course of corticosteroids before removing the FB.[1,2]

Rigid bronchoscope used to be the choice procedure in removing the FB in children; now flexible bronchoscopy is being safely and successfully used for extracting FB in children. Removal of an adult airway FB requires both skill and experience to minimize the complications. Success rate also depends on the skill and expertise of a bronchoscopist rather than the type of bronchoscope used, rigid or flexible. Successful performance of the bronchoscopist must allow to transfer know-how ability and prowess to the younger pulmonologists to the true spirit of pulmonary medicine, keeping high standards in the procedure and safety of the patient while imparting knowledge. The actual technique involved in removing FB using flexible bronchoscopy has an advantage over rigid one, being operational with local anesthesia, where the patient remains under conscious sedation, which permits preservation of cough reflex that actually itself assists in FB removal. However, airway is not secured during the flexible FOB procedure. But experience has shown that patients can tolerate bronchoscope under conscious sedation and may not necessarily require complete sedation and control over ventilation. In a *rare* instance, if respiratory distress occurs, easy securing of the airway can be achieved by placing an ET, through which FB can be extracted. In case deeper sedation is required, laryngeal mask airway can be used for reasonable airway control during flexible bronchoscopy.[6,7]

Most important precaution in removing FB from the airway is not to push it distally to the airways, "focally balloon" is quite useful to dislodge the FB and to help in bringing it proximally into the trachea before actually attempting its removal. Balloon then inflated helps in putting the FB from the bronchial subsegment to trachea. Once in the trachea, the use of a basket or forceps helps in removing the FB. For a small, soft, simple, and friable FB, some workers have encouraged the patient to sit and cough up once the FB comes in upper trachea and hence appreciated a highly successful yield. Regarding the removal of a FB from the airway, let this be made clearer that FB is never removed through the working channel of a bronchoscope. Once the FB is adequately captured by basket or forceps, and then the three (bronchoscope, grasping instrument, and FB) are removed simultaneously with a constant eye on the FB, which is always kept in the center of the airway. Always remove FB using oral approach of bronchoscopy, as there is always a chance of losing the FB in the nasal passages. In case of endotracheal intubation, the ET has to be withdrawn in conjunction with the bronchoscope with secured FB, followed by reintubation promptly. FB extraction using optical versus non-optical forceps offers no added advantage.[10]

Hemoptysis is a rare complication during FB removal from the airways and admittedly can be better controlled with a rigid bronchoscope.

But the fear of massive bleeding from the airways should not be the reason to prefer the use of rigid to flexible bronchoscope in removing FB from airways. Removal of a sharp FB is a definite challenge that requires special skill, art, and patience. The art lies in locating the sharp edge of the FB, and it is the free sharp end that is grabbed and then FB is removed. Holding the FB from another end will expectedly complicate, as the sharp end is likely to be caught in the mucosa.

In case of large FB or tissue-impacted FB, the laser may be used to break the FB or vaporize the granulation tissue, as is the case. This is followed by the same procedure with similar precautions, following all the set guidelines, and this actually holds the key to the successful removal of FB from the airway without or with minimum complications. Despite the variable and non-specific presentation of FB aspiration, the radiographic evaluation is often useful in clinching the diagnosis. Therapeutic flexible bronchoscopy has become the gold standard in recognizing and locating the FB in the airways. Safe and successful removal of an airway FB through bronchoscope under local anesthesia in recent years has seen pulmonary medicine excelling in the present era of medicine. Advanced bronchoscopy with aided improved imaging technology has helped in decreasing morbidity and mortality from non-asphyxiating FBs in the airways, although the incidence of FB aspiration has not decreased. Death rates have been stable for the last 5 years; the incidence of deaths due to bronchotracheal FBs has been 1.2 per 10,000 in the United States in 1998. A decline in FB aspiration episode after fifth year of age may find an ascendance again in the fourth decade of life; and most of these asphyxiating events occur at home (41%), in restaurants (29%), and in nursing homes or mental hospitals (14%).[11–13]

Non-asphyxiating events are, however, seen in children, and 75%–85% of events occur in children under 15 years of age. In adults, it is after the sixth decade of life that such an event is observed and that too possibly due to the factors such as alcohol intoxication, sedative drugs, loose dentition, senility, mental retardation, Parkinson's disease, seizure, trauma, or under the effect of general anesthesia.

Classical triad of cough, wheezing, and choking is present only in a few number of patients following FB aspiration. If a large asphyxiating object occludes larynx, an acute attack of cough, hoarseness, choking, and gagging is observed. Sometimes, even the patient is unable to speak and cyanosis develops. Heimlich maneuvers recommended for the expulsion of F13. But if the FB is aspirated beneath the cords into subglottic or tracheal area, bouts of cough with inspiratory stridor are noted. F8 if passes into either of the bronchus, minimal symptoms or unilateral or localized wheezing may be the only clinical finding. 10%–20% in laryngotracheal, 30%–40% in left bronchus, and 40%–70% in right bronchus, FB aspiration in the airway is reported. Unlike children, FB aspiration in adults is mostly non-asphyxiating. Site of impaction often determines the clinical symptomatology, which can be symptom free (1%) or with symptoms such as wheezing (1%), choking (3%), chest pain (4%), breathlessness (16%), fever (21%), hemoptysis (21%), or cough (81%). Non-specificity in symptoms often leads to misdiagnosis, and diagnosis is made even after — one or two decades of FB aspiration. In that situation, recurrent pneumonia, obstructive emphysema, bronchial stenosis, bronchiectasis, pneumothorax or pneumomediastinum, bronchopleural fistulae, chronic lung disease, recurrent hemoptysis, pleural effusion or empyema, and even osteomyelitis of rib are faced as delayed complications of FB aspiration.

A variety of FBs can be aspirated. These may be organic or inorganic substances. Dental crowns, pins, or coins are commonly seen. Endotracheal appliances, ET segment, or dental prostheses and drugs (pills)[14] are commonly seen in adults. Even hypodermic needles have been reported in drug addicts. Corns, seeds, beans, and chicken or fish bone are commonly seen in adults as compared to children where nuts, seeds, and pen appliances are mostly aspirated. As discussed, various objects with varying shapes and structure pose every time a new challenge to the bronchologist who has to individualize his or her approach each time, depending on the type of FB, peripheral tissue reaction, and area of impaction of FB in the airways.

Chest radiogram offers diagnosis in radiopaque FBs. Other radiological signs such as air trapping atelectasis, pulmonary infiltrates, and shift of mediastinum do pointer toward FB aspiration. CT scan, ultrasound scan, and fluoroscopy also help in certain cases. In the present times, flexible bronchoscopy remains the gold standard in identifying and localizing FB in the airway. Gustav Kilian in 1897 was the first to remove FB, using a rigid bronchoscope. The success rate increased gradually over a period of more than half a century to the tune of 99% and with the complication rate getting reduced to only 0.2% and the fatality rate being less than 0.1%. Flexible bronchoscopy by Shigeto IKeeda in 1968 revolutionized the care of pulmonary patients. Doubt was raised at the initial stage over its safety but with expertise and advancement, flexible bronchoscopy has not only achieved a performance status of almost 99% in the United States in the present times, where it was initiated only as a diagnostic tool, but also has become an accepted therapeutic procedure, giving 86%–100% results in removing airway FBs. Multiple accessories have been devised to be applied to use with the flexible bronchoscope, such as grasping forceps, balloon catheters, Dormia basket, fish-net basket, multipronged snares, magnet extractor, cryoprobe, and neodymium–yttrium–aluminum garnet (Nd:YAG laser).

The bronchoscopic removal of airway FB is a state of the art that requires observing all the necessary precautions and following the step-by-step guidelines to achieve higher success and minimize the rate of complications. These three-handed procedures require trained assistants and associates to achieve the best and that can only be achieved when the bronchoscopist preplans his operation and performs patiently while keeping his eagle eye on the target till last. In case of failure, surgical extraction may be sought, since the management of FB is a teamwork of pulmonologists, thoracic surgeons, and anesthetists, who always complement each other. It should never be taken lightly, as hypoxia may result and ultimately may prove fatal.

Table 9: Contraindications for bronchoscopic procedures

— Severe refractory hypoxemia
— Hemodynamic instability
— Uncontrolled coagulopathy
— Recent myocardial infarction
— Unstable angina

Therapeutic bronchoscopy

Bronchoscopy is an important diagnosis as well as a therapeutic tool in managing certain inflammatory, infectious, and malignant disorders of the respiratory system. Nearly half of bronchoscopies account for therapeutic procedures. Nearly 50%–75% of bronchoscopies are done to remove retained secretion, 12% for hemoptysis, and less for endotracheal intubations. Frequently, diagnostic and therapeutic bronchoscopies are performed simultaneously. Other therapeutic indications include:

1. Removal of mucous plug which is not being cleared by other non-invasive techniques.
2. Dilation of stricture or stenosis.
3. Debulking of endotracheal abnormal tissues to maintain airway lumen.
4. Draining an abscess or cyst.
5. For procedures such as brachytherapy, cryotherapy, electrocautery, and so on.
6. Closure of chronic bronchopleural fistula, using glue, coils, or mechanical device.

Hemoptysis

Bleeding can be stopped by endobronchial tamponade, fibrin precursor application, iced saline, and epinephrine. If bleeding is >200 mL/24 hours, rigid bronchoscopy is preferred to avoid dangerous and fatal complications such as asphyxiation, as a rigid bronchoscope can provide both a laser suction device as well as a balloon-tipped catheter to tamponade the bleed. n-Butyl-cyanoacrylate glue can also be injected, using a video bronchoscope. Apart from the topical vasoconstrictors or coagulants, cryotherapy or electrocautery can also be used for endobronchial embolization with a si icon spigot is helpful.

Foreign body removal

Rigid bronchoscope is ideal for the extraction of tracheobronchial FB, especially in children and in case the foreign body is a larger one. Flexible bronchoscopes with newer ancillary equipment such as wire basket, biopsy forceps, and retrieval forceps to grasp and remove larger FBs in the proximal airways are being successfully used. What is most important is to remove the FB along with the flexible bronchoscope, keeping the FB in the middle of the scope and keeping an eye on the FB, so that it is not lost while being extracted.

Tracheobronchial stents

Endobronchial stents are used when there is airway obstruction, often caused by malignant lesions. They help not only in relieving the obstruction of airways but also in preventing respiratory failure. Stents of different shapes and sizes are more useful in diseases affecting trachea or bronchi rather than airway diseases involving lobar or distal bronchi. Silicone stents are better suited for benign and malignant lesions of airways, whereas covered metallic stents are useful in malignant airway stenosis. Silicone stents are essentially placed, manipulated, and removed by using rigid bronchoscope, whereas metallic stents can be inserted by flexible bronchoscope or fluoroscopic guidance. Complications with silicone stents include migration of stent and inspissation of thick mucus within the stent lumen. Uncovered metallic stents should be never bought and replaced. Uncovered metallic stents should never be inserted in an airway with malignant lesions because cancerous growth through wire mesh negates the benefit of placement of the stent. Self-expandable metallic and alloys stents and hybrid stents are also being used. Ideal stent is yet to come. Biodegradable stents and those which can deliver chemotherapeutic and radioactive substances are being researched.

Dilatation of airway stenosis

Rigid bronchoscope when repeatedly passed using gradually increasing diameter bronchoscopes helps in dilatation of the trachea and main stem bronchus. Shorter stenosis can be dilated with balloon through flexible or rigid bronchoscope. The procedure is effective in stenosis of intrinsic origin rather than of extrinsic nature and has to be repeatedly done in most of the patients having chronic benign strictures. Short-length membranes or web-like lesions involving short lengths of airways are effectively dilated. Surgery or stent therapy is essential for transmural strictures and long-segment strictures of airways. Rigid bronchoscopy is also indicated in massive hemolysis, laser bronchoscopy, central airway obstruction, and stent placement and removal.

Laser therapy

It is performed using Nd:YAG laser, both for benign and malignant tumors, to relieve symptoms of airway obstruction, rather than curing the neoplasm. Results are more than 90%, and they are obtained quickly with rigid rather than flexible bronchoscopes. Complications include hemorrhage, pneumothorax, and pneumomediastinum. The cost of equipment and the need for specialized training to perform with laser are major hurdles. Laser therapy is not useful in the peripheral airway even for visible lesions except when there is a postobstructive pneumonia where the patient cannot undergo surgical resection.

Brachytherapy

Bronchoscopic delivery of radiation from within the airway lumen to relieve airway obstruction caused by a malignant tumor is called brachytherapy. This is attempted as palliative treatment in those who had full dose external beam radiation, and the response is good in nearly 60% of patients, lasting for a few weeks or months. Brachytherapy alone is less effective as compared to external radiotherapy. Complications are seen in 6%–8% of cases, mostly fistulae formation between airways and other thoracic structures. In high-dose radiation patients, serious hemorrhage, causing massive hemoptysis may occur. The role is mainly palliative. Studies that have included external radiotherapy and brachytherapy did not observe any improvements in survival. Brachytherapy has been reported to improve cough, dyspnea, and hemoptysis related to lung cancer by varying degrees from 20% to 80%. In inoperable cancers at an early stage, brachytherapy alone can give a response rate of 60%–80% and 5-year survival rates vary widely between 30% and 80%.

Contraindications of therapeutic FOB brachytherapy include the following:

1. Tumors directly involving the major vessels.
2. Fistulas involving the airways.
3. High-grade tracheal obstruction: Brachytherapy can lead to post-treatment edema and complete obstruction.

Phototherapy

Intravenous administration of hematoporphyrin derivative followed by putting on light on the airway malignant tumor through a bronchoscope for several minutes at an appropriate wavelength results in the production of toxic oxygen radicals as a result of chemical reaction when hematoporphyrin derivatives fluoresce. Complete response is seen in nearly half of the patients and sustained for at least 1 year. Sunburn on skin affected by bright light, hemoptysis, and thick necrotic expectoration are the commonly encountered complications. Further therapeutic bronchoscopy may be required to clear this pseudomembrane of thick necrotic materials. It is useful in treating stump recurrence and in providing preoperative help in advanced lung cancer.

Electrocautery

Alternating electrical current is bronchoscopically delivered to coagulate and vaporize endobronchial lesions, using Argon plasma coagulator, both with rigid or flexible bronchoscope. Almost 55%–75% of patients get symptomatic relief from airway obstruction. Instrument and electrocautery probes are not costlier and thus it is a good alternative to expensive laser therapy. Endobronchial fire and electric shock to the patient or the operator are the complications that can occur. Argon plasma coagulation is superior to laser therapy and electrocautery, achieves better hemostasis, can be used both with rigid and flexible bronchoscopes, and has less than 10% of complications.

Cryotherapy

Repeated cycles of cold application followed by thawing using liquid nitrogen or nitrous oxide to achieve 80°C temperature, applied through cryphobes via a rigid or flexible bronchoscope helps in causing cold-induced death of malignant cells. This can be applied to treat smaller polypoid lesions, visible in the distal airway. Cryotherapy is not costly, and subjective relief of airway obstruction is achieved in more than three-fourths of the cases where it is used for benign as well as malignant lesions. Complications are few and rare, but therapy requires longer duration and repeated freeze–thaw cycles. So repeated bronchoscopy is not preferred for most of the patients.

Bronchoscopic resection of airway lesion

Rigid bronchoscopy is preferred for bronchoscopic resection of large neoplastic growths of trachea and mainstem bronchus to provide palliative therapy for the immediate relief of airway obstruction. Severe bleeding is the major complication, often controlled by tamponading the bleeding points with the rigid bronchoscope itself. Prevention of hypoxemia eventually reduces cardiac arrhythmias, which is the most commonly encountered complication of bronchoscopy.

Navigation bronchoscopy

Combined with radial EBUS to target peripheral cancers, using radiofrequency ablation electrodes is being used. This is being used in bronchial asthma to reduce the reactive smooth muscle airway, especially in uncontrolled severe or persistent asthma. The process involves using controlled thermal energy, causing frictional heating resulting in protein denaturation and desiccation.

Bronchoscopic lung volume reduction

The National Emphysema Treatment Trial has confirmed the efficacy of the bronchoscopic lung volume reduction (BLVR) trial. Most of these patients with gross emphysema are sick and may not be eligible for major surgeries. BLVR has shown improved exercise tolerance, lung functions, survival, and health-related quality of life. This could be an important alternative to open lung volume reduction surgery or lung transplantation, which have been the mainstay of treatment of gross emphysema.

Devices for BLVR	Mechanisms
Endobronchial valve devices	They allow air circulation in only one way. Air can be exited from the target segment, but cannot re-enter during inspiration, leading to deflation of the emphysematous areas. Endobronchial Valve for Emphysema Palliation Trial (VENT) was a prospective, multicenter randomized trial that evaluated the safety and efficacy of endobronchial valve in patients with advanced heterogeneous emphysema. Though there was some improvement, it did not reach statistical significance.
Reduction coils	Made from nitinol wires. Retract and fold the parenchyma causing lung volume reduction. Improves clinically relevant outcomes, such as 6-minute walk test, lung functions, and exercise capacity.

(*Continued*)

Devices for BLVR	Mechanisms
Biologic sealant	Made from synthetic polymeric foam sealant. Collapses areas of emphysematous lung. Improves clinically relevant outcomes, such as 6-minute walk test, lung functions, and exercise capacity.
Thermal vapor ablation	Delivery of the steam water vapor at a precise temperature leading to localized inflammation in the target segment and permanent collapse and fibrosis.

Bronchial thermoplasty

Bronchial thermoplasty delivers heat to the airway walls in a controlled manner helping to reduce airway smooth muscle mass, thus reducing airway constriction and improving asthma symptoms and control. A radiofrequency electrical generator and a catheter with four-electrode basket at the tip is used for the purpose, delivering energy every 5 mm intervals from beyond the bronchoscopy visual range to the proximal bronchi. The complete treatment period may extend to around 2 months. Three sessions 3 weeks apart are used: first and second sessions are used to treat each lower lobe separately and both upper lobes are treated during the third session.

The main indications are severe persistent asthma in spite of maximal medical treatment. The main contraindications are an implantable electronic device, unable to tolerate the procedure due to severe comorbid conditions, and forced expiratory volume >65%. It is important to realize that there can be asthma exacerbations in the immediate postoperative period. Over long term, there are reductions in acute asthma attacks and improved quality of life. GINA guidelines have recently recommended them under Step 5 treatment category. Long-term benefits of bronchial thermoplasty have been confirmed over 5 years. Eighty percent reduction in hospital visits and a 30% reduction in severe asthma attacks have been observed in severe persistent asthma after thermoplasty.

Role of bronchoscopy in ICU patients

Introduction

FOB has attained a significant place in ICU, both for diagnostic and therapeutic indications. It provides prompt diagnosis in critically ill patients in ICU where specific and effective treatment decisions when urgently taken are always rewarding. It must be kept in mind that these patients in ICU are either having immunodepressed status or having poor cardiorespiratory functions. Hence, FOB in ICU is fundamentally different from routine bronchoscopy. Since potential risk factors are weighed against expected yield value, the adept bronchoscopist has to work to perfection with insertion technique on critically ill patients with ventilator settings. And the beneficial results have to overweigh the risks involved in each patient, for which bronchoscopist has to be specially trained and experienced, who can perform on critically ill patients in ICU with safety, expediently and correctly, with best outcome and without complications.

Indications

Diagnostic FOB can be performed in case of newer or non-resolving lesions on chest X-ray film. This can also be done to assess airway patency or take sample for the culture of microorganisms. FOB is indicated in hemoptysis. It is also used in procedures like BAL, TBNA, TBLB, and double-sheath brush biopsy of central airways. This is also used to diagnose ventilator-associated pneumonia.

Therapeutic indications of FOB in critically ill patients in ICU include tracheobronchial toilet to mobilize or clear secretions, to resolve atelectasis, to assist difficult intubation, to confirm proper positioning of ET and TT, to guide percutaneous TT, airway hemorrhage or hemoptysis, and in removing FB in the airways.

Preparation and premedication

Since FOB is going to adversely affect cardiorespiratory functions, the attending interventionalist must consider the possible cardiorespiratory dysfunctions which are ought to be faced and may be directly related to the ultimate major complications of the procedure. Arterial hypoxia is the most common derangement that occurs during and after the FOB procedure. Possible mechanisms responsible for this include airway occlusion by the bronchoscope, induced bronchospasm, created V/Q imbalance, and increased airway resistance.

In critically ill ICU patients, the PaO_2 drop during or following FOB is three to six times greater than that occurs in routine bronchoscopy, which is usually 5%–10%. Nevertheless, the change in $PaCO_2$ is minimal. Cardiac complications that are commonly encountered include tachycardia and arrhythmias, which may occur due to decreased $PaCO_2$ irritation of affordances in the airways and stimulation of the vagus nerve during bronchoscopic insertion.

Bronchoscopy should be done only if definitely indicated. Routine investigations must include platelet count and coagulation profile. Avoid bronchoscopic procedure if platelet count is below 20,000, and lung biopsy is not to be attempted if platelet count is less than 60,000. Minimum starvation of 6 hours is essential to avoid the risk of aspiration. To keep the procedure and avoid airway injury as well as to minimize complications such as respiratory depression, hypotension, and cardiac arrhythmias, premedication with sedative, atropine, and local anesthesia is very useful.

Contraindications: Again, the value of conducting FOB in a critically ill patient in the ICU must be rationally weighed for the relative (added) risks against the (absolute) possible benefits from the expected diagnostic yield. And in case relative risks become potential threats to the expected results of the procedure, FOB is contraindicated in those sick patients in ICU, avoiding the overutilization of this procedure. Nevertheless, there are certain absolute contraindications, where insertion of FOB cannot be justified; these are cases of malignant arrhythmias, severe refractive hypoxemia, or rapidly worsening hypercapnia. Procedure FOB is an effective tool but being underutilized for want of proper training. This is otherwise, a safe procedure that needs to be done expediently and correctly. Bronchoscopist must position themselves to carry out FOB smoothly, with a look on all monitors. The 3-D procedure must have additional skilled nursing staff to monitor vital signs and management of the ventilator, who ensure smooth and keep on passing information to the bronchoscopist regarding vital parameters. Continuous monitoring of ventilators, pulse oximetry, and cardioscope is done along with the conventional method of transnasal or oral route, which is used for the insertion of a brochoscope in a non-intubated patient. For those who are incubated and are on a ventilator, insertion of FOB is done through TT/ET tube, for which the minimum diameter of the tube should be 8 mm to allow smooth maneuvering of the bronchoscope. Otherwise, reintubation with a larger tube can be done for doing the bronchoscopy, or FOB can be inserted from outside by passing the tube. For those patients on the ventilator with IMV/SIMU or cPap, MV mode is disconnected for some time to insert FOB. And if the patient is on the mandatory mode of a ventilator and cannot be afforded to disconnect, then a sealed T-tube connection is utilized, to keep one part for the ventilator and another for introducing FOB. Ventilator must be re-set before performing bronchoscopy as FOB is going to increase peak airway pressure, end-expiratory pressure, and other ventilator pressures by three times and also causes the reduction in expired tidal volume. Complications are more with PEEP following bronchoscopy, and postprocedural care demands resetting of oxygen support that is required to be increased for 4–6 hours, along with intensive monitoring and a close watch for complications such as hemorrhage, and pneumothorax is required, more vigilantly as compared to routine bronchoscopy. Chest X-ray has to be done for any kind of new lesion or change in the early lesion. Nearly half of bronchoscopic procedures on critically ill patients in ICU are done for diagnostic purposes, and almost one-third of these are meant for therapeutic effects, while 10%–15% of FOB are done both for diagnostic and therapeutic purposes, significantly influencing the management and outcome in these patients.

Complications: FOB is an effective diagnostic and therapeutic tool in critically ill patients in ICU, when judiciously used and is a safe procedure in expert hands. However, complications are more in critically ill patients as compared to routine FOB and can occur in 10% of patients. Tachycardia and mild hypoxia are seen in almost all the patients, the degree of hypoxia varying from patient to patient, requiring a higher F10 to control the symptoms. Other cardiac arrhythmias such as bradycardia, atrial ectopics, AF, VPBS, temperature rise in fever can be seen in more than 10% of patients, mostly elderly patients. Hemorrhage is a commonly faced complication in almost one-third of cases, mostly in those tissue biopsy has been conducted; the risk is much higher in those with thrombocytopenia and pulmonary hypertension. In less than 5% of cases, pneumothorax can occur more so in patients of PEER. Mortality is very rare if all the precautions are taken, guidelines are followed, and life parameters are monitored.

Comments: FOB is a safe procedure in the hands of an expert bronchoscopist. The coordinated effort of the intensivist, attending physician, and interventional pulmonologist can improve diagnostic yield and management outcomes in critically ill patients in ICU. Each patient must be individually assessed for FOB and indicated, definite guidelines have to be followed for carrying out bronchoscopy for improved diagnostic yield and therapeutic attempts only when risk–benefit ratio tilts in the favor of patients within an acceptable range so that each bronchoscopic outcome (may be diagnostic or therapeutic) is rewarding. All the life parameters need to be strictly monitored in these critically ill patients in ICU to reduce both morbidity and mortality. Thus, underutilized safer tools should be optimally used for rewarding results. At the same time, constant evaluation of pathogens and consumed antibiotic patterns is important in lieu of the rising trend of multidrug-resistant injections in ICU.

References and suggested readings

1. Ikeda S, et al. FOB. Keio J Med. 1968;17:1–1.
2. Ernst A, Silvestri GA, Johnstone D. American College of Chest Physicians. Interventional pulmonary procedures: guidelines from American College of Chest Physicians. Chest. 2003;123:1693–1717.

3. Rand IAD, Blaikley J, Booton R, Chaudhuri N, Gupta V, Khalid S, Mandal S, Martin J, Mills J, Navani N, Rahman NM, Wrightson JM, Munavvar M; British Thoracic Society Bronchoscopy Guideline Group. BTS guide lines on diagnostic flexible bronchoscopy in adults: accredited by NICE. Thorax. 2013;68:i1–i44.
4. Khan GQ, Bhatia RS. FOB. IN: RS Bhatia, GO Khan, ed. Pulm Med. Pee Pee Publ. 2007;1:1–5.
5. Bhatia RS, Sibia SS. Therapeutic use of FOB. Lung India. 1994;12:138–139.
6. Bhattacharya P, Mukerjee A. Role of FOB in the diagnosis of pulmonary TB. IN: RS Bhatia, ed. Tuberculosis. Pee Pee Publ. 2007;14:78–81.
7. Koul PA. Bronchoscopy where it helps. Med Update; API. 2016;26:978–984.
8. Kumar R, et al. Bronchoscopy in immediate diagnosis of smear negative TB. Pneumonol Alergol Pol. 2014;82:410–414.
9. Vaidya PJ, et al. The evolution of FOB from historical. 2015;32:208–210.
10. Bilaceroglu S, Chhajed P. TBNA-a diagnostic tool in routine bronchoscopy. JAPI. 2005;53:797–802.
11. Bilaceroglu S, et al. TBNA-Asia-pacific experience. J Bronchol. 2004;11: 206–214.
12. Colt HG, et al. Bronchscopy in North America-the AAB survey. J Bronchol. 2000;7:8–25.
13. Harrrow EM, et al. Utility of TBNA in staging of bronchogenic carcinoma. Am J Respir Crit Care Med. 2000;161:601–607.
14. Hermens FHW, et al. Diagnostic yield of TBNA in patients with mediastinal lymph node enlargement. Respiration. 2003;70:631–635.
15. Gupta D, et al. Endobronchial ultrasound guided transbronchial needle aspiration vs. conventional TBNA in the diagnosis of sarcoidosis. Chest. 2014;46:547–556.
16. Cetinkaya E, et al. Diagnostic value of TBNA by Wang 22-gauge cytology needle in intrathoracic lymphadenopathy. Chest. 2004;125:527–531.
17. Bilaceroglu S, et al. TBNA in diagnosing intrathoracic lymphadenitis. Chest. 2004;126:259–267.
18. Chokhani R. TBNA in the diagnosis of respiratory disease. Nepal Med Coll. 2004;6:24–27.

19. Holty J, et al. Accuracy of TBNA for mediastinal staging of ySCLC a meta analysis. Thorax. 2005;30.
20. Diacon AH, et al. Utility of ROSE of TBN aspirates. Respiration. 2005;72:182–188.
21. Shankar S, et al. CT guided transthoracic fine needle aspiration versus transbronchial fluoroscopy-guided needle aspiration in pulmonary nodules. Acta Radiol. 1998;39:395–399.
22. Kramer H, Groen HJM. Current concepts in the mediastinal lymph node staging of NSCLC. Ann Surg. 2003;238:180–188.
23. Vaidya PJ, et al. Endobronchial ultrasound guided TBNA in lung cancer diagnosis and staging. Expert Rev Respir Med. 2015;9:45–53.
24. Herth F, et al. Conventional vs endobronchial ultrasound guided TBNA-a randomised trial. Chest. 2004;125:322–325.
25. Herth FJ, et al. Transbronchial and transesophageal ultrasound aspiration of enlarged medistinal lymph nodes. Am J Respir Crit Care Med. 2005;171:1164–1167.
26. Rintoul RC, et al. Endobronchial and endoscopic ultrasound guided real time fine needle aspiration for mediastinal staging. Eur Respir J. 2005;25:416–421.
27. Annema JT, et al. Endoscopic ultrasound guided fine needle aspiration for diagnosis of sarcoidosis. Eur Respir J. 2005;25:405–409.
28. Ma GK, et al. TBNA & PET in the diagnosis of lung cancer. J Branchol. 2004;11:237–241.
29. Annema JT, et al. Towards a minimally invasive staging strategy in NSSLC-analysis of PET positive mediastinal lesions by EUS-FNA. Lung Cancer. 2004;44:53–60.
30. Hsu LH, et al. TBNA guided integrated PET & CT. J Bronchol. 2005;12:76–80.
31. Becker HD, et al. Bronchoscopic biopsy of peripheral lung lesions under electromagnetic guidance-a pilot study. J Bronchol. 2005;12:9–13.
32. Schwarz Y, et al. Electromagnetic navigation during flexible bronchoscopy. Respiration. 2003;70:516–522.
33. Schieppati E. Le puncion mediastinal a traves del espolon traqueal. Rev Argent Med Assoc. 1949;663:497.
34. Reynolds HY. State of the art. Am Rev Respir Dis. 1987;135:250–263.

35. Helmer RA, Hunnigahake GW. Broncho alveolar lavage in the non compromised patient. Chest. 1990;96:1184–1190.
36. Klech H, Pohl W. Technical recommendation and guidelines for broncho alveolar lavage report of the European Society of Pneumonology Task Group on ML. Eur Respir J. 1989;2:561–565.
37. Xaubet A, Rodrigeuz-Roisin R, Bombi IA. Correlation of broncho alveolar lavage and clinical and functional findings in asbestosis. Am Rev Respir Dis. 1986;133:848–854.
38. Sestini P, Rotto II L, Gotti G. BAL diagnosis of bronchoalveolar carcinoma. Eur J Respir Dis. 1985;66:55–57.
39. Reynolds HY. Interstitial lung diseases; classification, definition and correction between clinical and histologic staging of interstitial lung disease. Semin Respir Dis. 1984;6:–9.
40. Garcia JGN, Parham N, Kiilam D. Bronchoalveolar lavage fluid evaluation in rheumatoid arthritis. Am Rev Respir Dis. 1986;133:450–454.
41. Haslam PL, Furton CWC, Luboszek A. Bronchoalveolar lavage fluid cell counts in cryptogenic fibrosing alveolitis and their relation to therapy. Thorax. 1986;35:328–339.
42. Bauwer W, Gomy MK, Baumann HR. T Lymphoctyte subsets and immunoglobulin concentration in bronchoalveolar lavage of patients with sarcoidosis. Am Rev Respir Dis. 1985;132:1060–1065.
43. Milburn L, Prentice HG, Dubois RM. Role of bronchoalveolar lavage in evaluation of pneumonitis in receipts of bone marrow transplants. Thorax. 1987;42:766–772.
44. Stover DE, White DA, Romani PA. Diagnosis of pulmonary disease in AJDS. Am Rev Respir Dis. 1984;130:559–572.
45. Bhatia RS. BAL indications and present status. Lung India. 1984;XII:27–29.
46. Turner JF, et al. Rigid bronchoscopy. J Bronchol. 2000;7:171–176.
47. Cassol V, et al. Foreign body in children's airways. J Pneumol. 2003 May 29/June.
48. Limper AH, Parkash UBS. Transbronchial foreign bodies in adults. Am Intern Med. 1990;112:604–609.
49. Sen MK, Suri JC. Therapeutic bronchoscopy. Ind J Chest Dis Allied Sci. 2000;42:167–179.

50. Bittercourt PFS, Camragos PAM. Aspiracoao de corp estranhos. J Paediatr. 2002;77:9–18.
51. Prakash UBS. Advances in bronchoscopic procedures. Chest. 1999;116: 1402–1408.
52. Asmatullah, et al. Endoscopic removal of the tracheobronchial foreign bodies at a peripheral hospital. J Postgrad Med Inst. 2004;18(3):447–452.
53. Hilmi OJ, et al. A randomized control trial of surgical task performance in rigid bronchoscopy: foreign body extraction with optical versus non-optical forceps. Cli Otolaryngo All Sci. 1999;24:499–501.
54. Martinot A, et al. Indications for flexible versus rigid bronchoscopy in children with suspected foreign body aspiration. Am J Respir Crit Care Med. 1997;155:1676–1679.
55. Tietjen PA, et al. Aspiration emergencies. Clin Chest Med. 1994;15:117–135.
56. Dhadke SV, et al. Foreign body in left maize bronchus. JAPI. 2015;63:70–71.
57. National Safety Council. Deaths due to unintentional injuries. 1999. Available at: http://www.nsc.org.
58. Sindhu VA, et al. Tablet in the bronchus. JAPI. 2014;62:63–69.
59. Killian G. Meeting of the society of physicians of Freiburg; Dec 17, 1897. Munchen Med Wscher. 1898;45:378.
60. Schellhase DE. Paediatric flexible bronchoscopy. Curr Opin Pediatr. 2002;14:327–333.
61. Fang YF, et al. FOB with multiple modalities for foreign body removal in adults. PLOS One. 2015.
62. Herth F, Becker HD. Endobronchial ultrasound in the airways and mediastinum. Monaldi Arch Chest Dis. 2000;55:36–45.
63. Liewad F, et al. Comparison of virtual and fibroptic bronchoscopy. Thor Cardiovas Surg. 1998;46:364–364.
64. Kewalramani N, Nene A. Haemoptysis due to tracheal diverticulum. JAPI. 2016;64:93–94.
65. Brown KL, Shefler A, Cohen G, DeMunter C, Pigott N, Goldman AP. Near fatal grape aspiration with complicating acute lung injury successfully treated with extracorporeal membrane oxygenation. Pediatr Crit Care Med. 2003;4(2):243–245.

66. Sinha S, Guleria R. Laser therapy. IN: M. Panja, ed. PG Med; API. 2003;17:185–191.
67. Sheski FD, Mathur PN. Cryotherapy, electro-cautery and brachytherapy. Clin Chest Med. 1999;20:123–138.
68. Cortese DA, et al. Photodynamic therapy for early stage squamous cell carcinoma of lung. Mayo Clinic Proc. 1997;72:595–602.
69. Homasson JP, Bell J. Endotracheal electrocautery. Semin Respir Clin Care Med. 1997;18:535–543.
70. Prakash UBS. Bronchoscopic resection of surgically resectable tracheobronchial neoplasms. J Branch. 1996;3:85–87.
71. Khan GO, Hassan G. Complications of FOB-experience of 1542 procedures. IN: RS Bhatia, GQ Khan, ed. Pulm Med. Pee Pee Publ. 2007;18:152–165.
72. Gupta AA, et al. Indications of FOB. Lung India. 2015;32:211–215.
73. Vaidya PJ, et al. Endobronchial ultrasound guided transbronchial needle aspiration. J Cancer R There. 2013;9:549–551.
74. Davies L, et al. Cardiovascular consequences of FOB. Eur Respir J. 1997;10:695–698.
75. Sidman JD, et al. Management of acute pulmonary haemorrhage in children. Laryngoscope. 2001;111:33–35.
76. Lichten Stein DA. Lung ultrasound in critically ill. Ann Intensive Care. 2014;4:1.
77. Chhared PN, et al. Ultraflex stents for the management of airway complications in lung transplant recipients. Respirology. 2003;8:59–64.
78. Mehta, AC. Don't loose the forest for the trees: satisfaction and success in bronchoscopy. Am J Respir Crit Care Med. 2002;116:306–307.
79. Khan GQ, Hassan G. Complications of FOB-experience of 1542 procedures. IN: RS Bhatia, GQ Khan, ed. Pulmonary Medicine. Pee Pee Publ. 2007;18:152–165.
80. Charu J. Emergence of resistant bacterial infection in Indian ICU. IN: M. Panja, ed. PG Med; API. 2013;27:572–575.

https://doi.org/10.1142/9789811271410_0009

9 Medical thoracoscopy

Medical thoracoscopy is an important but as yet underutilized diagnostic and therapeutic procedure, especially in developing countries that carry the highest need. Using a rigid or a semirigid thoracoscope, the pleural space is visualized. Its primary role is diagnostic, though therapeutic applications are possible such as the application of talc in the pleura for pleurodesis. It is performed by respiratory physicians with interventional training. The primary indication is the work-up of undiagnosed exudative pleural effusions.

Thoracoscopies were performed more than a 100 years ago, and it is one of the most important investigations into pleural diseases. It is usually a safe procedure with few complications when properly done. It can be performed in the operation theater (OT) or in the endoscopy room.

Indications

Some of the common indications are listed in Table 1. The most common indication would be to evaluate an undiagnosed pleural effusion, which is a common problem. Even after thoracentesis and/or closed pleural biopsy, about 25%–40% of pleural effusions remain undiagnosed. The accurate diagnosis of pleural effusion is quite challenging for the chest physician. Tuberculous pleural effusion is one of the important considerations in an undiagnosed pleural effusion. The difficulties arise due to several factors. Pleural fluid staining for AFB is virtually always negative. Pleural fluid cultures are positive for *Mycobacteria* in <25% of cases. High ADA levels in the background of lymphocytic effusions are used to diagnose tuberculous effusions, but these are elevated in malignant effusions as well which also

Table 1: Common indications and contraindications

- Pleural effusions of unknown etiology
- Recurrent pneumothorax
- Evaluating chest trauma
- Lung biopsy
- Talc pleurodesis
- Early empyema

have lymphocyte predominance. Positive predictive value of ADA is as low as 15% in low-prevalence regions. ADA as the sole method of diagnosis of tuberculosis (TB) carries a risk of missing drug-resistant TB, which is an increasingly frequent scenario in countries with high rates of TB. Therefore, there is a need for additional tools to help in confirming the diagnosis and medical thoracoscopy is an important tool to fulfill that need. But it is to be noted that medical thoracoscopy/pleuroscopy is an invasive procedure and the risk/benefit ratio must be considered. It needs a careful evaluation of the patient as well as of the indications and contraindications of the procedure.

Another important indication is in the evaluation and management of parapneumonic effusions. Pleural effusions are a common finding in patients with pneumonia, and more than 40% of patients with bacterial pneumonia develop parapneumonic effusions. Treatment with antibiotics leads to resolution in most patients, but some patients develop a more fibrinous reaction, with the presence of frank pus in the most severe cases leading to empyema thoracis. The common causes or complications of diseases as well as iatrogenic procedures leading to empyema are pulmonary infection, surgery, trauma, esophagal perforation, complications of thoracentesis/chest tube placement, subdiaphragmatic infection, spontaneous pneumothorax secondary to a ruptured infective focus in the lungs (pyogenic or tubercular), and septicemia. The common indications and contraindications are listed in Table 1.

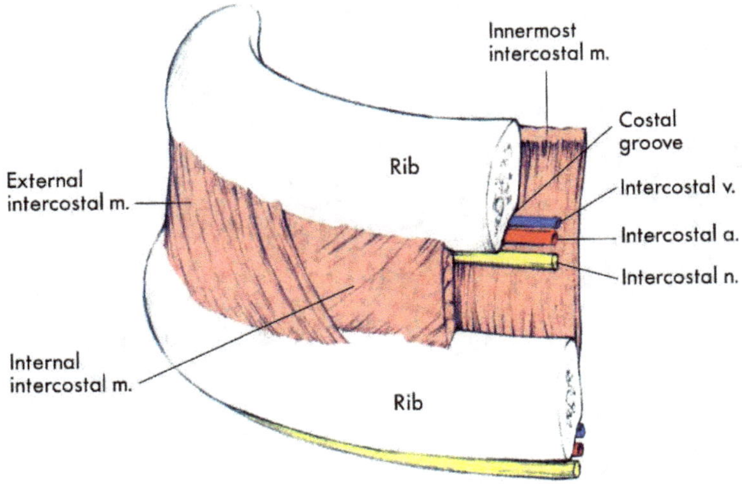

Figure 1: Blood vessels.

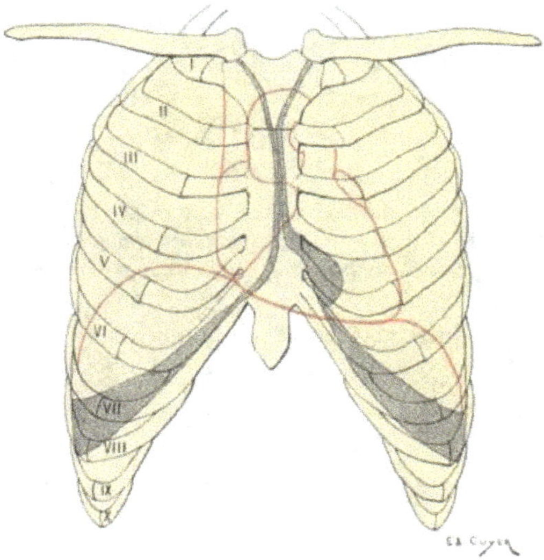

Figure 2: Position of the diaphragm.

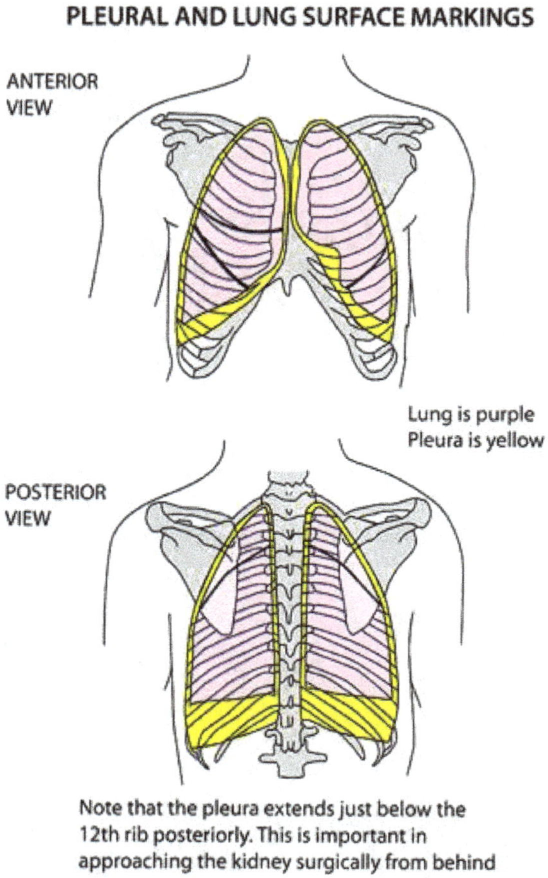

Figure 3: Pleural and lung surface.

Absolute

- Size of free pleural space <6–10 cm usually due to extensive adhesions
- Uncorrectable bleeding disorders

Relative

- Respiratory insufficiency requiring ventilatory support
- Pulmonary arterial hypertension
- Intractable cough

- Hypoxemia
- Bleeding and coagulation disorders
- Unstable cardiovascular status

Procedure

The procedure can be performed in the OT, endoscopy suite, or a clean room. The room ideally should consist of a thoracoscopy table, which is a simple operating table with facilities for height adjustment; oxygen source and suction equipment; cardiorespiratory monitors: pulse oximetry, NIBP/electrocardiogram (ECG) recording, and ECG monitoring; full resuscitation facilities; trolley to hold all instruments and facilities to display patient's radiographs.

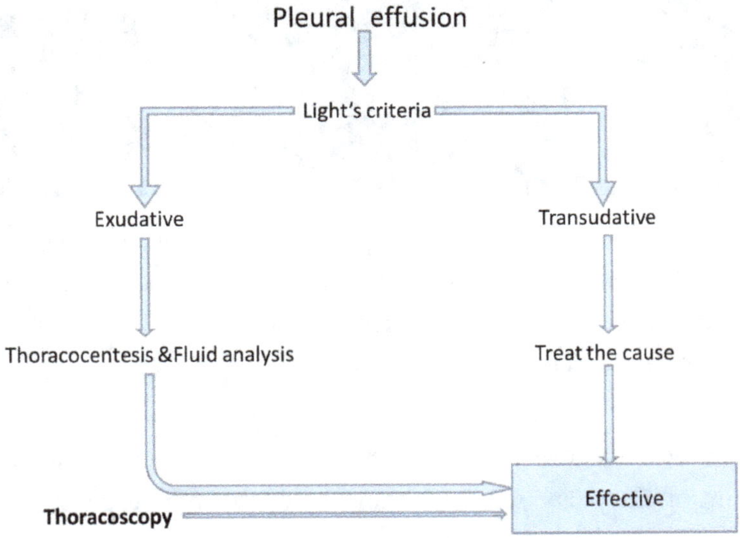

Equipments

It is important to have a good light source for the thoracoscope ideally xenon lamps. The thoracoscopic telescopes can be either rigid or semirigid instruments. While the rigid thoracoscope allows for a larger biopsy specimen, especially hard lesions, and better vision, the semirigid thoracoscope

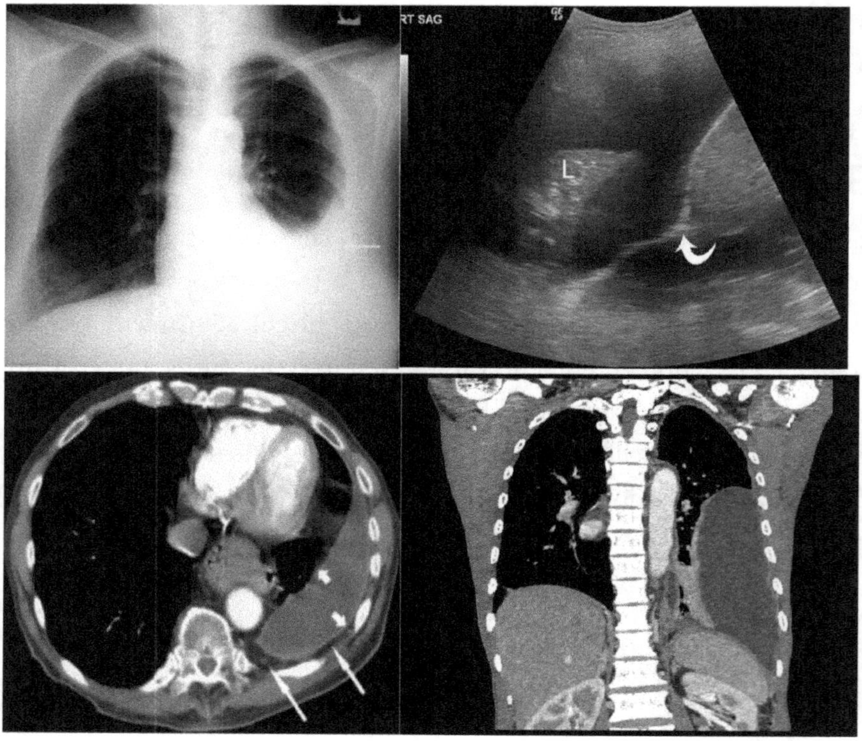

Figure 4: Chest X-ray shows left-sided pleural effusion. Silhouette sign is positive for the left hemidiaphragm and left cardiac border. Ultrasonography shows a non-septated pleural effusion. Computed tomographic (CT) scan shows an encysted pleural effusion.

is easy to use and allows easily for lateral vision and vision in areas around the point of entry. The semirigid thoracoscope is more expensive and is prone to damage (fragile) than the rigid scope and has smaller working channels, and biopsies in some areas can be difficult. A trocar is important to insert the scope into the thoracic cavity and rigid scopes need a larger trocar. But a larger trocar leads to patient discomfort and need for general anesthesia, while the semirigid scopes need a smaller trocar and can be performed under local anesthesia and intravenous analgesics. A conical shape trocar is preferable. Usual medical thoracoscopes are 5–7 mm and

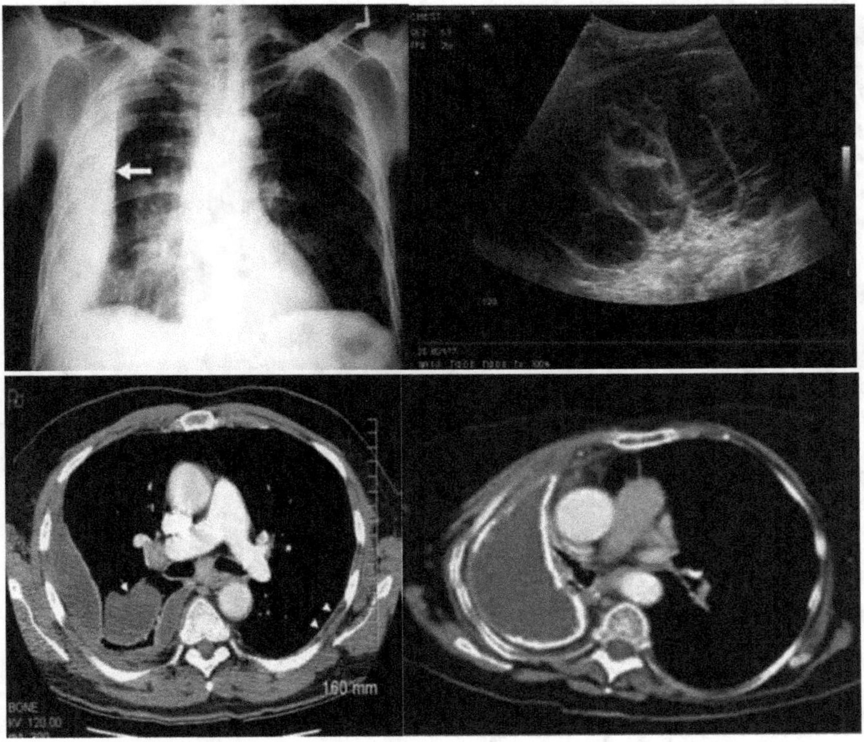

Figure 5: Chest X-ray shows a right-sided encysted pleural effusion, which was confirmed to be empyema. Ultrasonography shows a complex septated pleural effusion. CT scan shows multiple encystments in the right pleural space, pleural thickening, split pleura sign, and pleural enhancement on contrast.

a conical-shaped trocar can be ideal to prevent damage to the nerves and vessels during insertion into the thoracic cavity.

It is important to have a good suction system, and all the pleural fluid needs to be removed before exploration and biopsies. Patient monitoring includes oxygen saturation, pulse, blood pressure, and ECG. For diagnostic thoracoscopy, usually one port of entry is sufficient. Two ports may be needed when dealing with areas that are hard to access or there is a need to use electrocautery. The second port can be located in one intercostal space superior or inferior to the first entry.

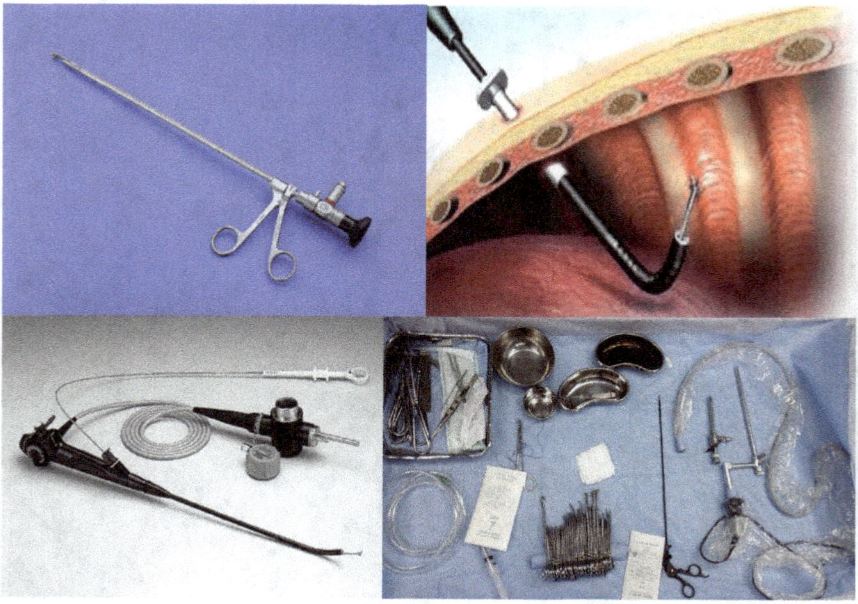

Figure 6: Various accessories in thoracoscopy.

Thoracoscopy technique

Patient preparation

Medical thoracoscopy is safe and simple when the thoracoscopist has good training and understands the endoscopic anatomy of the thorax. Difficulties arise due to the limited field of vision. The important steps in the preparation of the patient include the following:

Explain the procedure in simple language to the patient. There is a need to discuss with the patient whether they prefer local anesthesia with intravenous analgesia or general anesthesia. Patients will have less anxiety and cooperate better when they understand the procedure and what is expected of them.

Patient performance status

It is important to thoroughly evaluate the patients who are undergoing the procedure and whether they are fit for the procedure. Some of the patients

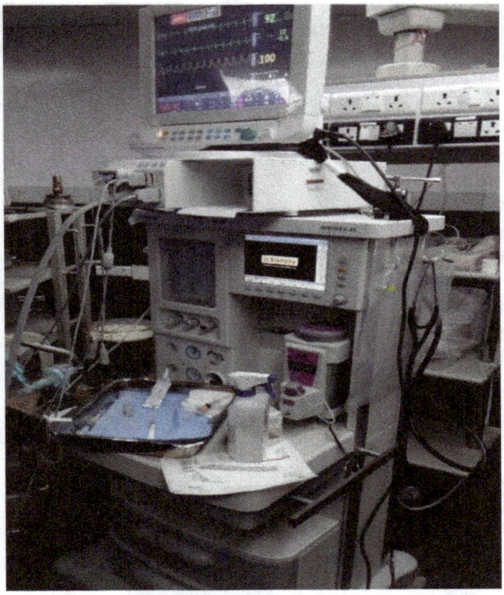

Figure 7: Monitors.

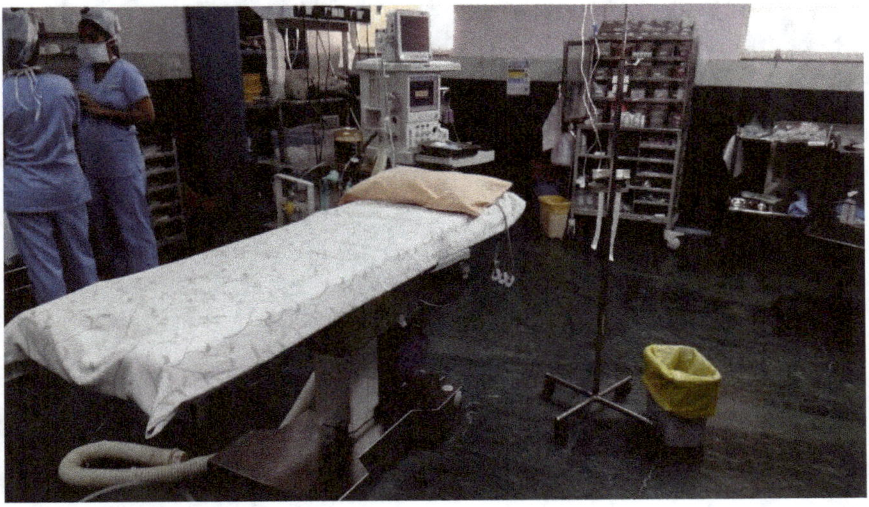

Figure 8: Operating table.

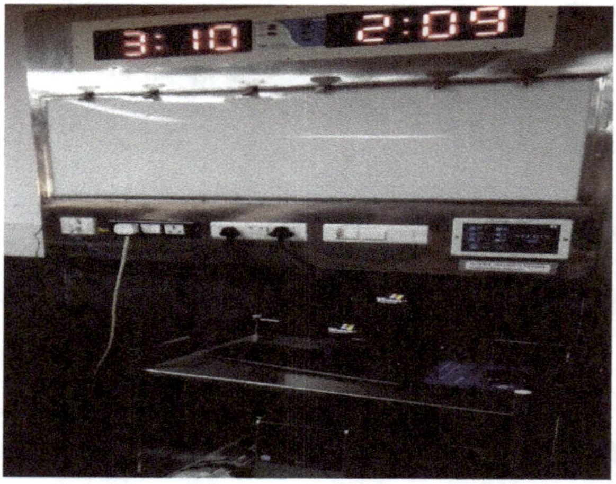

Figure 9: Radiographs display.

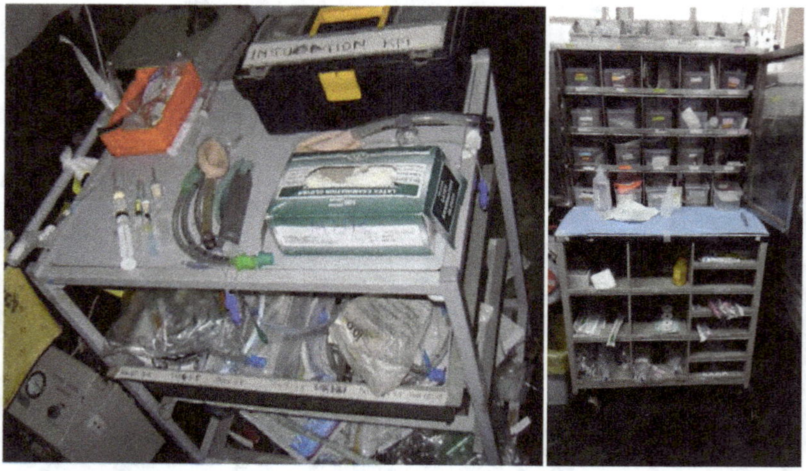

Figure 10: Resuscitation equipments and drugs.

may be cachexic, whether they have hypoproteinemia, drug allergy, whether they have severe cough or dyspnea when the procedure and exploration may become more difficult and result in a greater risk of complications such as subcutaneous emphysema.

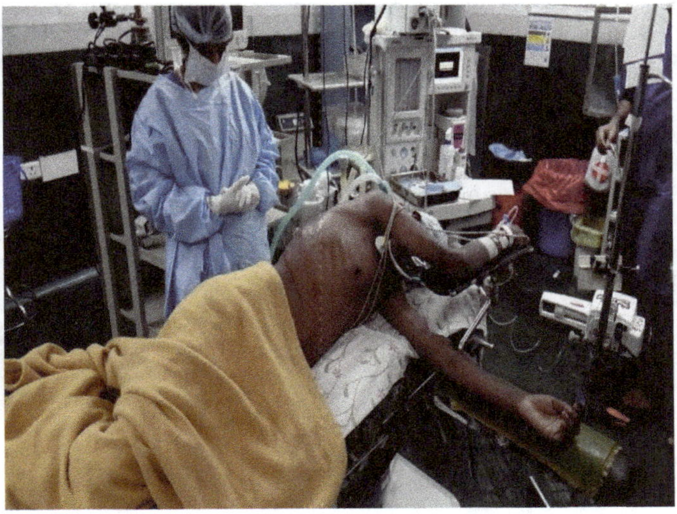

Figure 11: Position of patient.

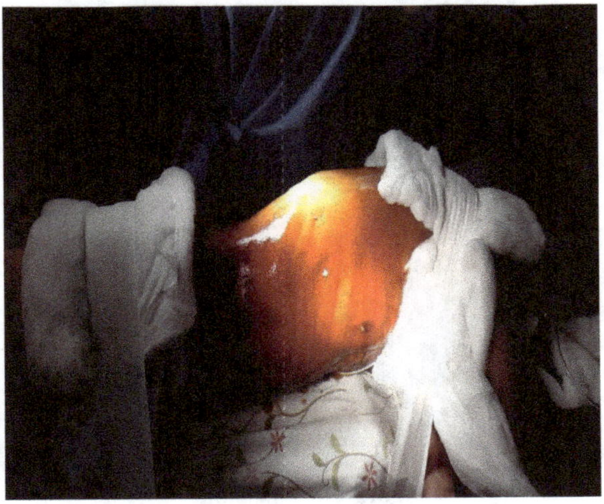

Figure 12: Painting.

Evaluation prior to thoracoscopy

Radiological examination including a chest X-ray posteroanterior and corresponding lateral view of the affected hemithorax is mandatory. This helps to identify the ideal port of entry and identify any pathology in the

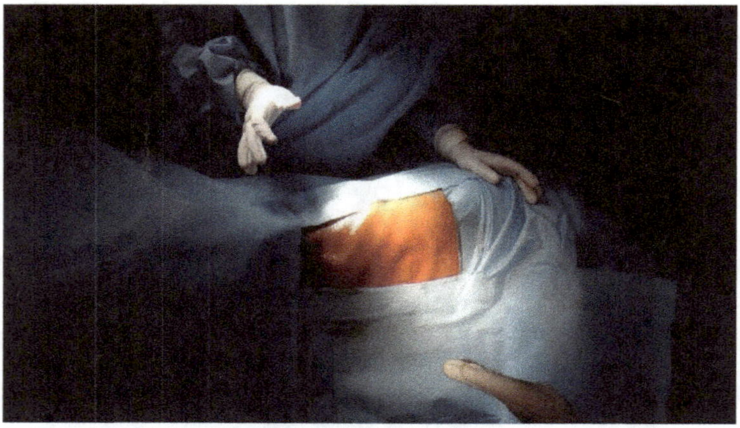

Figure 13: Draping.

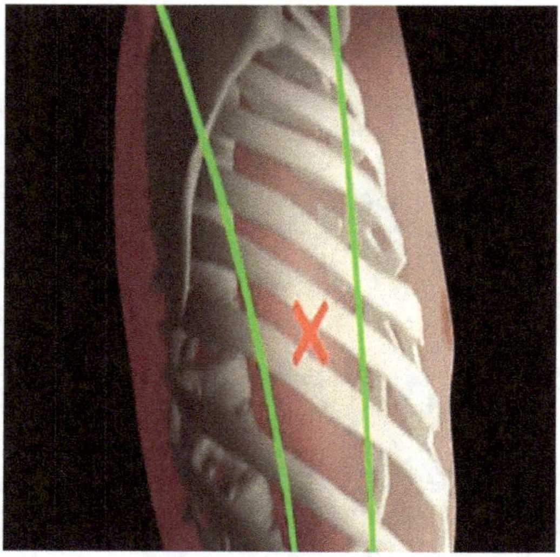

Figure 14: Incision.

other hemithorax. Bilateral lung pathologies increase the risk of acute respiratory failure, especially during the induction of pneumothorax during the thoracoscopy. Imaging also gives us an idea of the size of the pleural effusion.

Some experts suggest the induction of a pneumothorax a few hours or even 1 day before thoracoscopy, which may help to reduce blood flow

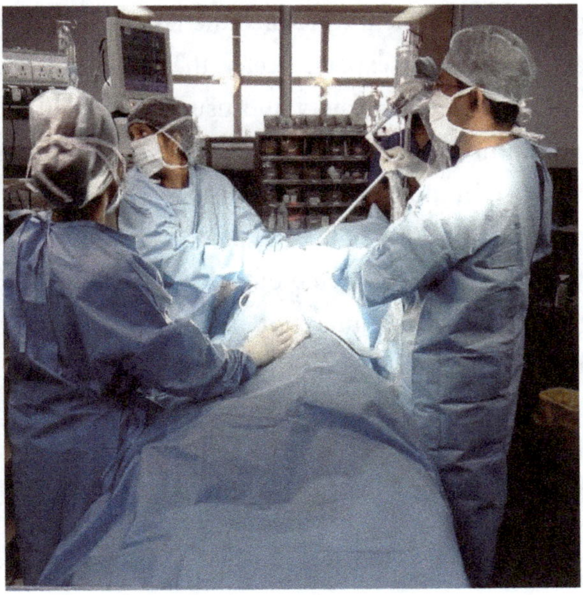

Figure 15: Position of the assistants.

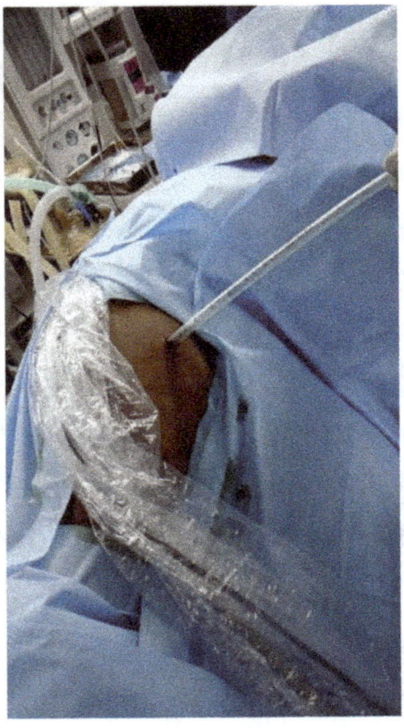

Figure 16: Post-procedure care.

in the lung periphery and help to reduce the risk of damage to the lung during thoracoscopy. Most experts prefer the direct introduction of a blunt trocar into the thoracic cavity and usually carry little risk if there is a sufficient amount of pleural fluid. A contrast CT scan is essential and is usually performed in most cases these days. Cardiac evaluation with an ECG and echocardiography, coagulation profiles, and arterial blood gases are necessary. It is important to rule out cardiac diseases such as unstable angina, recent myocardial infarction, CCF, and when present, thoracoscopy should not be attempted. Patients with significant hypoxia and hypercapnia (>55 mmHg) should be carefully handled or the procedure deferred until they are stable.

A complete blood count should be performed, and thoracoscopy is contraindicated in patients with pancytopenia or coagulation disorders. If platelets are below 60,000/mm^3, the procedure is to be postponed. It is important to ask whether the patient is on any regular medications such as aspirin or anticoagulants, which may prolong the bleeding time.

Thoracoscopy premedication

It is important for adequate preoperative preparation. Adequate chest physiotherapy, inhaled or nebulized bronchodilators, and antibiotics are needed. In a patient with acute dyspnea due to chronic obstructive pulmonary disease, steroids for a few days may be helpful. The common premedication includes 0.4–0.8 mg of atropine (intramuscular), just prior to the procedure, which is useful to avoid vasovagal reactions. Intravenous midazolam is useful, and sedatives include a narcotic (morphine, pethidine, or fentanyl) and a benzodiazepine. If the procedure is likely to be lengthy, general anesthesia is preferred. In subjects at the risk of pulmonary embolism, heparin is advised during their hospital stay.

Post-procedure care

The chest drain removal can be done "on the table" if it is a diagnostic procedure, and in 3–6 days if it is a therapeutic procedure. There is a need for

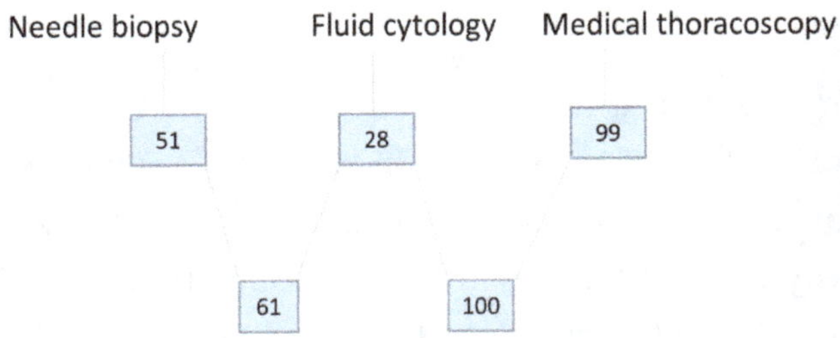

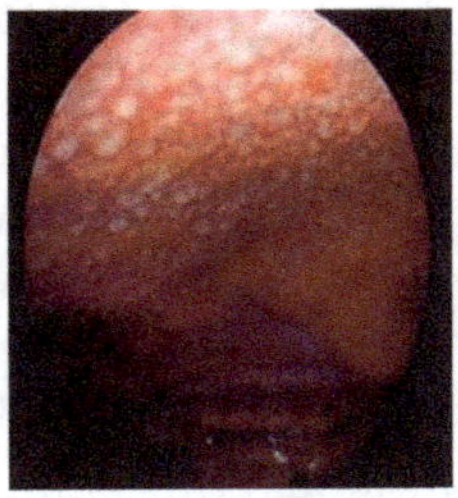

Figure 17: Tuberculous pleural effusions.

Tuberculous pleural.

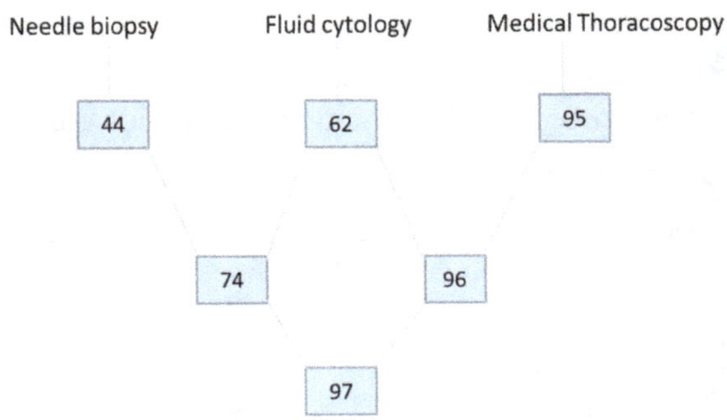

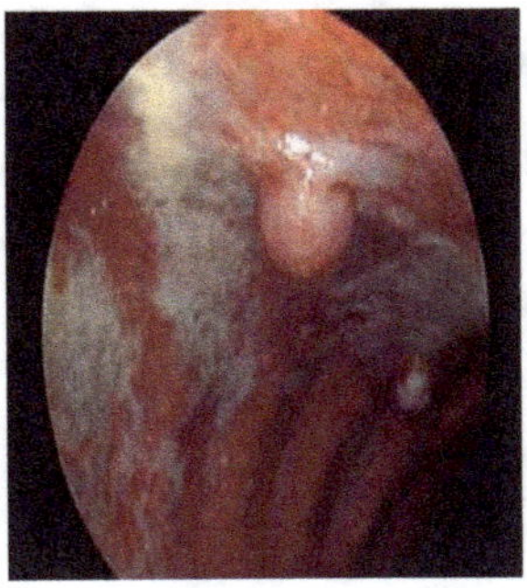

Figure 18: Malignant pleural effusions.

Malignant pleural.

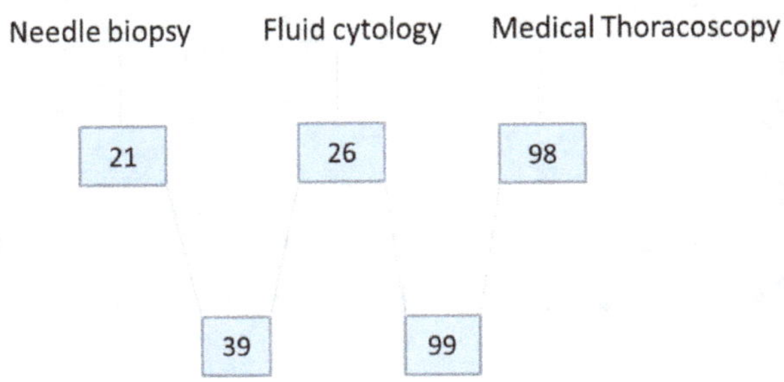

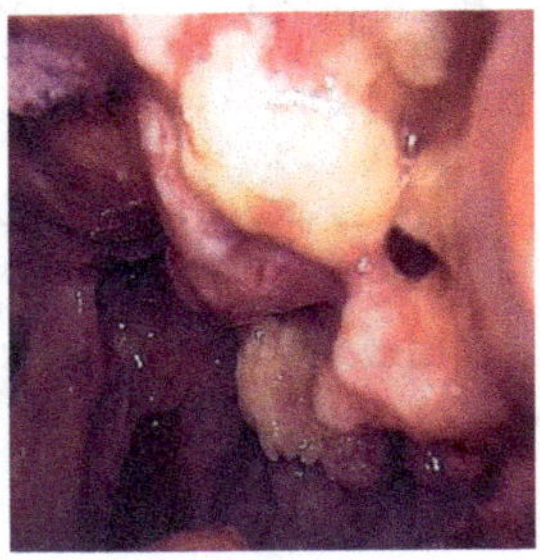

Figure 19: Mesothelioma effusion.

Mesothelioma.

a negative suction pressure to drain the pleural fluid and about −20 cms of H_2O can be applied. It is important to assess the patient clinically and radiologically prior to the removal of the drain. Once the follow-up results are obtained, definitive treatment can be commenced. It is important to never forget radiotherapy to incision sites in the case of malignant pleural mesothelioma.

Safety

Overall, medical thoracoscopy is a safe procedure. Data from 47 studies show the death occurred in 16/4,736 cases (0.34%, 95% CI 0.19% to 0.54%). Of these studies, 28 were of diagnostic thoracoscopy — 0/2,421 (0%, 95% CI 0% to 0.15%). The 19 studies involving talc poudrage gave a combined mortality of 16/2,315 (0.69%, 95% CI 0.40% to 1.12%).

Complications

Major complications

Thoracoscopy is generally a safe procedure. The incidence of major complications in a large study was 86 out of 4,736 cases (1.8%, 95% CI 1.4% to 2.2%). The common major complications are listed below:

- Empyema
- Hemorrhage
- Port site tumor growth
- Bronchopleural fistula
- Postoperative pneumothorax/air leak
- Pneumonia

Minor complications

The incidence of minor complications was about 177 out of 2,411 cases (7.3%, 95% CI 6.3% to 8.4%) in a large study. The common minor complications are listed below:

- Subcutaneous emphysema
- Minor hemorrhage
- Operative skin site infection
- Hypotension during procedure
- Raised temperature
- Atrial fibrillation

Training in thoracoscopy

Three main levels of training in thoracoscopy have been defined. Level 1 training would equip the medical professional to manage large pleural effusions, may undertake smaller effusions as experience increases, biopsy of the parietal but not the visceral pleura, and perform therapeutic talc insufflation. Level 2 training would equip them to additionally perform visceral pleural biopsy, lung biopsy, lysis of adhesions and lavage in the setting of a loculated or infected pleural space, talc pleurodesis in patients with secondary pneumothorax unsuitable for general anesthesia/VATS and perform sympathectomy. Level 3 training would equip them to cover all VATS techniques (eg, lung resection), which is currently the province of the thoracic surgeon. The technical skills are best learned under the direct supervision of an experienced thoracoscopist, and the manual dexterity, confidence, and expertise vary from physician to physician. It is difficult to specify a minimum number of procedures necessary to obtain the skill or to maintain competence. However, a minimum of 20 procedures is desirable to achieve sufficient familiarity with the instrumentation and interpretation of normal and pathological thoracoscopic findings. Procedural competence can probably be maintained if about 10–12 thoracoscopies are performed yearly.

References and suggested readings

1. Mondoni M, Saderi L, Trogu F, Terraneo S, Carlucci P, Ghelma F, Centanni S, Sotgiu G. Medical thoracoscopy treatment for pleural infections: a systematic review and meta-analysis. BMC Pulm Med. 2021 Apr 20;21(1):127. doi: 10.1186/s12890-021-01492-9. PMID: 33879116; PMCID: PMC8056545.
2. Ranganatha R, Tousheed SZ, MuraliMohan BV, Zuhaib M, Manivannan D, Harish BR, Manjunath PH, Hibare KR, Kumar H, Sagar C, Annapandian VM. Role of medical thoracoscopy in the treatment of complicated parapneumonic effusions. Lung India. 2021 Mar–Apr;38(2):149–153. doi: 10.4103/lungindia.lungindia_543_20. PMID: 33687009; PMCID: PMC8098890.

3. Sumalani KK, Rehman U, Akhter N, Rizvi NA. Use of medical thoracoscopy for retrieval of broken intrapleural catheter. Turk Thorac J. 2021 Mar;22(2):179–181. doi: 10.5152/TurkThoracJ.2021.19120. Epub 2021 Mar 1. PMID: 33871344; PMCID: PMC8051304.
4. Chang JY, Mehran RJ, Feng L, Verma V, Liao Z, Welsh JW, Lin SH, O'Reilly MS, Jeter MD, Balter PA, McRae SE, Berry D, Heymach JV, Roth JA; STARS Lung Cancer Trials Group. Stereotactic ablative radiotherapy for operable stage I non-small-cell lung cancer (revised STARS): long-term results of a single-arm, prospective trial with prespecified comparison to surgery. Lancet Oncol. 2021 Oct;22(10):1448–1457. doi: 10.1016/S1470-2045(21)00401-0. Epub 2021 Sep 13. PMID: 34529930; PMCID: PMC8521627.
5. Mehta AA, Shafi TM, Nambiar A, Pavithran K. Diagnostic utility of medical thoracoscopy in T cell lymphoblastic lymphoma presenting with pleural effusion. Respir Med Case Rep. 2020 Dec 11;32:101322. doi: 10.1016/j.rmcr.2020.101322. PMID: 33425676; PMCID: PMC7776927.
6. Wang H, Tang H, Fang Y, Tan L, Yin J, Shen Y, Zeng Z, Zhu J, Hou Y, Du M, Jiao J, Jiang H, Gong L, Li Z, Liu J, Xie D, Li W, Lian C, Zhao Q, Chen C, Zheng B, Liao Y, Li K, Li H, Wu H, Dai L, Chen KN. Morbidity and mortality of patients who underwent minimally invasive esophagectomy after neoadjuvant chemoradiotherapy vs neoadjuvant chemotherapy for locally advanced esophageal squamous cell carcinoma: a randomized clinical trial. JAMA Surg. 2021 May 1;156(5):444–451. doi: 10.1001/jamasurg.2021.0133. PMID: 33729467; PMCID: PMC7970392.
7. Yong Z, Dingding W, Kaiyun H, Yichao G, Yanan Z, Junmin L, Shen Y, Shuangshuang L, Peize W, Jinshi H. Thoracoscopy for esophageal diverticula after esophageal atresia with tracheo-esophageal fistula. Front Pediatr. 2021 May 4;9:663705. doi: 10.3389/fped.2021.663705. PMID: 34017810; PMCID: PMC8129005.
8. Zhang L, Xie T, Fu Y, Wu H. Assessment and review of treatment for secondary spontaneous pneumothorax using medical thoracoscopy-assisted argon plasma coagulation in association with autologous blood pleurodesis. Ther Adv Respir Dis. 2021 Jan–Dec;15:1753466620986390. doi: 10.1177/1753466620986390. PMID: 33573519; PMCID: PMC7887667.

9. An G, Zhang Y, Chen N, Fu J, Zhao B, Zhao X. Opioid-free anesthesia compared to opioid anesthesia for lung cancer patients undergoing video-assisted thoracoscopic surgery: a randomized controlled study. PLoS One. 2021 Sep 23;16(9):e0257279. doi: 10.1371/journal.pone.0257279. PMID: 34555043; PMCID: PMC8460000.
10. Gao S, Wang C, Yu X, Teng T, Shang Y, Jia J, Dong L, Zhao L, Liu S, Chu N, Huang H. Xpert MTB/RIF Ultra enhanced tuberculous pleurisy diagnosis for patients with unexplained exudative pleural effusion who underwent a pleural biopsy via thoracoscopy: a prospective cohort study. Int J Infect Dis. 2021 May;106:370–375. doi: 10.1016/j.ijid.2021.04.011. Epub 2021 Apr 15. PMID: 33845198.
11. Bonhomme O, Heinen V, Detrembleur N, Corhay JL, Louis R, Duysinx B. Probe-based confocal laser endomicroscopy for pleural malignancies diagnosis. Respirology. 2021 Feb;26(2):188–195. doi: 10.1111/resp.13945. Epub 2020 Oct 1. PMID: 33001538; PMCID: PMC7891618.
12. Maesen B, Bidar E, Luermans JG, Maessen JG. Ablation of persistent atrial fibrillation: the added value of hybrid. Eur J Cardiothorac Surg. 2021 Jul 30;60(2):231–232. doi: 10.1093/ejcts/ezab170. PMID: 33842938; PMCID: PMC8327200.
13. Korzeniewska-Koseła M, Gątarek J, Bestry I, Opoka L, Klatt M, Langfort R, Augustynowicz-Kopeć E, Orłowski T. Tuberculosis diagnosed by thoracic surgeons. Pol Arch Intern Med. 2021 Aug 30;131(7–8):633–642. doi: 10.20452/pamw.16020. Epub 2021 May 31. PMID: 34057343.
14. Cattoni M, Rotolo N, Mastromarino MG, Cardillo G, Nosotti M, Mendogni P, Rizzi A, Raveglia F, Siciliani A, Rendina EA, Cagini L, Matricardi A, Filosso PL, Passone E, Margaritora S, Vita ML, Bertoglio P, Viti A, Dominioni L, Imperatori A. Chronic chest pain and paresthesia after video-assisted thoracoscopy for primary pneumothorax. J Thorac Dis. 2021 Feb;13(2):613–620. doi: 10.21037/jtd-20-2860. PMID: 33717534; PMCID: PMC7947510.

https://doi.org/10.1142/9789811271410_0010

10 Airway disease pharmacology

The key groups of drugs that are relevant for the management of airway diseases include bronchodilators, short-acting beta-2 agonists (SABAs), short-acting anticholinergics (SAMAs), long-acting beta-2 agonists (LABAs), long-acting anticholinergics (LAMAs), methylxanthines, phosphodiesterase inhibitors, inhaled corticosteroids, and their various combinations. Oral and parenteral corticosteroids are reserved for the management of acute exacerbations of asthma and chronic obstructive pulmonary disease (COPD) and in very rare cases need to be used frequently. Recently, there is a surge in the availability of biologics as the understanding of the pathogenesis of asthma has improved for a more personalized approach. The table given below provides an overview of the various drugs available in this group, their dosages, adverse effects, combinations available, their mechanism of action, and the newer biologics.

Short-acting beta-2 agonists		
Name	Dose	Adverse effects
Fenoterol	100–200 μg (MDI), 2.5 mg (PO)	Headache, cough, dizziness Hypokalemia, immediate hypersensitivity reactions, bronchospasm Tremor, itching Muscle cramps
Levalbuterol	45–90 μg (MDI), 0.1, 0.21, 0.25 (mg/mL)	
Salbutamol (albuterol)	90, 100, 200 μg (MDI, DPI) 2, 4, 5, 8 mg (PO)	

(*Continued*)

Short-acting beta-2 agonists		
Name	Dose	Adverse effects
Terbutaline	500 µg (DPI) 2.5, 5 mg (PO)	
Long-acting beta-2 agonists		
Arformoterol	0.0075 mg/mL	Tremor, headache, nervousness, weakness Paradoxical bronchospasm, hypokalemia, urticarial, angioedema, nasopharyngitis Myopathy, blurred vision, numbness, hoarseness, rapid heartbeat, throat irritation
Formoterol	4.5–9 µg (DPI)	
Indacaterol	75–300 µg (DPI)	
Olodaterol	2.5, 5 µg (SMI)	
Salmeterol	25–50 µg (MDI and DPI)	
Anticholinergics		
Short acting		
Ipratropium bromide	20, 40 µg (MDI)	Dry mouth, nausea, headache, urinary retention, constipation, sore throat, muscle pain
Oxitropium bromide	100 µg (MDI)	
Long acting		
Aclidinium bromide	400–800 µg (DPI and MDI)	Sore throat, myopathy, headache, dry mouth, difficulty in urinating, heat stroke Tachycardia and atrial fibrillation, angioedema, depression, conjunctivitis
Glycopyrronium bromide	15.6, 50 µg (DPI)	
Tiotropium	2.5–5 µg (SMI)	
Umeclidinium	62.5 µg (DPI)	

Methylxanthines		
Aminophylline	0.4 mg/kg/hour (max — 400 mg/day)	Fever with cold, dyspnea, gastrointestinal bleeding, tachycardia, atrial fibrillation, headache, vomiting, diarrhea, seizures, rashes, insomnia
Theophylline	0.2 mg/kg/hour (max — 100–600 mg [PO])	
Acebrophylline	100 mg twice daily	
Phosphodiesterase-4 inhibitors		
Roflumilast Cilomilast	500 µg (PO) 15 mg BID	Diarrhea, vomiting, dyspepsia, weight loss, headache, abdominal pain, depression
Long-acting beta-2 agonist + anticholinergic (LABA/LAMA)		
Formoterol/aclidinium	12/400 µg (DPI)	
Formoterol/glycopyrronium	6.6/14.4 µg (MDI)	
Indacaterol/glycopyrronium	27.5/15.6 µg (DPI)	
Vilanterol/umeclidinium	25/62.5 µg (DPI)	
Olodaterol/tiotropium	5/5 µg (SMI)	
Short-acting beta-2 agonist + anticholinergic (SABA/SAMA)		
Fenoterol/ipratropium	50/20 µg (SMI)	
Salbutamol/ipratropium	100/20 µg (SMI), 75/15 (MDI)	

(*Continued*)

Long-acting beta-2 agonist + corticosteroids		
Formoterol/ beclomethasone	6/100 (MDI and DPI)	
Formoterol/budesonide	4.5/160 (MDI), 4.5/80 (MDI), 9/320 (DPI), 9/160 (DPI)	
Formoterol/mometasone	10/200, 10/400 µg (MDI)	
Salmeterol/fluticasone	5/100, 50/250, 5/500 (DPI)	
Vilanterol/fluticasone	25/100 (DPI)	
Triple combination		
Fluticasone/ umeclidinium/vilanterol		
Beclomethasone/ formoterol/ glycopyrronium		

Mechanism of action

Beta-2 receptor agonist

Stimulation of beta-2 adrenergic receptors results in the activation of cytoplasmic G proteins, which in turn activates adenylyl cyclase resulting in the production of cyclic adenosine monophosphate (cAMP). cAMP catalyzes the activation of protein kinase A (PKA), which is involved in the inhibition of Ca^{2+} release from intracellular stores, reducing Ca^{2+} entry into the cell, and sequestering intracellular Ca^{2+} causing smooth muscle dilation.

Management of asthma involves SABAs and LABAs. The short onset of action of salbutamol is attributed to its hydrophilic nature. Formoterol is moderately lipophilic, thereby forming a depot in the cell membrane, which also accounts for its greater selectivity for beta-2 receptors compared to salbutamol. The onset of action of salmeterol is slower than formoterol and salbutamol.

Stimulation of these receptors causes activation of Na^+–K^+–ATPase causing gluconeogenesis, producing insulin, and resulting in the decrease in potassium levels.

Anticholinergic

Excessive stimulation of the parasympathetic nervous system leads to bronchoconstriction and increased mucus secretions. Anticholinergics induce relaxation of smooth muscles by reversible and competitive inhibition of M_1, M_2, and M_3 receptors, thereby blocking the effects of endogenous Ach.

Among the various cholinergic drugs available, only ipratropium and tiotropium are approved for the management of asthma.

Ipratropium has a short duration of action requiring three to four doses per day, whereas tiotropium is a long-acting anticholinergic with once-daily dosing. This is attributable to its slow dissociation from M1 and M3 receptors, which are primarily involved in bronchoconstriction and mucus secretion by Ach. Tiotropium dissociates rapidly from the autoinhibitory M2 receptors.

Tiotropium is also shown to reverse goblet cell hyperplasia and attenuate goblet cell metaplasia induced by interleukin-13 (IL-13).

Aclidinium, glycopyrronium, and umeclidinium are the drugs that are approved for COPD but not for asthma.

Monoclonal anti-IgE antibody

Omalizumab binds to immunoglobulin E (IgE) and prevents the binding of IgE to FcεRI (high-affinity IgE receptor) on basophils and mast cells, thereby reducing the amount of free IgE that is available to trigger the allergic cascade. Treatment of atopic subjects with omalizumab resulted in a marked downregulation of FcεRI receptors on basophils.

IgE binds to the receptors FcεRI and CD23 on basophils and mast cells triggering the allergic cascade. Omalizumab, a monoclonal antibody, binds to IgE, thereby preventing the interaction between IgE and the receptors inhibiting mast cell and basophil activation and blocking IgE binding to CD23 on B cells and antigen-presenting cells.

Mechanism of action of corticosteroids

Corticosteroids act by binding to the cytoplasmic glucocorticoid receptor (GR), which allows the activation of GR–corticosteroid complex. GR combines with another GR to form a dimer at DNA sites called glucocorticoid response elements (GREs). This GR complex can lead to the regulation of preventing inflammatory gene expression in four different mechanisms. Changes in the histone deacetylation 2 (HDAC2) activity can regulate the inflammatory gene expression and corticosteroid function.

Phosphorylation and nitration of specific tyrosine residues in HDAC2 induced by oxidative stress reduce HDAC2 activity. Nitration of HDAC2 leads to ubiquitination and proteasomal degradation, which results in enhanced inflammatory gene expression and a reduction in corticosteroid sensitivity. Reversal of corticosteroid sensitivity by kinase inhibitors, phosphorylation of amino acid leading to the upregulation of HDAC2 activity, thereby restoring the corticosteroid actions and reducing the inflammatory response.

The anti-inflammatory mechanisms by which the corticosteroids act is by increasing the number of adrenergic beta-receptors and improving receptor responsiveness to beta-2 stimulation, which results in bronchodilation. It also reduces mucus production and hypersecretion.

Adverse events

Increased hepatic glucose output and decreased peripheral glucose utilization results in insulin-resistant diabetes mellitus. Long-term use increases the risk of hypertension and diminished capacity for wound healing. Decreased reabsorption of calcium by the kidney leads to secondary hyperparathyroidism and retardation of bone growth, which leads to osteoporosis. Increased appetite and increased need for insulin result in weight gain, abnormal fat deposition and typical cushingoid features. Though steroids have some mood elevator activity, in some patients they can trigger psychosis. Cataract formation is accelerated, increased intraocular pressure and very rarely macular edema which can lead to sudden loss of vision and blindness. Skin changes are common, though less serious such as thinning of the skin, striae, acne vulgaris (predominantly in the face and truncal in older subjects), color changes, and hirsutism. In children, there may be a growth retardation.

Inhaled corticosteroids are usually associated with local effects rather than systemic effects, which are common in oral corticosteroid therapy. They include loss of taste, hoarseness of voice, weak voice, and oral candidiasis, which is florid in some cases. When doses exceed 1,500 μg/day, on long-term use, adrenal suppression is reported, though its clinical significance is yet to be ascertained. Higher doses may also lead to an increased risk of adverse events associated with oral steroid use, such as glaucoma, cataracts, osteoporosis, skin thinning, purpura in high doses, and growth retardation in children.

Oral corticosteroids	Dose
Prednisone, methylprednisolone, prednisolone	➢ >12 years old — 40–80 mg/day in one or two divided doses ➢ <12 years old — 1–2 mg/kg/day in two divided doses, maximum 60 mg/day
Inhaled corticosteroids	Dose
Beclomethasone dipropionate	40 and 80 μg/actuation (hydrofluoroalkane) HFA MDI, 120 actuations
Budesonide	90 or 180 μg/dose DPI, Flexhaler, 200 doses, 200 and 500 μg ampoules, 2 mL each
Ciclesonide	80 or 160 μg/actuation HFA MDI
Flunisolide	250 μg/actuation CFC MDI, 100 actuations 80 μg/actuation HFA MDI, 120 actuations

(*Continued*)

Fluticasone propionate	44, 110 and 220 μg/actuation HFA MDI, 120 actuations, 50, 100, and 250 μg/dose DPI, Diskus, 60 doses
Mometasone furoate 9	110 and 220 μg/dose DPI, twisthaler, 14, 30, 60, and 120 doses

Methylxanthines

Methylxanthenes are potent bronchodilators with anti-inflammatory properties.

They act by non-selective inhibition of phosphodiesterase isoenzymes resulting in increased cyclic AMP and cyclic guanosine monophosphate concentration, which in turn results in bronchial smooth muscle relaxation. It also inhibits the adenosine and stimulates catecholamine release.

Phosphodiesterase inhibitors (PDE4 inhibitors)

PDE4 inhibitors suppress the release of inflammatory signals such as cytokines. Roflumilast decreases the release of inflammatory mediators from neutrophils, the expression of adhesion molecules on T lymphocytes, and the release of cytokines such as IL-1β or tumor necrosis factor (TNF)-α from a variety of cell types. Roflumilast reduces oxidative stress and improves mucociliary clearance, mitigating mucociliary malfunction. MUC5AC is the predominant mucin gene expressed in healthy subjects and is increased in patients with asthma or COPD. Selective PDE4 inhibition also decreases MUC5AC expression in cultured epithelial cells in the human airway and in human bronchial tissue. The accumulation of cAMP due to PDE4 inhibition is associated with anti-inflammatory and antifibrotic effects, and a direct effect of roflumilast on smooth muscle relaxation is found to be idiosyncratic. This is due to roflumilast's high selectivity for PDE4, and human airway smooth muscle contains several PDEs.

Mast cell inhibitors

Mast cell stabilizers prevent the release of mast cell mediators such as histamine through the stabilization of the mast cell membrane. These agents are most effective when used prior to antigen exposure. Mast cell stabilizers limit the flux of calcium across the mast cell membrane, thus preventing degranulation and release of vasoactive substances. Medications in this group include sodium cromoglycate 4%, lodoxamide tromethamine 0.1%, and the newer mast cell stabilizers: pemirolast potassium 0.1% and nedocromil sodium 2%. Cromolyn sodium reportedly inhibits chemotaxis, activation, degranulation, and cytotoxicity of neutrophils, eosinophils, and monocytes. Lodoxamide and cromolyn sodium may also have effects on type 2 helper T-cells (Th2), which have been implicated in the pathogenesis of VKC. In addition to preventing mast cell degranulation, mast cell stabilizers may inhibit leukocyte activity. They may also dampen mediator release from mast cells, basophils, eosinophils, and neutrophils.

Mast cells are known to produce many molecules that cause inflammation, but only a few mediators or their stable breakdown products (metabolites) have been found reliably elevated in episodes of MCAS and measurable in commercial laboratory tests. Increases in serum mast cell tryptase and in urine levels of *N*-methylhistamine, 11B-prostaglandin F2α, and/or leukotriene E4 are the only useful tests in the diagnosis of MCAS.

Leukotriene inhibitors

Exposure to allergens results in the generation of cysteinyl leukotrienes (cysLTs), specifically LTs C_4, D_4, and E_4. The mobilization of Ca^{2+} from intracellular and extracellular reservoirs leads to the activation of cytosolic phospholipase A_2, as well as other types of PLA_2 enzymes causing arachidonic acid cleavage and ultimately the formation of cysLTs.

The cysLTs then bind to receptors cysLTR1 and cysLTR2 of which the former is found in the human airway including airway smooth muscle cells and airway macrophages and on other proinflammatory cells including eosinophils and certain myeloid stem cells causing chronic eosinophilic airway inflammation, bronchoconstriction, bronchial hyperresponsiveness, mucus hypersecretion, and airway remodeling. Montelukast and zafirlukast are orally active compounds for the cysLT$_1$ receptor, thereby relieving symptoms of asthma.

Monoclonal anti-IgE antibody

Omalizumab binds to IgE and prevents the binding of IgE to FcεRI (high-affinity IgE receptor) on basophils and mast cells, thereby reducing the amount of free IgE that is available to trigger the allergic cascade. Treatment of atopic subjects with omalizumab resulted in a marked downregulation of FcεRI receptors on basophils.

Immunoglobulin E binds to the receptors FcεRI and CD23 on basophils and mast cells triggering the allergic cascade. Omalizumab, a monoclonal antibody, binds to IgE, thereby preventing the interaction between IgE and the receptors inhibiting mast cell and basophil activation, and blocking IgE binding to CD23 on B cells and antigen-presenting cells.

Newer agents

Interleukin-4 (IL-4)

- Pascolizumab

Interleukin-13 (IL-13)

- Lebrikizumab
- Tralokinumab

Interleukin-4R alpha (IL-4R alpha)

- Pitrakinra

Blocking IL-4 activity or IL-4 expression

Blocking specifically IL-4 has been addressed by administering soluble IL-4R, monoclonal antibodies, or antisense technology.

Soluble IL-4R

Soluble IL-4R (sIL-4R) is a naturally occurring secreted form of IL-4R that contains the extracellular portion of the IL-4Rα chain but lacks the transmembrane and cytoplasmic domains. sIL-4R functions as a decoy receptor by binding IL-4 and neutralizing it, without mediating cellular activation. In a murine asthma model, sIL-4R significantly inhibited AHR and IgE production when administered at the time of sensitization. Moreover, sIL-4R also reduced late-phase pulmonary inflammation, by blocking endothelial VCAM-1 expression, airway eosinophil infiltration, and mucus hypersecretion (but not AHR), when administered during allergen challenge, suggesting that blocking IL-4 could provide clinical benefit, even after full sensitization to an allergen.

Anti-IL-4 monoclonal antibody

Another approach to block IL-4 was the use of a humanized anti-IL-4 mAb (pascolizumab; Biopharma, Winchester, UK). Pascolizumab was generated as a murine mAb (3B9) with specificity for human IL-4, which was subsequently humanized to reduce immunogenicity. Anti-IL-4 reduced IgE production and AHR in murine asthma models. An in vitro study demonstrated that pascolizumab effectively neutralized IL-4 bioactivity in human cell lines and inhibited Th2 cell-related processes, such as IL-5 synthesis and induction of IgE production.

Blocking IL-13 activity

The predominant role of IL-13 in goblet cell hyperplasia, airway wall remodeling, and AHR has led to blocking strategies with anti-IL-13 mAbs.

Lebrikizumab, an IgG4 humanized mAb to IL-13, has been tested in both subjects with mild asthma and subjects with uncontrolled asthma by monthly subcutaneous administration for up to 6 months. Within the working hypothesis that anti-IL-13 therapy would benefit patients with a pretreatment profile consistent with IL-13 activity, patient subgroups were prespecified according to their baseline Th2 status (assessed with total IgE levels, blood eosinophil count, and the serum levels of periostin, a matricellular protein that is secreted by bronchial cells in response to IL-13). Lebrikizumab significantly improved prebronchodilator forced expiratory volume in 1 second (FEV_1) by 5.5% at week 12, and a subgroup of patients with high periostin levels had even a relative increase in FEV_1 of 8.2% compared with placebo. This suggests that measuring serum periostin levels in individuals with asthma could be used as a biomarker to identify potential responders toward lebrikizumab and that anti-IL-13 therapy can be targeted to susceptible patients. However, lebrikizumab treatment did not result in a significant improvement in secondary outcomes, such as asthma symptom scores or exacerbation rates.

Tralokinumab (CAT-354), another IgG4 humanized anti-IL-13 mAb, has been demonstrated to be potent in preclinical models and to be safe in both healthy volunteers and subjects with asthma.

Blocking IL-4 receptor-α activity or expression

Recombinant human IL-4 (pitrakinra)

Pitrakinra is a recombinant form of human IL-4 with two functional mutations at positions 121 (arginine to aspartic acid) and 124 (tyrosine to aspartic acid). Pitrakinra has a high affinity for the IL-4Rα chain and acts as a competitive receptor–antagonist that blocks both IL-4- and IL-13-dependent responses by inhibiting the binding of IL-4 and IL-13 to the IL-4Rα receptor complexes. The effectiveness of such an approach was initially tested in a murine asthma model, using a murine IL-4 mutant protein (mouse IL-4 receptor antagonist, mIL-4Ra) and showed inhibition of allergen-induced Th2 cytokine production, eosinophilic inflammation, goblet cell hyperplasia, AHR, and allergen-specific IgE. Also, local transgenic overexpression of mIL-4Ra in the lungs by intratracheal administration of the *IL-4Ra* gene on a plasmid attenuated airway inflammation and regulated the Th1/Th2 balance in mice.

Anti-IL-4 receptor-α monoclonal antibodies

AMG 317 (anti-IL4Rα), a humanized mAb directed toward human IL-4Rα, has become an alternative approach to tackle the biological redundancies between IL-4 and IL-13. AMG 317 (Amgen) not only prevents binding of IL-4 to IL-4Rα but also prevents signal transduction by IL-13. Preclinical studies in mouse asthma models using murine anti-IL-4Rα demonstrated reduced pulmonary inflammation, AHR, and goblet cell hyperplasia.

In Phase I and II trials, the pharmacokinetics and pharmacodynamics of AMG 317 were evaluated using single and multiple dosing by the intravenous or subcutaneous route. Sustained subcutaneous dosing of AMG 317 over several months was shown to reduce total serum IgE levels. The Phase II study in patients with moderate-to-severe asthma demonstrated that AMG 317 was safe and well tolerated. No clinical efficacy was demonstrated across the overall group of patients, but AMG 317 treatment did lead to significant clinical improvement in patients with higher baseline Asthma Control Questionnaire symptom scores.

Mepolizumab

Dose: 100 mg/mL

Mepolizumab is an interleukin-5 (IL-5) antagonist (IgG1 kappa). IL-5 is the major cytokine responsible for the growth and differentiation, recruitment, activation, and survival of eosinophils. Mepolizumab binds to IL-5 with a dissociation constant of 100 pM, inhibiting the bioactivity of IL-5 by blocking its binding to the alpha chain of the IL-5 receptor complex expressed on the eosinophil cell surface. Inflammation is an important component in the pathogenesis of asthma. Multiple cell types (e.g., mast cells, eosinophils, neutrophils, macrophages, lymphocytes) and mediators (e.g., histamine, eicosanoids, leukotrienes, cytokines) are involved in inflammation. Mepolizumab, by inhibiting IL-5 signaling, reduces the production and survival of eosinophils.

Benralizumab

Dose: 1 mg/ml

IL-5 induces an eosinophil-mediated inflammatory response by binding to the IL-5 receptor (IL-5R) expressed in eosinophils, basophils, and some mast cells. Benralizumab, unlike IL-5 low-affinity binding, binds with high affinity to the domain I of the α-chain of IL-5R and blocks its signaling and the proliferation of IL-5-dependent cell lines. On the other hand, benralizumab is an afucosylated antibody in the CH2 region which gives it a high affinity for the FcγRIIIa on natural killer cells, macrophages, and neutrophils. This binding triggers a magnified apoptosis response in eosinophils via antibody-dependent cell-mediated cytotoxicity.

Dupilumab

Dose: 150 mg, 200 mg, 300 mg

Dupilumab is a fully human mAb inhibitor of IL-4 and IL-13 approved for use in patients with asthma and elevated eosinophil levels. As both IL-4 and IL-13 are critical in the initiation Th2-mediated inflammation, it was proposed that dupilumab may be beneficial in the treatment of atopic dermatitis.

Mucolytics

Classic mucolytics

- *N*-acetylcysteine (NAC)

Administration of NAC dissociates mucin disulfide bonds and other disulfide bond cross-linked gel components which are responsible for the viscoid nature of the respiratory mucus, thereby reducing its viscosity. NAC also has antioxidant effects which may protect the airways from free radical damage. However, NAC is acidic and has an irritant effect when inhaled. Nacystelyn (NAL), the lysine salt of acetylcysteine, exerts mucolytic and antioxidant activity and has a neutral pH in solution making it an interesting alternative.

Dose: Solution for inhalation: 1–10 mL of 20% solution every 6–8 hours or 2–20 mL of 10% solution every 2–6 hours.

Oral: 600 mg once daily to twice daily.

- Erdosteine

The drug reduces the viscosity of mucus with the same mechanism as described above. It produces an active metabolite, N-thiodiglycolyl-homocysteine which produces antioxidant effects during the respiratory burst of human PMNs, due to the presence of an SH group. Erdosteine has also been demonstrated to inhibit bacterial adhesion to epithelial cells.

In addition, the drug might also exert an antitussive effect due to its anti-inflammatory properties via the improvement of mucociliary clearance and the reduction of chemokines from epithelial cells. In COPD patients who smoke, erdosteine has also been observed to reduce the levels of reactive oxygen species and cytokines (IL-6 and IL-8) in peripheral blood and bronchial secretions, respectively. The drug has metabolic products that interfere with the metabolism of methionine, hence is contraindicated in subjects suffering from liver cirrhosis and deficiency of the cystathionine-synthetase enzyme.

Dose: 300 mg twice daily for maximum 10 days.

Duration of therapy longer than 10 days has been reported, however, that must be considered as an off-label use.

- Carbocysteine

Carbocysteine lysine salt monohydrate and its mucolytic efficacy is related to its capacity to replace fucomucins by sialomucins, thereby reducing mucus viscosity. Carbocysteine also inhibits the TNF-α-induced overexpression of sialyl-Lewis epitopes in mucins secreted by patients suffering from various respiratory diseases, such as chronic bronchitis, asthma, and cystic fibrosis (CF). Furthermore, CLS increases Cl^- secretion in rabbits, an effect that might contribute to the overall mucoregulatory action.

Dose: Initial daily dosage of 2,250 mg carbocysteine in divided doses, reducing to 1,500 mg daily in divided doses when a satisfactory response is obtained. For example, two capsules three times a day reducing to one capsule four times a day.

Peptide mucolytics

- Dornase alfa

Patients with CF experience chronic bacterial lung infections causing infiltration of neutrophils which on degeneration release DNA, increasing the viscosity of the sputum, and the patient's ability to clear it. Dornase alfa, a recombinant human deoxyribonuclease I, hydrolyzes the extracellular DNA in the sputum greatly decreasing viscoelasticity and improving the mucociliary clearance of the sputum and FEV_1 in patients with CF.

Dose: 2.5 mg via inhalation twice daily.

- Gelsolin and thymosin β4

Actin being the most prevalent cellular protein in the body plays a vital role in maintaining the structural integrity of cells. It polymerizes to form F-actin which contributes to the viscoelasticity of expectorated CF sputum.

Both gelsolin and thymosin β4 are recognized to specifically depolymerize F-actin polymers in CF sputum, therefore reducing its viscosity; however, these agents need to be further evaluated in clinical trials.

Non-destructive mucolytics

- Dextran and heparin

Mucin is a polyionic tangled network, and the charged nature of the oligosaccharide side chains helps to hold this network together as a gel. Non-destructive mucolytics dissociate or disrupt this polyionic oligosaccharide mucin network by a mechanism termed "charge shielding."

A trial conducted showed the safety of heparin at the dose of 50,000 IU administered twice daily for 2 weeks in CF adults; however, data on efficacy still need to be established.

Drug	ADRs
Classic mucolytics	Hypersensitivity, fixed drug eruption, hypotension, headache, tachycardia, tinnitus, rash, fever
Peptide mucolytics (dornase alfa)	Conjunctivitis, dysphonia, dyspnea, pharyngitis, laryngitis, rhinitis, dyspepsia, rash, urticarial, pyrexia
Non-destructive mucolytics	Data not available

References and suggested readings

1. Balsamo R, Lanata L, Egan CG. Mucoactive drugs. [online] Err.ersjournals.com. 2010. Available at: https://err.ersjournals.com/content/errev/19/116/127.full.pdf [Accessed 1 May 2019].
2. Gillissen A, Jaworska M, Orth M, Coffiner M, Maes P, App EM, Cantin AM, Schultze-Werninghaus G. Nacystelyn, a novel lysine salt of N-acetylcysteine, to augment cellular antioxidant defence in vitro. PubMed — NCBI. [online] Ncbi.nlm.nih.gov. n.d. Available at: https://www.ncbi.nlm.nih.gov/pubmed/9135855 [Accessed 1 May 2019].
3. Dal Negro RW. Erdosteine: antitussive and anti-inflammatory effects. — PubMed — NCBI. [online] Ncbi.nlm.nih.gov. 2008. Available at: https://www.ncbi.nlm.nih.gov/pubmed/18185958 [Accessed 1 May 2019].
4. Pdr.net. Pulmozyme (dornase alfa) dose, indications, adverse effects, interactions. [online] PDR.net. n.d. Available at: https://www.pdr.net/drug-summary/Pulmozyme-dornase-alfa-1336 [Accessed 1 May 2019].
5. Cramer GW, Bosso JA. The role of dornase alfa in the treatment of cystic fibrosis. — PubMed — NCBI. [online] Ncbi.nlm.nih.gov. 1996. Available at: https://www.ncbi.nlm.nih.gov/pubmed/8792953 [Accessed 1 May 2019].
6. Rubin, B. Mucolytics, expectorants, and mucokinetic medications. [online] Rc.rcjournal.com. n.d. Available at: http://rc.rcjournal.com/content/respcare/52/7/859.full.pdf [Accessed 1 May 2019].
7. Patents.google.com. US6339075B1 — Use of dextran and other polysaccharides to improve mucus clearance — Google Patents. [online]. n.d. Available at: https://patents.google.com/patent/US6339075 [Accessed 1 May 2019].

8. Serisier D, Shute J, Hockey P. Inhaled heparin in cystic fibrosis. [online]. 2006. Available at: https://erj.ersjournals.com/content/27/2/354 [Accessed 1 May 2019].
9. Macciò A, Madeddu C, Panzone F, Mantovani G. Carbocysteine: clinical experience and new perspectives in the treatment of chronic inflammatory diseases. — PubMed — NCBI. [online] Ncbi.nlm.nih.gov. 2009. Available at: https://www.ncbi.nlm.nih.gov/pubmed/19239402 [Accessed 1 May 2019].
10. Koehler P, Bassetti M, Chakrabarti A, et al. Defining and managing COVID-19-associated pulmonary aspergillosis: the 2020 ECMM/ISHAM consensus criteria for research and clinical guidance. Lancet Infect Dis. 2021;21(6):e149–e162. doi: 10.1016/S1473-3099(20)30847-1.
11. Sheahan TP, Sims AC, Zhou S, et al. An orally bioavailable broad-spectrum antiviral inhibits SARS-CoV-2 in human airway epithelial cell cultures and multiple coronaviruses in mice. Sci Transl Med. 2020;12(541):eabb5883. doi: 10.1126/scitranslmed.abb5883.
12. Gadgeel S, Rodríguez-Abreu D, Speranza G, et al. Updated analysis from KEYNOTE-189: pembrolizumab or placebo plus pemetrexed and platinum for previously untreated metastatic nonsquamous non-small-cell lung cancer. J Clin Oncol. 2020;38(14):1505–1517. doi: 10.1200/JCO.19.03136.
13. Laidlaw TM, Bachert C, Amin N, et al. Dupilumab improves upper and lower airway disease control in chronic rhinosinusitis with nasal polyps and asthma. Ann Allergy Asthma Immunol. 2021;126(5):584–592.e1. doi: 10.1016/j.anai.2021.01.012.
14. Reck M, Rodríguez-Abreu D, Robinson AG, et al. Five-year outcomes with pembrolizumab versus chemotherapy for metastatic non-small-cell lung cancer with PD-L1 tumor proportion score ≥ 50. J Clin Oncol. 2021;39(21):2339–2349. doi: 10.1200/JCO.21.00174.
15. Lange P, Ahmed E, Lahmar ZM, Martinez FJ, Bourdin A. Natural history and mechanisms of COPD. Respirology. 2021;26(4):298–321. doi: 10.1111/resp.14007.

https://doi.org/10.1142/9789811271410_0011

11 Rising respiratory problems and suggested preventive measures

Introduction

The prevalence of respiratory problems has greatly increased in the last two decades. The escalation may be due to more awareness and health orientation or availability of new diagnosis facilities and specialist services in pulmonary sciences clubbed with critical care management, but there has been a significant rise, especially in the nontuberculous pulmonary disorders. Apart from usual causes such as infections, tobacco-related, dietary, and constitutional factors which have been considered as important etiological culprits, air pollution creating environmental factors has been attributed to be most significantly contributing to many disorders of the chest. In addition to the occupational or ambient exposure to chemicals and industrial pollutants including automobile pollutants, in the recent years, acquired immunodeficiency syndrome (AIDS)-related, tobacco-induced, drug-induced iatrogenic, and traumatic pulmonary disorders have also been increasingly seen.

Respiratory diseases were earlier diagnosed in medical outpatient department with the help of stethoscope, assisted with routine blood tests, chest X-ray, and sputum analysis. Chest medicine in this country was considered virtually synonymous with tuberculosis (TB). The development and growth of pulmonology in recent years into an important medical subspecialty has brought forth a battalion of investigations, such as bronchoscopy and bronchoalveolar lavage analysis, spectroscopy, blood gas analysis, pulmonary scintiphotography, interventional radiology, high-resolution computed tomography (HRCT), magnetic resonance imaging, and pleural and lung biopsy. The actual rise in respiratory diseases is, therefore, partly attributed to the advancement in diagnostic facilities, availability of specialized services, and increased awareness among physicians about the existence of certain pulmonary disorders.

Environmental pollution

A significant part has been played by environmental pollutants in the present rise in respiratory disorders.[1–7] Industrial or domestic burning of fuel and automobile exhaust pollute the atmosphere with air pollutants, such So, No SPM, CO, and PO (polycyclic organic matter). Excessive and inefficient burning of fuel is leading to global warming called the greenhouse effect as reflected excess of CO_2 reduced stratospheric ozone and increased fluctuations in the climate. In addition, women are exposed to the large scale of air pollution in the ill-ventilated kitchens, produced from the burning of poor-quality coal, wood, cow dung, and kerosene during domestic cooking.

The hazardous occupational exposure to various pollutants in the coal mine, rock crushers, silica asbestos, and cloth-making industries is responsible for acute and chronic lung disorders. More than 2,000–2,400 metric tons of air pollutants are liberated into the atmosphere in a busy city that has an automobile share of nearly 60%, industrial contribution of 30%–35%, and domestic share of 5%–10%. The synergism between these environmental pollution and undernutrition, smoking, and dusty occupation is known to contribute to a rise in respiratory diseases, aggravated by exhaustive frequent local travel through a dusty automobile exhaust vitiated atmosphere. The United Kingdom has vowed to cut down atmospheric CO_2 by 50% in the coming decade. Kyoto treaty has not targeted sufficiently to address the problem. Wind and wave power will *be* used to achieve the target, and California, USA, joins the same issue and plans to take steps for the green land effect. India's health interests may hopefully get a stimulus.

Diesel exhaust alters airway fluid polymorphs and delays the clearance of soot particles and lung collagen. SO_2 and NO_2 decrease the resistance to bacterial and viral infections, thereby increasing the severity and duration of it Ihess. In addition, SO_2 increases airway hyperactivity, leading to airway obstruction, increased susceptibility to lung infections, and precipitation of acute asthmatic attacks. NO_2 possibly' causes long-term effects such as interstitial alveolitis, and high levels of SPM inhalation lead to hemorrhagic pneumonitis in animals and frequent colds and chronic productive cough in man. PAH, POM, benzene, and aldehyde absorption is increased if SPM levels are increased in the inhaling air, which in turn enhance carcinogenicity. Lung cancer is 1.5 times more with diesel fumes exposure, since the size of particles expelled after combustion is less than 1 μm in 90% of cases and causes damage in the form of epithelial metaplasia, bronchial plaques, and carcinogenesis through its toxic irritants and carcinogenic substances, and CO_2 in the atmosphere is 25% more than it used to be a century ago. CO_2 level of 208 ppm in 1990 was increased to 306 ppm in 1997 and is expected to reach 660 ppm in 2025. The rise in global temperature — greenhouse effect if rises by 10% more shall have a deteriorating effect on the population. Power cut and use of industrial and home generators for life comforts — the release of gas used for refrigerators and air conditioners and agony to it.

Oxidants such as O_2, aldehydes, and NO induce respiratory inflammation and epithelial injury. Chronic ozone exposure leads to obstruction in the small airway near the centriacinar junction. Further indoor pollution is equally responsible for sick building syndrome. Fashion of indoor games, overuse of computers, video, and CD playing facilities, switch over to indoor sleeping patterns, artificial cooling facilities such as cooler and air conditioners, and spending of 50% of their lives (-the ladies), more so with the ill-ventilated kitchens have produced more of respiratory illness, especially in children and ladies, as is evident from the rise in the symptoms of postnasal drip and bronchial asthma by 5%, cough in 10% chronic bronchitis in 20%–30%, and dyspnea in 50% of patients. Periodic attacks of rhinosinusitis, nasobronchial allergy, and wheezing chests are commonly seen in practice where air pollution caused by threshers' use to procure grains is a precipitating factor. In the younger age group, acute respiratory tract infections have shown a rising trend possibly because of indoor pollution and passive smoking, aggravated further by vitamin A deficiency, low birthweight babies (lack of pre- and postnatal care), malnutrition (lack of health education) and improper breastfeeding (urbanizing fashion effect). A person normally inhales 10,000 L of air/day and is likely to get in contact with various irritants, allergens, and infectants. His or her right to inhale fresh air should not be vesicated by man-created pollutants. All MS study in the recent past clearly reveals that an increase of 39% of acute asthma cases and 38% of other respiratory diseases have increased over a period of 2 years. Delhi government has decided to run compressed natural gas (CNG) buses and phase out all diesel vehicles gradually. Also pollution-free vehicle certificates are made mandatory.

Nearly 40,000 people die due to air pollution in America. In India, no such data are available. But cities like Mumbai, Kolkata, Ahmedabad, Kanpur, Nagpur, and Delhi have been facing this problem of rising air pollution, with Delhi being the dirtiest. Thanks to the Delhi Government for taking measures against automobile exhaust pollution by shifting to CNG and ordering the phased removal of diesel vehicles older than 10–15 years. Ludhiana had been declared polluted having 893/$\mu g/m^3$ of SPM by a report city from Punjab Pollution Control Board, Patiala. Late chief minister immediately ordered for cutting down industrial pollution and asked for submitting a compulsory plan for the prevention of water and air pollution through industrial wastes. Alas, only 626 industries could adopt accepted modes. More than 1,200 industries are still causing water pollution and more than 2,200 industries are causing air pollution. Nearly 300 industries have been issued notices to comply with the orders, otherwise would face closure. Political will, people's support, and professional participation are essential for the success of environmental health schemes. Only recently, Deputy Commissioner of Ludhiana has ordered to start CNG buses for public transport numbering 100 *each*, but was able to phase out only 40–50 three-wheelers. Although 6,000 three-wheelers are permitted in the city, 25,000 are running on the roads, adding to air pollution. "Chetna Lehar* has started to use school children to inform them about such polluting vehicles. Should this prove fruitful time will tell.

Infections

Community-acquired pneumonia has been one of the most common respiratory infections worldwide, one of the leading causes of hospitalization, and one of the most common causes of premature death. Though microbiological diagnosis is lacking in more than 50% of cases, *Streptococcus pneumonia*, followed by other organisms, such as *Mycoplasma pneumoniae*, Influenza A virus, and *Haemophilus influenzae* are commonly found as culprits. Less commonly implicated organisms are *Legionella pneumophila*, *Staphylococcus aureus*, and *Chlamydia psittaci*. The trend is ever-rising with changing sensitivity to antimicrobials at times, requiring intensive care as chances of mortality are — three to six times, and treating with a single antibiotic that must cover *S. pneumonia* till reports is awaited. Bacterial infections are responsible for acute exacerbation in 40% of cases in chronic obstructive pulmonary disease (COPD), while viral infections contribute to 30% of cases.

Human immunodeficiency syndrome (HIV) disease

AIDS is the great waster upon the community. The infection is dreaded, tie complications are horrible and chest infections including TB are increasingly seen in these patients. The risk of TB in HIV infection increases by 100 times in endemic areas with old-infected foci due to depressed cell-mediated immunity. The most common complication in all stages of immunosuppression of HIV disease is TB, which is found in 70%–80% of HIV-positive cases in South Africa. In this giant pander — since 1990, the Tambaram TB Sanatorium has seen 3,8941 new TB cases in 1992 which grew to 103,635 in 2001. In a recent US report, China has been listed as a major Asian country to suffer from HIV infection due to the lack of government's commitment, improper health care, unsatisfactory preventive measures, and insufficient local resources. In North India, Punjab has been listed as the leading state in harboring HIV diseases, followed by Haryana and Himachal Pradesh; thus, an alarming situation of an uprise in HIV-related opportunistic respiratory infections should send tremor signals in the health management circles.

At the term of the century, newer opportunistic infections affecting the respiratory system have also emerged such as *Rhodococcus equi* and *Chlamydia pneumoniae* in patients with HIV. The century in the end has also seen zoonotic infections, such as human ehrlichiosis, rodent-borne Hantavirus, and infection from the nasal discharge of sick horses causing equine acute respiratory syndrome. Immunosuppressive therapy has produced complications that lead to a rise in infections such as bacterial pneumonia, cytomegalovirus pneumonia, and other viral infections such as herpes simplex virus and respiratory syncytial virus. Candida and Aspergillus fungal infections have risen in these patients and so there is an increased susceptibility and occurrence of *Pneumocystis carinii* infection.

Drugs

There had been 100,000 deaths in the United States in 1988 due only to medical mistakes. Indiscriminate use of corticosteroids has led to the precipitation or aggravation of various infections including respiratory infections.

Activation of pulmonary TB has been found in 6.5% of cases with the use of corticosteroids. Unsupervised corticosteroids given for certain pulmonary disorders, many a time, complicate other respiratory infective diseases, thus acting as a double-edged sword. This may partly be attributed to illiteracy or ignorance of the patients that they do not report to the attending physicians and go on taking the drug for their relief, forgetting that self-medication is dangerous and ultimately land in complications. Let us do our part of duty as physicians and use these drugs judiciously and for a required period with an educative advice to patients who come for follow-up and gradually taper off, thus working within the latest level of management.

Other drugs that may cause pulmonary disorders include antibiotic drugs, antimalarials, tranquilizers and sedatives, antiarrhythmics, antihypertensive, analgesics, and antiinflammatory drugs. Recently, a rising trend of increased cough and precipitation of asthmatic bronchitis have been observed with angiotensin-converting enzyme inhibitors. Reports of beta-blockers effects and aspirin-induced bronchospasm are documented. Pulmonary disorders due to cytotoxic drugs which are being used extensively in chemotherapy have also been increasingly observed in these patients being treated for a variety of malignancies.

Cases with precipitation of acute bronchial asthma with aerosol therapy have been noted where accompanying gas been found to be culprit. Knowledge about the same shall help in an immediate stopping of using the inhaler. Penicillin and its derivative are also notorious for giving rise to such kind of drug-induced bronchial disorder. Increased use of methotrexate in various malignant and connective tissue disorders as well as in resistant bronchial asthma has been documented for an alveolar and interstitial reaction in the lungs. The same is also seen when bleomycin and busulfan are used. Increased pulmonary vascular disorders are observed when antiarrhythmic drugs in cardiology and when phenytoin and carbamazepine in neurology are used. NFT also produces similar effects. Aspirin has been the culprit due to its significant use in routine and especially in cardiology in producing pulmonary hemorrhage that has also been observed by use of the pills by women (for contraception). A lot number of these cases go unnoticed, and many more remain undocumented.

Drug-induced systemic lupus erythematosus involving pleura and causing pleural fibrosis have been documented in recent years by use of protocol, methysergide, bromocriptine, and ergotamine. The iatrogenic morbidity and mortality showing all during March and April 2000 in Israel during doctors' strike should not surprise. Mediastinal pseudo lymphadenopathy has recently been recorded with the use of phenytoin and even with methotrexate. Documentation of cases of drug-induced eosinophilic lung disease has been tremendous, attributed to drugs like sulfonamides, penicillin, NFT, thiazide, and tricyclic antidepressants. Enhanced use of narcotics and opium derivatives in rural areas has led to wheezing chests, especially in adults.

Other factors

The rising trend of respiratory disorders has also been attributed to decreased body resistance to fight against infections due to undernutrition and improper dietary pattern, lack of regular exercise and changing life-style, and exposure to unnecessary autoexhaust and tobacco smoke (passive effect) in cities and exposure to toxic agroinsecticides in rural areas. Even resistant bacterial chest infections have emerged, possibly because of improper use of antimicrobials for an inappropriate period in an inadequate dose. A rise in asthma cases has been observed in these years, and a rising prevalence from 1.2% to 6.2% in adults has been recorded. The Indian data show a significant increase from 0.6% to 3.4%. The incidence of chronic bronchitis in smoking-related cases has been around 42%. Air pollution–related chronic bronchitis has risen by 2–25 times in reports from different areas, depending on the environmental pollution. Similarly, high prevalence of cough and dyspnea patients in 13% of nonsmokers has been found in patients in Mumbai, being attributed to increasing industrial pollution.

Pulmonary edema due to chemicals, vegetables, drugs, or fragrance spray; humidifier lung disease due to improperly cleaned coolers; and malignant chest disorders in arsenic and nickel polish industrial workers have been observed. Various allergic inflammatory, interstitial, infective, malignant, and obstructive small airway occupational diseases are showing a rising trend. Clinical profile of chronic airflow limitation in patients attending a tertiary care center in India reveals that two-thirds of the cases have bronchial asthma, more than 15% have COPD, less than 15% have obliterative bronchiolitis (OB), more than 5% have bronchiectasis, and more than 1% have occupational airway disease. COPD patients are tobacco inhalers, almost 85% smoke bidies, more than 90% of OB cases are post infections, almost 80% are post-TB an Indian study compared to otherwise infections and collagen disorders in India and post-transplant OB in the west fever airflow limitation is seen in more than one-third of cases of COPD, almost one-third of cases of bronchiectasis, more than one-fifth of cases of asthma and more than half the number of cases of OB.

Almost 15% of cases with COPD, OB, and bronchiectasis develop pulmonary hypertension, while pulmonary hypertension is missing in asthma patients although two-thirds of cases have CAL and one-fifth have severe CAL. Tobacco is the common cause of CAL in COPD, while respiratory infections form an important cause of OB, where past TB-OB is the most common in almost 80% of cases.

In Ludhiana we have found a rising trend in allergic, infective, inflammatory, and airflow obstructive disorders by 2½ times. Even TB has a high prevalence among migrant laborers. The number of patients of TB has risen from one case per month to — one to four cases per week in an OPD clinic. So is the rise in MDR-TB, mostly a secondary type of drug resistance. The risk of getting TB has increased from 3% in 1986 to more than 50% in 1996 and is alarmingly increasing.

Technology[8,9]

Improved diagnostic facilities have improved the diagnostic yield of non-tuberculous respiratory diseases such as sarcoidosis, connective tissue disorders in lungs, pulmonary metastasis, neoplastic lung disorders, and airflow obstructive pulmonary disorders. Newer diagnoses of lymphomas, malignant neurogenic tumors, and malignant thymomas of mediastinum have been documented because of better techniques and hence better therapeutic modalities are planned. Advancement of technology in the form of HRCT helps in determining the characteristic abnormality in fibrotic, granulomatous, and cystic lung disease and tumors and also in determining the activity of the disease and optimal site for biopsy. A rising trend of 4.2–31 cases/10,000 patients admitted in a chest ward and an increase of 414 cases/annum to 658 cases/annum in just 5 years owes much to better diagnostic techniques and some extent to a rising trend of the disease due to certain etiological factors such as smoking and air pollution. Since primary lung cancer in early 60s was rare or very infrequent, a rising trend of bronchogenic carcinoma by 9–10 folds in average smokers and more than 20 folds in heavy smokers narrates the story by itself.

In case of sarcoidosis, which used to be a rare disease in India, 40 cases in even years in 1987, increased through diagnostic facilities by 1–2 cases per week at PGI, Chandigarh explains better diagnostic facilities. Bronchoscopy and transbronchial biopsy have shown a rise in bronchogenic carcinoma from — two to three cases per month to one case per week. Increased documentation of aspergillosis through antibodies and HRCT peaks of enhanced disease awareness and improved diagnostic technology. The incidence of pickup of interstitial lung disease has increased due to easy availability of autoantibody profiles. An uncommon sarcoidosis a decade back is being diagnosed — one to two cases per month with the use of transbronchial biopsy. The awareness of diseases like sleep apnea has pressed for opening of sleep laboratory.

Trauma

Chest problems following chest trauma due to peronalshufie, accident, automobile collision injuries. terrorist's blasts, and police's countr crime action injuries have *been* rising seen during these years. The thrill in speed adds to grievous chest injuries many a times both blunt and penetrating, requiring skilled cardiothoracic management along with interaction of surgeons, pulmonologists, anesthetisis. intensive care physicians and physiotherapists.

In developed countries in the 3 Cs pattern, mortality from car accidents leads ahead of coronary heart disease and cancers, as compared to developing nations, where cancers and car accidents are trying to take the side. In recent years, there is an increase in chest injuries by 25% causing pneumothorax, hemothorax, and injury to great vessels further aggravated by 10%–20% due to chest complications arising out of associated polyfracture and spinal injuries requiring early surgical intervention and ventilatory support. The potential risk of fat embolism and thromboembolism that proves fatal adds the risk of 10% in mortality due to acute respiratory distress syndrome. I affogenic complications have also been increasingly seen due to increased use of chest tubes being inserted in small nursing homes unlike earlier days when insertion of intercostal chest tube was considered only the domain of hospital. Similarly, more and more number of cases of mediastinitis have been documented due to injuries and instrumental by inexperienced endoscopists. At least 10% of patients on ventilators suffer from ventilator-assisted pneumonia. A rising trend in nosocomial pneumonia has been observed in the last few years.

Prevention

a. Steps for the prevention of air pollution:

Since none of the classical pollutants with exception of particular has yet been found in influencing mortality, a strong evidence of relationship between the level of fine particulars and cardiopulmonary illnesses exists, and research and prevention are directed towards its mechanism.

Catalytic converters to be used in new cars (Euro II and III Models). Benzene contents are to be brought down from 3% to 5% to less than 10%, and the sulfur content of diesel is to be brought down from 0.25% to less than 0.1%.

Use of four-stroke engines

Regular check for air pollution of old vehicles, and vehicles older than 10–15 years to be phased out (Government action is evident from the number of vehicles, that is, 30–40 per month has increased to 70–90 per day for air pollution vehicles).

Legislative force to achieve goals for improved air quality

Better traffic management through the avoidance of congestion at peak hours by diversion of traffic and building of new flyovers (bridges). Delhi has taken the lead, and Ludhiana, my city, is gearing up.

Education for ventilated kitchens, safe fuel utilization promoting outdoor games, and avoiding overplaying video games in closed congested rooms.

Avoiding the use of toxic agroinsecticides and covered use of grain thrashers.

b. Antitobacco steps:

Abstinence from tobacco saves 100% from lung cancer and prevents 15%–20% of exacerbation in COPD. Separate scheme plan for tobacco-free atmosphere should be entrusted with responsibility, and answerable to accountability.

Public education and implementation of court's order for prohibition should be result-oriented and time-bound.

Government participation to mobilize other sources of income and not from tobacco and tobacco products at the cost of public health.

The right to inhale clean air by nonsmokers should not be snatched. Supreme Court's order on tobacco ban in public places should be strictly implemented.

c. For occupational disorders:

The government suggested guidelines and safety measures to be strictly followed, and all related legalities to be implemented with strict vigilance and application to prevent occupational respiratory disorders.

Regular inspection of working places especially in silica, talc, coal, and asbestos industries; regular medical check-up of the workers; and shifting of workers' place, duty hours, and even job, shifting to some other department on suspecting minimal signs of developing disease of the respiratory system. Improvement of general health through dietary supplements and educating against smoking.

Radiation-induced chest disorders can be reduced by following guidelines strictly.

d. Infections:

Timely suspecting and instituting proper antibiotic can save 10%–20% of cases of nosocomial pneumonia. Early diagnosis and urgent treatment of CAP at least prevent exacerbation of symptoms in COPD in 50% of cases.

Proper treatment, proper use of drugs, and for a proper duration under medical supervision. Improving environmental sanitation and vaccination cover.

Curb should be on overuse or ill-use of corticosteroids since a large number of cases of dissemination of infection including TB and potential risk of development and metastasis of malignancy owe to immunosuppressive therapy.

HIV

Improving moral values and making people religious to cut down polygamy and educating through deaddiction camps and using safe blood for transfusion to prevent the spread of HIV disease and its related chest disorders.

DOT for TB to be strictly implemented.

HAART to be given to selected patients, CD cells >200/mm^3 is safe.

Trauma

Promoting humanism in police and sending message through public awareness camps to cut down terrorism and crime-related chest injuries.

Chest tube insertion and endoscopic instrumentation by experienced persons only.

Ventilatory-assisted pneumonia can be prevented by EMI-recumbent positioning maintaining adequate endotracheal tube cuff pressures, continuous subglottic aspiration, and use of nasogastric tube to avoid gastric overdistension.

e. Lifestyle and exercise:

Promotion of a healthy lifestyle through regular exercise and breathing exercise training to bring down allergic inflammatory and even infectious respiratory disorders, at least by 20%–25%. Unfortunately, Ludhiana city with a population of nearly 30 lakhs could hardly see 3,000 people going for morning walks or exercising in parks.

Sedentary habits, excessive fatty dietary intake, and regular use of pills (in women) may be responsible for a marginal rise in peripheral vascular disease and pulmonary thromboembolism.

Early chest physiotherapy in patients of polyinjuries, ventilatory support, or cardiothoracic surgery.

Accidents

Display of proper sign boards and proper roads can cut down road accidents. Unfortunately India has 10% of the total global roads, out of which only 1% is safe. Punjab Government is gearing up in this direction.

Driver's capability for a safe drive, people's participation in highway traffic use of seat belts, and use of proper signals can cut down chest injury accidents. Mobile traffic vans have recently been started by Haryana Police. Additionally, they shall help to bring out the injured from the accidental vehicle and are equipped with cutting machines, first-aid team, and mobile ambulance to take the injured to nearby hospitals.

For antiterrorist waves and police-created chest injuries, a peace plan, negotiation, and humanistic approach can only be requested. Medical check-ups of criminals in police remand should be enforced.

Drugs

Mushroom sale of opium and related product should be checked.

Indiscriminate use of corticosteroids should be avoided.

Drugs should be judiciously used and finding an offendant to the respiratory system should be immediately stopped, thus aiming at increasing healthy life, rather than increasing mere life expectancy. Let us all participate to curtail the rising trend in the diseases and disorders of the chest. We all physicians with tunnel vision can carve a niche and travel even in the most curved path to work together for a healthy community. After all, we are also part of it.

Summary[10–13]

A rising trend in respiratory problems has been observed in the last two decades. The Irish Times reported that respiratory diseases are found to be 200% higher. Apart from the actual rise in diseases such as bronchial hypersensitivity, airflow obstructive disorders, and infective diseases of lungs including TB, there has been a tremendous effect on the evaluation of neoplastic diseases as well. The rise in bronchitis, asthma, emphysema, respiratory infection, and lung cancer has *been* attributed to air pollution due to tobacco smoke, agroinsecticides, aeroallergens, autoexhaust, and environmental pollution from incomplete burning of fuels in houses and industries. By 2020, India alone is likely to account for 18% of the 8.4 million tobacco-related deaths. And the real tragedy of COPD is that it is preventable by cessation of tobacco smoking. The rise in infections, especially pulmonary TB, has *been* attributed to the rise in HIV disease in the late decade. Post-traumatic lung injuries have been attributed to increased terrorist activities, blasts at public places, police excesses, and automobile accidental injuries.

A variety of lung disorders have been increasingly described due to increased knowledge about the disease since there is growth and development of pulmonology as a super specialty as well as advancement in the diagnostic facilities in pulmonary sciences. Programs directed and preventive measures suggested towards reducing air pollution from wood fires and incomplete industrial combustion, improving quality of diesel exhaust emission, and developing cleaner modes of transport have been suggested. Preventing allergic and infective chest disorders through bringing about lifestyle changes, self-safety from the modern plague (AIDS), and minimizing or initiating a chain of iatrogenic complications. Decreased body resistance and immunosuppressive effect make people more susceptible to various chest infections including community-acquired pneumonia in which the risk to get hospitalization is aggravated treatment with improper antibiotic treatment given with an inadequate dosage and for an insufficient period. This practice is common in rural areas, where people fall prey to unqualified doctors. Nosocomial infections have also been on the rise in hospitalized patients. Again appropriate urgent measures including appropriate antimicrobial therapy have shown a decrease in mortality by 10%–20%.

Half of what a rich man eats keeps him going and the other half keeps his doctor going. Preventive measures start from reverting to traditional living and eating habits, regular exercise, antipollution stringent measures, a clean transportation system, safe driving within rules and speed limits, safety measures applied, first aid and ambulance shifts to trauma center in case of accidents, proper use of drugs, minimal hospital stay, and avoidance of tobacco, check on opium products and narcotics and restricting the use of open grain threshers and toxic agroinsecticides through education and administrative actions.

Tobacco smoking

Introduction

Smoking is a social evil, and most of the smoking (tobacco)–related lung diseases including COPD and lung cancer are dose dependent, where a cumulative dose of tobacco determines the risk. Pack-year (PY) like parameters have been used to express the exposure to tobacco smoke, where PY means one packet of cigarettes or 20 g of tobacco smoked every day over a course of 1 year. The variability in the number of cigarettes or bidies in the Indian market brings a nonuniformity and *hence* smoking index is used where the number of bidies or cigarettes smoked per day in relation to the number of years (duration) of smoking is accounted. Also there is a difference among the brands in showing differences in the total particulate matter because of nonuniformity and clinical analysis of different laboratories.

Cigarette smoking is a major risk factor for CHD, stroke, lung cancer, and COPD and is even correlated with enhanced mortality from pulmonary TB. Chewing tobacco is associated with similar risks as smoking. However, it has been observed that spirometric measurements show pulmonary physiological abnormalities such as bronchial hypersensitivity may reverse in those with higher smoking index. This is further confirmed by experimental, clinical, and epidemiological studies that a relationship exists between cigarette smoking and a wide range of respiratory diseases. Smoking is not only responsible for lung cancer but also directly linked with enhanced morbidity and mortality from other nonneoplastic respiratory diseases such as chronic bronchitis, emphysema, cor pulmonale, and respiratory infections. US Surgeon General's reports on smoking had, therefore, rightly concluded that cigarette smoking is the largest avoidable cause of death and disability in the United States.

Smoking effects on pulmonary anatomy and physiology

Structural changes include increased mucous formation due to hypertrophy and hyperplasia of mucous glands of large airways. Sputum production is increased, mainly because of the tar contents of cigarettes. Small airways get inflamed; there is hyperplasia of goblet cells and airways get closed because of intraluminal mucous formations. Experimental studies have demonstrated that tobacco smoke damages the tight junction of airway epithelium and facilitates epithelial permeability. This is further supported by the fact that abnormal permeability decreases after cessation of smoking. The abnormal permeability enhances the absorption of inhalant toxins and other aerosols resulting in exaggerated bronchial hyperresponsiveness to inhaled methacholine in both symptomatic and nonsymptomatic smokers. The damage caused to alveolar walls by smoking leads to centrilobular emphysema. This may result in increased influx of neutrophils, which release neutrophil elastase and also activate alpha-1 antiprotease.

Functional changes due to tobacco smoking result from small airway diseases, manifested by an increased closing volume and closing capacity. Small airway dysfunction can occur even in asymptomatic patients. In advanced cases, expiratory flow rates are reduced and the forced expiratory volume in 1 second (FEV_1) can be used as a predictor of the development of obstructive airway disease. Discontinuation of smoking reverses theta!! in FEV_1 similar to nonsmokers, in patients before the age of 40 years.

Chronic bronchitis and emphysema

It is now an established fact that COPD is a smoking-related disease. The pattern is similar in female smokers in the west. The prevalence of chronic bronchitis is high among Indian smokers. Various studies conducted in Mumbai, Northern India, Orissa, and Andhra Pradesh have shown similar rising trends of COPD among smokers. Airway obstruction and increased production of phlegm are commonly seen in smokers, and the airway obstruction reversibility becomes difficult in susceptible smokers. The response to treatment is poor among bronchial asthma patients compared to smoking patients. A steep fall in forced expiratory volume is observed in smokers with hyperbronco reactivity.

Environmental tobacco smoke

Passive smoking or environmental tobacco smoke (ETS) is involuntary or secondary smoking that causes impairment in lung functions and thus exposes the innocents to higher rates of respiratory illness and chronic airway disease. ETS has been associated with lung cancer and bronchial asthma in children and is also responsible for the increased severity of the disease. ETS adversely affects the treatment of asthmatic patients. Airway obstruction worsens due to reflex stimulation of parasympathetic pathways by smoke particles. ETS increases bronchial responsiveness even in non-asthmatic patients, and the respiratory symptoms are more pronounced in these patients. It has been observed that wives of smokers have increased bronchial reactivity to inhaled bronchoconstrictor aerosols due to increased epithelial permeability, which starts with increased absorption of most of the tobacco combustion by-products that these subjects inhale in the company of smoking husbands. This would explain partially the prevalence of chronic respiratory disease and lung cancers in nonsmoking subjects, especially the women in our country.

Parental smoking badly affects and exacerbates respiratory diseases in children. The rate of lower respiratory illness in children has been found to be linearly related to maternal smoking. There is twice the risk of pneumonia and bronchitis among the children of smoking parents during the first year of life. Heavy smoking during pregnancy may have a direct effect on the offspring's subsequent lung functions. Asthmatic children of smoking mothers have lower expiratory low rates than those of nonsmoking mothers. These observations emphasize the adverse effects of exposure to ETS in children.

Exercise tolerance is reduced by smoking even in asymptomatic subjects. The effects are observed even with a single bidi or cigarette smoking. And this reduction goes further in bronchitis patients if smoking is continued due to increased levels of carboxyhemoglobin. Lung infections such as pneumonia and influenza are enhanced in smokers. Postoperative complications are more in smokers. Smoking is an important cause of spontaneous pneumothorax. In synergism with certain occupational exposures such as coal mine dust, grain, and cotton or wool dust, smoking can produce airway obstruction following chronic bronchitis. Significant airway obstruction can be produced by tobacco smoke in silica workers. It increases the risk of lung cancer following chronic occupational exposure in these workers.

Tobacco and 5"P"

Tobacco affects 5"P", that is, poverty, people, politics, policies, and professionals (medical). Although the effects of tobacco are known to all and everyone, it has not been possible to eradicate this social evil because of its unique power that is enjoyed worldwide. Those who favor this evil are virtually involved in its cultivation and processing. Tobacco cultivation does not require intensive irrigation and the income generated to the disciplinary operation among themselves. They must realize that their duty and contribution does not end with disease management alone; they need to extend their responsibility towards the community as well as towards opinion makers of the society to create and develop a healthy atmosphere.

An epidemic of tobacco-related cancers, vascular, heart, and lung diseases including obstructive lung disorders can only be prevented by creating a national coalition of doctors, teachers, religious leaders, and opinion makers to work sincerely in this direction. Those who are afraid of political bosses for their pressure and distance experience would lose the battle by default. The political people are our people, they can be made to understand the gravity of damages caused by tobacco. They can be explained the health effect of tobacco-free environments. They need to be siressed that this can only be achieved through their help and by their action. After all, politicians are also responsible people, they are also open to arguments and pressure and the suggestions which are purely based on medical facts and meant simply for the community well-being. They must be made assured of the ugly heads of tobacco products which are projecting and becoming fashion of every house. They will surely confirm to lend their hand of help to save three million deaths every year that are occurring because of tobacco — the social evil. Can we dream of such a tobacco-free society where no one, not even bollywood star, politician or common man would bow before these tobacco people? Let us not compromise with the health of the people at least!

References and suggested readings

1. Bhatia RS, Vijayan VK. Tobacco and health: what can medical profession do? Lung India. 1994;12:178–185.
2. Pais P, et al. Increased risk of acute myocardial infarction associated with beedi and cigarette smoking in Indians. Ind Heart J. 2001;53:731–735.

3. Bhatia RS. Smokeless tobacco: a challenging smoke. JAPI. 1994;42:344. 1995;1261.
4. Bhatia RS, Sibia SS. ST–T wave change with tobacco snuff as tooth paste. JAPI. 1993;41:668.
5. Chhabra SK, et al. Patterns of smoking in Delhi and comparison of chronic respiratory morbidity among beedi and cigarette smokers. Ind J Chest Dis All Sci. 2001;43:19–26.
6. Bhatia RS. Rise in respiratory problems and their prevention. IN: S Das, ed. Med Update; API. 2003;13:260–267.
7. Bhatia RS. Cardiopulmonary manifestations of tobacco. IN: BB Thakur, ed. Med Update; API. 2000;10716–10718.
8. Kant S, Bhatia RS. Lung cancer. Lucknow, India: JBS Foundation. 2017.
9. Raj M. Air pollution and health hazards. Envir Poll. 2000;1:3–17.
10. Behera D, et al. Passive smoking, domestic fuels and lung functions in North Indian children. Ind J Chest Dis All Sci. 1998;40:89–98.
11. Juidal SK, Vij A. Health effects of air pollution. Med Update; API. 2016;26:969–977.
12. Bhatia RS. Respiratory disease pattern in a private clinic in Ludhiana. Lung India. 1995;13:125–126.
13. Bhatia RS, Singhal M. Bronchial asthma: current trend. Med Update. 1996;817–818.
14. Bhatia RS. Pan masala: why not ban it. JAPI. 1989;37:244.
15. Gupta BK, et al. Cardiovascular risk factors in tobacco chewer — a controlled study. JAPI. 2007;55:27–31.
16. Gothi D, et al. Clinical profile of disease causing chronic airflow obstruction in a tertiary care centre in India. JAPI. 2007;55:551–555.
17. Sharma P. Nicotine quantity and packing disclosure is smoked and smokeless tobacco products in India. 2015;47:440–443.
18. RS Bhatia, Kant S. COPD. Foundation. 2014.
19. Rose MJ, et al. Role of smoking as a modifiable risk factors as a modifiable risk factor in diabetic nephropathy. JAPI. 2016;64:34–38.
20. Johi SR. Tobacco free India — save our childrens. JAPI. 2006;54:605–02.
21. Bhatia RS. Disease of small airway of lung. JIACM. 2001;2:222–224.
22. Bhatia RS. Community acquired pneumonia; emerging aetiology with implications of therapy. IN: YP Munjal, ed. PG Medicine API. 199. 13:275–282.

23. Bhatia RS. HIV and TB: where we stand? IN: SB Gupta, ed. Med Update; API. 2002;12:1180–1193.
24. Vijayan VK. Drug induced resp. diseases. IN: S Chanderekhran, ed. Med Update; API. 1993;3:177–188.
25. Bhatia RS. Enalpril precipitating an attack of asthmatic bronchitis. JAPI. 1994;42–506.
26. Bhatia RS, et al. Diet, disease, drugs: has the change lead to a change? J Diab Assoc India. 1996;36:31–54.
27. Bhatia RS. Humidifier disease. Lung India. 1994;12:198–200.
28. Bhatia RS. ARI in children: our exphence. IN: K Jagadeean, et al., ed. Update Med and Surg. RCPS Glassgow. 1998;162–168.
29. Shankar PS. HRCT of lungs. IN: BC Banal, ed. PG Med. API. 1997;11: 353–359.
30. Jindal SK, Gupta D. Diagnosis and management of sarcoidois: current trend. IN: BC Bansal, ed. PG Med; API. 1997;11:347–352.
31. Gupta A, Prakash C. Ind J Med Res. 2006;14:254–257.
32. Bhatia RS. Rising trend in pulmonary disorders-reasons and remedies. Chest Med. Lucknow: Arora Publ. 2005;4:23–34.
33. Bhatia RS. Tuberculosis and AIDS. JAPI. 2000;48:613–616.
34. Udwadia ZF. The burden of undiagnosed airflow obstruction in India. JAPI. 2007;55:547–549.
35. Aydogdu MO, Altun E, Chung E, et al. Surface interactions and viability of coronaviruses. J R Soc Interface. 2021;18(174):20200798. doi: 10.1098/rsif.2020.0798.
36. Malik C, Khanna S, Jain Y, Jain R. Geriatric population in India: demography, vulnerabilities, and healthcare challenges. J Family Med Prim Care. 2021;10(1):72–76. doi: 10.4103/jfmpc.jfmpc_1794_20.
37. Mills MV. The use of osteopathic manipulative treatment in the newborn nursery and its effect on health in the first six months of life: a retrospective observational case-control study. Complement Ther Clin Pract. 2021;43:101357. doi: 10.1016/j.ctcp.2021.101357.

https://doi.org/10.1142/9789811271410_0012

12 Asthma

Learning objectives from this chapter

1. Understand the burden of asthma in the community.
2. Understand the protective and risk factors for asthma; some risks are preventable and some are not.
3. Understand the various cells and mediators involved in asthma.
4. Understand the structural changes in asthma and early (reversible) and late (irreversible) changes.
5. Understand the clinical features, diagnostic modalities and their usefulness, and differential diagnosis (asthma mimickers).
6. Understand the treatment options and how to select them (based on case studies).

Introduction and epidemiology

Asthma is a very common cause of morbidity and mortality in the world. It affects a large proportion of the population across all ages and genders in both developing and developed countries across the world. In many western countries, the prevalence has reached more than 30% in children. New Zealand, Australia, and the United States have the highest number of asthma prevalence, followed by Europe. Asia has the least number of asthmatics, but many countries in Asia have been observing an increasing trend in the prevalence of asthma. Most studies in India that have been conducting multiple surveys have observed an increasing trend. The largest survey among children in the world is the ISAAC study which was conducted more than a decade back and is being repeated across the world again as the Global Asthma Network study at present (2018–2019). Equivalent large surveys in the world for adults are lacking, though there are large surveys in different countries like the NHANES in the United States, the ECRHS in the Europe, and INSEARCH in India.

Risk factors

Genetics

The key risk factors are the close and complex interactions between the host's genetics and the environment. Studies have been so far unable to pinpoint the exact genetic susceptibilities or the key environmental determinants. It is unlikely to be unraveled in the near future. More than 100 different asthma susceptibility genetic polymorphisms have been identified in different studies and even whole genome screening of large populations has been unable to identify genetic polymorphisms that have stood the test of reproducibility across different populations and ethnicities. Probably the strongest and the oldest of the genetic polymorphisms identified that has stood the test of time has been the ADAM33. Even this gene has multiple polymorphisms (more than 30 have been associated with asthma) that need closer study in different populations that is yet to be conducted.

Common genetic polymorphisms associated with asthma			
Abbreviation	Gene name	Abbreviation	Gene name
ADAM33	Disintegrin and metalloproteinase domain 33	ORMDL3	Orosomucoid 1-like 3
SOD1	Superoxide dismutase 1	iNOS; NOS2	Nitric oxide synthase
CBR1	Prostaglandin-E(2) 9-reductase	CCL5	CC chemokine ligand 5
GSTT1	Glutathione S-transferase	ALOX 15	Arachidonate 15-lipoxygenase

(*Continued*)

(*Continued*)

Common genetic polymorphisms associated with asthma			
Abbreviation	Gene name	Abbreviation	Gene name
TIMP1	Tissue inhibitor of metalloproteinase 1	CMA1	Mast cell chymase 1
CYSLTR1	Cysteinyl leukotriene receptor 1	PTGER2	Prostaglandin E receptor 2
KIT LG	Kit ligand precursor	ADRB2	Beta-2 adrenergic receptor
SPINK5	Serine protease inhibitor Kazal type 5 precursor	PAF1	Peroxisome assembly factor 1

Environment

Many different environmental characteristics influence asthma development. These are important in "switching on" the asthma genes. Asthma genes are fixed features of an individual and cannot be changed. Environmental influences, which have the potential to be modified, are therefore key determinants for preventing or delaying the development of asthma. Therefore, the need to understand these environmental influences at the present time is urgent. Unlike the cardiologists, the respiratory physicians are far behind in both the scope and scale of research into these environmental influences. They know exactly how much salt reduction or intensity of exercise would impact lowering the blood pressure. All the risk factors that have been so far identified have been association studies and in almost all of them the causation is still unclear and the effects of modification are unclear. For example, longer breastfeeding, which is more common in the rural population, is found to be protective in most studies. But if an urban woman were to breastfeed her child for 2 years, what is the risk reduction in the incidence of asthma in her child? It would take decades of research for a clearer picture to emerge and to answer these questions.

Protective factors	Risk factors
Breastfeeding for a longer time	No breastfeeding/infant foods
Rural lifestyle	Western lifestyle
Large family size	Atopy
Diet rich in fiber	Comorbid allergies — rhinitis, atopic dermatitis, food allergy
Gut microbiome	Age, gender, race
Physical activity	Tobacco smoke
Close contact with large farm animals (cattle)	Air pollution (ambient, indoor)
	Infections (especially certain viral)
	Stress
	Obesity
	Maternal smoking
	Pets — some studies (cat)
	Occupational exposures
	High load of allergen exposure during the first year of life, especially dust mites

Pathogenesis

The exact pathogenesis and the exact sequence of gene–environment interactions are still not clear. However, considerable research into certain steps involved in the pathogenesis has given good insight. Two main groups of asthma can be considered. The most common is atopic asthma and then we have non-atopic asthma. The first important step in the pathogenesis of atopic asthma is the development of sensitization to allergens, which is called the intermediate phenotype. The allergens which are mostly inhaled are taken up by the antigen-presenting cell in the airway mucosa. Depending on the presence of available mediators in the airway milieu, the outcome would be the development of tolerance by producing immunoglobulin M (IgM) and immunoglobulin G (IgG) antibodies or the development of sensitization by producing immunoglobulin E (IgE) antibodies. The various mediators and their pathophysiologic effects in worsening or ameliorating allergic inflammation are listed below.

Mediator	Pathophysiologic effects
Mediators that increase allergic inflammation	
IL-4	Promotes Th2 differentiation B-cell isotype switching to IgE Increases chemokine secretion from airway epithelium
IL-5	Migration, maturation, and survival of eosinophils
IL-9	T-cell and mast cell growth factor Airway hyperresponsiveness Leads to elevated IgE Mucus hypersecretion
IL-13	Promotes airway inflammation Mucus hypersecretion Subepithelial fibrosis Secretes eotaxin Increases airway hyperresponsiveness
IL-17	Produced by Th-17 cells and ILC2 Recruits neutrophils into airways Steroid insensitivity Airway remodeling Mucin hypersecretion
IL-25	Produced by airway epithelial cells Promotes Th2 cytokines Airway remodeling
IL-33	Promotes Th2 differentiation that is independent of IL-4, STAT6, and GATA3 Increases IL-5 and IL-13 production Chemoattractant for Th2 cells Increases eosinophil survival

(*Continued*)

Mediator	Pathophysiologic effects
	Maturation of mast cells Airway remodeling Steroid resistance
TSLP	Thymic stromal lymphopoietin Derived from epithelium Increase in antigen-presenting cells promoting Th2 deviation along with IL-33 Inducing Th9 and Th17 differentiation Airway remodeling Regulation of ILC2 Suppression of T regulatory cells
IL-6	Produced by epithelial cells, macrophages, and inflammatory cells On exposure to allergens, RS virus, pollutants Promotes Th2 differentiation Inhibits Th1 differentiation Mucus production Matrix deposition Protease release from granulocytes
IL-2	T-cell activation Non-allergic asthma Reduces steroid responsiveness Increases glucocorticoid receptor beta-subunit
IL-11	Secreted from epithelium. Profibrotic (along with TGF-beta and IL-17) Steroid responsive
TGF-beta	Macrophages, epithelial cells, and eosinophils, profibrotic Promotes type I and III collagen in subepithelial region — remodeling Not responsive to steroids

(*Continued*)

(*Continued*)

Mediator	Pathophysiologic effects
CRTH2	Chemoattractant receptor TH2 Receptor for prostaglandin D2 Increases chemotaxis of Th2 cells, eosinophils, and basophils
GATA3	Transcription factor expressed in Th2 cells Essential for the expression of IL-5 Possible role for expression of IL-4 and IL-13
ROR alpha	Transcription factor expressed in Th2 cells Essential for the expression of IL-5 Possible role for the expression of IL-4 and IL-13
STAT-6	Signal transducer and activation of transcription factors Very important in Th2 differentiation
Protective mediators that reduce allergic inflammation	
IL-10	From T regulatory cells, dendritic cells Potent anti-inflammatory and immunosuppressive cytokine IL-10 is increased on administering steroids and immunotherapy
IFN-gamma	IFN-gamma is a cytokine required for innate and adaptive immunity Counterregulates IL-4 Associated with neutrophilic asthma and steroid resistance
IL-12	Dendritic cells Reduce allergic inflammation Controls antigen-driven Th2 and Th17 responses
IL-22	T-cell, ILC-derived cytokine Proinflammatory with IL-17 Anti-inflammatory without IL-17
STAT-4	Signal transducer and activation of transcription factors Very important in Th1 differentiation
ALX/FPR2	Lipoxin A4 receptors Inhibits NK and ILC2 Lipoxin A4 reduces the severity of asthma

Various cells of the immune system are relevant for developing tolerance or developing allergies and asthma. The key cells and their functions are listed below:

Cells	Pathophysiologic effects
Airway epithelium	Maintains barrier function. Epithelial damage due to virus infections, and pollution could be one of the primary initiating factors in the development of clinical allergy.
Dendritic cell	Important as the antigen-presenting cell. Releases IL-33, IL-25, and TSLP. Interacts with naive T-cell via MHC II for differentiation into Th2 cells.
Th0	These are CD4 cells classified based on their cytokine profile and functions. Can differentiate into Th1 or Th2.
Th1	Th0 differentiates into Th1 in the presence of IL-12 from macrophages. Th1 pathway is protective against allergy. Produces IgM and IgG on exposure to any new antigen.
Th2	Th0 differentiates into Th2 in the presence of IL-4. Th2 releases IL-5 (eosinophil maturation and survival) and IL-13, which affects B cells to "switch" to IgE production.
ILC2	Similar to Th2 cells, lymphoid morphology lacks specific antigen receptors. Express CRTH2 receptors. Secretes IL-5 and IL-13. Promotes airway inflammation.
B cells and plasma cells	Key cells in all aspects of adaptive immune responses. Responsible for the production of IgE antibodies.

(*Continued*)

(*Continued*)

Cells	Pathophysiologic effects
Eosinophil	Important cell in asthma. Eosinophilic inflammation can occur in the airways via two pathways: a. Allergens — dendritic cells (IL-33, IL-25, and TSLP) — Th0 — Th2 differentiation — IL-5 — eosinophilic inflammation. b. Pollutants, microbes — macrophages and natural killer cells — ILC2 cells — IL-17 and TSLP-driven production of IL-5 — eosinophilic airway inflammation.
Basophil	Important in asthma. Correlates well with histamine and late-phase mediators in asthma. Associated with fatal asthma.
Mast cell	Important for immediate/early phase response. Secrete histamine, PGD2, and LTC4.
Neutrophil	Relevant for neutrophilic asthma — an important phenotype characterized by severe treatment-resistant asthma. Reversible neutrophilic asthma is seen in smokers, exposed to indoor air pollutants, which turns eosinophilic once these triggers are removed.

Pathology

Initial pathologic changes in the acute phase are those of a type I hypersensitivity reaction. This leads to mucosal swelling and bronchospasm of the airway smooth muscles and due to recurrent exposures to the allergen and noxious stimuli, chronic inflammation sets in. This leads to various structural changes in the airways and is accompanied by changes in the clinical picture. A summary of the structural changes and the clinical features are enumerated in the box below:

Structural changes	Clinicians perspective
Airway epithelial denudation Subepithelial fibrosis Increased smooth muscle mass Mucosal edema Chronic inflammatory infiltrate with eosinophils, basophils, mast cells, neutrophils, T cells Increased activated fibroblasts and myofibroblasts Vascular changes	Low lung functions Poor response to treatment Disease progression Airway remodeling Persistent airflow limitation Accelerated decline in lung functions Increased bronchial hyperresponsiveness

Clinical features

The clinical features of asthma in a typical case would be cough with thick white sputum unless infected, wheezing, and dyspnea especially in more severe asthma. The symptoms are variable and respond spontaneously or to treatment. In most subjects, symptoms are worse at night than at daytime unless in those who have occupational asthma or asthma due to outdoor allergens. In some cases, symptoms may be limited only to cough (cough variant asthma). The signs include increased respiratory rate, use of accessory muscles of inspiration and expiration, tachycardia, hyperinflated lung fields, hyperresonant on percussion, rhonchi or in severe cases "silent chest," cyanosis, inability to speak a few words or only gesticulation and altered consciousness.

Diagnosis

The diagnosis of asthma is usually straightforward for the pulmonary physician, but not always so. There are cases when the diagnosis is difficult. The common tools that are used for the diagnosis of asthma are good history, clinical examination, pre- and post-bronchodilator spirometry, peak flow monitoring, and in some cases bronchial challenge test. The details of these are listed below:

History	Comorbid allergies such as rhinitis. Family history of allergies. Seasonal symptoms. Seasonal exacerbations. Specific and consistent triggers known to cause a type I hypersensitivity reaction. Quick response to medications.
Clinical examination	Rhonchi. Crepitation may be more dominant in young children. Allergy crease, allergic shiners.
Spirometry	200 mL and 12% improvement in forced expiratory volume in 1 s (FEV_1) after 400 μg of salbutamol.
Peak flow monitoring	Diurnal variation of greater than 20%.
Broncho provocation test Histamine Methacholine Exercise Cold air Hypertonic saline (All the above are not associated with a late-phase reaction and are much safer.) Specific allergen (most dangerous as there is a risk for severe reaction and late-phase reaction as well.)	Generally done when spirometry is normal, but symptoms suggestive of asthma. Methacholine is most commonly used. A 20% drop in FEV_1 is indicative. If there is no drop of FEV_1 by 20% even after 16 mg/mL of methacholine, the test is considered negative and the chance of asthma is highly unlikely at present time. Contraindicated if FEV_1 is below 70% predicted.

Differential diagnosis

There are various asthma mimickers that may obfuscate the diagnosis even for the well-trained physician. Therefore, a high index of suspicion is always needed to think of other diagnoses that may mimic asthma. A detailed history and relevant investigations are warranted. Some common causes are listed below:

Organic disorders	Functional disorders
COPD	Vocal cord dysfunction
Bronchiectasis including cystic fibrosis	Habit cough
Bronchiolitis	Hyperventilation syndrome
ABPA	Panic attacks
Pulmonary embolism	
Lung cancer	
Congestive heart failure	
Hypersensitivity pneumonitis	
Sarcoidosis	
Churg–Strauss syndrome	
Foreign body (children)	
Primary immune deficiency (children)	
Ciliary dyskinesia (children)	
Gastroesophageal reflux disease	
Microaspirations	
Obstructive sleep apnea	
Drug reaction	
Tracheomalacia and laryngomalacia	
Laryngeal web	

Treatment

The mainstay of treatment revolves around adequate patient education and counseling, appropriate pharmacotherapy, allergy avoidance, personal monitoring using a peak flow meter, and in some selected cases immunotherapy. The goal of treatment is said to be met if the subject does not have any daytime and nighttime symptoms, have normal lung functions, normal decline in lung functions in adults and normal lung development in children, no absence from school or work due to asthma, no adverse effects from medications, no emergency room visits, no oral steroid use for managing exacerbations, and no rescue medicine use.

Patient education is the most important aspect of asthma management that helps to overcome simple deficiencies that would otherwise lead to recurrent asthma exacerbations. Most of the subjects do not use inhaled steroids regularly and not in the proper dosage; inhaler technique is inappropriate and has poor coordination. It is always prudent to have the patient demonstrate the inhaler technique in front of you to confirm the proper technique. The language needs to be simple so that the subject can understand the principles of treatment.

Pharmacotherapy remains the mainstay of asthma treatment. The key classes of medications include bronchodilators (rescue medications) and anti-inflammatory medications including inhaled steroids (preventive medications). All these drugs, their dosage, mechanisms of action, and adverse events have been discussed in detail in Chapter 11. Guidelines recommend a stepwise approach to treatment based on the severity of asthma. GINA guidelines and the NAEPP (USA) are good guidelines to follow. Other guidelines are the British Thoracic Society (BTS) and the NICE guidelines. Other national recommendations are generally based on this evidence. GINA guidelines is the most widely followed in the world and recommends five steps of asthma treatment based on the asthma severity. In step 1, one could consider giving low-dose inhaled corticosteroid (ICS), whereas in step 2 one should give low-dose ICS. Other controller options in step 2 are leukotriene receptor antagonists (LTRAs) or even low-dose theophylline. For step 3, low-dose ICS + LABA is the most recommended, while other options include medium- to high-dose ICS, low-dose ICS + LTRA. Step 4 includes medium- to high-dose ICS + LABA as the most recommended and other options include adding tiotropium, LTRA, or theophylline. Step 5 includes all of the step 4 medications and the following as add-on treatments depending on the availability and the cost:

anti-IgE (omalizumab), anti-IL-5 (mepolizumab, reslizumab), anti-IL-5 receptor (benralizumab), oral corticosteroids, and bronchial thermoplasty.

Allergy avoidance is an important part of asthma management. Sensitization to specific allergens can be identified by either the skin prick test (SPT) or serum-specific IgE. SPT is the preferred method since it gives far more important information as compared to serum-specific IgE, which only measures free IgE in the blood and that may or may not be clinically reactive. On the other hand, the SPT measures IgE fixed to the mast cells in the skin and the two IgE antibodies have to be positioned close to each other to elicit a positive SPT, which is, therefore, likely to be clinically more relevant. A good history after the SPT is needed to understand whether the sensitized allergen is indeed clinically relevant.

Complications and risk of death

Asthma is known to be associated with severe morbidity and even mortality. Most of the deaths occur in low and middle-income countries, mostly due to the lack of proper diagnosis and treatment. There are certain features associated with the risk of death from asthma. The most important of these are the following: (1) previous severe asthma attack needing care in the intensive care unit (ICU) and or needing ventilator support; (2) in the last 1 year, three or more visits to the casualty/emergency room for asthma exacerbations; (3) in the last 1 year, two or more hospital admissions for the management of asthma; (4) using two or more rescue medication canisters (SABA) per month; (5) poor perceivers of symptoms and severity of asthma; (6) serious mental health issues and psychosocial problems; (7) illicit drug users; and (8) subjects with poor adherence to asthma medications and asthma action plan.

Key messages

1. Asthma is a common disease among all age groups in the world, and the prevalence and severity of asthma seem to increase over the last few decades.

2. Though the diagnosis seems to be straightforward in many cases, physicians should learn to identify and diagnose atypical cases.
3. A person with lung functions more than 100% predicted can have uncontrolled asthma!!
4. Some asthmatics with predominant mucosal edema may not show immediate bronchodilator reversibility but may show reversibility after appropriate treatment.
5. Allergic rhinitis is one of the most important comorbidities of asthma, and aggressive treatment of allergic rhinitis can prevent asthma in some cases.
6. Even subjects with mild asthma can have a sudden attack leading to hospital admission or death and therefore no asthmatic should be neglected for adequate counseling.
7. ICSs form the mainstay of anti-inflammatory treatment of asthma, and the current recommendation includes the addition of LABA to ICS even for milder cases.
8. Never forget to consider asthma mimickers, especially when the presentation is atypical or there is inadequate or poor response to treatment.
9. The key to successful asthma management in a given case is complete patient education, which should be considered at par with guideline-based management of appropriate medications, adequate dosage, and adequate duration.

Suggested readings

Global Initiative for Asthma. Global strategy for asthma management and prevention. 2019. Available at: www.ginasthma.org.

Scottish Intercollegiate Guidelines Network (SIGN) 50 handbook. Available at: www.sign.ac.uk.

Health Improvement Scotland. BTS/SIGN British Guideline for the management of asthma. 2016. SIGN 153.

Asthma: diagnosis, monitoring and chronic asthma management, NICE nG80, 2017 Nov. Available at: https://www.nice.org.uk/guidance/ng80.

Asthma: diagnosis and monitoring of asthma in adults children and young people. NICE NG 80, Methods, evidence and recommendations. 2017 Nov. Available at: https://www.nice.org.uk/guidance/ng80/evidence/full-guideline-asthma-diagnosis-and- monitoring-pdf-4656178047.

Chronic Asthma Management. NICE NG 80, Methods, evidence and recommendations. 2017 Nov. Available at: https://www.nice.org.uk/guidance/ng80/evidence/full-guideline-chronic-asthma-management-pdf-4656179345.

Case study

Case 1.1. Acute asthma BTS

Case study: Case studies in the management of acute asthma

History: K.D., a 25-year-old girl, is a known case of bronchial asthma for 2 years, presented to the emergency department with complaints of dyspnea and coughing that has progressively worsened during the past 2 days. She is unable to speak in complete sentences; her mother gives the history of use of levosalbutamol + ipratropium bromide inhaler greater than two times a week for the last 1 month. She has had — three to four nighttime awakenings and has experienced mild limitations while undergoing her gym training. She also gives a history of taking a 5-day course of antibiotics 1 week back for her cough. She had been admitted for 5 days with similar complaints 10 months ago.

Physical examination: The patient is tachypneic, anxious, with the use of accessory muscles of respiration. She finds it difficult to speak even a few words. She is conscious, oriented, with a good respiratory effort. K.D.'s vital signs are as follows: respiratory rate, 32 breaths/minute; blood pressure, 130/90 mmHg; heart rate, 129 beats/minute; temperature, 98.6°F, SpO_2 by pulse oximetry is 89% at RA. Chest is hyperinflated with bilateral polyphonic rhonchi.

Question 1: How would you classify the severity of her acute asthma?

Question 2: What investigations would you immediately ask for in the emergency room (ER)?

Question 3: Does this case need admission or can be discharged after treatment in the ER?

K.D.'s investigation reports are as follows:

1. Peak flow meter at the ER showed a peak expiratory flow rate (PEFR) of 80 L/minute. Peak flow of less than 100 is an indication for admission.
2. Chest X-ray: Shows hyperinflated lung fields with no evidence of pneumonia or mucus plugging.
3. ABG: pH — 7.35, PaO_2 — 59 mmHg, $PaCO_2$ — 38 mmHg, HCO_3 — 20 mEq.
4. Complete blood count (CBC): It showed raised total counts with elevated neutrophils and eosinophils.
5. Spirometry: Once she is stable, spirometry has to be done before discharge. FEV_1 >80% and FEV_1/FVC ratio is normal.

Question 4: Is there a change in the classification of asthma severity after investigations?

Treatment plan: After evaluation, the ER resident initiated oxygen (O_2) to maintain SpO_2 of 90% and 2.5 mg of salbutamol by nebulizer every 20 minutes for three doses. After the initial treatment, K.D. claims some subjective improvement and appears to be more comfortable.

Question 5: Would you like to evaluate her treatment plan? What changes would you recommend? Is salbutamol via pMDI and spacer equally effective as a nebulizer in this case? Would you recommend intravenous beta-agonists rather than through a nebulizer?

In her case, apart from the O_2 and albuterol, she should also be started with ipratropium bromide of 0.5 mg via an oxygen-driven nebulizer and prednisolone tablets 40–50 mg/day or intravenous hydrocortisone 100 mg four times a day.

She felt better after 4 hours and her nebulization with both salbutamol and ipratropium bromide was continued every 6 hours, along with parenteral steroids. Her peak flow returned to her best value of 410 L/minute by 24 hours. She was monitored closely for the next 24 hours with peak flow meter monitoring every 6 hours, which varied between 250 and 410 L/minute.

Question 6: Is she ready for discharge? What would her discharge medications be?

Discussion of the case

Question 1: How would you classify the severity of her acute asthma?

Answer: Life-threatening asthma.

A patient is said to have ***acute severe asthma*** if *any one of the following* criteria is satisfied: inability to complete a full sentence in one breath, PEFRs 33%–50% predicted, respiratory rate ≥25 breaths/minute and heart rate ≥110 beats/minute. A patient with severe acute asthma is said to have ***life-threatening asthma*** if *any one of the following* is present: altered consciousness, poor respiratory effort, cyanosis, exhaustion, arrhythmias, hypotension, silent chest, SpO_2 <92%, peak expiratory flow (PEF) <33% predicted or best value of the patient, PaO_2 <8 kPa, and normal $PaCO_2$. It is classified as ***near-fatal asthma*** if the $PaCO_2$ is raised or the patient needs mechanical ventilation with elevated inflation pressures.

Question 2: What investigations would you immediately ask for in the ER?

Answer: Two immediate investigations needed in the ER are chest X-ray and ABG.

Chest X-ray is indicated in a patient presenting to the ER in the following situations: *life-threatening asthma*, suspected pneumonia, suspected pneumothorax or pneumomediastinum, needs mechanical ventilation, or there is a poor response to treatment.

ABG is indicated in a patient with a *SpO_2 <92%* since there is a chance of hypercapnia, which significantly increases the chance of death during an acute asthma attack. ABG is also indicated *in any case of asthma with features suggesting life-threatening asthma*. Hypercapnia cannot be identified by pulse oximetry measurements.

Question 3: Does this case need admission or can be discharged after treatment in the ER?

Answer: This case needs to be admitted to the hospital.

The criteria and indications for admissions when a case with acute asthma presents to the ER are as follows: *any life-threatening asthma* or near-fatal asthma, features of acute severe asthma persists in spite of initial management in the ER, pregnancy, presentation at night, adherence is poor, living alone, asthma attack despite using steroid tablets at the onset of symptoms, previous near-fatal asthma and has psychological problems.

Question 4: Is there a change in the classification of asthma severity after investigations?

Answer: No, it is still classified as life-threatening asthma due to $PaCO_2$ levels just below normal.

Question 5: Would you like to evaluate her treatment plan? What changes would you recommend?

The following changes are needed to provide ideal treatment:

a. Oxygen: Enough oxygen should be given to maintain SaO_2 levels of 94%–98% and not 90%. Oxygen can be given via nasal cannula, face mask, or venture mask. Some patients may find face masks troublesome and claustrophobic. Some patients may breathe only through the mouth and then nasal cannula may be less effective. Unlike in COPD, high concentrations of oxygen can be given in asthma. Even when pulse oximeter is not available, if the clinical signs are suggestive of acute severe asthma, oxygen may be given.

b. Bronchodilators: When asthma is *life-threatening*, salbutamol should be used only via a nebulizer, preferably an *oxygen-driven nebulizer*. When the patient has life-threatening asthma, they may desaturate when salbutamol is given through an air-driven nebulizer. For other asthma attacks, pMDI with spacer is equally effective as a nebulizer. Meta-analysis studies have confirmed that there is no advantage of giving beta-agonists through an intravenous route as compared to the nebulizer. To drive an oxygen-driven nebulization, the minimum oxygen flow is 6 L/minute. Most hospitals do not have the facility for continuous nebulization, which is better than the bolus nebulization routinely followed in most hospitals. Continuous nebulization of salbutamol is given usually at 5–10 mg/hour. There is no added advantage in using high-dose bolus such as 10 mg.

c. Ipratropium bromide: Using ipratropium bromide in addition to salbutamol is more effective than using salbutamol alone. Add 0.5 mg every 6 hours to salbutamol and can be mixed together, which should be used in subjects with life-threatening asthma. The other indication is an insufficient response to nebulized beta-agonists alone.

d. Steroids: Should be started as soon as possible. Oral steroids are as good as parenteral steroids. Prednisolone 40–50 mg/day or hydrocortisone 400 mg/day can be used. It helps to reduce the duration of hospitalization as well as mortality.

Question 6: Is she ready for discharge? What would her discharge medications be?

Answer: No, she is not yet ready for discharge.

The discharge criteria according to BTS recommendations are the following:

She should be on discharge medications for at least 12–24 hours. She is still on parenteral steroids and nebulized bronchodilators. DISCHARGE CRITERIA NOT MET.

Her peak flow rates should be >75% predicted or her best and the diurnal variation needs to be less than 25% — Though she has reached 410 L/minute, which is her best, she has another value at 250 L/minute, and thus her diurnal variation is 39%. DISCHARGE CRITERIA NOT MET.

She needs to be started on inhaled steroids and LABA combination and needs to be stable for 24 hours on oral steroids before discharge.

She needs to be given a peak flow meter and a written asthma action plan before discharge.

Her inhaler technique needs to be assessed and needs regular medication counseling.

She needs to see her doctor 2 days from the day of discharge from the hospital.

If she is not under the care of a respiratory physician, should see one within 4 weeks.

Key messages from BTS guidelines for the management of acute severe asthma

High-dose inhaled β2-agonists is the first-line agent of choice in patients with acute asthma and should be administered as early as possible. Spacer and pMDI is equivalent to nebulized salbutamol in acute asthma but not in acute severe life-threatening asthma or near-fatal asthma when oxygen-driven nebulized salbutamol must be used.

Steroids should be given in adequate doses in all cases of acute asthma attack either orally or parenterally.

Nebulized ipratropium bromide (0.5 mg 4–6 hourly) in addition to nebulized β2-agonist such as salbutamol should be given for patients (a) with acute severe or life-threatening asthma and (b) who have a poor initial response to β2-agonist nebulized therapy.

Supplementary oxygen should be given to any patient who has hypoxemia with acute severe asthma. Enough oxygen should be given to maintain an SpO_2 level of between 94% and 98%. In case pulse oximetry is not available, oxygen must be used.

Case 1.2. Chronic asthma

Case study: Chronic asthma

History: L.P. is a 13-year-old boy weighing 42 kg and is 150 cm tall. He was diagnosed with asthma 1 year back and was prescribed SABA-only treatment. He complained of waking up at night due to cough and daytime symptoms for at least twice a week. He also complained of shortness of breath while climbing a few steps. He gives a history of hospitalization due to exacerbation 3 months back. He has been taking more than 10 puffs of his SABA per day.

When asked to demonstrate his inhaler technique, it is found that he is not able to follow the steps as directed. He does not have any other comorbidities. However, his family history shows that his father is a known case of COPD and is a chronic smoker exposing the child to tobacco smoke.

Physical examination: On auscultation L.P. has diffuse expiratory wheezes. His vital signs are normal.

Investigations:

1. Spirometry: His FEV_1 is 65% predicted before the use of albuterol and improves to 80% predicted 15 minutes after the use of the SABA revealing significant reversibility.
2. CBC: Normal.

Question 1: Is it necessary to reconfirm the diagnosis of asthma in this patient?

Answer: Yes, it is necessary to reconfirm the diagnosis.

This is important to avoid overtreatment and miss other important diagnoses. The variability of symptoms and airflow limitation must be assessed.

If the patient has variable respiratory symptoms and variable airflow limitation, the diagnosis of asthma is established.

If the patient has variable respiratory symptoms without variable airflow limitation, a bronchodilator reversibility test should be repeated. If the test is normal, an alternative diagnosis should be considered.

If the patient has few respiratory symptoms, normal lung function, and no variable airflow, a bronchodilator reversibility test should be repeated. If symptoms emerge and lung function falls, asthma is confirmed. However, if there is no change in symptoms or lung function at the lowest controller, then the controller should be stopped and the patient must be monitored for 12 months.

Persistent shortness of breath and persistent airflow limitation requires stepping up of controller medication for 3 months followed by reassessment.

Question 2: How would you assess the patient's asthma control and severity?

Answer: Asthma control

According to the GINA symptom control tool, L.P. has uncontrolled asthma.

Level of asthma symptom control			
In the past 4 weeks, has patient had	Well controlled	Partly controlled	Uncontrolled
Daytime symptoms more than twice/week? Yes O No O Any night waking due to asthma? Yes O No O Reliever needed more than twice/week? Yes O No O Any activity limitation due to asthma? Yes O No O	**None of these**	**1–2 of these**	**3–4 of these**

Other methods available for assessing symptom control include the following:

1. Simple Screening Tools: Primary Care Asthma Control Screening Tool, 30-s Asthma Test.
2. Categorical Symptom Control Tools: Consensus-based "Royal College of Physicians Three Questions" tool which asks about difficulty sleeping, daytime symptoms, and activity limitation due to asthma in the previous month. Asthma APGAR tool is another example.
3. Numerical Asthma Control Tools: Asthma Control Questionnaire (ACQ) and Asthma Control Test (ACT) involve a set of questions that are scored.

Lung function to assess asthma control

Answer: L.P. has uncontrolled asthma and is at the risk of asthma exacerbation.

Patients with a low FEV_1 (especially <60%) are at higher risk of exacerbation, irrespective of symptoms.

An increase in FEV_1 >12% and 200 mL from baseline in a patient taking controller treatment or in a patient who has taken SABA within 4 hours or LABA within 12 hours suggests uncontrolled asthma.

Severity

Question 3: What are the risk factors in L.P.?

Answer: Uncontrolled asthma symptoms, incorrect inhaler technique, exposure to smoking and one episode of exacerbation in the last 12 months, low FEV_1, high BD reversibility are the risk factors for further flare-ups and persistent airflow limitation in this patient.

The presence of the following factors should be assessed:

1. Risk factors for exacerbation
   a. Uncontrolled asthma.
   b. Medication: High SABA use, inadequate or nor prescribed ICS, poor adherence, and incorrect inhaler technique.
   c. Comorbidities: Obesity, chronic rhinosinusitis, gastroesophageal reflux disease (GERD), food allergy, and pregnancy.
   d. Exposure: Smoking, allergen exposure, and air pollution.
   e. Context: Major psychological or socioeconomic problem.
   f. Lung function: Low FEV_1 and high bronchodilator reversibility.
   g. Others: Blood eosinophilia and elevated FENO.
   h. Ever intubated or in ICU for asthma.
   i. One or more severe exacerbations in the last 12 months.
2. Risk factors for developing persistent airflow limitation
   a. History: Preterm birth, low birth weight and greater infant weight gain, and chronic mucus hypersecretion.

b. Medications: Lack of ICS treatment.

c. Exposures: Tobacco smoke, noxious chemicals, and occupation exposures.

d. Investigations: Low initial FEV_1, sputum or blood eosinophilia.

3. Risk factors for medication side effects

a. Systemic: Frequent OCs, long-term, high-dose, and/or potent ICS, also taking P450 inhibitors.

b. Local: High dose or potent ICS, poor inhaler technique.

Question 4. What steps need to be taken to improve L.P.'s care?

Answer: SABA-only treatment that the patient is receiving is not recommended for any level of asthma. L.P. has uncontrolled asthma, and his therapy needs to be optimized. He must be started with budesonide 200 μg and formoterol fumarate dihydrate 6 μg, powder for inhalation 1 puff twice a day (controller) and as a reliever.

According to GINA-2019, SABA-only treatment is not recommended in adults and adolescents as strong evidence suggests as it increases the risk of exacerbations and asthma-related death and that adding any ICS reduces the risk.

Options for the management of this patient include the following:

1. Treatment with the combination of low-dose ICS-LABA (fluticasone + formoterol/vilanterol/salmeterol, beclomethasone/budesonide/mometasone + formoterol) as maintenance treatment with as-needed SABA as reliever or
2. Low-dose ICS-formoterol as a maintenance and reliever regimen (beclomethasone/budesonide + formoterol) have shown to significantly reduce exacerbation in patients with one or more exacerbations in the previous year. (Hence, the treatment of choice for this patient) or
3. Low-dose ICS plus LRTA or low-dose sustained-release theophylline.

Question 5: How frequently would you monitor the patient? What are the elements that you would monitor? (p. 45)

Answer: Patients with asthma should be reviewed regularly to monitor their symptom control, risk factors, and occurrence of exacerbation, as well as to document the response to any treatment changes. For most controller medications, improvement begins within days of initiating treatment, but the full benefit may be only evident after 3–4 months.

Asthma control, adherence, and inhaler technique should be assessed at every visit. The frequency of visits depends on the patient's initial level of control, their response to treatment, and their level of engagement in self-management. Ideally, patients should be seen 1–3 months after starting treatment and every 3–12 months thereafter.

Question 6: How will you train L.P. in the self-management of asthma?

Answer: The essential components of effective guided self-management education are the following:

1. Self-monitoring of symptoms and/or peak flow: Since there is a change in L.P.'s treatment, he must monitor changes in the PEF, which will help him in assessing the response and early detection of exacerbation.
2. Written asthma action plan: (General) It shows how to make short-term changes to their treatment with changes in their symptoms and/or PEF and how and when to access medical care.
3. Regular review by health care provider:
    a. Asking the patient if they have any concerns. Adolescents may be seen separately from the parents to address sensitive issues and identify beliefs and behaviors that could be barriers to optimal treatment.
    b. Assessing asthma control by reviewing symptoms, PEF diary, asking about the action taken by the patient in a particular situation, and so on.

c. Assessing treatment issues like watching the patient use inhaler, asking about medication adherence and barriers, and reviewing and updating the action plan.

Case 1.3. Difficult-to-treat asthma

Case study: Difficult-to-treat asthma

Mr. R.G. is a 73-year-old retired school teacher from a well-to-do family. He visits your clinic with complaints of shortness of breath, nighttime awakenings for more than once a month, and chest tightness. His family history is unremarkable. He has never smoked or taken any recreational drugs. He drinks alcohol socially.

He is a known case of type 2 diabetes mellitus and hypertension since 10 years on T. metformin 1,000 mg twice daily and T. telmisartan 40 mg twice daily. He takes "painkillers" on and off from the pharmacy for his joint pain.

He had a history of asthma since 15 months with one severe exacerbation 7 months back. During this period he was initially treated with *Levosalbutamol rescue inhaler — three to four times a week*. He continued to have uncontrolled asthma as defined by the GINA and was started with *fluticasone 125 µg 2 puffs twice a day*. He remained symptomatic with the need to use his rescue inhaler — three to four times a week. His treatment was then escalated to *fluticasone propionate 250 µg + salmeterol 50 µg 2 puffs twice a day*. A spirometry was performed with FEV_1 70% of predicted and 13% improvement post-BD. R.G. visits your clinic with similar complaints.

Question 1: What is the current diagnosis of the patient? Does the patient have severe asthma?

Answer: The diagnosis of this patient is "difficult-to-treat asthma." The patient cannot be classified to have severe asthma unless contributory factors such as inhaler technique and adherence have been addressed.

Difficult-to-treat asthma is asthma that is *uncontrolled despite GINA Step 4 or 5 treatment* (e.g., medium- or high-dose ICS with a second controller; maintenance oral corticosteroid) or that requires such treatment to maintain good symptom control and reduce the risk of exacerbations. It does not mean a "difficult patient." In many cases, asthma may appear to be difficult to treat because of modifiable factors such as incorrect inhaler technique or poor adherence, tobacco smoking or comorbidities, or even if the diagnosis is incorrect.

Severe asthma is the subset of difficult-to-treat asthma. It means asthma that is uncontrolled despite adherence with maximal optimized therapy and treatment of contributory factors or that worsens when high-dose treatment is decreased.

Question 2: What steps do you plan to take next?
Answer: A set of investigations is required to rule out other common causes like cardiac disease, GERD, and bronchiectasis.

Investigations:

- **Spirometry**: Initial FEV_1 72% of predicted with greater than 200 mL and 12% improvement post-BD.
- **CBC**: White blood cells: 6,667 cells/mm^3, eosinophils: 6%.
- **Electrocardiogram and echocardiogram**: WNL.

Additional investigations:

- **Computed tomography (CT)**: Normal lung parenchyma with no scarring or bronchiectasis.
- **CT sinus**: Sinonasal polyposis+.
- **Upper gastrointestinal endoscopy**: Normal.
- **ENT opinion**: Normal vocal cord evaluation.

After confirming the diagnosis, the next step is to look for modifiable risk factors.

On questioning, R.G. admits of being forgetful and frequently missing his medications lately. He also confides taking less than the prescribed puffs as his friend told him that it was unnecessary and taking steroids on regular basis could "harm" him. This is a clear case of poor medication adherence due to unintentional (forgetfulness) and intentional (concerns about side effects) factors.

The patient needs to be given a method for reminding inhalers (setting an alarm in the morning and evening) and counseled about the critical importance of long-term controller therapy with steroids. Assuring him that adherence to the regimen could help him control asthma and provide a chance to step down ICS, educating him about the difference between oral steroids and the recommended inhaled steroids, which have very minimal and non-threatening side effects like cough, dysphonia, oral thrush which could be easily managed if they do occur.

Poor medication adherence in asthma

1. Factors contributing to poor adherence in asthma

- **a.** Medication/regimen factors
    - **i.** Difficulty using inhaler device (e.g., arthritis)
    - **ii.** Burdensome regimen
    - **iii.** Multiple different inhalers
- **b.** Unintentional poor adherence
    - **i.** Misunderstanding about instructions
    - **ii.** Forgetfulness
    - **iii.** Absence of a daily routine
    - **iv.** Cost
- **c.** Intentional poor adherence
    - **i.** Perception that treatment is not necessary
    - **ii.** Denial or anger about asthma or its treatment
    - **iii.** Inappropriate expectations
    - **iv.** Concerns about side effects (real or perceived)
    - **v.** Dissatisfaction with health care providers

vi. Stigmatization
vii. Cultural or religious issues
viii. Cost

2. **Identification of poor medication adherence in clinical practice**
   a. Ask empathetic questions
   b. Check medication usage and pharmacy refills
   c. Use devices with dosage counters
3. **Examples of successful adherence interventions**
   a. Shared decision-making for medications/dose choice
   b. Inhaler reminders, either proactively or for missed doses
   c. Prescribing low-dose ICS once daily instead of twice daily
   d. Home visits for a comprehensive asthma program by an asthma educator

Question 3: After your thorough counseling session, you told R.G. to review after 3 months. However, he comes to your clinic just after 1 month of his previous visit. He assures you that he has been following his treatment regimen as directed but with only mild improvement in the symptoms, which troubles him more than thrice a week and sleep disturbance more than twice a week. With only a slight impairment of lung functions can this case be called as a "severe asthma." What is your plan of action?

Answer: A subject can have severe asthma even with a lung function of 100% predicted. So, this case can be now classified as severe asthma. The patient's inflammatory phenotype (type 2 or non-type 2) should be assessed. The patient should also be asked for additional investigations.

FeNO: 20 ppm.
Allergy skin test: Negative.
Total IgE: 20 IU/mL.
Blood eosinophil: 600/μL.

The patient has evidence of type 2 inflammation and should be now considered for add-on biologic type-2 targeted treatment.

Type 2 inflammation is found in ~50% of people with severe asthma. The possibility of refractory or type 2 inflammation should be considered if any of the following are found while the patient is taking high-dose ICS or daily OCS:

- Blood eosinophils ≥150/μL.
- FeNO ≥20 ppb.
- Sputum eosinophils ≥2%.
- Asthma is clinically allergy driven.
- Patients requiring maintenance OCS may also have underlying type 2 inflammation.

Consider repeating blood eosinophils and FeNO up to three times before assuming asthma is non-type 2, on the lowest possible OCS dose.

Question 4: Is the patient eligible for an add-on type-2 targeted biologic? If yes, which one would you consider?

Answer: Yes, the patient is eligible for an add-on biologic. In view of a low total IgE and negative SPTs and high blood eosinophils, he should be started with mepolizumab (anti-IL-5), 100 mg subcutaneous injection 4-weekly for at least 4 months, rather than omalizumab.

Criteria for add-on type-2 targeted biologic:

- Affordability and availability.
- Patients with exacerbation and poor symptom control on high-dose ICS-LABA who
  - have eosinophilic or allergic biomarkers or
  - need maintenance OCS.
- Consider cost, frequency, dosing, route, and patient preference.
- Consider local payer eligibility criteria and predictors of response when choosing between therapies.

Drug	Patient eligibility	Predictors of good response
Anti-IgE ▪ Omalizumab	▪ Sensitization on skin prick testing or specific IgE ▪ Total serum IgE and weight within the dosage range ▪ Exacerbations in last year	▪ Blood eosinophils ≥260/μL++ ▪ FeNO ≥20 ppb + ▪ Allergy-driven symptoms + ▪ Childhood-onset asthma +
Anti-IL-5/anti-IL-5R ▪ Mepolizumab ▪ Benralizumab	▪ Exacerbations in last year ▪ Blood eosinophils ≥300/μL	▪ Higher blood eosinophils +++ ▪ More exacerbations in the previous year +++ ▪ Adult-onset asthma + ▪ Nasal polyposis ++
Anti-IL-4R ▪ Dupilumab	▪ Exacerbations in last year ▪ Blood eosinophils ≥150/μL or FeNO ≥25 ppb	▪ Higher blood eosinophils +++ ▪ Higher FeNO +++

Question 5: R.G. enters your clinic for your review after 4 months. You are delighted to know that he is responding well to your treatment. R.G. wants to know if he should still continue taking all the drugs.

Answer: R.G. has to continue mepolizumab at least for a total of 12 months. Biologics can be withdrawn only when he remains well-controlled on medium-dose ICS + LABA therapy. However, conversion of high-dose fluticasone + salmeterol inhaler to medium dose could be attempted after 3–6 months if he remains stable.

If the patient has a good response, consider the following:

1. Oral treatments: Reducing or stopping OCS should be considered first due to its adverse effects.
2. Inhaled treatments: ICS + LABA dose can be reduced after 3–6 months, but not stopped completely.
3. Biologic treatments: Generally, in a patient with good response, a trial of withdrawal of biologic should not be considered until after at least 12 months of treatment, and only if asthma remains well-controlled on medium-dose ICS therapy, and (for allergic asthma) there is no further exposure to a previous well-documented allergic trigger.

Case 1.4. AIA

Case study: Aspirin-induced asthma

History: T.J. is a 31-year-old woman who had a known case of asthma since childhood presented to the EMD with complaints of shortness of breath, rhinorrhea, nasal congestion, and exacerbation of asthma since morning. Her sister gives a history of T.J. consuming T. aspirin 150 mg in the morning for headache and she developed the symptoms within 1 hour after taking the tablet. T.J. is on regular medications levosalbutamol and ipratropium bromide inhaler. Her sister claims that T.J. had developed this kind of reaction for the first time and gives a safe history of aspirin use before. Her sister also gives the history of T.J. having a common cold 15 days ago.

Physical examination: The patient is conscious, oriented, and able to talk in words rather than sentences. Loud wheezing sounds are heard, and she is tachypneic and is using accessory muscles of respiration. Suprasternal retractions are present. Nasal polyps are present. Her vitals are as follows: respiratory rate: 35 breaths/minute; blood pressure: 90/60 mmHg; heart rate: 126 beats/minute; SpO_2: 88% at RA. Rhonchi are heard.

Question 1: Why did she react to the drug, if she was tolerant to aspirin before?

This might be a case of aspirin-induced asthma. Aspirin exacerbated respiratory disease (AERD) is an inflammatory condition characterized by the triad of asthma, rhinosinusitis, and sensitivity to aspirin. AERD is also known as Samter triad, aspirin triad, aspirin-induced asthma, aspirin-sensitive asthma, and aspirin-intolerant asthma. AERD is an acquired disorder that usually peaks around the third or fourth decade of life, for this reason, the patients usually do not report any previous history of rhinitis or asthma following the consumption of aspirin or other non-steroidal anti-inflammatory drugs (NSAIDs).

Question 2: How would you confirm she has aspirin-induced asthma? What diagnostic tests and investigations are to be carried out?

She is suspected to have aspirin-induced asthma because typically the symptoms occur within a few minutes to hours following the ingestion of aspirin, which is seen in this patient's case. Clinical presentation of aspirin-induced asthma is rhinorrhea, nasal congestion, wheezing, shortness of breath, exacerbation of asthma after ingestion of aspirin or other NSAIDs, and the presence of nasal polyp.

Aspirin-induced asthma should be suspected when the following exist:

1. A history of exacerbation of asthma after ingestion of aspirin.
2. Chronic and intractable nasal congestion and watery rhinorrhea, especially if specific IgE tests are negative.
3. Nasal polyposis.
4. Total or near-total opacification of the sinus cavities as demonstrated by CT scan.

(Healthy sinuses on radiographs and CT scan demonstrate the likelihood of having aspirin-induced asthma is low. Evidence of IgE-mediated upper and lower airway diseases has a low incidence of aspirin-induced asthma.)

We can confirm her case as aspirin-induced asthma by performing an aspirin challenge.

Investigations:

CBC: Showed elevated eosinophil counts.

Question 3: What is the management plan for her?

For asthma, standard therapies including ICSs with or without a long-acting beta-agonist and as needed short-acting beta-agonist to be prescribed in accordance with the established asthma guidelines. Individuals with aspirin-induced asthma occasionally require systemic corticosteroids in addition to their regular maintenance therapy.

Leukotriene inhibitors, such as zileuton, which inhibits 5-lipoxygenase and leukotriene receptor antagonists, such as montelukast and zafirlukast are used to treat aspirin-induced asthma.

Omalizumab is an anti-IgE monoclonal antibody. It is reported to be beneficial in the treatment of patients with AERD, even though the primary pathophysiologic disturbance of leukotriene overproduction and the adverse reaction to aspirin ingestion are not thought to be IgE-mediated. Omalizumab is currently indicated for use in severe asthma.

For the management of chronic rhinosinusitis, intranasal corticosteroids should be used. Intranasal corticosteroids have also been associated with a reduction in polyp regrowth and improved control of rhinitis symptoms.

Surgical management: Patients with AERD are more likely to have the recurrence of nasal polyposis following surgery than patients with other forms of nasal polyposis. Surgical benefits seem to be preserved when performed in conjunction with aspirin desensitization. Aspirin desensitization is usually performed 1 month after surgery so as to avoid the risk of postoperative epistaxis from platelet inhibition. Aspirin therapy is not known to shrink the existing polyp burden, but it does seem to prevent polyp regrowth, with an overall reduction of half in the use of systemic corticosteroids and improvement in rhinitis and asthma.

Question 4: What is aspirin desensitization? Is it recommended?

Challenge versus desensitization

Graded drug challenge entails cautious administration of increasing doses of medication. Such challenges are not intended to induce drug tolerance.

Drug sensitization, also referred to as temporary induction of drug tolerance, is performed when there is a high likelihood of drug hypersensitivity and the medication is necessary for patients.

Both graded challenge and desensitization are used in the diagnosis and treatment of AERD. Graded challenge may be performed alone to simply confirm or refute the diagnosis of AERD. However, challenge and desensitization are routinely combined in AERD for diagnostic and therapeutic purposes; these terms are often used interchangeably.

Candidate selection

Appropriate candidates should include those with poorly controlled symptoms despite standard therapies, frequent need for systemic corticosteroids, regrowth of nasal polyps, and/or indication for aspirin or other NSAIDs for the treatment of comorbid conditions.

Absolute contraindications should be assessed including pregnancy, unstable asthma, FEV_1 less than 60% predicted, and aspirin-specific contraindications such as gastric ulcers and bleeding disorders.

Prechallenge considerations

It is vital to ensure that patients are medically stable and optimized for desensitization to minimize the impact of reactions when they occur.

- Patients with active infections, allergic rhinitis, and gastroesophageal reflux should be treated with appropriate pharmacologic and non-pharmacologic interventions prior to desensitization.
- For asthma, it is recommended that all patients continue their current controller medications. This may include ICSs with or without a long-acting beta-agonist, as well as oral corticosteroids if indicated.
- FEV_1 should be at least 60% of predicted values.

- If the patient is not already taking leukotriene-modifying drugs, this should be started at least 1 week prior to desensitization. Patients on leukotriene-modifying drugs premedication tend to have less severe bronchospasm during the challenge.
- Nasal decongestants and oral antihistamines should be withheld 1 week prior to desensitization to allow the clinician to adequately assess if an upper airway reaction occurs.
- It is suggested that those with nasal polyps undergo sinus surgery prior to aspirin desensitization.
- On the day of desensitization, it should be confirmed that the patient used their asthma controller medications and leukotriene-modifying drugs that morning.

Aspirin desensitization

Small incremental dosage causes decreased leukotriene production, down-regulates cysteinyl leukotriene receptors, and reduces histamine and tryptase release from mast cells.

Oral and inhalational agents have been used for NSAID challenge, and both are effective.

In general, patients are treated with incremental doses of aspirin over set time intervals. After a positive response to aspirin and subsequent

Oral aspirin challenge in patients with suspected AERD			
Time	Day 0 (or 1)*	Day 1 (or 2)	Day 2 (or 3)
8 am	Placebo	20–40 mg	100–160 mg
11 am	Placebo	40–60 mg	160–325 mg
2 pm	Placebo	60–100 mg	325 mg

*A placebo challenge can be conducted the week before. Alternatively, if the patient's baseline FEV_1 is the same as their prior best value and they have not used their albuterol rescue inhaler in the past week, you can skip 1 day placebo challenge. If a patient has not reacted to 325 mg of ASA, they will not react to 650 mg. Therefore, if no reaction occurs in 3 hours after ASA of 325 mg calls it a negative challenge.

recovery, the dose at which the response occurred is repeated until no reaction occurs and the dose is increased until a maximum dose is reached. The desensitized state only exists as long as regular aspirin continues to be administered, an interruption of 1–5 days returns the patient to a desensitized state.

1. Measure FEV_1 every hour and wait for 3 hours between doses.
2. FEV_1 should be at least 1.5 L and >60% of predicted.
3. Reactions can be
   a. Naso-ocular alone.
   b. Naso-ocular and ≥15% decline in FEV_1.
   c. Lower respiratory reaction only (FEV_1 declines by 20%).
   d. Laryngospasm with or without a, b, c.
   e. Systemic reactions: hives, flush, gastric pain, hypotension.
4. Aspirin desensitization:
   a. After a reaction has been treated and resolved, go to b.
   b. Repeat the ASA-provoking dose.
   c. If no reaction, continue to escalate the doses.
   d. At 325 mg of ASA, desensitization is always completed.
   e. Give 650 mg as the first dose and then treat with 650 mg twice daily.

Intranasal NSAID challenge

Parenteral ketorolac can be diluted in saline and administered intranasally as an NSAID challenge to diagnose AERD. Patients received increasing doses of intranasal ketorolac at 30-minute intervals. In countries outside the United States, aspirin-lysine is available for bronchial or nasal inhalation. Similar to the ketorolac challenge, the procedure involves administering increasing doses of aspirin at 30-minute intervals.

Advantages to bronchial/nasal challenge

- Symptoms induced by bronchial or nasal challenge tend to be less severe and more quickly reversible relative to oral challenges.
- Bronchial/nasal challenges can be performed more quickly.
- Nasal administration is safer for patients whose FEV_1 precludes oral challenge.

Disadvantages to bronchial/nasal challenge

- There is some evidence that challenge with these agents may be less sensitive as compared with oral challenge, thus leading to potential false-negative results.
- Nasal inhalation cannot be done in patients with complete or severe nasal obstruction secondary to polyposis.

Desensitization begins with an increasing number of sprays of intranasal ketorolac administered at 30-minute intervals. Following a dose of 7.56 mg of ketorolac (6 sprays), desensitization proceeds with oral aspirin dosing. Two consecutive doses of 60 mg aspirin are administered 90 minutes apart. The patient is then observed for an additional 3 hours prior to discharge. After returning on day 2, 150 mg of aspirin is given, followed by a final dose of 325 mg 3 hours later. Again, the patient is observed for 3 hours prior to discharge. Reaction at any time during desensitization confirms NSAID sensitivity.

Time	Dose of ketorolac (in mg) or oral aspirin (in mg)
Day 1	
08:00 am	Ketorolac 1.26 (1 spray in one nostril)
08:30 am	Ketorolac 2.52 (1 spray in each nostril)
09:00 am	Ketorolac 5.04 (2 sprays in each nostril)
09:30 am	Ketorolac 7.56 (3 sprays in each nostril)
10:30 am	Aspirin 60
12:00 pm	Aspirin 60

(*Continued*)

(*Continued*)

Time	Dose of ketorolac (in mg) or oral aspirin (in mg)
03:00 pm	Instructions and discharge
Day 2	
08:00 am	Aspirin 150
11:00 am	Aspirin 325
02:00 pm	Instructions and discharge

Question 5: What would be her patient counseling points?

- Should be advised to avoid aspirin and products containing aspirin.
- Acetaminophen or salsalate are recommended for headaches and relatively minor pain.
- Patients with aspirin-induced asthma can also safely take sodium salicylate, salicylamide, choline magnesium trisalicylate, benzydamine, chloroquine, azapropazone, and dextropropoxyphene.

Case 1.5. Asthma in pregnancy

Case study: Asthma in pregnancy

J.Y., a 25-year-old woman, is a non-smoker and is a known case of asthma since childhood presented to the clinic with complaints of gradual onset of wheezing, cough, and chest tightness for the last 4 weeks and claims that the symptoms worsen at night. She is 24 weeks pregnant with her first child. She gives a history of minimal relief from the use of her reliever inhaler. She has no complaints of fever or pain.

On examination, she is able to communicate in words, with an occasional cough. Diffuse wheezes and rhonchi are heard on auscultation and she is tachypneic. Her vitals are as follows: respiratory rate: 29 breaths/minute, heart rate: 89 beats/minute, SpO_2: 91% at room air, pulsus paradoxus present, FEV_1 >80%.

Her ABG shows hyperventilation with a subsequent respiratory alkalosis (pH:7.42,$pCo2$:30 $mm\ Hg$,$pO2$:95 $mm\ Hg$,$bicarbonate$:28 mEq/L).

Question 1: What changes can be seen in the pulmonary function during pregnancy?

In pregnancy, there is an increase in oxygen consumption by 20% to support the increased maternal metabolic rate.

Functional residual capacity — the amount of air remaining in the lungs during normal breathing is decreased by 17%–20%; residual volume — the air remaining in the lungs after maximal expiration is decreased by 20%–25%; tidal volume — the air displaced between inhalation and exhalation with no extra effort is increased by 30%–50%; expiratory reserve volume — the air that can be further pushed out at the end of normal expiration is decreased by 5%–15%; minute volume/ventilation — the volume of air inhaled in 1 minute is increased by 30%–50%.

FEV_1 and PEFR are not changed during pregnancy and therefore can be used for assessing pulmonary function during pregnancy.

$PaCO_2$ is generally low during pregnancy due to hyperventilation. The ABG is altered during pregnancy, and respiratory alkalosis is presented.

$$pH{:}7.4\text{–}7.45, PaCO_2{:}28\text{–}32\ mmHg, PaO_2{:}greater\ than\ 100\ mmHg,$$
$$HCO_3{:}18\text{–}31\ mEq/L$$

Question 2: What will be the differential diagnosis?

Every pregnant woman with asthma who develops worsening breathlessness has to be evaluated for conditions, such as pulmonary embolism, pneumonia, and pulmonary edema.

Pulmonary embolism typically presents with an acute respiratory distress with or without tachycardia, cough, chest pain, and hemoptysis. Signs of leg swelling may be present. Pneumonia also presents with shortness of breath in the setting of productive cough, pleuritic chest pain, and fever. In asthma patients, pneumonia can trigger an exacerbation. Pneumonia can be distinguished by an increased white blood cell count, and infiltrate on chest X-ray is observed. Pulmonary edema can be confirmed by chest X-ray.

J.Y. was evaluated to rule out pulmonary embolism, pneumonia, and pulmonary edema.

Her chest X-ray was found to be normal, and her complete hemogram was also normal

$$[Hb:11.5\frac{gm}{dL}(11-14);WBC:6930\frac{cells}{mm^3}(4{,}000-11{,}000);$$

$$DLC{:}N{:}86.8\%(40\text{–}75),L{:}\ 09\%\ (20\text{–}40),M{:}3.8\%\ (2\text{–}8),$$
$$E{:}0.1\%\ (0\text{–}4),B{:}0.3\%\ (0\text{–}1);$$

$Platelet:1.83\frac{lakhs}{mm^3}(1.5-4.0);RBC:4.04\frac{million}{mm^3}(4.5-5.5)$], this confirms no pulmonary edema and pneumonia in her case.

D-dimer levels are raised in normal pregnancy, particularly in the second and third trimesters. Clinical prediction rules used in the non-pregnant population, such as the modified Wells score are not validated for use in pregnancy due to poor positive predictive values. There is a pregnancy-specific scoring system (the "LEFT" rule) to predict the likelihood of a diagnosis of DVT: (1) left leg presentation, (2) ≥2 cm calf circumference difference, and (3) first-trimester presentation. It is suggested that all pregnant women with suspected pulmonary embolism should undergo bilateral duplex ultrasound scanning of the lower limbs prior to any objective testing for pulmonary embolism. This is because treatment for both conditions — DVT and pulmonary embolism — is the same and if DVT is detected in the ultrasound, then it would avoid further testing and subsequent radiation exposure to both mother and the fetus from CT pulmonary angiography.

If the Doppler ultrasound test is, then all patients should be referred for CT pulmonary angiography. All neonates exposed to iodinated contrast in utero should have their thyroid function tested in the first week of life because of the risk of contrast-induced hypothyroidism can occur. Other investigation can be ECG. In one study, ECG abnormalities were seen in approximately 40% of pregnant women with acute pulmonary embolism.

These changes include T-wave inversion, evidence of right heart strain, and the classic $S_1Q_3T_3$ pattern.

In J.Y.'s case, she has no complaints of unilateral left leg swelling or pain and her chest radiography is normal. In the chest radiography, one can identify the abnormal features that can be attributed to pulmonary embolism, which include pulmonary edema, pleural effusions, and focal opacities.

Based on her presentation and examination, she was diagnosed with an exacerbation of asthma likely triggered by pregnancy.

Question 3: What are the effects of pregnancy on maternal asthma?

1. Hormonal influences:

   Increases in maternal hormones during pregnancy may contribute to physiological changes that result in improved asthma.

   For example, progesterone may contribute to improved asthma via increased minute ventilation or smooth muscle relaxation. Alternatively, progesterone-induced changes in beta-2 adrenoreceptor responsiveness and airway inflammation and airway inflammation may contribute to worsening asthma during pregnancy.

2. Maternal inflammation and immune function:

   During pregnancy, there are alterations in the maternal immune system, which are important to ensure a successful pregnancy, including a suppression of cell-mediated immunity and the development of a predominantly Th2 cytokine environment.

   It has been shown that the placenta has a high Th2:Th1 cytokine ratio. It is found that this Th2:Th1 predominance was significantly greater in placental samples collected from women with asthma who did not use ICS treatment during pregnancy, suggesting that the Th2 environment of pregnancy may be further enhanced when the mother has asthma. This may contribute to worsening asthma in some women.

3. Influence of fetal sex:

   It has been suggested that maternal asthma symptoms may be influenced by the fetus. Beccroft et al. reported that more mothers of girls reported shortness of breath, nocturnal waking, and worsening of cough and asthma, in general. While mothers of boys were more likely to report an improvement in asthma during pregnancy. Dodds et al. also reported fewer asthmatic women pregnant with boys required steroids for treatment (14%) compared to asthmatic women pregnant with girls (20%) suggesting better-managed asthma in the women pregnant with a male fetus.

Question 4: How will you manage asthma in pregnancy?

Immediate management:

- Measurement of FEV_1/PEFR.
- Give supplemental inhaled O_2 to keep oxygen saturation >94% in order to prevent maternal and fetal hypoxia.
- Administer inhaled albuterol via nebulizer with oxygen every 20 minutes up to three doses in the first hour.
- If no improvement is seen or if severe exacerbation, give intravenous or oral corticosteroids.
- Continuous external fetal monitoring for those >24 weeks of gestation.
- Provide ample hydration with intravenous fluids, if oral intake is not possible.

According to the BTS-SIGN (Scottish Intercollegiate Guidelines Network) guidelines, drug therapy should be given for a non-pregnant patient with acute asthma including nebulized beta-2 agonists and early administration of steroid tablets. In severe cases, intravenous beta-2 agonists, aminophylline or intravenous bolus magnesium sulfate can be used. The risk of harm to the fetus from severe or chronically undertreated asthma outweighs any small risk from the medications used to control asthma.

GINA guidelines suggest the use of ICS, beta-2 agonists, and montelukast or theophylline is not associated with an increased incidence of fetal abnormalities. The use of ICS reduces the risk of exacerbation of asthma during pregnancy.

Pharmacological treatment:

- ICSs, short- or long-acting beta-2 agonists and theophylline do not increase the risk of maternal or neonatal outcomes, such as pre-eclampsia, fetal congenital malformations, low birth weight, or preterm delivery. Therefore, good asthma control remains the aim during pregnancy.
- ICSs are the standard anti-inflammatory therapy for asthma.
- The safety of LABA prescribed alone in the absence of ICSs is controversial with respect to asthma control and thus they should always be used together with an ICS.
- Theophylline is safe in pregnancy at recommended doses. However, plasma levels need to be monitored as the protein binding of theophylline is affected during pregnancy.
- Oral corticosteroids have been shown to increase the risk of fetal cleft lip or palate in the first trimester. However, this risk is small (<0.3%); therefore, oral corticosteroids can be prescribed when required but should be used with caution.
- Leukotriene modifiers can also be used in mild-to-moderate asthma and are known to have a good safety profile.

Acute exacerbation during labor and delivery is uncommon, but bronchoconstriction may be induced by hyperventilation during labor and should be managed by SABA.

Neonatal hypoglycemia may be seen, especially in preterm babies, when high doses of beta-2 agonists have been given within the last 48 hours prior to delivery.

Treatment for acute exacerbation:

Inhaled albuterol every 20 minutes should be established followed by the administration of oral or intravenous corticosteroids. Nebulized ipratropium bromide at 0.25–5 mg every 30 minutes for three doses should also be added to this regimen, if the patient has an FEV_1 less than 40% or initially does not respond to albuterol.

A biophysical profile, including a non-stress test for reactive fetal heart rate, measurement of the amniotic fluid volume by ultrasound, observation for the presence of gross movements, fetal breathing movements, and fetal heart tones should be performed.

Evaluation of the initial therapy should be done every 30–60 minutes and decision regarding admission or discharge should be done after 4 hours of the initial evaluation. If the patient responds well and is discharged, then 5–10 days course of prednisone should be prescribed to prevent early recurrence of symptoms.

Question 5: When is hospitalization recommended?

Hospitalization is indicated in patients who have a moderate to severe exacerbation or do not respond to the initial therapy and if oxygen saturation remains <95% at room air, if FEV_1/PEFR are persistently below 70%, or if there is evidence of fetal compromise.

ICU admission or intubation is indicated in those with life-threatening asthma who is not responding to bronchodilators and corticosteroids. Indications include a pCO_2 >40 mmHg on ABG, mental status changes, maternal exhaustion, respiratory acidosis, or fetal distress.

Systemic administration of epinephrine should be avoided during pregnancy because of its teratogenic effects and placental and uterine vessel vasoconstriction.

Terbutaline can be administered subcutaneously, 0.25 mg every 15–30 minutes for three doses, if the bronchoconstriction does not improve.

Intravenous magnesium sulfate 1–2 g over 30 minutes can be considered in severe acute asthma exacerbation.

The other conditions that may aggravate asthma such as allergic rhinitis and GERD should be aggressively treated. Intranasal corticosteroids are the therapy of choice for allergic rhinitis due to their limited systemic effects. Second-generation antihistamines can be safely used, but combinations with pseudoephedrine are contraindicated due to potential fetal side effects.

Question 6: When can a patient be discharged?

Patients whose FEV_1 or PEFR measurements are ≥70% sustained for 60 minutes after the last treatment, no distress, and reassuring fetal status may be discharged.

Medication regimen after an acute asthmatic episode should continue treatment with SABAs 2–4 puffs every 3–4 hours, as needed. Oral corticosteroids 40 mg total daily for 3–10 days and an ICS should be initiated or continued.

References and suggested reading

1. Moore WC, Kornmann O, Humbert M, et al. Stopping versus continuing long-term mepolizumab treatment in severe eosinophilic asthma (COMET study). Eur Respir J. 2022;59(1):2100396. Published 2022 Jan 6. doi: 10.1183/13993003.00396-2021.
2. Corren J, Pham TH, Garcia Gil E, et al. Baseline type 2 biomarker levels and response to tezepelumab in severe asthma. Allergy. 2022;77(6):1786–1796. doi: 10.1111/all.15197.
3. Gaspar-Marques J, van Zeller M, Carreiro-Martins P, Chaves Loureiro C. Severe asthma in the era of COVID-19: a narrative review. Pulmonology. 2022;28(1):34–43. doi: 10.1016/j.pulmoe.2021.04.001.
4. Menzies-Gow A, Hoyte FL, Price DB, et al. Clinical remission in severe asthma: a pooled post hoc analysis of the patient journey with benralizumab. Adv Ther. 2022;39(5):2065–2084. doi: 10.1007/s12325-022-02098-1.
5. Sher LD, Wechsler ME, Rabe KF, et al. Dupilumab reduces oral corticosteroid use in patients with corticosteroid-dependent severe asthma: an analysis

of the phase 3, open-label extension traverse trial. Chest. 2022;162(1):46–55. doi: 10.1016/j.chest.2022.01.071.

6. Menzies-Gow A, Steenkamp J, Singh S, et al. Tezepelumab compared with other biologics for the treatment of severe asthma: a systematic review and indirect treatment comparison. J Med Econ. 2022;25(1):679–690. doi: 10.1080/13696998.2022.2074195.
7. Fritzsching B, Contoli M, Porsbjerg C, et al. Long-term real-world effectiveness of allergy immunotherapy in patients with allergic rhinitis and asthma: results from the REACT study, a retrospective cohort study. Lancet Reg Health Eur. 2021;13:100275. Published 2021 Nov 30. doi: 10.1016/j.lanepe.2021.100275.
8. Kindi ZA, McCabe C, McCann M. Impact of nurse-led asthma intervention on child health outcomes: a scoping review. J Sch Nurs. 2022;38(1):84–97. doi: 10.1177/10598405211003303.
9. Bateman ED, Price DB, Wang HC, et al. Short-acting β_2-agonist prescriptions are associated with poor clinical outcomes of asthma: the multi-country, cross-sectional SABINA III study. Eur Respir J. 2022;59(5):2101402. Published 2022 May 5. doi: 10.1183/13993003.01402-2021.
10. Chatkin J, Correa L, Santos U. External environmental pollution as a risk factor for asthma. Clin Rev Allergy Immunol. 2022;62(1):72–89. doi: 10.1007/s12016-020-08830-5.
11. Suzuki Y, Aono Y, Akiyama N, et al. Involvement of autophagy in exacerbation of eosinophilic airway inflammation in a murine model of obese asthma. Autophagy. 2022;18(9):2216–2228. doi: 10.1080/15548627.2022.2025571.
12. Sunjaya AP, Allida SM, Di Tanna GL, Jenkins C. Asthma and risk of infection, hospitalization, ICU admission and mortality from COVID-19: systematic review and meta-analysis. J Asthma. 2022;59(5):866–879. doi: 10.1080/02770903.2021.1888116.
13. Allen H, Price OJ, Hull JH, Backhouse SH. Asthma medication in athletes: a qualitative investigation of adherence, avoidance and misuse in competitive sport. J Asthma. 2022;59(4):811–822. doi: 10.1080/02770903.2021.1881968.
14. McIntosh MJ, Kooner HK, Eddy RL, et al. Asthma control, airway mucus, and ^{129}Xe MRI ventilation after a single benralizumab dose. Chest. 2022; 162(3):520–533. doi: 10.1016/j.chest.2022.03.003.

https://doi.org/10.1142/9789811271410_0013

13 COPD

Introduction

Chronic obstructive pulmonary disease (COPD) is one the most important causes of mortality and morbidity in the world. It is the fourth leading cause of death in the world and is projected to be the third leading cause of death by 2020. In India, it is already the second leading cause of death after ischemic heart disease. It is also one of the diseases whose prevalence and mortality have been increasing in spite of the advances in medical care due to the prevalence of risk factors that have shown no signs of abating. The present prevalence of the disease is due to exposures a few decades ago. It causes millions of deaths globally each year, and it roughly accounts for 6% of all causes of death globally.

Definition

The GOLD guidelines have defined COPD as a common, preventable, and treatable disease, characterized by persistent respiratory symptoms and airflow limitation that is due to airway or alveolar abnormalities usually caused by significant exposure to noxious particles or gases. The important aspect that this definition emphasizes is its preventability and treatability.

Causes

Many of the causes of COPD are well known, but many remains to be understood. There are host factors that probably include a genetic predisposition, increased airway responsiveness to noxious stimuli, poor lung growth in childhood, or accelerated decline of lung functions in adulthood.

The other key interaction of the host factors is with the environment. Many of the host factors cannot be avoided, but the environmental factors can be controlled. The two most factors include tobacco smoking and air pollution, which is both indoor (biomass fuel cooking and heating) and outdoor (ambient air pollution).

Risk factors	Description
Environmental factors	
Tobacco smoke	Contains nearly 4,000 noxious particles and gases. At least 10 pack-years of smoking is required to confer a risk. Smoking in any form is a risk (cigarette, beedi, waterpipe, cigar). Additional marijuana may accentuate the risk. Passive smoke (environmental tobacco smoke) also is a risk. Smoking in pregnancy may cause poor lung growth in utero.
Indoor air pollution	Wood, crop residues, and dung are called biomass fuels. Women who cook with biomass fuels are especially at high risk. A biomass exposure index of at least 60 is needed to confer risk. Poorly ventilated dwellings add to the risk.
Outdoor air pollution	Contributes to the particle load and gaseous injury in the lungs. PM 1, 2.5, 10 along with NO_2, O_3, SO_2, and black smoke cause risk. Though the association with causing COPD is weak, significant association with COPD morbidity, lung function declines, hospital admissions and deaths.
Occupational exposure	Organic (agricultural and others) and inorganic dust, fumes, and chemicals. Associated with more gas trapping and emphysema.

(*Continued*)

Risk factors	Description
Host risk factors	
Genetics	Hereditary alpha 1 antitrypsin deficiency (protease inhibition). MMP-12 (matrix metalloproteinase 12) (elastase activity). GSTCD (glutathione S-transferase C terminal domain) (lung repair). TGF-2B (transforming growth factor 2 B) (lung repair). SOX 5 (sex determining region Y box 5) (lung development). HHIP (Hedgehog-interacting protein) (lung development). BICD1 (bicaudal D homolog 1) (telomere length — lung aging). IL-6 R (interleukin 6 receptor) (inflammation). HDAC (histone deacetylase) (gene expression). THSD4 (thrombospondin, type I, domain containing 4) (nicotine dependence). GSTO2 (glutathione S-transferase) (arsenic biotransformation). FAM13A (family with sequence similarity 13 A1) (oxidative stress).
Age	COPD presents usually after the age of 50 years, though in some cases earlier, especially, if actively looked for by spirometry of asymptomatic individuals Some studies have suggested that COPD is an accelerated aging of the lung because COPD lung (airways and parenchyma) mimics the lung of the very old.
Gender	In countries, where men smoke more than women, COPD predominates in men. In countries, where biomass exposure is very common, the rates of COPD in women may be similar to that of men. Some studies suggest that women may be more susceptible to tobacco smoke than men.

(*Continued*)

(*Continued*)

Risk factors	Description
Socioeconomic status (SES)	Poor SES is one of the important causes though the pathway involves nutrition, increased indoor and outdoor pollution, crowding and infections, and possibly a higher burden of smoking.
Lung growth	Insults occur at all ages including during the gestation period. The study by Lange observed two main groups. Lung functions reached normal levels, but then had an accelerated decline, seen in 50% of subjects with COPD. Lung functions did not reach normal levels and also had an accelerated decline, seen in 50% of subjects with COPD.
Asthma	Asthma was observed in the Burden of Obstructive Lung Diseases (BOLD), European Community Respiratory Health Survey (ECRHS), and the Tucson studies as one of the most important risk factors. Risk worsens in subjects who had uncontrolled asthma. It is associated with an accelerated decline in lung functions.
Chronic bronchitis	It is defined as cough for more than 3 months in a year for 2 or more years (Medical Research Council, UK). Associated with the increased risk for COPD — Fletcher study. Associated with the frequency and severity of COPD acute exacerbations.
Infections	History of severe respiratory infections in childhood is a risk. Tuberculosis has been observed as a risk (BOLD study).

Pathogenesis

Many key mediators and cells are involved in the pathogenesis, some are common to asthma, and many are different. The most important of them are listed in the table below.

The key pathogenetic mechanisms involve

1. an increase in oxidative stress or a decrease in antioxidant reserve or both.
2. an increase in protease activity or a decrease in antiprotease protection or both.

Mediator	Pathophysiologic effects
	Risk factors
IL-8	Chemotactic — neutrophils, $CD8^+$ cells. Neutrophil degranulation. Expressed in airway epithelium. Associated with acute exacerbation COPD. Growth-related oncogene has a similar effect as IL-8 in COPD.
TNF-alpha	Proinflammatory cytokine. Chemoattractant for neutrophils. Associated with weight loss. Hypoxia activates TNF-alpha.
MCP-1	Monocyte chemoattractant protein 1. Monocytes differentiate into macrophages (lung levels are 5–10 fold higher in COPD). Macrophages recruit neutrophils.
Neutrophil elastase	Serine proteinase. Responsible for emphysema (degrade extracellular matrix). Bronchial squamous metaplasia. Reduced mucociliary clearance.
SLP1 and elafins	Secretory leucocyte proteinase inhibitor produced by airway mucosa. Potent antiproteinases (NE), alarmins. Defensin peptides — antimicrobial effect. Increased exposure to LPS, IL-1, TNF.
PR-3	Proteinase-3 from neutrophils along with cathepsin G. Degrade airway mucin, damage airway epithelium, and decrease mucociliary clearance.
MMP-9	Responsible for homeostasis and turnover of extracellular matrix. Secreted by neutrophils and macrophages. Degrades collagen, elastin, and gelatin. NE cleaves MMP-9 from pro-MMP-9. NE cleaves TIMP from MMP-9.

(*Continued*)

(*Continued*)

Mediator	Pathophysiologic effects
NOX-1, NOX-2	NADPH oxidase is usually latent. From neutrophils, macrophages, and epithelium. Generate reactive oxygen species on exposure to cigarette smoke.
MPO	Myeloperoxidase. From neutrophil and macrophage. Important in bacterial killing. Drives inflammation and tissue oxidation. Inhibitor stopped emphysema progress. Small airway remodeling and pulmonary hypertension.
MAPK	Mitogen-activated protein kinases are critical for airway inflammation. Cytokine activation. Increases MMP-9 and IL-8 in lungs.
NF-kB	Oxidative stress increases transcription factor NF-kB. Increases TNF-alpha and IL-8.
PRR	Pathogen recognition receptors. Pathogen-associated molecular patterns and cell interaction. TLR-4 Gram-negative bacteria. TLR-2 Gram-positive bacteria.
P2X7	Purinoceptor 7. ATP receptor binding to extracellular ATP (pattern recognition receptor). Mediated cigarette smoke-induced inflammation.
NLRP3 and caspase 1	Protein complex (inflammasome)–activating caspase 1 and the release of mature forms of IL-1 beta and IL-18. Nucleotide-binding domain, leucine-rich containing family, pyrin domain-containing-3. combination of proteins (inflammasome). Cysteine-aspartic proteases, enzymes playing a role in programmed cell death (apoptosis).
	Protective factors
Nrf2	Nuclear factor erythroid 2-related factor (Nrf2). Transcription factor. Catabolism of oxidants. Synthesis of reducing factors.

(Continued)

Mediator	Pathophysiologic effects
	Regeneration of oxidized cofactor. Antioxidant proteins.
Sirtuin 1 Sirtuin 6	Antiaging molecules. Promotes genetic stability. Reduced in COPD patients due to excessive reactive oxygen species. SIRT 6 is important in DNA repair, telomere structure, and anti-inflammatory agent (Pi3K/AKT pathway).
GPx, CAT, SOD	Glutathione peroxidase, catalase, superoxide dismutase. Converts H_2O_2 to harmless water and oxygen Reduces reactive oxygen species.
PPAR gamma	Peroxisome proliferator–activated receptor gamma. Transcription factor. Agonists attenuate TLR-mediated inflammation due to cigarette smoke.
Siglec 14	Sialic acid–binding lectin on innate cells. Granulocytes and monocytes. Gram-negative bacteria contain sialic acids. Less Siglec proteins lead to attenuated response to bacteria. Higher concentrations of Siglec proteins lead to an increase in proinflammatory cytokines and worsening of COPD exacerbations.
HDAC2	Histone deacetylase 2. Nuclear enzyme. Anti-inflammatory effect of corticosteroids is by recruiting HDAC to the nucleus. Switches "off" inflammatory genes activated by NF-kB. Reduced by oxidative and nitrative stress. Increased by theophylline, resveratrol, and curcumin.

There is a long-standing interaction between the protective factors and the risk factors in the background of the host genetics that determines whether there is a development of COPD and what would be the severity of COPD. The steps can be briefly summarized as follows:

Lung antioxidant and antiprotease reserves + genetics	*Environmental insults* Tobacco smoke, biomass fuels, chemicals and fumes, organic and inorganic dusts, other indoor pollutants such as mosquito coils (one equivalent to 100 cigarettes), dhoop stick (one equivalent to 1,000 cigarettes), and agarbathies/incense sticks (one equivalent to 5 or more cigarettes)
Antioxidants *superoxide dismutase, albumin, vitamin C, vitamin E, mucin, glutathione peroxidase, and glutathione synthetase*	*Oxidant stress* O^{2-}, H_2O_2, *HOCL, NO,* $ONOO^-$ *Proteases (PR3, MMP-9, NE)*
Reduced capacity of the lung to defend itself from damage due to insults	Increased oxidant stress Reduced antiprotease reserves (elafin, SLPI, AAT1)
Lung inflammation (macrophages, neutrophils)	
Long-term injury to the airways	Long-term injury to the parenchyma
Death of airway epithelial cells Reduced mucociliary clearance Bacterial colonization and recurrent infections Mucus hypersecretion Mucus gland hyperplasia Increased Reid index Smooth muscle hypertrophy Airway fibrosis Fixed airway obstruction	Loss of small airways leading to air trapping Decreased parenchymal elasticity Destruction of the lung parenchyma Therefore, reduced structural support of the small airways that have no cartilage and are kept open by the elastic recoil of the alveoli Permanent enlargement of the alveoli Bulla formation and development of bullous areas (dead space) Protease degradation of extracellular matrix
Chronic bronchitis	**Emphysema**

Pathology

The most important features include permanent changes in the airways and the lung parenchyma as described above. These changes can continue even after cessation of smoking since the activated alveolar macrophages, which are the most important inflammatory cell in COPD along with neutrophils continue to oversecrete various inflammatory mediators for 10 years after smoking is stopped. The key changes are goblet cell hyperplasia, increased chronic inflammatory cells in the airways, increased mucus in the airway lumen, increased Reid index, smooth muscle hypertrophy, dilation, and destruction of the alveolar spaces with the resultant increase in dead space. There is peribronchiolar and interstitial fibrosis in COPD patients, due to the chronic inflammation and release of profibrogenic growth factors. Small airway inflammation is present, and the common inflammatory cells are Th1, Th17, and ILC3 cells. In some cases of COPD, eosinophils, ILC2, and Th2 cells may be present as well.

Clinical features

The main clinical features are cough and sputum in the initial stages followed in later stages by wheezing, chest tightness or heaviness, dyspnea on exertion which progresses to dyspnea at rest at a variable pace. Chronic cough can be present with or without sputum though in subjects with chronic bronchitis sputum would be a usual feature and may be absent in subjects who have a predominant emphysema. Dyspnea is persistent with little variability, worse on exertion, and may not respond well to treatment. Usually, the age of presentation is above the age of 40 years, though most patients present above the age of 50 or even 60 for the first time to the physician. It is important to ask for the history of exposure to risk factors and whether it was for a sufficiently long duration (e.g., cooking with biomass fuels for 5 hours a day for 5 years may not cause COPD; a biomass index of 60 is needed to increase the risk of chronic bronchitis; cooking for 3 hours a day for 20 years or 4 hours a day for 15 years is necessary). For smoking, at least exposure to 10 pack-years is necessary to have an increased risk of COPD. Additional features include fatigue, weight loss (an important poor prognostic feature), cough syncope, rib fractures, and the presence of other comorbidities such as ischemic heart disease, obstructive sleep apnea, and metabolic syndrome.

Diagnosis

The diagnosis of COPD has three important arms. The first includes the presence of various symptoms described previously. The second is the presence of risk factors for a sufficient duration. In this background, COPD is then confirmed by spirometry which shows a forced expiratory volume in 1 s/forced vital capacity (FEV_1/FVC) ratio of less than 0.7. In the early stages, FEV_1 may be normal, but later, it is inevitably reduced. All subjects undergoing spirometry must undergo postbronchodilator spirometry 15–20 minutes after a 400 μg of salbutamol or 160 μg of an anticholinergic like ipratropium bromide or both combined. It is important that the spirometry satisfies the American Thoracic Criteria. When a fixed criterion of less than 70% of FEV_1/FVC ratio is used, we tend to overdiagnose COPD in the elderly and underdiagnose COPD in the young. To overcome this deficiency, many researchers use the lower limit of normal (LLN) values which is more suitable, but data are not available for LLN in many populations. The present FEV_1/FVC ratio that is used is independent of any reference value for the given population. The GOLD guidelines recommend a fixed level of <0.7 for the diagnosis of COPD. Additionally, the newer versions of the GOLD guidelines correctly recommend not to use a single measurement of FEV_1/FVC ratio for confirming COPD if the ratio is between 0.6 and 0.8. In such situations, repeat measurements are warranted as the values can change in the subsequent measurements as has been discussed in the asthma chapter. In the event that the first spirometry showed a ratio of <0.6, COPD can be confirmed. Unlike in asthma, the degree of reversibility of airflow limitation is not important in COPD.

Classification and assessment of COPD

The key features of COPD assessment by the clinician include the degree of health impairment (symptoms, dyspnea scores), level of airflow obstruction, the risk for future exacerbations and complications, and the presence of other comorbidities. The degree of health impairment is assessed by the MMRC scores for dyspnea or the more comprehensive questionnaires such as St George's questionnaire (full or SGRQ C specific for COPD),

COPD assessment questionnaire (CAT), COPD control questionnaire can be used. The severity of airflow limitation is assessed by changes in FEV_1 and is categorized into four groups by the GOLD guidelines: Group 1, mild, FEV_1 >80% predicted; Group 2, moderate, FEV_1 50%–80% predicted; Group 3, severe, FEV1 30%–50% predicted; and Group 4, very severe, FEV_1 <30% predicted. The risks associated with future exacerbations are not very clear as FEV_1 is not found to be a very strong predictor. Generally, it is observed that as the stage of COPD worsens, the risk of exacerbation increases. COPD acute exacerbation (AE) is defined as a worsening of health status that results in additional treatment. It is classified as mild if only short-acting beta-agonists are sufficient, as moderate if antibiotics or oral steroids are needed, and severe if it necessitates emergency room visits or hospital admissions. The most reliable predictive factor is the previous history of exacerbations. Some studies have observed increasing sputum eosinophils as one of the predictive risk factors for AE. COPD is associated with multimorbidity, especially in later stages, which includes cardiovascular diseases, obstructive sleep apnea, metabolic syndrome, skeletal muscle dysfunction, osteoporosis, lung cancer and anxiety, depression, and cognition deficiencies.

Current COPD ABCD assessment tool

The GOLD guidelines recommend that every COPD patient be classified into one of the categories; ABC or D. This classification is dependent on the spirometry, MMRC dyspnea score (0–1 versus >2) or CAT score (<10 versus >10), and the risk for exacerbations (0–1 versus 2 or more or 1 with hospitalization). The table gives the details of the classification. The first step in COPD assessment is to confirm the airflow limitation (FEV_1/FVC ratio <0.7). The second step is to assess the severity of COPD by FEV_1 (mild to very severe described above). The third is to do the ABCD assessment. Unlike in earlier GOLD guidelines, FEV_1 is now not needed for the ABCD grading. The patients are now graded based on both FEV_1 and ABCD grading; for example, a person with a lung function of 45% with two hospital admissions in 1 year is graded as GOLD grade 3, group D.

GOLD grade	Description
A	MMRC dyspnea score 0–1 CAT score <10 Moderate or severe exacerbation 0–1 not leading to hospitalization
B	MMRC dyspnea score >2 CAT score >10 Moderate or severe exacerbation 0–1 not leading to hospitalization
C Till 2022	MMRC dyspnea score 0–1 CAT score <10 Moderate or severe exacerbation of 2 or more in 1 year. If there is 1, acute exacerbation leading to hospitalization
D Till 2022	MMRC dyspnea score >2 CAT score >10 Moderate or severe exacerbation of 2 or more in 1 year. If there is 1, acute exacerbation leading to hospitalization.
E From 2023	Moderate exacerbation of 2 or more in one year or if there is 1 or more AE leading to hospitalization

Investigations

The common investigations and their utility in evaluating COPD are listed in the table below:

Common investigations	Findings and clinical utility
Chest X-ray	Hyperinflated lung fields (Figure 1) Low-set flat diaphragm or in severe cases inverted diaphragm (Figures 2 and 3) Tubular heart (11 cm or less) (Figure 1) Prominent pulmonary artery (PA) (right PA >16 mm and left PA >14 mm suggestive of pulmonary hypertension (Figure 4)

(*Continued*)

Common investigations	Findings and clinical utility
	Peripheral pruning of vessels (Figure 4) Increased retrosternal air space (Figure 5) Bulla including tension bulla or bullous areas (Figures 2, 6, and 7) Can help to rule out comorbid conditions aggravating COPD or as a differential diagnosis of COPD (pneumonia, pneumothorax (Figures 8 and 9), pleural effusions, kyphoscoliosis, bronchiectasis among others)
HRCT scan	Not routinely recommended Can help to confirm paraseptal emphysema (Figure 10), centrilobular emphysema (Figure 11), or panacinar emphysema (Figures 12 and 13) Evaluation of bulla (Figure 14) and tension bulla (Figure 15) Comorbid conditions or complications such as spontaneous pneumothorax, especially when the patient already has a bullous disease Can help to confirm mild bronchiectasis In the evaluation of medical pneumonectomy, lung volume reduction surgery and lung transplantation
Spirometry	Pre- and postbronchodilator During first visit and follow-up to confirm the diagnosis, assess severity and therapeutic response
DLCO	Assesses the functional impact of COPD on gas exchange due to emphysema Indirectly gives an indication of air trapping (RV/TLC ratio >40% indicates air trapping)
Arterial blood gases (O_2) and oxygen saturation	To assess the need for oxygen therapy Evaluate oxygen desaturation during exercise and pacing
Exercise testing	6-minute walk test (unpaced) Shuttle walk test (paced) Very useful prognostic tool (lower walk distances are associated with a higher risk of mortality and poorer quality of life)

(*Continued*)

(*Continued*)

Common investigations	Findings and clinical utility
Other tests as indicated	Cardiac evaluation (electrocardiogram, echocardiogram) Sleep study
Alpha-1 antitrypsin levels	Deficiency is associated with gross emphysema in younger subjects (<40 years and non-smokers or smokers <10 pack-years) (Figure 16)

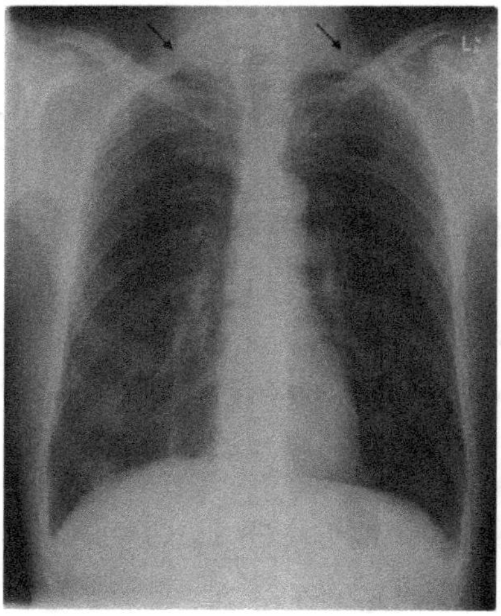

Figure 1: Tubular heart.

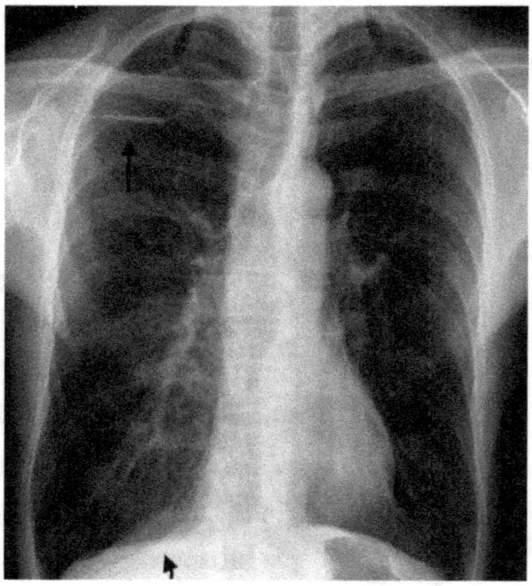

Figure 2: Bulla.

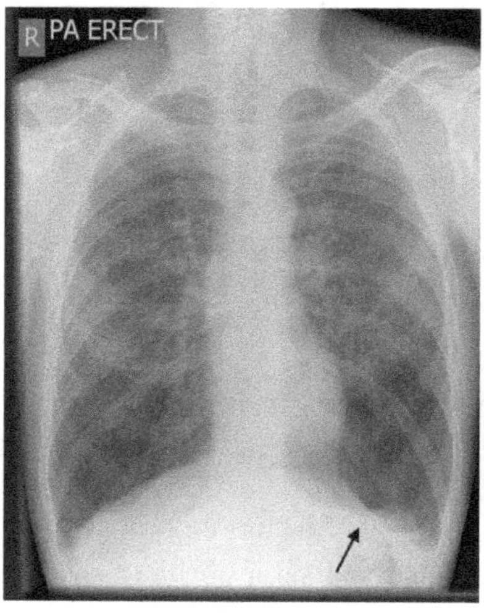

Figure 3: Panlobular emphysema.

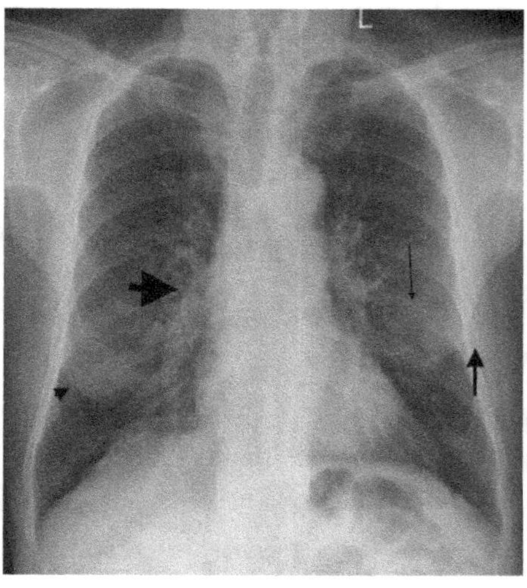

Figure 4: COPD with gynecomastia.

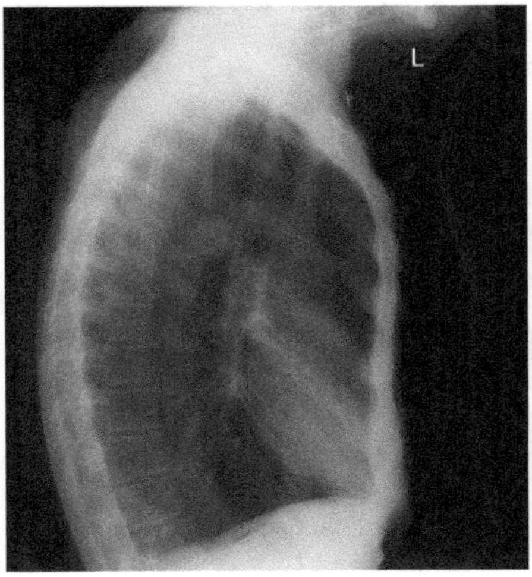

Figure 5: Retrosternal space widening.

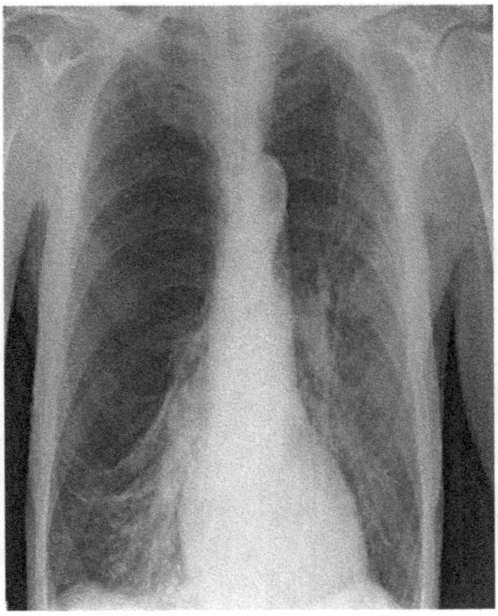

Figure 6: Large bullous area.

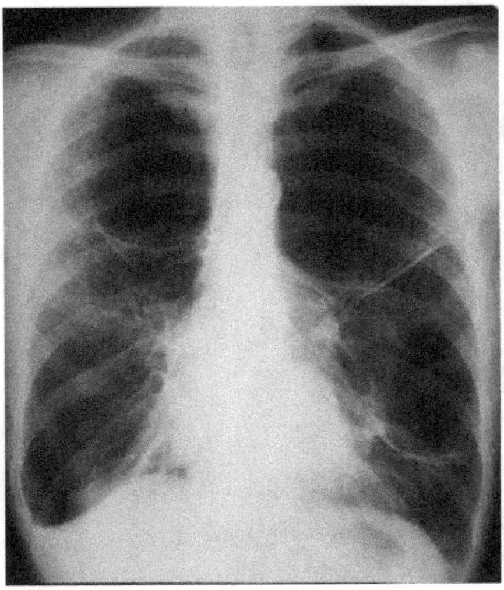

Figure 7: Tension bulla.

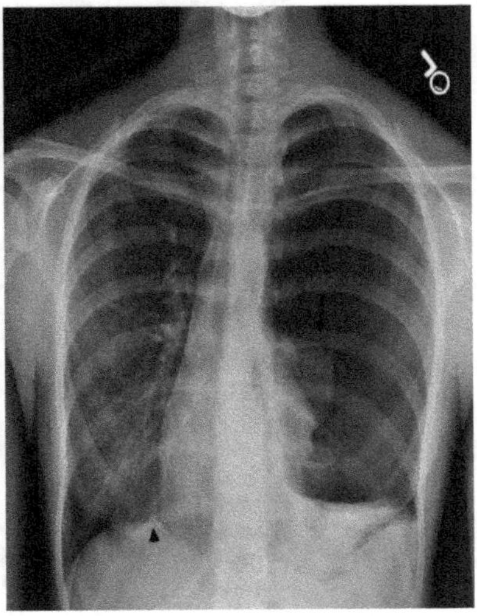

Figure 8: COPD with pneumothorax.

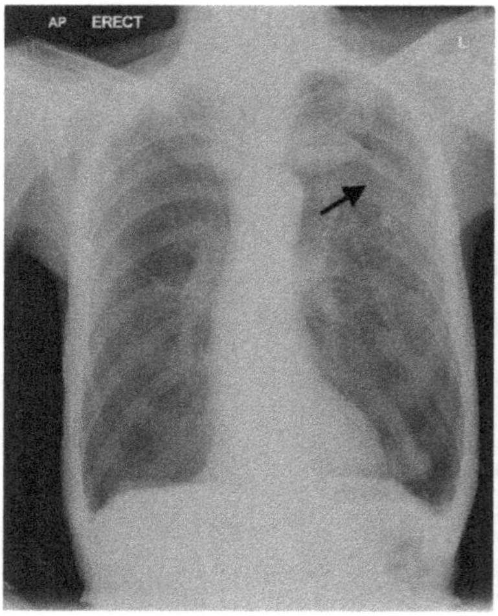

Figure 9: COPD with spontaneous pneumothorax.

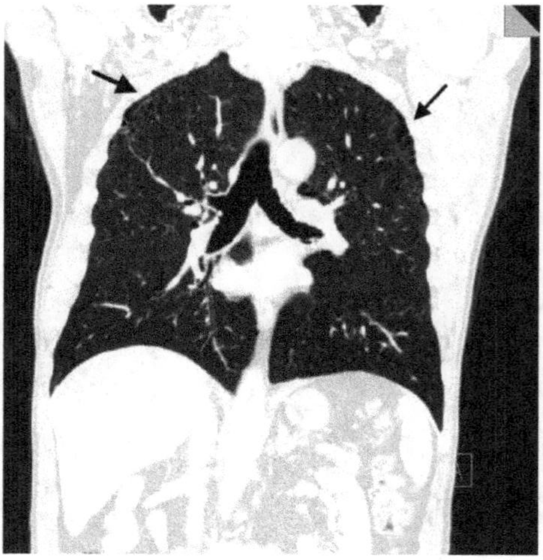

Figure 10: Parseptal emphysema.

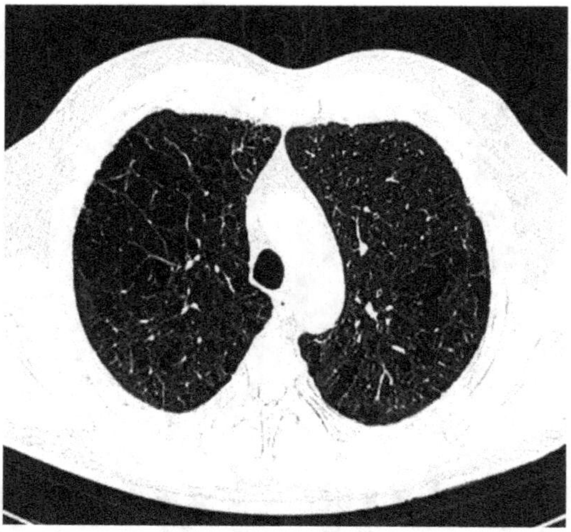

Figure 11: Cenrtrilobular emphysema.

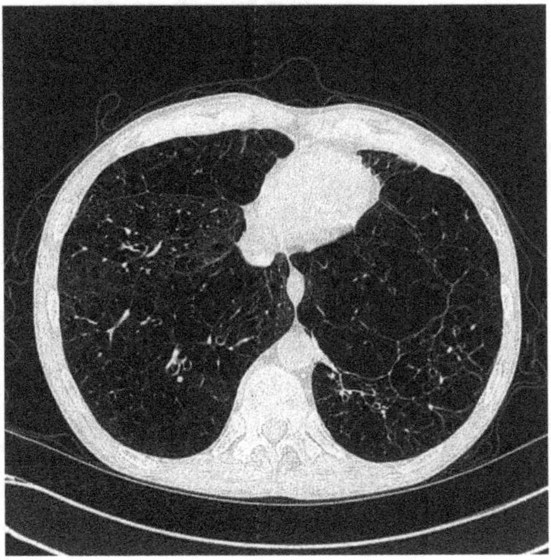

Figure 12: Panacinar emphysema — computed tomography.

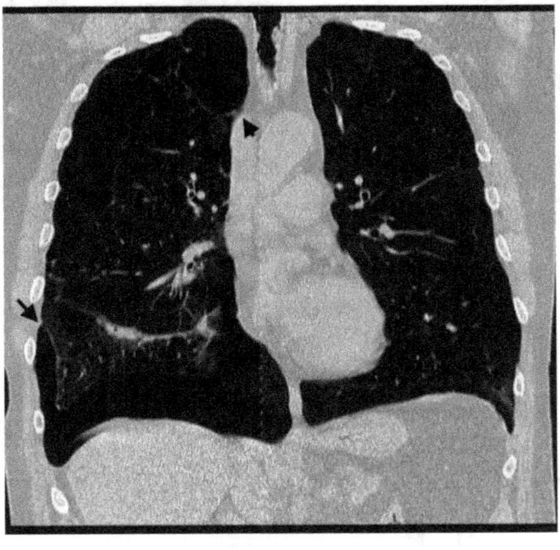

Figure 13: Panacinar emphysema with spontaneous pneumothorax.

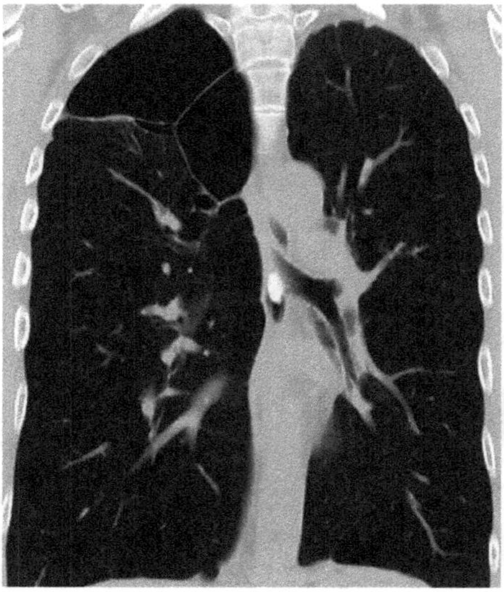

Figure 14: Evaluation of bulla.

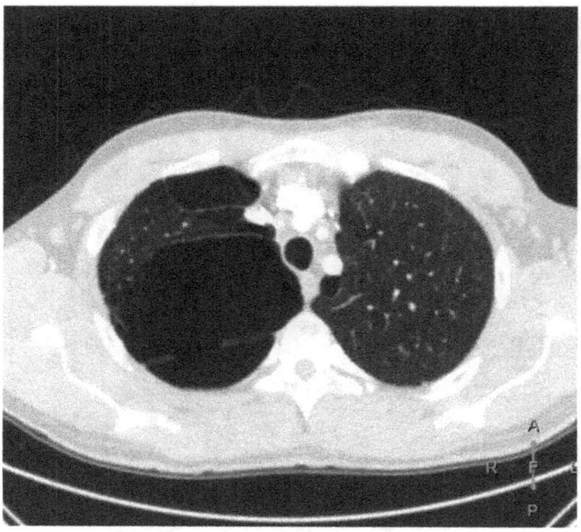

Figure 15: Bullous emphysema.

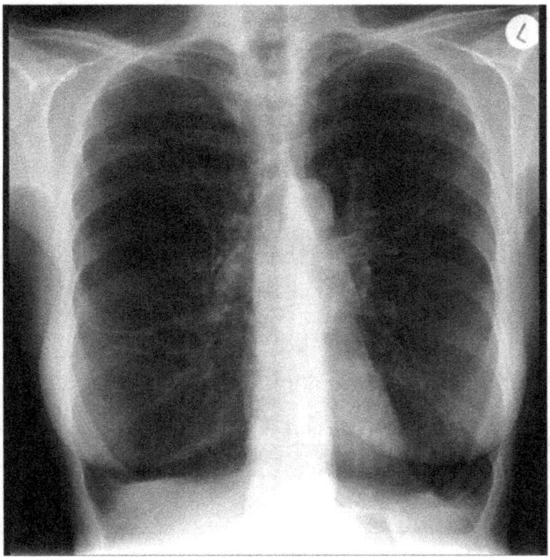

Figure 16: A case of Alpha-1 antitrypsin deficiency.

Differential diagnosis

The common differential diagnosis includes **asthma** (younger age of onset, atopic, seasonal variations, normal between attacks, comorbid allergic conditions such as rhinitis), **tuberculosis** (common in countries such as India, risk of tuberculosis in smokers is twice than that of the general population and in COPD, six times the risk of general population, chest X-ray abnormalities and confirmed by sputum AFB smear or CBNAAT), **congestive heart failure** (presence of cardiomegaly on chest X-ray, spirometry shows restriction and not obstruction, echocardiogram (ECHO) findings with dilated chambers and low ejection fraction suggestive, in suspected cases with normal ECHO, BNP, or pro-BNP is useful), **bronchiectasis** (large volumes of purulent expectoration, imaging can confirm), **obliterative bronchiolitis** (younger age, rheumatoid arthritis, or fume exposure may be present, non-smokers, after lung or bone marrow transplantation, CT on expiration shows areas of air trapping), **pan bronchiolitis** (Asian descent, non-smokers, CT shows centrilobular nodules and hyperinflated lungs, rapidly progressive downhill course). Other differentials may be reviewed from the asthma chapter.

Management

A complete management includes both pharmacological and non-pharmacological treatments. All the drugs that can be used in the management of COPD are discussed in a separate chapter on pharmacology in the management of airway disorders. The management protocols are selected based on the ABCD grading and enumerated in the table below.

Grade	Drugs recommended
A	Bronchodilator — beta-agonist (short-acting beta-agonist or long-acting beta-agonist [LABA]).
B	LABA or long-acting muscarinic agent (LAMA).
C	LAMA alone.
D	LAMA alone. LAMA + LABA (if CAT score is >20). LABA + inhaled corticosteroid (ICS) (if eosinophil counts are >300 cells/μL). In some cases, there may be a need for triple therapy (LABA, LAMA, ICS).
Other measures	Smoking cessation needs to be offered to all patients. Vaccination with influenza and pneumococcal vaccines is shown to reduce the risk for lower respiratory tract infections. Pulmonary rehabilitation is an important tool that is grossly underutilized. In patients with chronic respiratory hypoxemia, pulmonary hypertension, or cor pulmonale, long-term home oxygen may be considered. In patients with significant chronic hypercapnia, non-invasive ventilation may be considered to reduce hospitalizations. In selected cases, bronchoscopic or surgical interventions to reduce lung volumes or lung transplantation can be considered. Finally, in end-stage lung disease, palliative care can help to alleviate dyspnea (opiates, neuromuscular electrical stimulation). Nutritional support.

The follow-up of these patients should be done regularly, and the maintenance treatment will be the initial treatment if the patient does not have any symptoms or exacerbations. Otherwise, it depends on two important considerations. One is the presence of dyspnea and the other is exacerbation. The stepwise recommendations from the GOLD guidelines is as follows:

Key considerations	Recommended stepwise options (if no response, move to the step below)
Dyspnea	LAMA or LABA LABA + LAMA Consider LABA + ICS Consider changing molecules and adjusting dosage LABA + LAMA + ICS Consider additional causes of dyspnea
Exacerbation	LAMA or LABA LABA + LAMA Consider LABA + ICS LABA + LAMA + ICS (ICS will be useful especially if blood eosinophils >100 cells/μL) If eosinophils are below 100, consider roflumilast or macrolides

References and suggested readings

1. Serban KA, Pratte KA, Bowler RP. Protein biomarkers for COPD outcomes. Chest. 2021;159(6):2244–2253. doi: 10.1016/j.chest.2021.01.004.
2. van Bakel SIJ, Gosker HR, Langen RC, Schols AMWJ. Towards personalized management of sarcopenia in COPD. Int J Chron Obstruct Pulmon Dis. 2021;16:25–40. Published 2021 Jan 7. doi: 10.2147/COPD.S280540.
3. Tsutsui M, Gerayeli F, Sin DD. Pulmonary rehabilitation in a post-COVID-19 world: telerehabilitation as a new standard in patients with COPD. Int J Chron Obstruct Pulmon Dis. 2021;16:379–391. Published 2021 Feb 19. doi: 10.2147/COPD.S263031.

4. Gupta N, Malhotra N, Ish P. GOLD 2021 guidelines for COPD — what's new and why. Adv Respir Med. 2021;89(3):344–346. doi: 10.5603/ARM.a2021.0015.
5. Singhvi D, Bon J. CT imaging and comorbidities in COPD: beyond lung cancer screening. Chest. 2021;159(1):147–153. doi: 10.1016/j.chest.2020.08.2053.
6. Wu F, Burt J, Chowdhury T, et al. Specialty COPD care during COVID-19: patient and clinician perspectives on remote delivery. BMJ Open Respir Res. 2021;8(1):e000817. doi: 10.1136/bmjresp-2020-000817.
7. Halpin DMG, Criner GJ, Papi A, et al. Global initiative for the diagnosis, management, and prevention of chronic obstructive lung disease. The 2020 GOLD Science Committee report on COVID-19 and chronic obstructive pulmonary disease. Am J Respir Crit Care Med. 2021;203(1):24–36. doi: 10.1164/rccm.202009-3533SO.
8. Milne S, Li X, Yang CX, et al. Inhaled corticosteroids downregulate SARS-CoV-2-related genes in COPD: results from a randomised controlled trial. Eur Respir J. 2021;58(1):2100130. Published 2021 Jul 29. doi: 10.1183/13993003.00130-2021.
9. Yip KP, Stockley RA, Sapey E. Catching "early" COPD — the diagnostic conundrum. Int J Chron Obstruct Pulmon Dis. 2021;16:957–968. Published 2021 Apr 13. doi: 10.2147/COPD.S296842.
10. Yun R, Bai Y, Lu Y, Wu X, Lee SD. How breathing exercises influence on respiratory muscles and quality of life among patients with COPD? A systematic review and meta-analysis. Can Respir J. 2021;2021:1904231. Published 2021 Jan 29. doi: 10.1155/2021/1904231.
11. Vizza CD, Hoeper MM, Huscher D, et al. Pulmonary hypertension in patients with COPD: results from the comparative, prospective registry of newly initiated therapies for pulmonary hypertension (COMPERA). Chest. 2021;160(2):678–689. doi: 10.1016/j.chest.2021.02.012.
12. Mkorombindo T, Dransfield MT. COPD: coagulation-associated pulmonary disease? Respirology. 2021;26(4):290–291. doi: 10.1111/resp.14000.
13. Tu X, Donovan C, Kim RY, Wark PAB, Horvat JC, Hansbro PM. Asthma-COPD overlap: current understanding and the utility of experimental models. Eur Respir Rev. 2021;30(159):190185. Published 2021 Feb 16. doi: 10.1183/16000617.0185-2019.

14. Press VG, Myers LC, Feemster LC. Preventing COPD readmissions under the hospital readmissions reduction program: how far have we come? Chest. 2021;159(3):996–1006. doi: 10.1016/j.chest.2020.10.008.
15. Anderson M, Collison K, Drummond MB, et al. Peak inspiratory flow rate in COPD: an analysis of clinical trial and real-world data. Int J Chron Obstruct Pulmon Dis. 2021;16:933–943. Published 2021 Apr 12. doi: 10.2147/COPD.S291554.
16. Benlala I, Laurent F, Dournes G. Structural and functional changes in COPD: what we have learned from imaging. Respirology. 2021;26(8):731–741. doi: 10.1111/resp.14047.
17. Liu K, Yu X, Cui X, et al. Effects of proprioceptive neuromuscular facilitation stretching combined with aerobic training on pulmonary function in COPD patients: a randomized controlled trial. Int J Chron Obstruct Pulmon Dis. 2021;16:969–977. Published 2021 Apr 13. doi: 10.2147/COPD.S300569.

https://doi.org/10.1142/9789811271410_0014

14 Management of acute exacerbation of COPD in emergency and intensive care unit

Introduction

An acute exacerbation of chronic obstructive pulmonary disease (AECOPD) is characterized by an acute worsening of symptoms accompanied by most commonly a lung infection. In severe cases, an acute exacerbation may cause respiratory failure and death. Accurate diagnosis in a patient experiencing rapid deterioration of respiratory function may be confounded by underlying myocardial infarction, congestive heart failure, thromboemboli, or recurrent aspiration, which can simulate an exacerbation of COPD. For the emergency physician, primary importance should be directed toward identifying the underlying cause for breathlessness, clinically managing those patients exhibiting the signs of respiratory failure where noninvasive ventilation (NIV) or invasive mechanical ventilation is likely to be indicated, and coordinating emergency transport of these patients to areas capable of providing such support. Differential diagnosis and required diagnostic tests to be considered in acute-onset breathlessness in a COPD patient are given in Table 1.

Initial assessment

During the primary survey, the patient's work of breathing, oxygenation, mental status, and vital signs should be simultaneously assessed and addressed by immediate interventions when life-threatening abnormalities

Table 1: Differential diagnosis and required diagnostic tests

Decompensated heart failure	NT-proBNP, echocardiogram
Cardiac dysrhythmia	Electrocardiogram
Acute asthma	Spirometry
Pneumonia	Chest X-ray (CXR), C-reactive protein, procalcitonin
Pulmonary embolism (PE)	Computed tomography pulmonary angiogram with PE protocol
Acute myocardial infarction	Cardiac troponins
Pneumothorax	CXR, lung ultrasonography (USG)
Pericardial or pleural effusion	CXR, lung USG

are present. Sometimes, patients will present with obvious or imminent respiratory failure and require definitive airway management (e.g., endotracheal intubation) without any time for the physician to arrive at a provisional diagnosis. Caution must be taken in these cases to avoid, recognize, and treat the lung injury and prevent cardiovascular collapse that is associated with intubation and mechanical ventilation.

Diagnosis and assessment of severity

Patients with AECOPD commonly present to the emergency department (ED) or other acute care settings and may be unaware that they have COPD. Since EDs generally cannot perform spirometry regularly on patients with COPD, GOLD definition is difficult to apply in such scenarios for diagnosis and severity assessment. A prior diagnosis of COPD in a smoker over the age of 50 presenting to an ED with wheezing or breathing difficulty has been shown to be reliable for the diagnosis of AECOPD. A smoker or a patient with a previous smoking history being diagnosed as asthmatic is often incorrect, and these patients typically also have COPD. Whenever possible, postbronchodilator forced expiratory volume in 1 second (FEV_1) can be used to assess severity. The severity of airflow obstruction can then be classified as mild (FEV_1 ≥80% predicted), moderate (50%≤ FEV_1 <80% predicted), severe (30%≤ FEV_1 <50% predicted), and very severe (FEV_1 <30% predicted). Using the Anthonisen criteria, AECOPD can be classified clinically. The following are evaluated: increased sputum volume, increased sputum purulence, and dyspnea. Patients with type I have all three symptoms, patients with two symptoms are categorized into type II, and patients with one symptom are categorized into type III. Antibiotics and corticosteroids are advocated for type I and type II patients.

Management of AECOPD in ER

Management of acute COPD is aimed at relieving bronchospasm, treating infection/inflammation, identifying the cause(s) of the exacerbation, and maintaining adequate oxygenation. The treatment of a COPD exacerbation should occur concurrently with its diagnosis and evaluation. According to GOLD 2020 guidelines, the severity of acute exacerbation should be classified into the following:

a. No respiratory failure: respiratory rate (RR) 25–30 cycles per minute, no use of accessory muscles of respiration, no increase in $PaCO_2$, hypoxemia which improves on supplemental oxygen via venturi mask with fraction of inspired oxygen (FiO_2) 28%–35%, and no change in mental status.
b. Acute respiratory failure — non-life-threatening: RR >30 cycles per minute, use of accessory muscles of respiration, presence of hypercarbia ($PaCO_2$ 50–60 mmHg), hypoxemia which improves on supplemental oxygen via venturi mask with FiO_2 28%–35%, and no change in mental status.
c. Acute respiratory failure — life-threatening: RR >30 cycles per minute, use of accessory muscles of respiration, presence of hypercarbia ($PaCO_2$ >60 mmHg), hypoxemia which does not on supplemental oxygen via venturi mask with FiO_2 28%–35%, acute change in mental status, and presence of acidosis with pH <7.25.

Pharmacological management

Bronchodilators

Administration of bronchodilators is a first-line strategy for improving the lung physiology and symptoms of the patient with COPD exacerbation. The most common medication types used to treat the acute bronchospasm associated with AECOPD are short-acting β-agonists, such as salbutamol or albuterol, and anticholinergic agents, such as ipratropium bromide. Current consensus guidelines recommend increasing the dose and/or frequency of a patient's short-acting β-agonist regimen when treating an exacerbation with a dosing frequency increased up to every 20 minutes. Caution should be exercised to observe patients for signs of β-agonist toxicity (tremor and tachycardia). Although these agents are accepted widely as the initial treatment for both asthma and AECOPD, the reversibility of bronchospasm in patients with COPD exacerbation is quite limited. Nevertheless, early treatment focuses on bronchodilation for the relief of symptoms. It seems reasonable to use nebulizers in the acute setting, as dyspneic and elderly patients with COPD may have difficulty coordinating an inhaler and spacer during an exacerbation.

Corticosteroids

Corticosteroids are effective anti-inflammatory agents used in acute and chronic COPD. Cochrane meta-analysis data support the administration of corticosteroids in the treatment of AECOPD, especially in patients requiring hospitalization. Administration of systemic steroids to patients presenting with COPD exacerbation has been shown to improve FEV_1, reduce short-term treatment failure, and shorten hospital stay by helping to reverse some of the inflammatory response that contributes to airway hypersensitivity, bronchial obstruction, and worsened lung physiology. The most frequent adverse effect of steroids is hyperglycemia. Other adverse effects are possible, including skin changes, myopathy, psychiatric events, hypertension, decreased bone density, and immune suppression leading to serious infections. Since oral corticosteroids are as effective as intravenous agents, intravenous corticosteroids should be reserved for patients who are unable to have oral medications administered or are intubated. Optimal dose of steroids is still unclear with dose ranging from 30 to 40 mg of prednisolone or equivalent for 1–2 weeks to methylprednisolone 125 mg every sixth hourly in intubated patients. However, GOLD 2020 guidelines recommend a short course of steroids equivalent to 40 mg of prednisolone for 5 days.

Antibiotics

The most common cause of AECOPD is either viral or bacterial infection. Three bacterial pathogens, namely, *Streptococcus pneumoniae*, *Haemophilus influenza*, and *Moraxella catarrhalis*, are frequently implicated in AECOPD. *Pseudomonas aeruginosa* should be considered in patients with severe airway limitation, frequent administration of antibiotics (four courses in the last year), recent hospitalization, isolation of *P. aeruginosa* during a previous exacerbation or colonization during a stable period, and severe COPD exacerbations. Use of antibiotics has been shown to reduce mortality, lessen treatment failure, and reduce sputum production, especially in the severe category requiring hospitalization. The class of antibiotic to be administered depends on several factors and is summarized in Table 2.

Table 2: Antibiotics for COPD exacerbations

For patients who will be discharged from the emergency	For admitted patients or discharged patients who have recently failed a course of antibiotics
Macrolides	Respiratory fluoroquinolones
Doxycycline	Second- or third-generation cephalosporins
Trimethoprim/sulfamethoxazole	Beta-lactam/beta-lactamase inhibitor combinations
Second- or third-generation cephalosporins	

Adapted from Rowe et al. Expert Rev Resp Med. 2011;5(4):549–559.

Adjunct therapies

Methylxanthines act as nonselective phosphodiesterase inhibitors, although they also have been reported to have a range of nonbronchodilator actions. Available clinical trial data have failed to demonstrate the efficacy of methylxanthines for the treatment of AECOPD.

Heliox is a combination of helium (an inert gas) and oxygen, which has a lower density than air. The use of heliox in NIV reduces respiratory effort and auto-PEEP (positive end-expiratory pressure) but does not change outcomes like mortality or rates of intubation and invasive mechanical ventilation.

Nonpharmacological management: Respiratory support

Supplemental oxygen therapy

This is a key component of COPD management. Supplemental oxygen should be titrated to target saturation of 88%–92%. Aggressive oxygenation to target higher saturation is not recommended due to the risk of worsening respiratory acidosis. This is due to the worsening ventilation–perfusion mismatch rather than loss of hypoxic respiratory drive as thought earlier. Venturi masks are better as they offer more controlled and accurate oxygen delivery over nasal prongs.

High-flow oxygen therapy

High-flow nasal oxygen is a fixed-performance device delivering oxygen via the nasal interface at high rates of up to 60 L/minute and a fraction of inspired oxygen (FiO_2) of up to 100%. High rates of oxygen supplied are heated and humidified preserving the ciliary activity of the respiratory tract, reducing airway constriction, and decreasing the work of breathing. The flow generated also leads to PEEP, decreases hypercarbia, improved gas exchange, improved lung volume, and dynamic compliance. The evidence so far suggests HFNO use in severe COPD patients leads to a trend toward reduced intubation rates.

Ventilatory support

In patients whose acute exacerbation begins to overwhelm their physiologic reserves, hypercapnic respiratory acidosis ensues, which initiates a downward cycle of respiratory failure. To interrupt this vicious cycle, ventilatory support is necessary. In some patients, noninvasive positive pressure ventilation (NIPPV) may be employed, while some patients may require invasive positive pressure ventilation (endotracheal intubation).

NIPPV/NIV

The benefits of NIV have been well-demonstrated and include symptom improvement, correction of respiratory acidosis, decreased need for intubation, decreased length of hospital stay, and decreased mortality. NIV is preferred over invasive mechanical ventilation as the initial mode of positive pressure ventilation in AECOPD patients as the success rate is high (80%–85%). NIPPV increases transpulmonary pressure by applying supra-atmospheric pressure leading to lung inflation and decreased work of breathing, thereby unloading respiratory muscles.

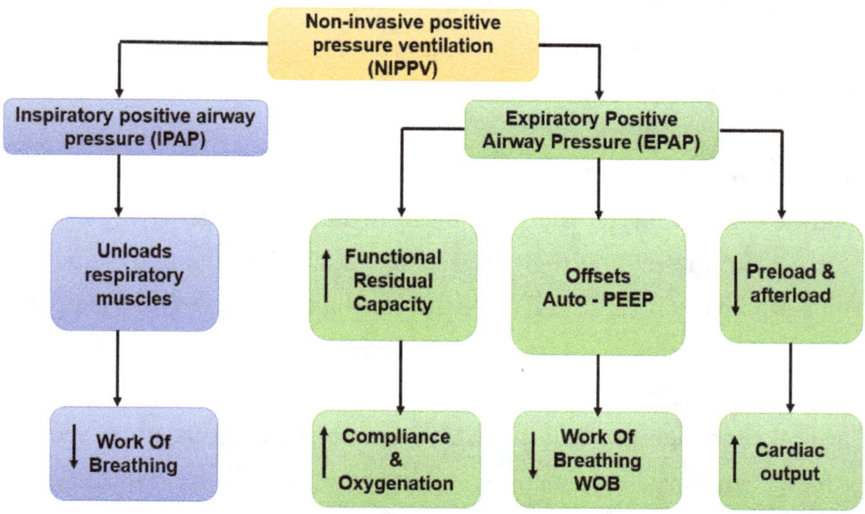

Figure 1: Beneficial effects of NIV.

Indications for NIV as per GOLD 2020 guidelines include the presence of at least one of the following:

- Respiratory acidosis (pH <7.35 with $PaCO_2$> 45 mmHg).
- Severe dyspnea with clinical signs suggestive of respiratory muscle fatigue, increased work of breathing or both, use of respiratory accessory muscles, paradoxical motion of abdomen, or retraction of intercostal spaces.
- Persistent hypoxemia despite supplemental oxygen therapy.

Bilevel positive airway pressure (BiPAP) is considered the first line in regard to the type of NIV used in the patient with AECOPD. This mode can be delivered by portable machines with different levels of positive pressure for inspiration (inspiratory positive airway pressure or IPAP) and expiration (expiratory positive airway pressure or EPAP).

Points to consider in setting up of BiPAP machine for a COPD patient are IPAP, EPAP, rise time, cycle variable, effect of leak, and trigger.

Table 3: Contraindications to NIPPV

Inability to tolerate the mask or use it effectively	Inability to protect the airway or coordinate breaths with the ventilator	Inability to tolerate possible aerophagia
Patient discomfort	Significant alterations in mental status/ obtundation	Recent gastrointestinal surgery
Craniofacial abnormalities or trauma	Hemodynamic instability (hypotension, dysrhythmias, hemorrhage)	
Facial hair, burns	Respiratory arrest/apnea	
Other skin abnormalities	Inability to clear secretions	

Adapted from Swadron S, et al. The acute presentation of chronic obstructive pulmonary disease in the emergency department: a challenging oxymoron. Emerg Med Pract. 2008;10:1–28.

Rise time: It is the time from the onset of inspiration to the achievement of peak flow. A faster rise time has been shown to unload respiratory muscles more completely. As the slope becomes flatter, the machine delivers lower flow rates, and the patient's work of breathing increases.

Cycle variable: It is the variable that decides switching from inspiration to expiration during ventilation. The common cycle variables are time, flow, and pressure. In time-cycled modes, ventilators use time criteria chosen by the clinician, and in flow-cycled modes, cycling occurs as the inspiratory flow decreases to a predetermined percentage of the peak inspiratory flow. Usually flow cycling is set at 25% or 35%, that is, once the flow reaches 25% or 35% of the peak inspiratory flow rate (PIFR), expiration valve opens, but in COPD patients, it is better to set flow cycling to 50% to prolong the duration of expiration.

Common modes available on BiPAP machines include the following:

Assist mode (spontaneous): Patient controls the beginning and the end of inspiration. The pressure is maintained as long as a minimal preset inspiratory flow is occurring. The end of inspiration occurs when the inspiratory flow reaches a predetermined percentage of the peak inspiratory flow.

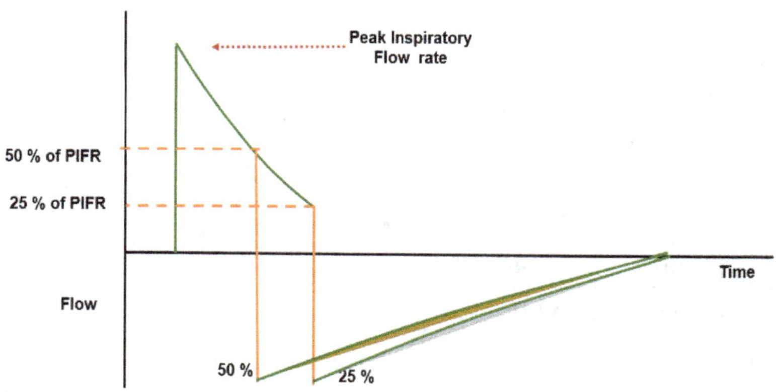

Figure 2: Flow cycling on spontaneous modes. Notice the increased expiratory time when flow cycling is set at 50% of the peak inspiratory flow rate (PIFR).

Assist mode (spontaneous/timed): In this mode, the patient controls the onset of inspiration, but the inspiratory length is regulated by the operator. The clinician must select an IPAP, inspiratory:expiratory (I:E) ratio, or an inspiratory time and an inspiratory trigger sensitivity and RR.

Timed mode: In this mode, all breaths are automatically delivered and set. The machine does not rely on the patient's breath-triggering effort. So, it is a machine-cycled and machine-triggered mode.

Suggested initial settings include IPAP between 8 and 10 cm H_2O and EPAP between 4 and 5 cm H_2O. These may be titrated based on patient tolerance and arterial blood gas (ABG) progress, with care to maintain a relative difference of IPAP greater than EPAP (this interval is also known as pressure support).

Subsequent adjustments include (based on ABG) increasing IPAP by 2 cm of H_2O in case of persistent hypercapnia and increasing both IPAP and EPAP by 2 cm of H_2O in case of persistent hypoxemia. The maximal IPAP should be limited to 20–25 cm of H_2O (to prevent gastric distension and patient discomfort), and maximal EPAP should be limited to 10–15 cm of H_2O.

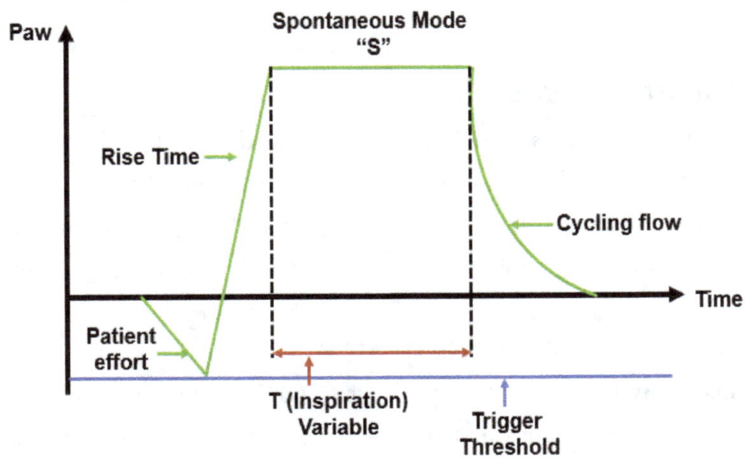

Figure 3: Typical pressure time scalar depicting variables when BiPAP is administered to a patient. (Credit: Dr. Jagadish Chandran, Consultant Critical Care Medicine, PSG Hospital, Coimbatore).

NIPPV with ventilator

Modern ventilators have noninvasive modes of ventilation incorporated into the software. The basic available modes are NIV with pressure support with CPAP and pressure control ventilation. Other advanced modes include proportional assist ventilation and average volume-assured pressure support. These advanced modes offer more safety in patients with additional comorbidities like neuromuscular disorders.

NIPPV delivered via ventilator is superior due to the presence of better flow sensors, presence of leak compensation, presence of backup ventilation (some modern BiPAP machines do have backup ventilation in case the patient stops breathing), detection of incomplete exhalation, and better monitoring due to larger display of scalars. Modern ventilators also have embedded software, which calculate resistance, airway pressures, percentage of leak, and actual I:E ratio due to patient's breaths which can useful for clinicians at the bedside in detecting NIV failure.

A trial of NIPPV should last not more than 2 hours, and if patients' symptoms are not improving and repeat ABG is worsening, then invasive mechanical ventilation should be considered. Prolonging NIV and delaying invasive mechanical ventilation in a worsening patient are shown to increase mortality.

Patient interfaces

The choice of interfaces to deliver NIPPV also determines the success of NIPPV. Various interfaces that are available include nasal masks, orofacial masks, full-face masks, total face masks, nasal pillow mask, mouthpiece, and helmets. The commonly used interfaces include full-face masks and helmets.

Disposition from emergency

Decisions to discharge or admit patients to the hospital with an AECOPD are complex. The following are the potential indications for hospitalization:

- Persistent respiratory failure despite bronchodilators.
- Presence of sudden severe worsening of respiratory dyspnea, decreased oxygen saturation, high RR, confusion, and drowsiness.

- Onset of new physical signs like cyanosis and peripheral edema.
- Presence of serious comorbidities (heart failure, arrythmias).
- Insufficient home support.

Management in intensive care unit (ICU)

Ventilatory management

Despite the clinical benefits of NIPPV with severe AECOPD, 20%–30% of patients will require intubation and mechanical ventilation. These patients have a poorer prognosis, with mortality rates between 20% and 73% and a mean life expectancy of one year.

The following are the indications for intubation: respiratory arrest, failure or contraindication to NIV, decreased level of consciousness (GCS ≤ 8), severe dyspnea with the use of accessory muscles and/or RR greater than 35 breaths per minute, hemodynamic instability, decreased level of consciousness, life-threatening hypoxemia, and severe acidosis (pH <7.25) and/or hypercapnia. The challenges in such patients are unique as they are often very hypoxic. Preoxygenation with NIPPV or high-flow oxygen has been proposed to remedy high-risk hypoxic patients with significant

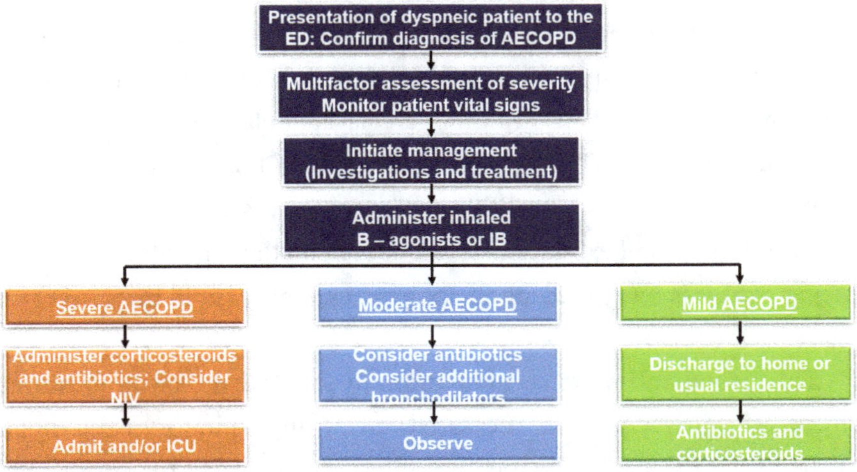

Figure 4: Suggested management approach to AECOPD in ER. (Adapted from Rowe et al. Expert Rev Resp Med. 2011;5(4):549–559.)

Table 4: Initial ventilator settings

Assist control mode	Most efficient at decreasing the work of breathing, more comfortable due to patient-triggered breaths
$FiO_2 = 1$	To counter the hypoxia and oxygen debt
Tidal volume 6–8 mL/kg	Excess tidal volume worsens dynamic hyperinflation
Inspiration: expiration ratio — 1:4 or 1:5	To allow sufficient time for exhalation
PEEP — 70% of the patient's intrinsic PEEP	To reduce work done on triggering breaths
Inspiratory flow: 80–100 L/minute	Higher flow allows for shorter inspiratory time and prolonged expiratory time

V/Q mismatch and shunt before sedation and paralysis and continuing its use through laryngoscopy, as this can extend the time before hypoxia occurs. Table 4 shows the initial ventilator settings in AECOPD patients after intubation.

Dynamic hyperinflation and auto-PEEP

Dynamic hyperinflation (DHI) refers to increased end-expiratory lung volume, and the pressure it exerts is called auto-PEEP. DHI can be predicted by observing for auto-PEEP or an elevated plateau pressure on the mechanical ventilator. The first indicator of DHI that can be seen on a mechanical ventilator is auto-PEEP, which represents an elevated alveolar pressure at the end of expiration. It can be seen on the ventilator flow-time tracing (which is more evident on applying expiratory hold maneuver) in Figure 5.

The second and more accurate indicator of DHI is plateau pressure, which is the airway pressure measured during an inspiratory pause/hold on the ventilator. A plateau pressure above 30 cm of H_2O is considered significantly elevated and correlates with complications of DHI. Peak

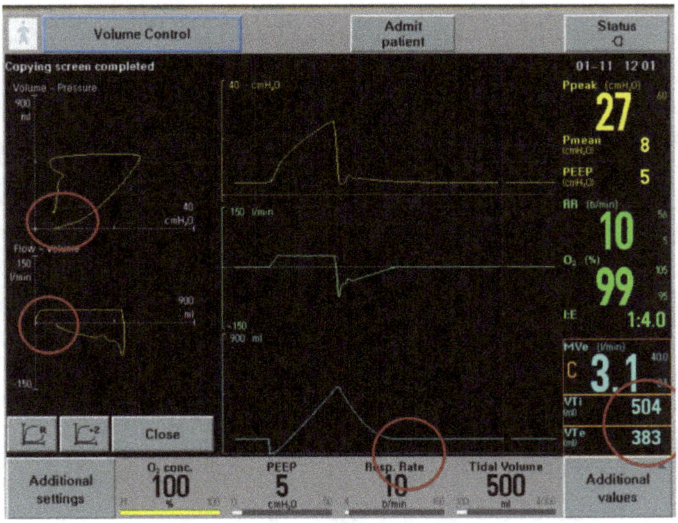

Figure 5: DHI (Credit: Dr. Shivakumar, assistant professor, SJMCH).

pressures on the ventilator do not correlate well with DHI and its consequences but should be kept under 50 cm of H_2O. A sudden rise in peak pressure is useful because it predicts endotracheal tube blockage, mucus plugging, and pneumothorax.

Causes of auto-PEEP in COPD patients are high resistance, low compliance, and incomplete time for exhalation. Auto-PEEP can also be worsened by errors in management like the use of small-sized endotracheal tubes and high tidal volume rate and RR, with shorter expiration time being set in a controlled mode of ventilation. The common problems while ventilating a COPD patient and its troubleshooting are given in Table 5.

Weaning from mechanical ventilation

Weaning a COPD patient from ventilation poses a unique set of challenges for the intensivist. There is now convincing evidence for the application of protocols to accelerate the process without increasing the failure rate as mechanical ventilation is associated with many side effects. In order to assess the readiness of patient's status for starting weaning, the following

Table 5: How to troubleshoot a COPD patient on a ventilator

Problem	Interventions to consider
High plateau pressure	• Consider pneumothorax • Increase inspiratory flow rate — shortens the inspiratory time • Decrease I:E ratio — prolongs the time for expiration • Sedate patient as needed to facilitate ventilation
Persistent hypoxia	• Aggressive suctioning • Ensure proper tube placement • Consider pneumothorax • Lung ultrasound — follow BLUE* (Bedside Lung Ultrasound in Emergency) protocol
Hypotension	• Decrease I:E ratio • Lung ultrasound — FALLS* protocol • Consider tension pneumothorax
PEA arrest	• General ACLS measures • Disconnect the endotracheal tube and apply manual pressure to chest if DHI is suspected

Adapted from Swadron S, et al. The acute presentation of chronic obstructive pulmonary disease in the emergency department: a challenging oxymoron. Emerg Med Pract. 2008;10:1–28.

*Refer to Lichtenstein D. FALLS-protocol: lung ultrasound in hemodynamic assessment of shock. Heart Lung Vessels. 2013;5:142–147.

need to be considered as the possible causes of ventilatory dependency and of difficult weaning (Table 6).

Table 7 summarizes the factors that predict successful weaning. Particularly in COPD, the use of noninvasive mechanical ventilation is recommended after extubation as it has been shown to reduce reintubation.

Nonventilatory adjunct therapies in ICU

Since critical illness is a highly catabolic state; nutrition should be adequately maintained. Excess carbohydrates in the diet should be avoided while maintaining adequate calorie and protein intake to avoid excess carbon

Table 6: Common causes of difficulties in weaning in a COPD patient

Gas exchange	• Ventilation–perfusion mismatch • Shunts (atelectasis, pulmonary thromboembolism)
Respiratory muscles	• Fatigue and muscle atrophy • Critical illness myopathy • Poor nutritional status due to COPD
Metabolism	• Overfeeding with excess CO_2 production • Electrolyte defects (hypokalemia due to beta-agonists, phosphate, magnesium deficiency)
Cardiovascular	• Left heart failure with acute lung edema • Pulmonary hypertension with right ventricle failure
Neurological	• Cortical dysfunction due to sedation and toxic — metabolic factors • Sleep apnea syndrome in obese COPD • Polyneuropathy of the critical patient • Severe restlessness and delirium

Adapted from Vicente EG, Almengor JS, Caballero LD, Campo JS. Invasive mechanical ventilation in COPD and asthma. Medicina Intensiva (English Edition). 2011 Jun 1;35(5):288–298.

Table 7: Factors predicting successful weaning

- pH >7.3
- Rapid shallow breathing index <100 (RR/tidal volume [L])
- Maximum inspiratory pressure > −20 to 30 cm H_2O
- P0.1 — occlusion pressure after 100 ms < 6 mbar
- Best diaphragmatic excursion on the right or left >25 mm
- Thickening fraction of the diaphragm during SBT >30%–36%
- Lung ultrasound score (LUS score) <13
- Capacity for inspiratory effort/cough
- No use of accessory muscles
- No relevant hyperinsufflation/auto-PEEP
- Normal cardiac output with good left ventricular systolic function

dioxide production to decrease the load on respiratory muscles. Factors like immobility, prolonged mechanical ventilation, and the use of corticosteroids will further add to muscle weakness. Hence, it is important to maintain good nutrition and physiotherapy. Bundled care is shown to reduce the incidence of ventilator-associated pneumonia, catheter-associated urinary tract infection, and central line–associated bloodstream infection rates. Attention should be given to prevent pressure ulcers and deep vein thrombosis (DVT). Pharmacological prophylaxis should be instituted for the prevention of DVT and pulmonary embolism in all AECOPD patients on invasive mechanical ventilation.

Summary

Short-acting beta-2 agonists, antibiotics, and corticosteroids remain the mainstay of pharmacological therapy in acute exacerbation of COPD. Coupled with nonpharmacological interventions like mechanical ventilation and weaning at the right time, good nutritional support, maintenance of electrolyte, and acid–base balances can lead to successful outcomes.

Case 1

Mr. SR is a 56-year-old gentleman with a history of diabetes for 10 years, current smoker with a smoking history of 35 pack-years, and COPD, on home BiPAP, now presents to the emergency room with increased sputum production with increased purulence for the past four days, increased shortness of breath despite BiPAP support, and worsening cough for the past two days. He says he is taking inhaled ipratropium and foracort 2 puffs twice a day, injection of human mixtard 20-0-18 units subcutaneously, tab metformin 500 mg twice a day, and tab vildagliptin 50 mg twice a day. He has been admitted twice to the hospital in the past four months for acute exacerbation of COPD and urinary tract infection. His nutritional status is poor with a body mass index of 18. He does not complain of fever, chest pain, or hemoptysis at present. His vitals include RR >45 cycles per minute, heart rate 132 beats per minute, blood

pressure of 90/30 mmHg, saturation of 82% on 15 L of oxygen, and temperature of 97.3°C. A quick clinical examination reveals cold peripheries and pedal edema, intercostal indrawing, paradoxical abdominal motion, and he is slow to respond.

Question 1: What is the next best step?

Answer: Mr. SR has AECOPD; the first goal is oxygen therapy as Mr. SR's saturation on 15 L of O_2 is 82%. We have to initiate NIPPV immediately starting with FiO_2 of 100% and gradually decreasing to target 92%. Hemodynamic stabilization has to be started simultaneously as SR is in septic shock as evidenced by wide pulse pressure. Fluid resuscitation should be cautious as he also possibly has right heart failure as evidenced by pedal edema. This can be confirmed by the point-of-care ultrasound (POCUS). His exacerbation should be medically managed with appropriate inhaler therapy which includes long-acting anticholinergic agents and short-acting beta-2 agonists and with inhaled corticosteroids. He is also a candidate for intravenous steroids. Antibiotic therapy is the next step with a stat dose of broad-spectrum antibiotic being administered in emergency as early antibiotic has shown to reduce mortality. A third-generation cephalosporin or a combination of beta-lactam–beta-lactamase inhibitor with antipseudomonal coverage is required as he has a history of recent hospitalization, and later based on cultures, including sputum, respiratory panel, and blood cultures, we can narrow the coverage.

POCUS in emergency shows right lower zone pneumonia, a normal left ventricular function with impaired right ventricular function (TAPSE-1.6 cm), and pulmonary hypertension with pulmonary artery systolic pressure of 55 mmHg. His ABG shows pH 7.19, $PaCO_2$ 65 mmHg, and PaO_2 56 mmHg on NIV. After a brief trial of NIV, there is no improvement in sensorium, and his RR increases to 55 cpm. A decision to institute invasive mechanical ventilation was made after speaking to the family.

Question 2: Explain how to proceed with intubation and invasive mechanical ventilation in this patient.

Answer: Rapid sequence intubation is preferred since all emergency intubation patients are considered to be full stomach and the risk of aspiration is more. Basic monitoring like electrocardiogram (ECG), NIBP, pulse oximeter, and capnography are required as the patient is significantly acidotic. Ventilator has to be checked and kept ready with circuit and filters. Preoxygenation should be done for 5 minutes with 100% oxygen by NIV mask. Induction and paralysis should be done with cardiostable drugs like injection fentanyl and midazolam combination or etomidate, and confirmation of tube placement should be done by capnography.

Question 3: What are the investigations you would do in this scenario in ER?

Answer: Apart from complete blood counts and tests for liver and renal functions, a 12-lead ECG is mandatory as the patient is diabetic. Incidence of ischemic heart disease in COPD patients is higher due to smoking-induced risks. Glucose levels should be monitored every 6–8 hours as the patient is in shock and has taken oral hypoglycemic agents; metabolism of these agents can be erratic leading to sudden hypoglycemia. Cultures and polymerase chain reaction panel should be directed toward the appropriate source respiratory in this patient. Computed tomography of the chest, although not mandatory, can be considered in this patient due to the suspicion of malignancy-induced weight loss.

After starting the patient on invasive mechanical ventilation, the patient was admitted to ICU. The following were the settings on the ventilator:

FiO_2-100%
Mode — Assist control
RR-24
PEEP — 8 cm of H_2O
Tidal volume — 500 mL

With the above settings, his intrinsic PEEP is 11 cm of H_2O and plateau pressure is 34 cm of H_2O. After half an hour in the ICU, his heart rate worsens to 140 cm of H_2O and blood pressure decreases to 80/60 mmHg. POCUS shows that his right heart function has worsened (TAPSE-1.1 cm).

Question 4: Explain the pathophysiology behind SR's deterioration and how do you rectify it?

Answer: Decompensated right ventricular failure secondary to DHI induced by inappropriate settings on the ventilator is the cause for his deterioration. In Mr. SR, who is a case of COPD, there is a setting of chronic pulmonary hypertension and right ventricle (RV) compensates by getting hypertrophied. Normally, RV has an innate but limited ability to undergo myocardial hypertrophy thus reducing wall tension and maintaining contractility for a finite period of time. But in this case, the inappropriate settings have caused an increase in pressure overload, which has led to worsening of right ventricular failure and DHI has caused decreased venous return leading to a drop in cardiac output which is seen as worsening hypotension and tachycardia. Immediate measure would be to disconnect SR from ventilator and allow complete exhalation. This should be followed by reducing RR to 12–14 breaths per minute, tidal volume to be kept 7 mL/kg of lean body mass, and ensuring sufficiently low I:E ratio (expiratory time should be at least four to five times the time constant of the patient. Time constant is the product of resistance and compliance which will be displayed on the ventilator).

Question 5: How do you treat right heart failure in SR?

Answer: Right heart failure in SR is acute on chronic. Factors contributing to acute worsening should be addressed to improve RV function. First would be to correct hypoxemia as oxygen is a potent pulmonary vasodilator. Employ the lowest plateau pressures through low tidal volume and PEEP in order to limit RV afterload and decrease in venous return. Avoid permissive hypercapnia to avoid hypoxic vasoconstriction and increase in pulmonary vasoconstriction. Hence, optimizing ventilator settings for a normal pH, optimal PEEP, and saturation of 92% is vital. Increasing RV contractility by the use of dobutamine or long-acting milrinone can be tried, especially after the septic shock component has settled. (Caution should be exercised while starting these agents as they can worsen distributive shock.)

Afterload reduction by selective pulmonary arterial dilation is also a crucial step in breaking the spiral of RV decompensation. Inhaled nitric oxide or inhaled epoprostenol can be tried, but there is no mortality benefit from the use of these agents. Once circulation is restored and patient has stabilized, excess volume can then be removed by diuretics, thereby reducing excess preload.

On day 5 of ICU stay, SR is still on invasive mechanical ventilation, intensivist's attempt to wean him off the ventilator has failed. His current treatment includes ceftriaxone 1 g intravenous twice a day, tab azithromycin 500 mg once daily, injection Lasix 20 mg twice a day, Inj human actrapid 8 units thrice a day, Inj pantoprazole 40 mg once daily, asthalin + ipratropium bromide inhalers 2 puffs twice a day, budesonide inhaler 2 puffs twice a day, and Inj heparin 5000 units subcutaneous twice a day. His shock has settled, and lung ultrasound shows persistent right lower lobe pneumonia with effusion. Investigations show persistent elevation of the total count, normalization of renal, and liver function tests are normal.

Question 6: Explain the factors that are contributing to delayed weaning in SR.

Answer: The following are the factors causing delayed weaning in SR: persistent lower lobe pneumonia with effusion might be due to inadequate initial antibiotic therapy (pseudomonal infection and infection by other multidrug-resistant organisms is common in COPD patients who have been recently hospitalized. Ceftriaxone and azithromycin do not cover these organisms). New-onset ventilator-associated pneumonia can also be a possibility. SR is on steroids and may not mount a fever.

The presence of effusion can act as a mechanical impediment for diaphragmatic excursion. Also, evaluation of the effusion is necessary to rule out empyema.

Poor nutritional status of SR means poor muscle mass. This coupled with mechanical ventilation which is known to cause deconditioning of respiratory muscles and diaphragm atrophy can lead to dependency on a ventilator. Use of steroids and muscle relaxants, mechanical ventilator, and shock on admission are all risk factors for critical illness polyneuropathy myopathy, which delays weaning.

After the escalation of antibiotics and removal of 1 L of exudative pleural effusion, SR is now tolerating spontaneous breathing trial on day 14. He is comfortable on FiO_2 40%, PS 14 cm of water, and PEEP 7 cm of water. His P0.1 is 4 mbar, and RSBI 78. His RV function is better with TAPSE-2.1, and he has a good cough reflex.

Question 7: How do you proceed with mechanical ventilation?
Answer: SR is now ready for extubation, although the pressure support on ventilator is high. Hence, despite having good indices of weaning (RSBI, P0.1), he is still at high risk of extubation failure due to the presence of chronic lung disease, poor muscle mass, and prolonged critical illness. He should be extubated onto NIV, and T-piece trial is inappropriate for him. Close monitoring over the next 2–3 days using ABG is necessary, and there should additional caution be exercised before deciding him to shift to step down unit.

Case 2

Ms. BC is a 45-year-old lady who is rushed to the emergency by neighbors in a state of unresponsiveness. The neighbors state that she lives

alone. She is seen smoking frequently since the past 10 years, but the neighbors are unaware of the history of pack-years. She was suffering from cough for three days and had difficulty in breathing for two days as per neighbors. She also complained of chest pain on the right side before loss of consciousness.

Question 1: What are the differential diagnoses to be considered in BC?
Answer:

1. AECOPD with pneumonia
2. Pulmonary embolism
3. Pneumothorax
4. Pleural effusion
5. Pulmonary edema (heart failure)
6. CVA
7. Acute coronary syndrome
8. Intoxication
9. Hypoglycemia

Question 2: How do you proceed to establish diagnosis in this patient?
Answer: Since history is grossly inadequate, physical examination and POCUS coupled with investigations is the only way to establish the diagnosis. Clinical examination should be quick and focused to narrow the diagnosis to one or two major systems like respiratory or cardiovascular. A normal random blood glucose rules out the diagnosis of hypoglycemia, and neurological examination can establish the diagnosis of CVA. ECG and point-of-care troponin tests help in establishing or ruling out acute coronary syndrome. For the rest of the differential diagnoses, POCUS is helpful. The BLUE and FALLS protocols should be followed.

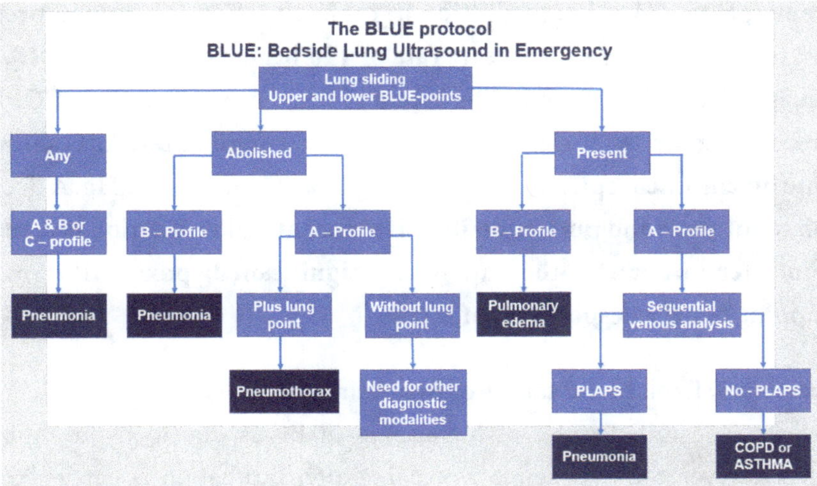

Adapted from Lichtenstein D. Breathe.2017 Jun;13(2):100–111. doi: 10.1183/20734735.004717.

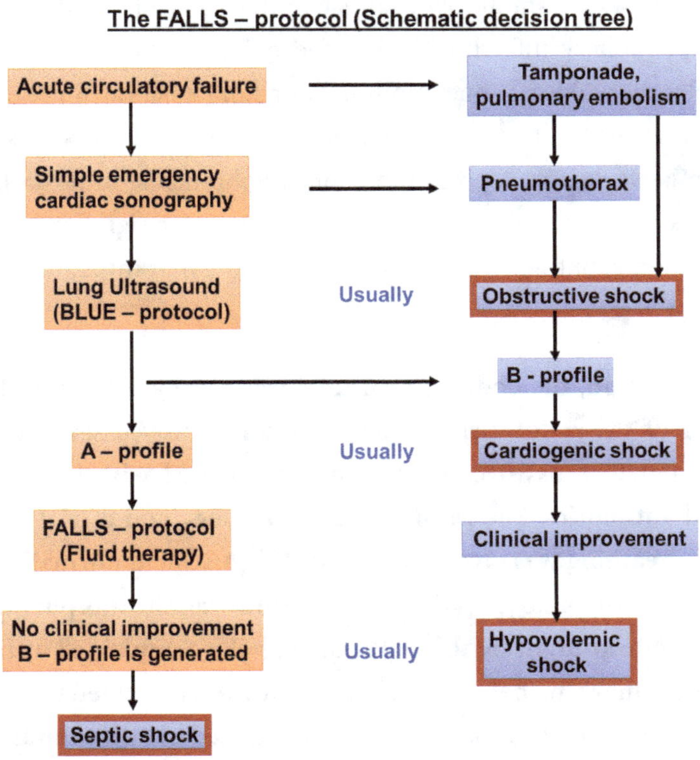

Adapted from Lichtenstein, D. FALLS-protocol: lung ultrasound in hemodynamic assessment of shock. Heart Lung Vessels. 2013;5:142–147.

In emergency room, her saturation in room air is 56% and blood pressure is 180/90 mmHg with heart rate of 120 beats per minute. POCUS is suggestive of COPD and a diagnosis of acute exacerbation of COPD is made. Her airway is clear, and she has poor cough reflex. ABG shows acute on chronic respiratory acidosis with $PaCO_2$ of 108 mmHg. A decision to intubate and put her on invasive mechanical ventilation is made. Soon after intubation, the patient has significant hypoxia with SpO_2 dropping to 36% despite FiO_2 of 100%.

Question 3: Explain the causes of hypoxemia in BC.

Answer: The initial cause of hypoxemia in BC is due to hypoventilation. However, the hypoxemia worsening after intubation is particularly concerning as now there is a shunt mechanism causing the worsening (hypoventilation is taken care of by invasive mechanical ventilation). The common causes for shunt (extracardiac in this particular case) are pneumonia, pulmonary infarction in massive pulmonary embolism, significant pulmonary edema, pneumothorax, or lung collapse. Since POCUS has already ruled out pulmonary edema and pulmonary embolism, and hypoxemia worsening is postintubation, endobronchial intubation causing lung collapse should be ruled out first. Another significant cause is pneumothorax, but it is unlikely to develop soon after intubation as DHI takes time to set in.

On examination, the endotracheal tube was fixed at 26 cm and repositioning of the endotracheal tube to 21 cm improved saturation. BC was ventilated in assist control mode and treated with bronchodilators and antibiotics. She regained consciousness, and a trial of spontaneous breathing was given after a day. Her ABG had normalized. She was planned for extubation the next day. However, she was put on assist control mode at night by the staff nurse as she complained of breathlessness. By morning before your rounds, you are informed that BC has cardiac arrest. On examination, you find reduced breath sounds on the

right side with a normal lung ultrasound with a plateau pressure of 42 on ventilator and she has pulseless electrical activity.

Question 4: What do you do next?

Answer: Causes of PEA are 5-Hs and 5-Ts, that is, hypoxia, hypotension, hypercarbia, H^+ ions-acidosis, hypothermia, toxins, tension pneumothorax, tamponade (cardiac), thrombosis (coronary), and pulmonary thromboembolism. In BC, there could be tension pneumothorax as suggested by high plateau pressure, normal ABG, and lung scan before. An immediate needle decompression in second intercostal space along the midclavicular line is necessary during the CPR. This should be followed by ICD placement after the return of spontaneous circulation.

An inquiry into the cause of the arrest reveals that the patient was ventilated overnight at a high rate and insufficient expiratory time causing DHI and tension pneumothorax. ICD placement has stabilized BC, and she does not suffer from any consequences of cardiac arrest like hypoxic encephalopathy as the duration of cardiac arrest was brief. A chest X-ray taken after ICD placement shows ICD in situ but multiple rib fractures secondary to CPR. Weaning was initiated after 48 hours. This time, however, she fails spontaneous breathing trial, and she is generating a low tidal volume. POCUS shows a profile on lung ultrasound with adequate lung sliding on both sides and a normal echocardiography (ECHO). Her ABG is normal except for potassium of 2.5 mEq/dL. How do you address this problem?

Answer: A normal lung scan and ECHO rule out cardiopulmonary causes for weaning difficulties as explained in Table 6. Weaning-induced cardiac dysfunction (an entity wherein cardiac dysfunction is unmasked after initiation of weaning) is also ruled out due to normal ECHO. Hypokalemia could be one of the reasons. This might be secondary to the use of beta-2 agonists, the dose of which can be tapered now due to decreased bronchospasm. Supplementing potassium will improve respiratory weakness.

Additional factor is the presence of pain due to rib fracture which prevents adequate ventilation. Analgesia to address pain should be started.

After correction of potassium and adequate analgesia, BC is now tolerating weaning on PS 5 cm of water. Her pneumothorax has resolved, and ICD has been removed. On day 7, intravenous steroids and antibiotics have been stopped with the continuation of inhaled bronchodilators. She is successfully extubated and is stable on 2 L of oxygen.

References and suggested readings

1. Halpin DMG, Criner GJ, Papi A, et al. Global initiative for the diagnosis, management, and prevention of chronic obstructive lung disease. The 2020 GOLD Science Committee report on COVID-19 and chronic obstructive pulmonary disease. Am J Respir Crit Care Med. 2021;203(1):24–36. doi: 10.1164/rccm.202009-3533SO.
2. Compagnon A, Nguyen L, Antoun Z, Stach B, Zanetti C, Le Guillou F. Management of acute COPD exacerbations in France: a qualitative survey in a private practice setting. PLoS One. 2021;16(1):e0245373. Published 2021 Jan 22. doi: 10.1371/journal.pone.0245373.
3. MacLeod M, Papi A, Contoli M, et al. Chronic obstructive pulmonary disease exacerbation fundamentals: diagnosis, treatment, prevention and disease impact. Respirology. 2021;26(6):532–551. doi: 10.1111/resp.14041.
4. Axson EL, Bottle A, Cowie MR, Quint JK. Relationship between heart failure and the risk of acute exacerbation of COPD [published online ahead of print, 2021 Apr 29]. Thorax. 2021;76(8):807–814. doi: 10.1136/thoraxjnl-2020-216390.
5. Lee RA, Centor RM, Humphrey LL, et al. Appropriate use of short-course antibiotics in common infections: best practice advice from the American College of Physicians. Ann Intern Med. 2021;174(6):822–827. doi: 10.7326/M20-7355.
6. Wu CT, Li GH, Huang CT, et al. Acute exacerbation of a chronic obstructive pulmonary disease prediction system using wearable device data, machine learning, and deep learning: development and cohort study. JMIR mHealth uHealth. 2021;9(5):e22591. Published 2021 May 6. doi: 10.2196/22591.

7. Ramakrishnan S, Janssens W, Burgel PR, et al. Standardisation of clinical assessment, management and follow-up of acute hospitalised exacerbation of COPD: a Europe-wide consensus. Int J Chron Obstruct Pulmon Dis. 2021;16:321–332. Published 2021 Feb 16. doi: 10.2147/COPD.S287705.
8. Teng W, Chen H, Shi S, Wang Y, Cheng K. Effect of bilevel continuous positive airway pressure for patients with type II respiratory failure due to acute exacerbation of COPD: a protocol for systematic review and meta-analysis. Medicine (Baltimore). 2021;100(2):e24016. doi: 10.1097/MD.0000000000024016.
9. Houchen-Wolloff L, Orme M, Barradell A, et al. Web-based self-management program (SPACE for COPD) for individuals hospitalized with an acute exacerbation of chronic obstructive pulmonary disease: nonrandomized feasibility trial of acceptability. JMIR mHealth uHealth. 2021;9(6):e21728. Published 2021 Jun 11. doi: 10.2196/21728.
10. Liang C, Mao X, Niu H, et al. Characteristics, management and in-hospital clinical outcomes among inpatients with acute exacerbation of chronic obstructive pulmonary disease in China: results from the phase I data of ACURE study. Int J Chron Obstruct Pulmon Dis. 2021;16:451–465. Published 2021 Feb 25. doi: 10.2147/COPD.S281957.
11. Alameda C, Matía ÁC, Casado V. Predictors for mortality due to acute exacerbation of COPD in primary care: derivation of a clinical prediction rule in a multicentre cohort study. Eur J Gen Pract. 2021;27(1):211–220. doi: 10.1080/13814788.2021.1959547.
12. Terraneo S, Rinaldo RF, Sferrazza Papa GF, et al. Distinct mechanical properties of the respiratory system evaluated by forced oscillation technique in acute exacerbation of COPD and acute decompensated heart failure. Diagnostics (Basel). 2021;11(3):554. Published 2021 Mar 19. doi: 10.3390/diagnostics11030554.
13. Takahashi Y, Watanabe N, Kamio N, Kobayashi R, Iinuma T, Imai K. Aspiration of periodontopathic bacteria due to poor oral hygiene potentially contributes to the aggravation of COVID-19. J Oral Sci. 2020;63(1):1–3. doi: 10.2334/josnusd.20-0388.
14. Tyagi D, Govindagoudar MB, Jakka S, Chandra S, Chaudhry D. Correlation of $PaCO_2$ and $ETCO_2$ in COPD patients with exacerbation on mechanical

ventilation. Indian J Crit Care Med. 2021;25(3):305–309. doi: 10.5005/jp-journals-10071-23762.

15. Mansfield KE, Mathur R, Tazare J, et al. Indirect acute effects of the COVID-19 pandemic on physical and mental health in the UK: a population-based study. Lancet Digit Health. 2021;3(4):e217–e230. doi: 10.1016/S2589-7500(21)00017-0.
16. Vestbo J, Waterer G, Leather D, et al. Mortality after admission with pneumonia is higher than after admission with an exacerbation of COPD. Eur Respir J. 2022;59(5):2102899. Published 2022 May 19. doi: 10.1183/13993003.02899-2021.
17. Yang T, Chen C, Chen Z. The CT pulmonary vascular parameters and disease severity in COPD patients on acute exacerbation: a correlation analysis. BMC Pulm Med. 2021;21(1):34. Published 2021 Jan 20. doi: 10.1186/s12890-020-01374-6.
18. Chen KY, Wu SM, Tseng CH, et al. Combination therapies with thiazolidinediones are associated with a lower risk of acute exacerbations in new-onset COPD patients with advanced diabetic mellitus: a cohort-based case-control study. BMC Pulm Med. 2021;21(1):141. Published 2021 Apr 29. doi: 10.1186/s12890-021-01505-7.

https://doi.org/10.1142/9789811271410_0015

15 Asthma–COPD overlap

Introduction

Asthma–chronic obstructive pulmonary disease (COPD) overlap (ACO) is the term used to describe patients with features of both asthma and COPD. It was observed in the Dutch hypothesis many decades ago that there are subjects who will have common features of chronic bronchitis and asthma and emphysema and asthma. It was recognized in various clinical studies that ACO is associated with a much greater number of acute exacerbations, hospital admissions in the wards as well as intensive care unit, and much higher use of public healthcare resources. There is little information on the ideal management strategies since most of the ACO subjects are excluded from clinical trials of asthma or COPD. There is now evidence that ACO itself has many phenotypes very similar to asthma and COPD, which are very heterogeneous disorders and have many phenotypes. More information is now available for both asthma and COPD targeting specific pathways and biologic mechanisms (endotypes).

Epidemiology

The prevalence of ACO is around 15%–20% of chronic asthma and COPD. As the subjects get older, physicians tend to diagnose COPD rather than asthma when there is fixed airflow limitation. In clinical studies that are based on spirometry criteria, among asthmatics, the prevalence of ACOS has ranged from 17% to 60% in non-smokers with severe asthma. Some features of incomplete reversibility of spirometry suggestive of fixed airflow limitation in asthmatics include male gender, older age, long duration of asthma especially childhood asthma, admission to hospital as a young child, atopy, eosinophilia in the blood or sputum, smokers, infrequent use of inhaled corticosteroids (ICS), sensitivity to non-steroidal anti-inflammatory drugs such as aspirin, and persistent low lung functions. In clinical studies based on spirometry among COPD subjects who had airway reversibility, the prevalence of ACO ranged from 24% in the ECLIPSE study to 52% in the UPLIFT study. In the Wellington study in New Zealand conducted on the general population, around 10% satisfied the criteria for ACO.

Definition of ACO

There is no consensus currently on the exact definition of ACO. Several organizations and investigators have defined ACO based on clinical spirometric and other criteria.

Criteria of Louie: Subjects with a physician diagnosis of asthma and COPD, atopy evidenced by allergic rhinitis or elevated immunoglobulin E (IgE), smoking history of greater than 10 pack-years, and fixed airway obstruction on postbronchodilator testing suggestive of COPD (forced expiratory volume in 1 second/forced vital capacity [FEV_1/FVC] <0.7). Other criteria included a reversibility of FEV_1 greater than 15% on postbronchodilator testing or 12% and 200 mL would be classified as minor criteria.

Spanish criteria: Subjects with COPD who had evidence of two or three major criteria that included: (1) a reversibility in FEV_1 on postbronchodilator testing of at least 15% and 400 mL, (2) elevated sputum eosinophil levels, and (3) previous history of asthma would be classified as ACO. Subjects with only one of the major criteria could be classified as ACO if they had two minor criteria: elevated serum total IgE, previous history of allergic rhinitis, previous reversibility in FEV_1 on postbronchodilator testing of greater than 12% and 200 mL on at least two occasions.

GINA–GOLD criteria: The GINA–GOLD document only described ACO and did not provide any definition. They described it as “ACOS is characterized by persistent airflow limitation with several features usually associated with asthma and several features usually associated with COPD."

Japanese criteria: This has the most stringent criteria for the diagnosis of ACO. The criteria include clinical and spirometric criteria. The characteristics that must be present (foundational) are age >40 years and fixed airflow limitation (FEV_1/FVC <0.7), the criteria used for COPD diagnosis. In addition, one of the following characteristics of COPD must be present: (1) smoking pack-years of greater than 10 pack-years or exposure to air pollution, (2) high-resolution CT having low attenuation scores typical of emphysema, and (3) a less than 80% DLCO. Along with the features of COPD, at least two features of asthma must be present: (1) age of asthma onset should be less than 40 years, (2) diurnal or seasonal variability in symptoms, and (3) fractional exhaled NO greater than 35 ppb. For patients who have only one feature of asthma, ACO can still be diagnosed If two additional features of asthma are present: (1) perennial allergic rhinitis, (2) postbronchodilator reversibility of FEV_1 greater than 12% and 200 mL, (3) increased total IgE, (4) increased specific IgE, and (5) increased peripheral eosinophilia of greater than 5% or absolute eosinophilia of greater than 300 cells/μL.

Pathophysiology

ACOS is diagnosed in subjects above the age of 40 years. There are differences in airway morphology and inflammation observed in patients with asthma, COPD, and ACO. Different clinical situations can lead to the development of ACO. One of them is childhood asthma, especially uncontrolled airflow limitation in early childhood can progress to ACO. Others include subjects with late-onset asthma who have significant smoking burden, subjects without any clinical symptoms but suffer from airway hyperresponsiveness can progress to chronic airflow limitation over time, subjects with small lungs due to various reasons including antenatal maternal nutritional deprivation, who are at higher risk of fixed airflow limitation. The major risk factors for the development of ACO are atopy and smoking (or equivalent risk factor for COPD such as biomass exposure and occupational exposure). The key pathophysiologic changes occur at the level of smooth muscle dysfunction and small airway inflammation. The smooth muscle abnormalities include smooth muscle hypertrophy and hyperplasia, bronchoconstriction, abnormal bronchial hyperresponsiveness, and inflammatory mediator release. The small airway changes include epithelial damage, mucosal edema, inflammatory cell infiltration, basement membrane thickening, inflammatory mediator release, and mucus hypersecretion.

The key differences between the pathophysiology of asthma, COPD, and ACO are listed in Table 1.

Table 1: The key differences between the pathophysiology of asthma, COPD and ACO

Variable	ACO	COPD	Asthma
Airway inflammation	Both eosinophils and neutrophils	Neutrophil predominant, except in some phenotypes	Eosinophil predominant, except in some phenotypes
	CD4 and CD8 T lymphocytes	CD4 and CD8 T lymphocytes	CD4 lymphocytes
	Mast cell	Alveolar macrophage	Alveolar macrophage
Smooth muscle	Hypertrophy and hyperplasia	Not a dominant feature	Hypertrophy and hyperplasia
Fibrosis	Peribronchiolar fibrosis	Peribronchiolar fibrosis	Basement membrane thickening
Emphysema	Emphysema can be seen	Emphysema common	No emphysema
Relevant cytokines	IgE, IL-4, IL-5, IL-13, IL-1, IL-8, IL-6, TNF-α, eotaxin, proteases, major basic protein	IL-1b, IL-8, IL-6, TNF-α, neutrophil elastase, proteinase-3, monocyte chemoattractant protein-1, matrix metalloproteinases, myeloperoxidase, mitogen-activated protein kinases	IgE, IL-2, IL-4, IL-5, IL-6, IL-9, IL-13, IL-17, IL-25, IL-33, TSLP, eotaxin, major basic protein, TGF-β

Adapted from Louie et al. Expert Rev Clin Pharmacol. 2013;6(2):197–219.

Clinical approach

With the differences in the current definitions, it is difficult for a clinician to make a clear diagnosis of ACO. It is important to understand the features of asthma and COPD and make the best judgment. Smoking and exposure to biomass and important risk factors that must be considered in a case of COPD. More research is needed to understand the threshold of these risk factors for ACO; for example, for the diagnosis of COPD at least 10 pack-years of smoking is necessary. Does the same hold good for ACO? The other important risk factor is asthma and both early-onset childhood asthma and late-onset asthma can be associated with ACO. The GINA–GOLD consensus document suggests the use of these steps.

The first is to confirm that the patient has a chronic airway disease. The second is a syndromic assessment of the diagnosis of three airway diseases: asthma, COPD, or ACOS. The third is performing spirometry to confirm the presence of chronic airflow limitation as well as postbronchodilator reversibility and understand the severity of the airflow limitation. The fourth is to start the treatment, and there are recommendations now on the ideal treatment for different ACO phenotypes. The fifth is to use additional investigations such as HRCT, FENO, peripheral and sputum eosinophilia, total IgE, specific IgE by skin prick testing, or serum-specific IgE for better phenotyping.

The GINA–GOLD recommends a checklist of characteristics that are suggestive of asthma and COPD and when there are similar number of features of asthma and COPD, the patient is said to have ACO (Table 2). One of the key issues with this recommendation is that every feature is given the same status. There is a need for further studies to understand the strength of each of these characteristics in the diagnosis of ACO. It is quite likely that exposure to smoking or biomass, fixed airflow limitation, and reversibility will be a few of the most important characteristics guiding the diagnosis.

Table 2: Characteristics of asthma, COPD, and ACO that aid in the diagnosis

Characteristic	ACO	Asthma	COPD
Normal FEV_1/FVC ratio postbronchodilator	Not compatible with diagnosis.	Compatible with diagnosis.	Not compatible with diagnosis.
FEV_1/FVC ratio <0.7	Needed for diagnosis.	May be seen. May improve with treatment unless there is airway remodeling.	Mandatory diagnosis.
FEV_1 > 80% postbronchodilator	Indicates mild disease.	Good control of asthma.	Indicates mild disease.
FEV_1 < 80% postbronchodilator	Decreasing FEV_1 indicates more severe disease. Risk factor for future risk acute exacerbations and mortality.	Decreasing FEV_1 indicates more severe disease. Risk factor for future risk acute exacerbations and mortality.	Decreasing FEV_1 indicates more severe disease. Risk factor for future risk acute exacerbations and mortality.
FEV_1 reversibility >12% and 200 mL	Is an important criterion for diagnosis.	Mandatory for diagnosis.	Can be seen in COPD in some cases.
FEV_1 reversibility >12% and 400 mL	Seen in some ACO phenotypes.	High likelihood of asthma.	Favours ACO.
Lung functions during asymptomatic or stable phase	Abnormal. Fixed airflow limitation.	Usually normal unless airway remodeling.	Abnormal. Fixed airflow limitation.
Family history of asthma	Can be present.	Present frequently.	Absent.
Allergic rhinitis	Can be present.	Present frequently.	Absent.

Age of onset	Usually diagnosis is made after the age of 40 years but can have childhood symptoms.	Usually childhood symptoms.	Starts after the age of 40 years.
Variations in respiratory symptoms	Variable, though persistent.	Highly variable, diurnal, and seasonal.	Continuous symptoms with some variability.
Natural course	Tends to progress with time.	Improves spontaneously or with treatment. Some cases develop fixed airflow limitations.	Progression is the rule.
Radiology	Hyperinflated lung fields.	Usually normal.	Hyperinflated lung fields.
Sputum cytology	Eosinophils and neutrophils.	Eosinophils usually, rarely neutrophils.	Neutrophils usually, in some cases, eosinophils.
Exacerbations	Frequent. More common than COPD.	Present. Risk substantially reduced with appropriate treatment.	Present. Comorbidities worsen the health status.
Corticosteroid responsiveness	Impaired.	High. Rarely impaired.	Impaired.
Tobacco smoke and biomass exposure	Usually present.	Not necessary for diagnosis.	Needed for diagnosis.
Systemic inflammation (IL-6, CRP)	Usual.	Not common.	Usual.
Hospitalizations and severe exacerbations	Common seen in 33% of subjects.	Rare.	Seen in around 18% of subjects.

Adapted from the GINA–GOLD document and Bateman et al.

ACO phenotypes

Clinical studies have identified heterogeneity in patients with ACO, and these phenotypes are useful to guide management and possibly influence the prognosis. Slightly different phenotypes of ACO have emerged from the studies of Lainez and Rhee. The important phenotypes and their characteristics from the Lainez classification are enumerated in Table 3. ACO phenotypes according to Rhee can be seen in Figure 1. In addition to other characteristics, differences in metabolites are observed between ACO and asthma and COPD, which is an important area of future research.

Management

There are hardly any good randomized clinical trials or meta-analysis of various medications for the management of ACO since the clinical trials on asthma and COPD have excluded ACO from their patient population. There are recommendations in the guidelines as consensus statements from expert groups based on the results from clinical trials of asthma and COPD.

Table 3: The important phenotypes and their characteristics from the Lainez classification

Characteristics	Phenotype A	Phenotype B	Phenotype C	Phenotype D
Symptom onset	Early onset before the age of 40 years	Late onset after the age of 40 years	Early onset before the age of 40 years	Late onset after the age of 40 years
FEV_1	<70% predicted	<70% predicted	>70% predicted	>70% predicted
MMRC scores	2 or more	2 or more	1 or less	1 or less
Body mass index	>25 kg/m^2	>25 kg/m^2	<25 kg/m^2	<25 kg/m^2
Pack-years of smoking	30 pack-years or more	30 pack-years or more	Less than 30 pack-years	Less than 30 pack-years
Emphysema on HRCT	Nearly two-thirds	Nearly two-thirds	Less than one-third	Less than one-third

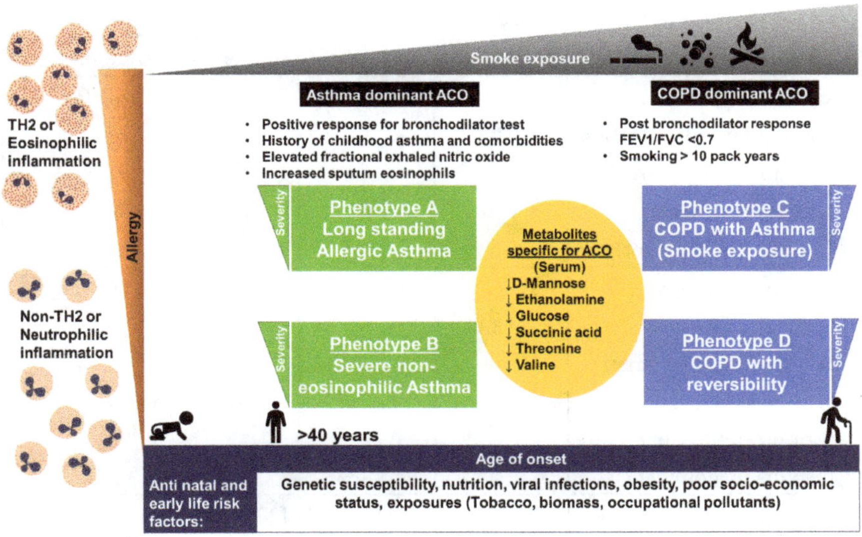

Figure 1: Phenotypes of ACO (modified from Rhee).

An important lesson learned from managing asthma and COPD patients that are useful in managing ACO is do not use LABA or LAMA alone in patients with ACO. Though they are useful in the management of COPD, they are detrimental when used alone in the management of asthma. The guidelines therefore recommend that for all patients with ACO, ICS must be included.

In subjects with ACOS, a subgroup with elevated sputum or blood or eosinophilia have a greater response to ICS. There is neutrophil-predominant inflammation in some patients with ACOS, which may not respond to ICS. Medications such as roflumilast that predominantly work in neutrophil-related pathways could be useful in ACOS. Subjects with greater cholinergic tone will benefit from anticholinergics such as tiotropium or glycopyrronium.

Based on the information on ACO phenotypes available, Rhee classified the subjects with ACO into four distinct phenotypes, where two were asthma predominant and two were COPD predominant. The possible management strategies are enumerated in Table 4.

Table 4: The possible management strategies

ACO phenotype	First choice	Add on — I	Add on — II	Add on — III
Lifelong allergic asthma -Eosinophilic inflammation Less or no smoke exposure Low or no emphysema (asthma predominant)	ICS + LABA	LAMA	LTRA	Anti-IgE
Severe non-eosinophilic asthma -Neutrophilic inflammation Less or no smoke exposure Low or no emphysema (asthma predominant)	ICS + LABA	LAMA	LTRA	Macrolide
COPD with a history of smoking and asthma -Eosinophilic inflammation High smoke exposure High emphysema (COPD predominant)	ICS + LABA	LAMA	LTRA	
COPD with reversibility -Neutrophilic inflammation High smoke exposure High emphysema (COPD predominant)	LABA + LAMA	ICS + LABA	ICS + LABA + LAMA	Add roflumilast Add macrolides

Conclusions and future research

The understanding of ACO needs further intense study as most of the clinical trials on asthma and COPD have excluded these subjects. Several phenotypes have been described even among subjects with ACO, and it is likely that these need to be studied and optimal pharmacotherapies for these phenotypes are likely to be different. There is a need for developing an algorithm for diagnosis, evaluation, phenotyping, and treatment of ACO.

References and suggested readings

1. Tu X, Donovan C, Kim RY, Wark PAB, Horvat JC, Hansbro PM. Asthma-COPD overlap: current understanding and the utility of experimental models. Eur Respir Rev. 2021;30(159):190185. Published 2021 Feb 16. doi: 10.1183/16000617.0185-2019.
2. Wu TD, Fawzy A, Kinney GL, et al. Metformin use and respiratory outcomes in asthma-COPD overlap. Respir Res. 2021;22(1):70. Published 2021 Feb 26. doi: 10.1186/s12931-021-01658-3.
3. Jung JY. Characteristics of asthma-COPD overlap according to various criteria. Tuberc Respir Dis (Seoul). 2021;84(1):87–88. doi: 10.4046/trd.2020.0157.
4. Barrecheguren M, Pinto L, Mostafavi-Pour-Manshadi SM, et al. Identification and definition of asthma-COPD overlap: the CanCOLD study. Respirology. 2020;25(8):836–849. doi: 10.1111/resp.13780.
5. Ahmedy F, Hayati F, Abdul Rahim SSS, Payus AO. A promising intervention for comprehensive pulmonary rehabilitation for asthma COPD overlap syndrome. Oman Med J. 2021;36(1):e232. Published 2021 Jan 31. doi: 10.5001/omj.2021.14.
6. Bircan E, Bezirhan U, Porter A, Fagan P, Orloff MS. Electronic cigarette use and its association with asthma, chronic obstructive pulmonary disease (COPD) and asthma-COPD overlap syndrome among never cigarette smokers. Tob Induc Dis. 2021;19:23. Published 2021 Apr 7. doi: 10.18332/tid/132833.
7. Orooj M, Moiz JA, Mujaddadi A. Letter in reply: a promising intervention for comprehensive pulmonary rehabilitation for asthma COPD overlap syndrome. Oman Med J. 2021;36(1):e234. Published 2021 Jan 31. doi: 10.5001/omj.2021.15.
8. Reddel HK, Vestbo J, Agustí A, et al. Heterogeneity within and between physician-diagnosed asthma and/or COPD: NOVELTY cohort. Eur Respir J. 2021;58(3):2003927. Published 2021 Sep 23. doi: 10.1183/13993003.03927-2020.
9. Queiroz APA, Fonseca FR, Rê A, Maurici R. Clinical, laboratory, and functional characteristics of asthma-COPD overlap in patients with a primary diagnosis of COPD. J Bras Pneumol. 2020;47(1):e20200033. Published 2020 Nov 6. doi: 10.36416/1806-3756/e20200033.

10. Hirai K, Tanaka A, Homma T, et al. Prevalence and clinical features of asthma-COPD overlap in patients with COPD not using inhaled corticosteroids. Allergol Int. 2021;70(1):134–135. doi: 10.1016/j.alit.2020.07.009.
11. Toyota H, Sugimoto N, Kobayashi K, et al. Comprehensive analysis of allergen-specific IgE in COPD: mite-specific IgE specifically related to the diagnosis of asthma-COPD overlap. Allergy Asthma Clin Immunol. 2021;17(1):13. Published 2021 Feb 4. doi: 10.1186/s13223-021-00514-9.
12. Kang J, Zheng J, Cai B, et al. Current situation of asthma-COPD overlap in Chinese patients older than 40 years with airflow limitation: a multicenter, cross-sectional, non-interventional study. Ther Adv Respir Dis. 2020;14:1753466620961699. doi: 10.1177/1753466620961699.
13. Ma P, Li S, Yang H, et al. Comparative RNA-seq transcriptome analysis on pulmonary inflammation in a mouse model of asthma-COPD overlap syndrome. Front Cell Dev Biol. 2021;9:628957. Published 2021 Mar 25. doi: 10.3389/fcell.2021.628957.
14. Dierick BJH, Flokstra-de Blok BMJ, van der Molen T, et al. Work absence in patients with asthma and/or COPD: a population-based study. NPJ Prim Care Respir Med. 2021;31(1):9. Published 2021 Feb 16. doi: 10.1038/s41533-021-00217-z.
15. Kaplan A, Cao H, FitzGerald JM, et al. Artificial intelligence/machine learning in respiratory medicine and potential role in asthma and COPD diagnosis. J Allergy Clin Immunol Pract. 2021;9(6):2255–2261. doi: 10.1016/j.jaip.2021.02.014.

https://doi.org/10.1142/9789811271410_0016

16 Bronchiectasis

Introduction

Bronchiectasis is defined as the permanent and abnormal dilation of the bronchi (morphological definition). In many countries, bronchiectasis is an important cause of morbidity and mortality. In western countries, cystic fibrosis is a very important cause of bronchiectasis, whereas in developing countries, causes such as postinfectious, particularly post-tubercular, sequelae are important. Bronchiectasis was first described by Laennec and is an important suppurative lung disease with multiple causes, pathologies, and clinical features. The incidence of bronchiectasis has been found to increase in different studies across the world, with a peak incidence at older ages in one study. Studies have found higher rates of bronchiectasis among Asians and women in general. These subjects have a high economic burden on themselves and the community with mortality rates of around 10% over a 4-year follow-up.

Types of bronchiectasis

Mainly classified similarly to the definition on *morphological* grounds.

- Cystic or saccular is the most severe form of bronchiectasis, with many cystic dilations in the airways. Entire segments or lobes may be involved. Easily diagnosed by the HRCT thorax.
- Varicose bronchiectasis (Figure 1), wherein the dilated segments alternate with constricted segments of the airways. Best diagnosed with the HRCT thorax.

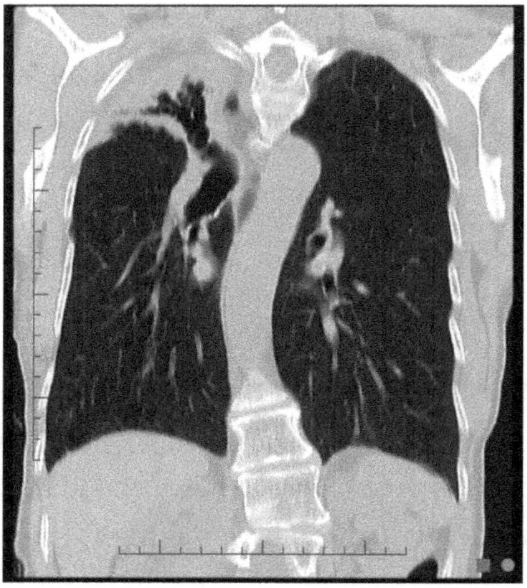

Figure 1: Varicose.

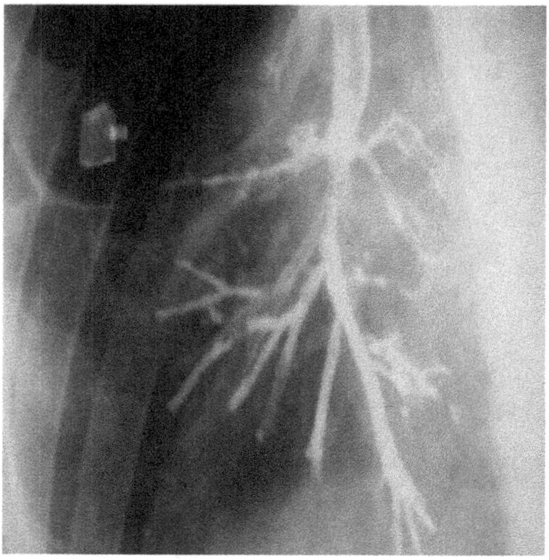

Figure 2: Normal bronchogram.

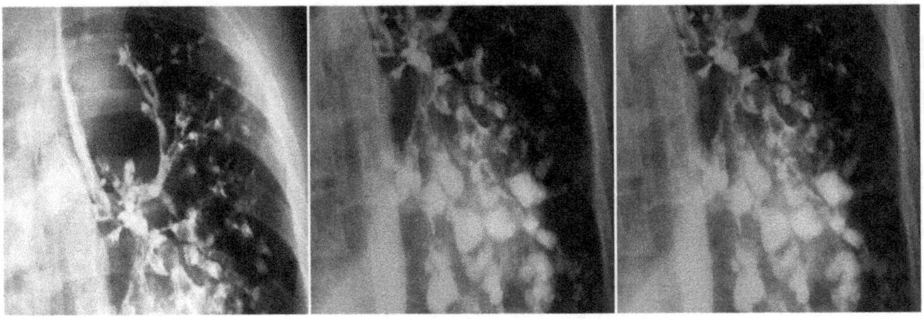

Figure 3: Series of images showing bronchiectasis in an abnormal dilation of the airways.

- Cylindrical or tubular, wherein the entire length of the airway is dilated. The best tool to diagnose this type of bronchiectasis is bronchogram, in which the size of the bronchi does not taper on branching. Most possible causes are postinfectious such as measles and diphtheria.

The other classification is according to the *etiology*, whether it is congenital or acquired. The classical examples of congenital bronchiectasis are cystic fibrosis and ciliary dyskinesia and of acquired bronchiectasis are post-tubercular and post-pneumonia bronchiectasis. In some cases of pneumonia, the airways may be dilated temporarily for up to 6 months which is called pseudobronchiectasis. Therefore, interpret bronchiectasis on HRCT within 6 months of a pneumonia carefully, and it may be useful to repeat it after 6 months to confirm the presence of true bronchiectasis.

Etiology of bronchiectasis

The common causes of congenital and acquired bronchiectasis are listed in the following table.

Congenital bronchiectasis	Acquired bronchiectasis
Cystic fibrosis	Postinfectious Tuberculosis
Ciliary dyskinesia (classical is Kartagener's syndrome)	Measles Diphtheria Human immunodeficiency virus
Mounier-Kuhn syndrome (or tracheobronchomegaly)	Other bacterial pneumonias Fungal (classical — *Aspergillus*)
William–Campbell syndrome with cartilage deficiency	Inhalational injury Smoke, gases
Marfan's syndrome	Collagen vascular diseases Rheumatoid arthritis
Young's syndrome	Sjogren's syndrome
Yellow nail syndrome	Foreign body Children (organic and inorganic)
Immunodeficiency syndromes	Elderly (dentures)
Job's syndrome	
	Inflammatory bowel disease
Alpha-1 antitrypsin deficiency	Crohn's disease Ulcerative colitis
	Aspiration
	Bronchial obstruction Benign tumors Malignant tumors Extraluminal obstruction (lymphadenopathy)

Pathogenesis

Bronchiectasis can be local or diffuse depending on the cause. Local mucosal injury, intraluminal (foreign body), intramural (benign tumor) or extraluminal obstruction (compression by enlarged lymph nodes), and localized infections (pneumonia, tuberculosis) usually leads to focused injury to that part of the airways. On the other hand, diffuse infections (viral), immunodeficiencies, ciliary dyskinesia, biochemical dysfunctions as seen in cystic fibrosis, and autoimmune defects such as rheumatoid arthritis generally lead to bilateral diffuse bronchiectasis. A congenital bronchiectasis mostly involves the left lung, whereas the acquired bronchiectasis involves the right lung initially, in early stages, and involves both lungs in later stages. The vicious cycle hypothesis proposes that impaired ciliary clearance of airway secretions due to any mechanism leads to bacterial colonization that invites neutrophils and their mediators into the airway lumen leading to the destruction of the cartilage causing bronchiectasis.

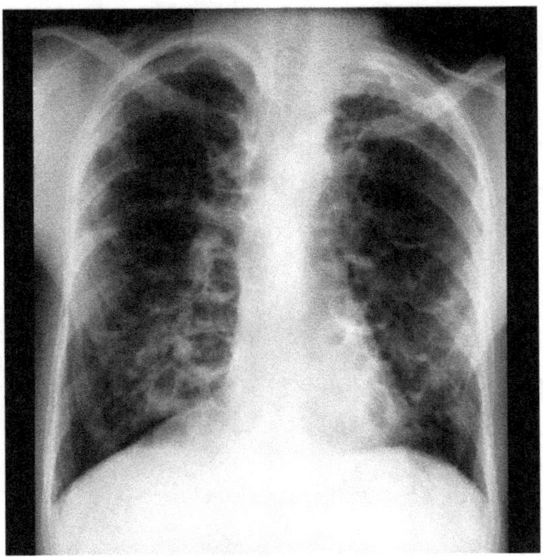

Figure 4: Bil bronchiectasis — X-ray.

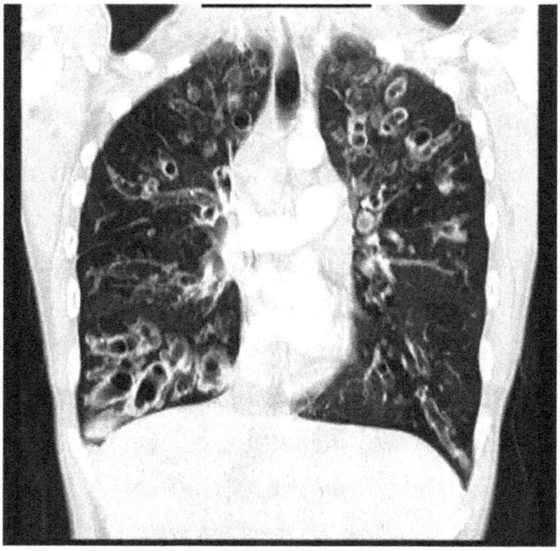

Figure 5: HRCT thorax of bilateral bronchiectasis.

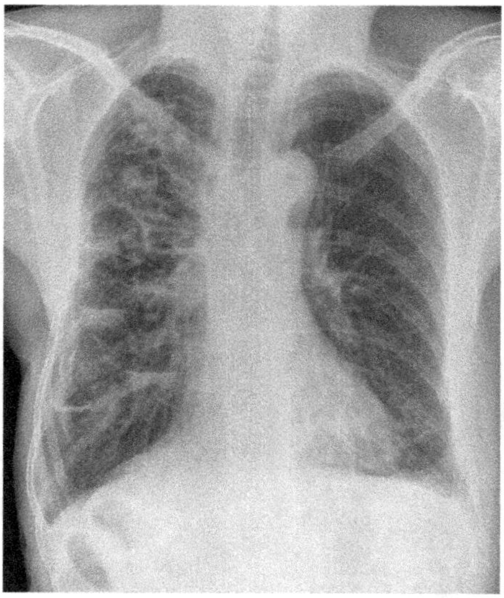

Figure 6: Cystic bronchiectasis — X-ray.

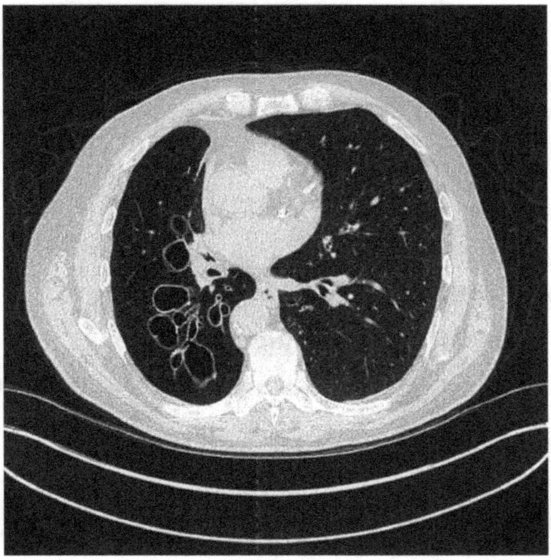

Figure 7: HRCT thorax of cystic bronchiectasis.

Cystic fibrosis

Mutations in the cystic fibrosis transmembrane conductance regulator (CFTR) are the underlying cause of CF. It is an autosomal recessive condition that is much more common in western countries. It usually presents in childhood, but sometimes it can present in adulthood for the first time. It may be associated with pancreatic dysfunction in some patients. The most common CFTR gene mutation is the ΔF508 mutation, which leads to the deletion of three nucleotides. This leads to the deletion of the amino acid phenylalanine in the 508th position in the CFTR protein, making it dysfunctional. More than 1,500 other mutations are known to cause CF. The CFTR protein is a chloride ion channel that is important in making sweat, mucus, and digestive juices. An increase in chloride in the airway secretions with loss of sodium from the sol layer of the mucus causes dehydration in the airway secretions and makes it thick and difficult to expectorate with a higher risk of infections. The thick secretions cause difficulty for cilia to function effectively. The cilia which beat usually in the sol layer now have to beat in the thicker and viscous gel layer due to the reduced sol layer, as a result of dehydration. Initially cystic fibrosis affects the upper lobes and later can be extensive. In later stages, the common organisms isolated are *Staphylococcus* or *Pseudomonas.*

Ciliary dyskinesia

Ciliary motility is one of the most important defense systems of the lung aiding in regular lung clearance. The mucus lining the airway mucosa is divided into the gel layer on the top and the sol layer on the bottom. The cilia usually beat in the much thinner sol layer, and the unidirectional movement is akin to rowing the boat. The classical case of ciliary dyskinesia is the "Kartagener's syndrome" which consists of sinusitis, bronchiectasis, and situs inversus or only dextrocardia and accounts for nearly half of all ciliary dyskinesia. It is inherited as an autosomal recessive disorder. The key defect is the absence or shortening of the dynein arms. Studies have identified the key defect to be a protein associated with the heavy chain in the dynein arm and the genetic defect located in the chromosome 5 p15-14, DNA H5. Many other defects are known including supernumerary microtubules or reduction in the number of microtubules in the cilia. The poor ciliary movement is associated with the retention of secretions, which leads to recurrent infections, and the proteases released by host defense cells such as neutrophils as well as the bacterial toxins lead to the destruction of cartilage over a period of time. Usually the lungs are normal at birth, and ciliary dyskinesia is present in children with recurrent lower respiratory tract infections or infections that do not respond easily to antibiotics.

Other causes

Immunodeficiency disorders cause recurrent lower respiratory infections and can end up causing bronchiectasis. These disorders may need to be worked up when the diagnosis of bronchiectasis cannot be elucidated.

Humoral immunodeficiencies related to IgG, IgM, and IgA have been commonly associated with bronchiectasis. Rarely, IgG subclass deficiency is also associated with bronchiectasis. Autoimmune and inflammatory disorders (rheumatoid arthritis, Sjogren's syndrome, Crohn's disease, and ulcerative colitis) that involve the lungs can cause bronchiectasis due to inflammatory destruction of the airway cartilage. Lung manifestations can be present sometimes before the clinical presentation of the autoimmune diseases. ABPA is a common cause of bronchiectasis which is classically central bronchiectasis. What is the reason for the central nature? It could be because of the large size of the fungal hyphae that elicit type I, III, and IV reactions in susceptible individuals that causes airway damage. In later stages, direct invasion of the airway wall and destruction have been reported. In the early stages, the damage is the result of various factors: mycotoxins and the host inflammatory response including neutrophil elastase and interleukins. Defective weakened collagen is the cause of cartilage weakening and bronchiectasis in Marfan's, William–Campbell, and Mounier-Kuhn syndromes. Patients with human immunodeficiency virus (HIV), especially in subjects with low CD4 counts, are prone to recurrent pyogenic, fungal, mycobacterial, and PCP infections that culminate in bronchiectasis. In children with HIV, the occurrence of lymphocytic interstitial pneumonia is associated with bronchiectasis. Long-standing asthma or chronic obstructive pulmonary disease (COPD) due to mucus hypersecretion, mucus plugging, recurrent infections, and chronic inflammation may cause bronchiectasis as has been seen in many studies. Brock's syndrome or middle lobe bronchiectasis is usually seen secondary to tuberculosis, and the important reasons for the involvement of the middle lobe bronchus are as follows: middle lobe bronchus originates at right angles to the right intermediate bronchus, it is the narrowest of all the lobar bronchi, it runs the longest intrapulmonary course of any lobar bronchi, and it is extensively surrounded throughout its course by lymph nodes which when enlarge causes bronchial obstruction leading to the stasis of secretions, recurrent infections, and bronchiectasis.

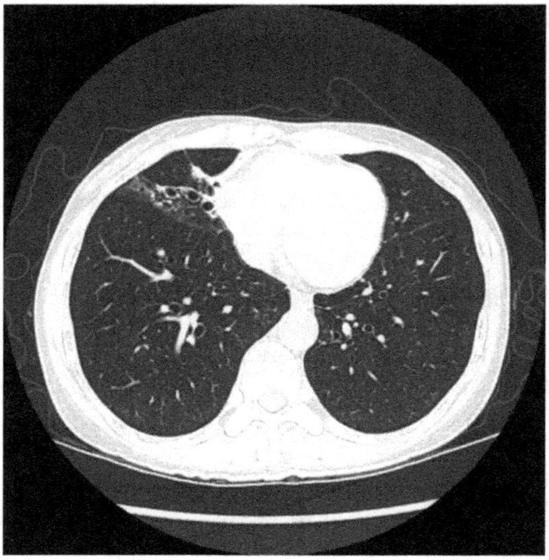

Figure 8: Middle lobe.

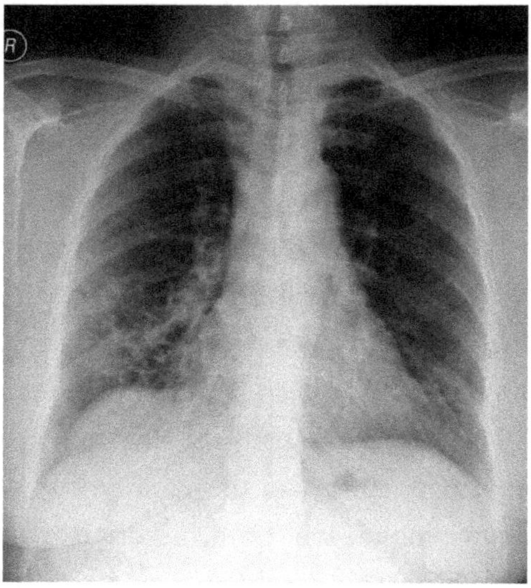

Figure 9: Middle lobe bronchiectasis.

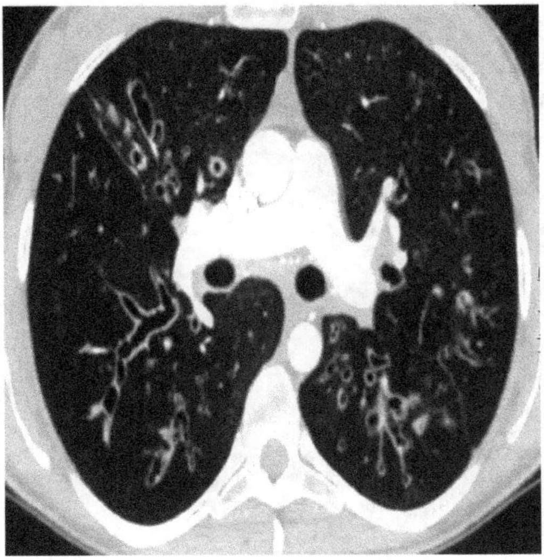

Figure 10: ABPA showing central bronchiectasis.

Clinical presentation

The classical clinical presentation of bronchiectasis includes copious foul-smelling purulent expectoration with a postural variation. Some bronchiectasis may have less purulent secretions or can be dry (bronchiectasis Sicca), which presents only with cough with or without hemoptysis. This is due to bronchiectasis being present only in the upper lobes of the lungs which drains due to the gravity unlike bronchiectasis in the lower lobes where natural gravity-assisted drainage is not possible. In later stages, dyspnea on exertion and progressing to dyspnea at rest is the rule. Many of these subjects with bronchiectasis will also have wheeze and may be mistaken for asthma or COPD. Hemoptysis can be sputum streaked with blood to massive hemoptysis if there is airway erosion during infection that leads to an arterial bleed. On clinical examination, clubbing may be prominent in some cases, but many cases of bronchiectasis can present without clubbing. Loss of lung volume may be an important feature of

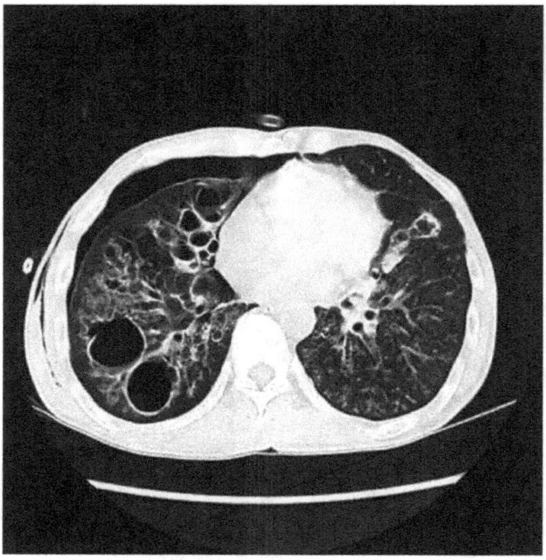

Figure 11: Bronchiectasis causing right-sided pneumothorax.

post-tubercular fibrosis associated with traction bronchiectasis. Crepitations are important localizing signs to suggest which lobes can be involved. Even a small bronchiectasis that may be seen only on HRCT and not on routine chest X-ray may cause generalized airway obstruction observed as bilateral rhonchi. In extensive cystic bronchiectasis, one may be able to auscultate a cavernous or even amphoric breath sounds.

Bronchiectasis is often characterized by exacerbations that increase in severity and frequency over time as the disease progresses. The O'Donnell's criteria for acute exacerbations of bronchiectasis include any four of the following symptoms: increase in quantity and purulence of sputum, increasing dyspnea, fever, increased cough, increased wheezing, radiological changes suggesting a new lesion, reduced pulmonary functions, lethargy, and decreased exercise tolerance; chest sounds such as crepitations have increased since when the subject was stable. Sometimes bronchiectasis can be associated with pneumothorax.

Investigations

The investigations for bronchiectasis are concerned with four main issues: structural, functional, microbiologic, and cause-specific. Structural investigations include chest X-ray and HRCT thorax that helps us to understand the extent of involvement (how many lobes are affected) and whether it is saccular, varicose, or cylindrical. The functional investigations include spirometry to assess the level of airway obstruction or restriction and its reversibility. As the disease worsens, one needs to investigate for hypoxia and hypercapnia (arterial blood gases). Studies evaluating bronchiectatic subjects with near-normal lung functions have shown that significant of them have increased bronchial hyperresponsiveness on methacholine challenge. Microbiologic evaluation includes the type of bacteria and their drug resistance. In the early stages of bronchiectasis, the common types of bacteria isolated in the early stage are *Streptococcus*, *Pneumococcus*, *Hemophilus*, and *Branhamella*. As the disease progresses, Gram-negative infections predominate, such as *Klebsiella*, *Proteus*, and *Serratia*. Later, *Staphylococcus*, which is very difficult to eradicate, and then the risk of death during an acute exacerbation increases. Lastly, difficult bacteria such as *Pseudomonas* and *Acinetobacter* are seen which are almost impossible to eradicate in subjects who also have structural and immunologic abnormalities that affect the normal host defense mechanisms. There is a high risk of significant morbidity and mortality from the third stage onward with *Staphylococcus*, *Pseudomonas*, and *Acinetobacter* infections. The cause-specific investigations include all the common causes: sputum AFB and GeneXpert TB PCR for mycobacterial infections; mucosal biopsy and electron microscopy studies for ciliary dyskinesia (easier way to study would include fresh semen analysis for sperm motility, and azoospermia may be seen in Young's syndrome); collagen vascular profile for rheumatoid arthritis; and Sjogren's, total IgA, IgM, and IgG for immunodeficiency disorders; imaging for Kartagener's syndrome; investigations for ABPA (discussed in a later chapter); sweat chloride test; CFTR gene mutation analysis; and bronchoscopy, especially when a radiolucent foreign body is suspected and may not be seen in routine imaging and fungal culture.

Management

The key goals enumerated in an excellent review by Barker remain the same even after it was published more than a decade and a half ago. The key goals are to limit, as far as possible, the further progression of the disease, reduce bacterial load leading to fewer acute exacerbations, manage acute exacerbations of bronchiectasis aggressively with early and appropriate introduction of antibiotics, some cases may need long-term antibiotic suppressive therapy, reduce airway inflammation, airway physiotherapy (bronchial toilet), and reduce viscosity and quantity of mucus. Hemoptysis should be managed according to its severity (discussed in a separate chapter), and surgical resection should be considered when the bronchiectasis is localized and is due to an acquired cause and is causing significant clinical morbidity.

Pharmacologic

1. Antibiotics: It is important that it is started early during the course of an exacerbation. Selection of an appropriate antibiotic is essential and not that difficult if the patient is on long-term follow-up in a single center, which has access to previous microbiologic reports. When the case is seen for the first time, empirical antibiotics can be started and modified based on the reports of culture sensitivity. Rapid drug sensitivity testing using polymerase chain reaction methods or liquid culture methods may soon become available and would immensely help the clinician. Depending on the severity of the exacerbation, oral or parenteral antibiotics can be chosen. Usual duration is 7–10 days but may need to be longer in some cases. Antibiotic suppressive therapy is used in some cases with a much longer duration of antibiotics. Oral erythromycin has been tried in the dose of 500 mg twice a day

for 8 weeks as well as quinolones. The various trials that have used macrolides are the EMBRACE trial (Effectiveness of Macrolides in patients with BRonchiectasis using Azithroymycin to Control Exacerbations), the BLESS trial (Bronchiectasis and Low-dose Erythromycin Study), and the BAT study (Bronchiectasis and Long-term Azithromycin Treatment). The key issue with long-term antibiotic use is the development of drug resistance. Some authors suggest alternating the antibiotics when suppressive therapy is planned, which can reduce the chance of drug resistance. Others have tried nebulized antibiotics; tobramycin at 300 mg per dose twice daily for 4 weeks had a beneficial effect on the microbiological load of *Pseudomonas*, but no functional effect on lung functions (many of them may have fixed airway obstruction, which may not respond to treatment, though there is a clinical improvement). A low-cost alternative is nebulized gentamicin at 40 mg twice daily. Nebulized antibiotics may lead to lesser systemic absorption and adverse events on long-term usage.

2. Antifungal and corticosteroids: This is advised for ABPA. Itraconazole at 200 mg twice daily for 16 weeks and once daily for the next 16 weeks along with corticosteroids had a better effect than corticosteroids alone.
3. *Mycobacterium tuberculosis*: The usual drug regimen is to be planned following the guidelines discussed in other chapters of this book.
4. *Mycobacterium avium* complex: Macrolides (azithromycin or clarithromycin), rifampicin or rifabutin, and ethambutol for 1 year after cultures have been negative are recommended.
5. Bronchodilators: inhaled (nebulized or via MDI/DPI).
6. Inhaled corticosteroids (ICS): Both for maintenance and during acute exacerbations. Both medium and high doses have been tried with variable benefits: reduction of sputum volume, sputum inflammatory mediators but not on lung functions, and number of acute exacerbations. Some adverse events such as osteoporosis and cataracts are higher on using long-term ICS, but the type of bacteria appears to be similar even in subjects using long-term ICS.

7. Oral corticosteroids: For acute exacerbations only as a short course.
8. Mucolytics: It has some benefits. Hydration with water is the best mucolytic. Others can be given (ambroxol, guaifenesin, bromhexine, acetylcysteine, carbocysteine, rhDNase, hypertonic saline).
9. Vaccinations: They are useful (influenza and pneumococcal).
10. Oral or inhaled indomethacin: It is not yet approved by FDA, and it reduces neutrophil mediators.
11. Long-term oxygen therapy as a palliative measure in cor pulmonale.

Non-pharmacologic

1. Pulmonary physiotherapy: This is the single most important therapeutic strategy that should be performed at least twice daily to delay the further progression of bronchiectasis and reduce the number of acute exacerbations. This is ideally performed under supervision but can be done at home with the "universal drainage" protocol that mainly drains the lower lobes. If the subject is elderly or debilitated or has knee pain or back pain, then this may not be possible. Then, the more traditional gravity-assisted postural drainage is essential. There are additional tools such as the chest vibrators (high-frequency chest wall oscillators) that can assist the subject in coughing and expectorating. Oral devices that apply positive expiratory pressure during expiration prevent the airways from collapsing and aid in expectoration.
2. Exercise: Other than the chest physiotherapy, regular exercise protocols are equally essential to increase the anaerobic threshold, thus improving exercise capacity, quality of life, and survival.
3. Surgery: It is indicated when there is a localized disease or difficult-to-treat localized MDR TB or MAC, difficult-to-control or recurrent massive or life-threatening hemoptysis, residual foreign body or tumor with a risk of progression to other segments in the same or contralateral lung over the course of the disease. In post-tubercular bronchiectasis that is localized, surgery can be curative.

References and suggested readings

1. McShane PJ, Naureckas ET, Tino G, Strek ME. Non–cystic fibrosis bronchiectasis. Am J Respir Crit Care Med. 2013 Sep 15;188(6):647–656.
2. Polverino E, Goeminne PC, McDonnell MJ, et al. European respiratory society guidelines for the management of adult bronchiectasis. Eur Respir J. 2017;50:1700629, 1–21.
3. Chalmers JD, Aliberti S, Blasi F. Management of bronchiectasis in adults. Eur Respir J. 2015;45:1446–1462.
4. Aliberti S, Lonni S, Dore S, et al. Clinical phenotypes in adult patients with bronchiectasis. Eur Respir J. 2016;47:1113–1122.
5. Barker A. Bronchiectasis. N Engl J Med. 2002 May 2;346(18):1383–1393.
6. Derbyshire EJ, Calder PC. Bronchiectasis-could immunonutrition have a role to play in future management? Front Nutr. 2021;8:652410.
7. Loebinger MR, Polverino E, Chalmers JD, Tiddens H, Goossens H, Tunney M, Ringshausen FC, Hill AT, Pathan R, Angyalosi G, Blasi F, Elborn SJ, Haworth CS; iBEST-1 Trial Team. Efficacy and safety of TOBI Podhaler in *Pseudomonas aeruginosa*-infected bronchiectasis patients: iBEST study. Eur Respir J. 2021;57(1):2001451.
8. Lee AL, Gordon CS, Osadnik CR. Exercise training for bronchiectasis. Cochrane Database Sys Rev. 2021;4(4):CD013110.
9. Sibila O. Reducing *Pseudomonas* sputum density in bronchiectasis. Eur Respir J. 2021;57(1):2003390.
10. Zhu L, Liu L. Coronary artery fistula and bronchiectasis: case report and literature review. Ann Palliat Med. 2021;10(7):8403–8412.
11. Horani A, Ferkol TW. Understanding primary ciliary dyskinesia and other ciliopathies. J Pediatr. 2021;230:15–22.e1.
12. Martinez-Garcia MA, Aksamit TR, Aliberti S. Bronchiectasis as a long-term consequence of SARS-COVID-19 pneumonia: future studies are needed. Arch. Bronconeumol. 2021;57(12):739–740.
13. Liu Y, Lu HW, Gu SY, Wang WW, Ge J, Jie ZJ, Jia JG, Gao ZT, Li J, Shi JY, Liang S, Cheng KB, Bai JW, Qu JM, Xu JF. Bronchoscopic airway clearance therapy for acute exacerbations of bronchiectasis. eBioMedicine. 2021;72:103587.
14. Inchingolo R, Pierandrei C, Montemurro G, Smargiassi A, Lohmeyer FM, Rizzi A. Antimicrobial resistance in common respiratory pathogens of chronic

bronchiectasis patients: a literature review. Antibiotics (Basel). 2021 Mar 20;10(3):326. doi: 10.3390/antibiotics10030326. PMID: 33804631; PMCID: PMC8003644.

15. Belli S, Prince I, Savio G, Paracchini E, Cattaneo D, Bianchi M, Masocco F, Bellanti MT, Balbi B. Airway clearance techniques: the right choice for the right patient. Front Med (Lausanne). 2021 Feb 4;8:544826. doi: 10.3389/fmed.2021.544826. PMID: 33634144; PMCID: PMC7902008.
16. Gruffydd-Jones K, Keeley D, Wildgoose J, Hill A. Managing bronchiectasis in adults in primary care: a clinical update. Br J Gen Pract. 2021 Mar 26;71(705):183–184. doi: 10.3399/bjgp21X715565. PMID: 33771804; PMCID: PMC8007266.
17. Williamson L. Living with bronchiectasis during the COVID-19 pandemic. Lancet Respir Med. 2021 Apr;9(4):343–344. doi: 10.1016/S2213-2600(21)00074-6. Epub 2021 Jan 28. PMID: 33516286; PMCID: PMC8547760.

https://doi.org/10.1142/9789811271410_0017

17 Small airway disease

Introduction

Small airways are non-cartilage caining airways less than 2 mm in internal diameter, the terminal bronchioles supply the secondary pulmonary lobule (10–25 mm in size), are purely conducting and lead to the respiratory bronchioles, which are both conducting and gas exchanging. Small airways are seen from eighth generation of airway branching and their number greatly increases with each subsequent branching. Small airways are usually called the "silent zone" of the lung. In the normal lung, they hardly contribute to airway resistance due to their large surface area. Small airway diseases, even minor ones, can cause a significant increase in airway resistance. In the peripheral small airways, the airflow is more laminar, unlike the large airways, where the airflow is turbulent.

Etiology and pathology

Small airways can be affected by disease either primarily or as a part of diffuse involvement of the lungs. The most common causes of small airway diseases (SADs) in the general population are asthma and chronic obstructive pulmonary disease (COPD). Both these diseases also involve the medium and large airways, and COPD also involves the parenchyma (emphysema) quite commonly. Other than these two groups of diseases, there are many less common causes of SADs. There are two main classifications based on histopathology. One group is inflammatory bronchiolitis and the other is fibrosing constrictive bronchiolitis. The common causes and pathology are given in the following table under the two headings.

Inflammatory cellular bronchiolitis	Constrictive bronchiolitis
Hypersensitivity pneumonitis (HSP) (Figure 1) Can be acute, subacute, or chronic. Exposure to pigeons, organic dust, chemicals, molds.	Childhood infections Mostly adenovirus infections. When it occurs before the age of 8 years can affect alveologenesis. Extreme form is the Swyer–James (Figures 2 and 3) or Macleod's syndrome or unilateral hyperlosage lung syndrome.
Panbronchiolitis (Asian panbronchiolitis, diffuse panbronchiolitis) Seen predominantly in Asians, mainly from Japan, and seen rarely in other populations. Exact cause is unclear.	Connective tissue diseases Most commonly rheumatoid arthritis. There could be a role for penicillamine, though many cases occur in the absence of this drug.
Aspiration bronchiolitis Acute aspiration leads to focal involvement in dependent areas, whereas chronic and recurrent aspiration leads to diffuse lung involvement. Hiatus hernia, esophagectomy with gastric pull through, swallowing difficulty, tracheaoesophageal fistula, elderly, dementia, bedbound, Parkinson's disease, and other neurological disorders impairing swallowing reflex.	Inhalational exposure Fire smoke, nitrous acid, nitrous oxide compounds, popcorn-flavoring agent.
Respiratory bronchiolitis and respiratory bronchiolitis with ILD (RB-ILD) Seen in smokers (features of both SAD and ILD).	Transplantation Lung transplantation. >3 months later, nearly 50% of patients have chronic allograft rejection manifestation.

(*Continued*)

Inflammatory cellular bronchiolitis	Constrictive bronchiolitis
Infectious bronchiolitis Viral (H1N1, adenovirus, parainfluenza), fungal (*Aspergillus*), bacterial, atypical bacteria (*Mycoplasma*), tuberculous mycobacterial and non-tuberculous mycobacteria. In children less than 2 years, bronchiolitis is most commonly due to rhinovirus or respiratory syncytial virus (RSV).	Transplantation Hematopoietic stem cell. 10% of subjects. Graft-versus-host disease. Skin, GIT can be additionally involved.
Follicular bronchiolitis Connective tissue disease (rheumatoid arthritis), human immunodeficiency virus, primary immunodeficiency diseases.	Diffuse idiopathic pulmonary neuroendocrine hyperplasia Proliferation of neuroendocrine cells. Located in the basement membrane of the bronchiolar epithelial cells. When it extends beyond, the epithelial basement membranes are called tumorlets: <5 mm and carcinoid: >5 mm.
Asthma Chronic inflammation in asthma extends across all the layers of the small airway: epithelium, submucosa, muscular layer, and the outer wall (peribronchiolar area). Eosinophils, $CD4^+$ cells, neutrophils. Higher mRNA expression of IL-4, IL-5, and eotaxin. Increased number of goblet cells and neutrophils are found in the small airways of subjects with fatal asthma.	COPD Chronic inflammation leads to fibrosis of the small airways that lead to air trapping. Some studies indicate that fibrosis occurs due to the release of transforming growth factor-beta and growth factors in response to smoking and is independent of inflammation.

(*Continued*)

(*Continued*)

Inflammatory cellular bronchiolitis	Constrictive bronchiolitis
COPD Small airways are significantly involved in COPD. Main inflammation is by $CD8^+$ lymphocytes. B lymphocytes are also present. Smooth muscle hypertrophy is common. Higher number of $CD8^+$ cells is associated with more severe SAD and airflow limitation	

Pneumonitis hyperlucent right lung (lower lobe)

Cellular bronchiolitis refers to any cellular infiltration of the bronchioles, and the cells may vary depending on the etiology of the bronchiolitis. Four main varieties of cellular infiltration are known. Follicular bronchiolitis has lymphoid hyperplasia with secondary germinal centers and is commonly

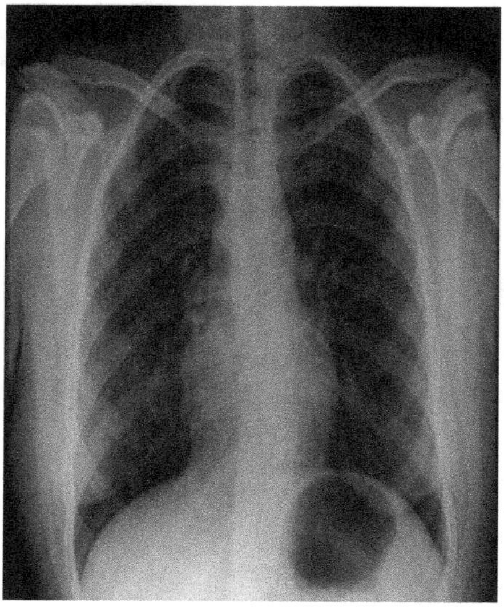

Figure 1: Hypersensitivity Swyer James syndrome.

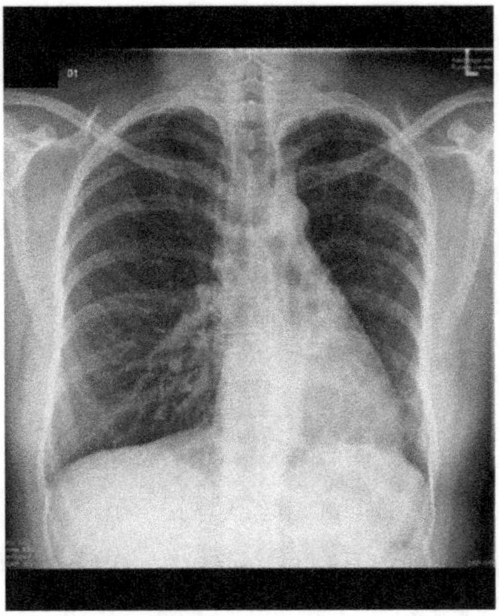 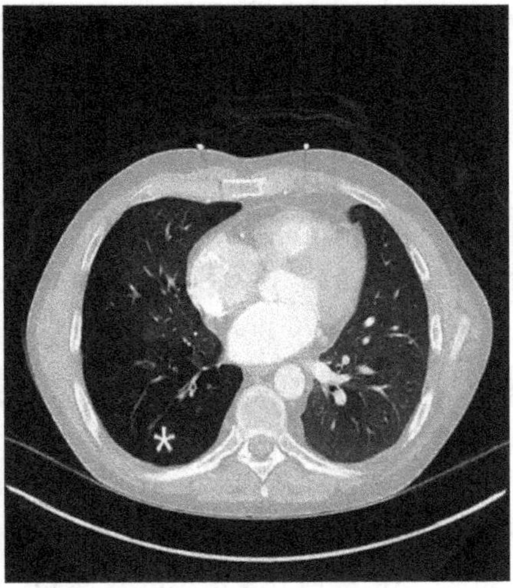

Figures 2 & 3: Chest X-ray and CT scan of Swyer James syndrome. Hyperlusent right lung (lower lobe).

seen in collagen vascular diseases (rheumatoid arthritis and Sjogren's syndrome), panbronchiolitis, hypersensitivity pneumonitis, and lymphoproliferative disease. The respiratory bronchiolitis is seen in tobacco smokers and has foamy pigmented macrophages in the small airways and may be associated with ILD (RB-ILD of smokers). The lymphocytic bronchiolitis has lymphocytes in the wall of the small airways and is seen in lymphocytic interstitial pneumonia, infections, and lung transplant rejection. The last group is diffuse panbronchiolitis (DPB), which has inflammation with the foamy macrophages in the small airway wall and is seen in Asian panbronchiolitis.

Two other types of bronchiolitis are commonly described. The first is the proliferative bronchiolitis with fibrotic buds in the small airways. This has been termed as bronchiolitis obliterans (BO), where the predominant clinical features are related to small airway obstruction. In many cases, these fibrotic buds extend into the alveoli. Then these are termed as BO with organizing pneumonia and the term is now modified as cryptogenic organizing pneumonia and the features are mainly related to the alveolar involvement with radiological shadows suggesting a pneumonia. The second is the constrictive bronchiolitis which has circumferential fibrosis in the submucosal and the peribronchiolar space leading to constriction and narrowing of the small airways. This is seen after lung or stem cell transplant, infections, inhalation and toxic fume exposure, and collagen vascular disease and a significant portion of them are idiopathic.

Clinical features

A very high degree of suspicion is needed for the diagnosis of SADs. Most of these patients will be misdiagnosed with asthma or COPD since the clinical presentation may be very similar to these two very common clinical conditions, and there is SAD in these subjects as well. These subjects present with cough, dyspnea which is exertional in early stages and progresses to dyspnea at rest later, wheeze, evidence of hyperinflated lungs on clinical examination similar to emphysematous lungs may be seen in some cases. Sputum is generally absent (since the small airways do not have any mucus-producing cells), unless medium and large airways are involved. Asian panbronchiolitis is commonly associated with sinusitis. It is important to assess all the comorbid conditions that are associated with SAD listed in the table above (etiology) including work-up for connective tissue diseases, human immunodeficiency virus, immunodeficiency disorders, and exposures to various irritants, both occupational and non-occupational.

The key to the suspicion of SAD as compared to other airway diseases is its speed of progress. Whereas COPD may take 20 years to develop respiratory failure and cor pulmonale, many conditions that cause SAD progresses rapidly and develop respiratory failure and cor pulmonale within a few years after the first onset of symptoms. However, at this stage, many of them are not reversible and therefore there is a need to be able to diagnose these cases early. When possible, they should be removed from the cause of disease, for example, mold-induced hypersensitivity pneumonitis. The source needs to be removed. In many cases, we have observed that it was due to the rotting wood in the tiled roofs and they continued to have symptoms and disease progression until they changed the house.

Many cases of infectious bronchiolitis, especially in children resolve spontaneously or with treatment in a few weeks. In other causes of bronchiolitis, the disease is slowly progressive and the presentation may be subacute or chronic with gradually increasing cough, wheeze, and shortness of breath.

On clinical examination, the findings may be similar to COPD with signs of hyperinflated lung fields. Both interstitial lung disease and SAD present with fine end-inspiratory Velcro crackles. Sometimes a subject with chronic heart failure may present with fine crepitations as well. It complicates the matter when patients with chronic heart failure have normal echocardiogram. In such situations, BNP or NT-proBNP is of value to identify the presence of heart failure, and symptoms and signs have resolved after the treatment of heart failure.

Investigations

The most important lung functions include lung functions and imaging studies to assess small airways. The key lung functions and imaging studies and their features are discussed in the table below. It would be useful to review older images and lung functions if available to understand the progression of the disease.

Test of small airways	Outcome measures
Flow at small airways	Spirometry FEF 50; FEF 25–75 Difference between SVC and FVC (small airway collapse during a forced maneuver)
Resistance at small airways	Impulse oscillometry R5
Inhomogeneity of ventilation distribution	Multiple breath nitrogen washout technique
Air trapping	RV/TLC ratio

(*Continued*)

(*Continued*)

Test of small airways	Outcome measures
HRCT thorax Needs both inspiratory and expiratory films	Centrilobular nodules Tree in bud appearance (Figure 4) Ground-glass pattern Mosaic attenuation (Figure 5) Increased air trapping and hyperlucent on expiratory films Bronchiolectasis

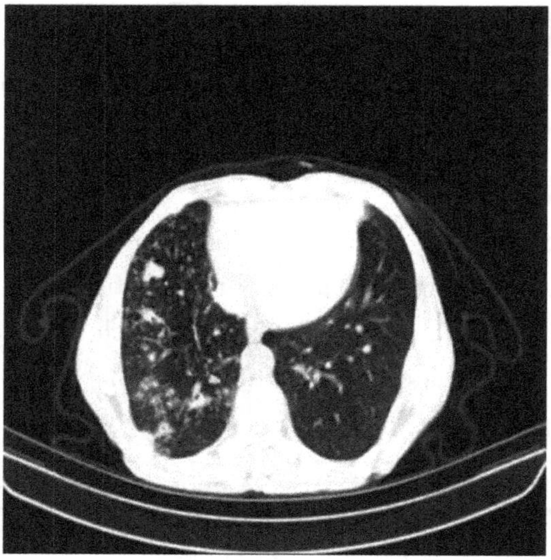

Figure 4: Centrinodular pattern with tree in bud.

Spirometry is a simple tool available to most chest physicians that can help to identify SAD. The most common variable used is the FEF 25–75. This is measured in the second half of the expiratory flow–volume curve and is effort independent. This measure correlates well with air trapping on computed tomography scan. It is important to note that SAD in asthma is eminently reversible, whereas in other conditions listed above including COPD, it is partially or poorly reversible even with treatment in later stages of the disease, when the pathology becomes irreversible. In the early stages,

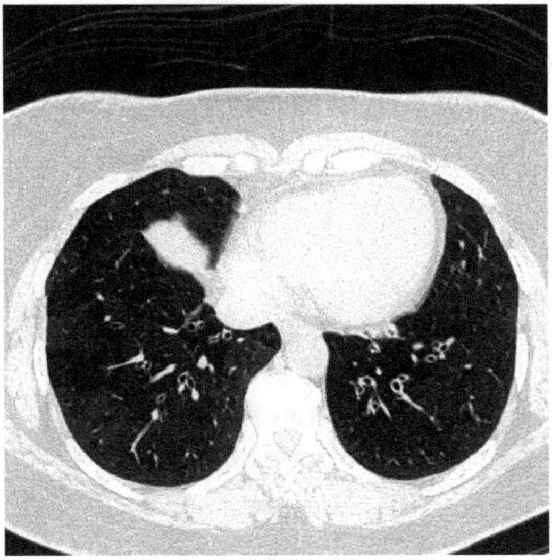

Figure 5: Mosaic attenuation.

there may be a slow resolution of the airway obstruction after treatment. The second most common method available to most chest physicians is the HRCT thorax. Routinely, the radiologist would not be performing inspiratory and expiratory films. Therefore, when SADs are suspected, the chest physician must explicitly ask for both inspiratory and expiratory films. The presence of areas of the lung that is still black suggests small airway obstruction and air trapping. The areas that remain black during expiration are the abnormal areas of the lungs, and the areas of the lung that become whiter suggest normal lungs. Unless there are both inspiratory and expiratory films, these findings cannot be detected. The other tool that is not commonly available to the chest physician is impulse oscillometry (IOS). The details of the IOS technique and its interpretation are dealt with in an earlier chapter. An increased peripheral resistance measured by increased R5 above 140% predicted would indicate SAD.

Management

The management depends on the etiology of bronchiolitis, which is quite diverse as discussed previously. Many subjects with viral bronchiolitis mainly need supportive treatment and some like RB-ILD need only smoking cessation as the main treatment strategy. Others like DPB need long-term treatment with macrolide antibiotics. Steroids and immunosuppressants are needed for others. Avoidance of inciting agents including organic dusts, chemicals, fumes, and inorganic irritants is a must. A summary approach to various SADs is given in the table below.

Diagnosis	Management options
RB-ILD early	Smoking cessation is sufficient. Steroids are of no value. Good prognosis.
RB-ILD late	Smoking cessation. Steroids may be necessary. Some sequelae may remain.
Diffuse panbronchiolitis	Generally, ends up in bronchiectasis, respiratory failure, and death. Low-dose macrolide is of benefit.
Cryptogenic organizing pneumonia (BOOP)	Steroids are of great benefit.
Constrictive bronchiolitis	Prognosis is varied: from slow progression to fulminant progression to respiratory failure and death. Only supportive therapy.
Follicular bronchiolitis	Good prognosis. Steroids and bronchodilators are of benefit.
Idiopathic acute and chronic bronchiolitis	Antibiotics and immunosuppressants.
Acute bronchiolitis in children less than 1 year of age (usually viral)	Good prognosis. Symptomatic treatment. Oxygen when there is hypoxia. Steroids are of benefit in some patients with croup.

For DPB, the mainstay of treatment is macrolide antibiotics. Treatment for DPB should be initiated at the earliest, as soon as the diagnosis is made. Late treatment may lead to irreversible sequelae. The first-choice macrolide treatment is erythromycin 400–600 mg/day. The other choices are clarithromycin at 200–400 mg/day and roxithromycin at 150–300 mg/day. All the above three are 14-ring macrolide antibiotics. Azithromycin, a 15-ring macrolide antibiotic, is also found useful. Macrolides with a 16-member ring (josamycin) are not useful in the management of DPB. After the initiation of treatment, one can expect some clinical response in 2–3 months and treatment should be continued for at least 2 years. It can be restarted if symptoms recur later. In some advanced cases, treatment needs to be continued for an even longer time. The main mechanism of action of macrolide antibiotics in DPB is not related to its antibacterial effects but to its effects on the neutrophils. After treatment with macrolide antibiotics, there is a substantial reduction in the number of neutrophils, neutrophil elastase, IL-8 (neutrophil chemoattractant) are all reduced. Mucus hypersecretion with copious sputum production is the hallmark of DPB and is reduced by macrolides, due to its suppressive effect on glycoconjugates from airway epithelial cells as well as blocking the chloride ions in the submucosa, thus reducing the watery secretions into the airway lumen. Macrolides also affect lymphocyte proliferation and reduce the nodular lesions that are rich in lymphocytes in DPB. At subtherapeutic levels, macrolides decrease the release of alginate from bacteria such as *Pseudomonas*. Alginate forms a biofilm that prevents antibiotic entry into the bacteria and protects them.

References and suggested readings

1. Polosukhin VV, Gutor SS, Du RH, Richmond BW, Massion PP, Wu P, Cates JM, Sandler KL, Rennard SI, Blackwell TS. Small airway determinants of airflow limitation in chronic obstructive pulmonary disease. Thorax. 2021 Nov;76(11):1079–1088. doi: 10.1136/thoraxjnl-2020-216037. Epub 2021 Apr 7. PMID: 33827979; PMCID: PMC8526883.

2. Maselli DJ, Yen A, Wang W, Okajima Y, Dolliver WR, Mercugliano C, Anzueto A, Restrepo MI, Aksamit TR, Basavaraj A, Aliberti S, Young KA, Kinney GL, Wells JM, San José Estépar R, Lynch DA, Diaz AA. Small airway disease and emphysema are associated with future exacerbations in smokers with CT-derived bronchiectasis and COPD: results from the COPDGene cohort. Radiology. 2021 Sep;300(3):706–714. doi: 10.1148/radiol.2021204052. Epub 2021 Jun 22. PMID: 34156303; PMCID: PMC8409101.
3. Owonikoko TK, Park K, Govindan R, Ready N, Reck M, Peters S, Dakhil SR, Navarro A, Rodríguez-Cid J, Schenker M, Lee JS, Gutierrez V, Percent I, Morgensztern D, Barrios CH, Greillier L, Baka S, Patel M, Lin WH, Selvaggi G, Baudelet C, Baden J, Pandya D, Doshi P, Kim HR. Nivolumab and ipilimumab as maintenance therapy in extensive-disease small-cell lung cancer: CheckMate 451. J Clin Oncol. 2021 Apr 20;39(12):1349–1359. doi: 10.1200/JCO.20.02212. Epub 2021 Mar 8. PMID: 33683919; PMCID: PMC8078251.
4. Remon J, Aldea M, Besse B, Planchard D, Reck M, Giaccone G, Soria JC. Small cell lung cancer: a slightly less orphan disease after immunotherapy. Ann Oncol. 2021 Jun;32(6):698–709. doi: 10.1016/j.annonc.2021.02.025. Epub 2021 Mar 15. PMID: 33737119.
5. Gadgeel S, Rodríguez-Abreu D, Speranza G, Esteban E, Felip E, Dómine M, Hui R, Hochmair MJ, Clingan P, Powell SF, Cheng SY, Bischoff HG, Peled N, Grossi F, Jennens RR, Reck M, Garon EB, Novello S, Rubio-Viqueira B, Boyer M, Kurata T, Gray JE, Yang J, Bas T, Pietanza MC, Garassino MC. Updated analysis from KEYNOTE-189: pembrolizumab or placebo plus pemetrexed and platinum for previously untreated metastatic nonsquamous non-small-cell lung cancer. J Clin Oncol. 2020 May 10;38(14):1505–1517. doi: 10.1200/JCO.19.03136. Epub 2020 Mar 9. PMID: 32150489.
6. Lange P, Ahmed E, Lahmar ZM, Martinez FJ, Bourdin A. Natural history and mechanisms of COPD. Respirology. 2021 Apr;26(4):298–321. doi: 10.1111/resp.14007. Epub 2021 Jan 28. PMID: 33506971.
7. Liu SV, Reck M, Mansfield AS, Mok T, Scherpereel A, Reinmuth N, Garassino MC, De Castro Carpeno J, Califano R, Nishio M, Orlandi F, Alatorre-Alexander J, Leal T, Cheng Y, Lee JS, Lam S, McCleland M, Deng Y, Phan S, Horn L. Updated overall survival and PD-L1 subgroup analysis of patients with extensive-stage small-cell lung cancer treated with atezolizumab, carboplatin, and etoposide

(IMpower133). J Clin Oncol. 2021 Feb 20;39(6):619–630. doi: 10.1200/JCO.20.01055. Epub 2021 Jan 13. PMID: 33439693; PMCID: PMC8078320.

8. Chukowry PS, Spittle DA, Turner AM. Small airways disease, biomarkers and COPD: where are we? Int J Chron Obstruct Pulmon Dis. 2021 Feb 18;16:351–365. doi: 10.2147/COPD.S280157. PMID: 33628018; PMCID: PMC7899307.
9. Reck M, Rodríguez-Abreu D, Robinson AG, Hui R, Csőszi T, Fülöp A, Gottfried M, Peled N, Tafreshi A, Cuffe S, O'Brien M, Rao S, Hotta K, Leal TA, Riess JW, Jensen E, Zhao B, Pietanza MC, Brahmer JR. Five-year outcomes with pembrolizumab versus chemotherapy for metastatic non-small-cell lung cancer with PD-L1 tumor proportion score ≥50. J Clin Oncol. 2021 Jul 20;39(21):2339–2349. doi: 10.1200/JCO.21.00174. Epub 2021 Apr 19. PMID: 33872070; PMCID: PMC8280089.
10. Schweitzer KS, Crue T, Nall JM, Foster D, Sajuthi S, Correll KA, Nakamura M, Everman JL, Downey GP, Seibold MA, Bridges JP, Serban KA, Chu HW, Petrache I. Influenza virus infection increases ACE2 expression and shedding in human small airway epithelial cells. Eur Respir J. 2021 Jul 1;58(1):2003988. doi: 10.1183/13993003.03988-2020. PMID: 33419885; PMCID: PMC8378143.
11. Cox NS, Dal Corso S, Hansen H, McDonald CF, Hill CJ, Zanaboni P, Alison JA, O'Halloran P, Macdonald H, Holland AE. Telerehabilitation for chronic respiratory disease. Cochrane Database Syst Rev. 2021 Jan 29;1(1): CD013040. doi: 10.1002/14651858.CD013040.pub2. PMID: 33511633; PMCID: PMC8095032.
12. Okuda K, Dang H, Kobayashi Y, Carraro G, Nakano S, Chen G, Kato T, Asakura T, Gilmore RC, Morton LC, Lee RE, Mascenik T, Yin WN, Barbosa Cardenas SM, O'Neal YK, Minnick CE, Chua M, Quinney NL, Gentzsch M, Anderson CW, Ghio A, Matsui H, Nagase T, Ostrowski LE, Grubb BR, Olsen JC, Randell SH, Stripp BR, Tata PR, O'Neal WK, Boucher RC. Secretory cells dominate airway CFTR expression and function in human airway superficial epithelia. Am J Respir Crit Care Med. 2021 May 15;203(10):1275–1289. doi: 10.1164/rccm.202008-3198OC. PMID: 33321047; PMCID: PMC8456462.
13. Qin S, Yu X, Ma Q, Lin L, Li Q, Liu H, Zhang L, Leng S, Han W. Quantitative CT analysis of small airway remodeling in patients with chronic obstructive pulmonary disease by a new image post-processing system. Int J Chron

Obstruct Pulmon Dis. 2021 Mar 2;16:535–544. doi: 10.2147/COPD.S295320. PMID: 33688178; PMCID: PMC7936712.

14. Spigel DR, Faivre-Finn C, Gray JE, Vicente D, Planchard D, Paz-Ares L, Vansteenkiste JF, Garassino MC, Hui R, Quantin X, Rimner A, Wu YL, Özgüroğlu M, Lee KH, Kato T, de Wit M, Kurata T, Reck M, Cho BC, Senan S, Naidoo J, Mann H, Newton M, Thiyagarajah P, Antonia SJ. Five-year survival outcomes from the PACIFIC trial: durvalumab after chemoradiotherapy in stage III non-small-cell lung cancer. J Clin Oncol. 2022 Apr 20;40(12):1301–1311. doi: 10.1200/JCO.21.01308. Epub 2022 Feb 2. Erratum in: J Clin Oncol. 2022 Jun 10;40(17):1965. PMID: 35108059; PMCID: PMC9015199.
15. Tanabe N, Shimizu K, Terada K, Sato S, Suzuki M, Shima H, Oguma A, Oguma T, Konno S, Nishimura M, Hirai T. Central airway and peripheral lung structures in airway disease-dominant COPD. ERJ Open Res. 2021 Mar 22;7(1):00672–2020. doi: 10.1183/23120541.00672-2020. PMID: 33778061; PMCID: PMC7983277.
16. Abdo M, Trinkmann F, Kirsten AM, Pedersen F, Herzmann C, von Mutius E, Kopp MV, Hansen G, Waschki B, Rabe KF, Watz H, Bahmer T. Study Group. Small airway dysfunction links asthma severity with physical activity and symptom control. J Allergy Clin Immunol Pract. 2021 Sep;9(9):3359–3368.e1. doi: 10.1016/j.jaip.2021.04.035. Epub 2021 Apr 27. PMID: 33930619.
17. Allwood BW, Byrne A, Meghji J, Rachow A, van der Zalm MM, Schoch OD. Post-tuberculosis lung disease: clinical review of an under-recognised global challenge. Respiration. 2021;100(8):751–763. doi: 10.1159/000512531. Epub 2021 Jan 5. PMID: 33401266.

https://doi.org/10.1142/9789811271410_0018

18 Allergic bronchopulmonary aspergillosis (ABPA)

Introduction

Aspergillus species is commonly present in both the indoor environment (leaky basement, bathrooms, house dust, and bed) and the outdoor environment (decaying vegetation, soil, swimming pool), and the exposure is universal.[1] In spite of the ubiquitous nature of the aspergillus, allergic bronchopulmonary aspergillosis (ABPA) is an uncommon disease in most parts of the world and generally needs a high degree of suspicion to ask for the relevant investigations to confirm the diagnosis.[1] Some individuals develop a hyperimmune response to aspergillus, and the spectrum of hypersensitivity reactions ranges from type I, III, and IV (Gel and Coomb's classification) in ABPA[1] to only type I reaction in asthma triggered by aspergillus and type IV alone in bronchocentric granulomatosis. ABPA is seen usually only in susceptible subjects with previous lung diseases such as asthma and cystic fibrosis (CF).[1] Hinson described ABPA in 1952 in a subject with asthma who had peripheral and sputum eosinophilia and infiltrates on the chest X-ray.[1] The spectrum of ABPA is large ranging from a mild disease to a destructive lung disease affecting the airways (bronchiectasis) and lung parenchyma (lung fibrosis).[1]

Other than ABPA, aspergillus can cause many different manifestations in the lungs. The milder forms include aspergilloma[1] due to the presence of aspergillus as a colonization in a preexisting bronchiectasis or a cavity, such as a post-tubercular cavity, which remains mostly with minimal symptoms, though on occasions when there is vasculitis, it can cause massive hemoptysis. Aspergillus-sensitive asthma[1] can be difficult to control in many asthmatics. Hypersensitivity pneumonitis[1] or extrinsic allergic alveolitis though reversible initially can lead to irreversible damage over the long term. Chronic necrotizing aspergillosis[1] is semi-invasive or locally invasive and is seen in patients with previous lung disease or immunosuppression. The most severe form is invasive aspergillosis,[1] spreading to all parts of the lung (airways, parenchyma, and can cause mycotic abscesses) and into the systemic circulation and can be rapidly life-threatening.

Classification based on staging of ABPA

ABPA is classified into five stages depending on the clinical, laboratory, and imaging studies: stage I — acute, stage II — remission, stage III — recurrence or exacerbation, stage IV — steroid-dependent asthma, and stage V — fibrotic lung disease.[1] The various characteristics of these five stages are discussed below. Usually, unless there is a high degree of suspicion or screening of all asthmatics and CF patients, the diagnosis is usually made in stage IV when the clinician finds it difficult to withdraw oral steroids in an asthmatic.

ABPA stage	Characteristic features
Stage I Acute stage	Patients present with acute asthma symptoms and has all the laboratory findings according to the major criteria and minor criteria discussed below, positive, unless treated (total IgE > 1,000), peripheral eosinophilia, serum precipitins, specific IgE for aspergillus (in-vivo or in-vitro tests), specific IgG for *Aspergillus fumigatus*, imaging findings, responds to treatment with oral corticosteroids (OCS) and or antifungals.
Stage II Remission	Resolution of symptoms, laboratory and imaging abnormalities discussed above for stage I. Maybe for months, years, or sometimes permanent.

(*Continued*)

ABPA stage	Characteristic features
Stage III Recurrence	Clinical, radiological, or laboratory features again become abnormal either in spite of the treatment or on withdrawal or reduction of treatment. Many cases with new radiological infiltrate are asymptomatic. This can lead to progressive lung damage. Very important to monitor closely. Total IgE every 2 months for 1 year at least. Intermittent chest X-rays.
Stage IV Steroid-dependent asthma	Asthma is refractory to other treatments. Need oral steroids on regular basis. Persistence or increase in imaging, laboratory, or clinical abnormalities in spite of treatment.
Stage V Fibrotic lung	Fibrosis in the lung leads to irreversible lung function abnormalities (both obstructive and restrictive), impaired spirometry, impulse oscillometry, diffusion defects. Bronchiectasis features both clinical and radiological.

Pathogenesis and pathology

The exact pathogenesis of ABPA is still unclear and involves type I, III, and IV hypersensitivity reactions. It is observed that ABPA occurs in subjects who have preexisting asthma or CF, but it does not occur in all subjects with asthma or CF.[1] Why only certain individuals are susceptible? It is clear that host factors are involved and not a load of exposure to aspergillus as observed in studies that the frequency of ABPA is similar in residents of both urban and rural areas.[1] Some studies have observed that there is an HLA linkage to ABPA: HLA DR2 and HLA DR5 increase the risk and HLA

DQ2 decreases the risk of ABPA.[1] In the HLA-DR2 locus, there are two alleles that can increase the risk for ABPA: DRB1*1501 and DRB1*1503 alleles.[1] The other host risk factors include the presence of CFTR mutations even in the absence of overt CF, interleukin 10 (IL-10) polymorphisms, and surfactant protein A polymorphisms. CFTR mutations may lead to thicker and more viscid mucus, whereas surfactant protein A polymorphisms are associated with increased growth of the aspergillus in the mucus due to reduced host defenses.[1] IL-10 polymorphisms are associated with impaired immune responses.[1]

The most important difference between ABPA and aspergillus-associated severe asthma is that in ABPA there is multiplication and growth of aspergillus within the airways, but these do not invade the bronchial epithelium, unlike a case of invasive aspergillosis.[1] The growth of these aspergillus releases many hyphae and spores (2–5 μm in size), which are taken up by the innate immune system, the ubiquitous antigen-presenting cells (APCs).[1] These cells communicate with the T lymphocytes via various systems akin to the many languages that we use for communication in the world. Depending on that, the cellular response differs. In ABPA, when the APCs with HLA DR2 or HLA DR5 markers present the aspergillus antigen to the T lymphocytes, there is a skew towards the TH2 lymphocyte response that leads to the secretion of aspergillus-specific IgE, along with aspergillus-specific IgG which is responsible for the immune complex reaction seen in ABPA and an eosinophilic inflammation of the airways.[1] The spores and hyphae also release various proteases that can cause direct damage to the airways leading to bronchiectasis. The airway inflammation is also accentuated due to the release of various inflammatory mediators such as IL-8, eotaxin, RANTES (regulated on activation, normal T cell expressed and secreted), monocyte chemoattractant protein-1, IL-8, and macrophage inflammatory protein-1α among others.[1] These cause severe eosinophilic inflammation with a $CD4^+$ TH2 response to aspergillus antigens, secreting various cytokines including IL-4, IL-5, IL-9, IL-10, and IL-13, which increases the growth and survival of eosinophils, proliferation of mast cells, and isotype switching of IgG to IgE.[1]

The most common pathologic finding in ABPA is mucoid impaction due to very thick and viscid mucus, which grows aspergillus. ABPA is one of the common causes of eosinophilic pneumonias. The other causes of eosinophilic pneumonias include Loeffler's syndrome, tropical pulmonary eosinophilia, acute eosinophilic pneumonia, chronic eosinophilic pneumonia, and Churg–Strauss syndrome.[1] There is parenchymal involvement as well with many cases having pulmonary fibrosis.

Clinical features

ABPA is mainly seen in two clinical settings[1]: one is in asthmatics and the second is in patients suffering from CF. A difficult-to-control asthmatic has recurrent exacerbations, is steroid dependent and has mucus plugging on imaging studies, brings out thick mucus plugs, and the presence of bronchiectasis needs to be evaluated for ABPA. The clinical features of ABPA in CF are similar to those seen in asthmatics, and the diagnostic criteria and treatment remain the same.

Diagnosis

The diagnostic criteria have changed recently and include both major and minor criteria listed in the table below.[1] These new criteria help to diagnose ABPA in the absence of classical radiological findings, which may be transient in early stages or eosinophilia, which may be absent when the asthmatic has been treated with oral steroids. Also, bronchiectasis is not listed in the criteria and ABPA can be diagnosed in the absence of bronchiectasis.

The characteristic radiological findings can be transient (consolidation that may be fleeting [earlier called as walking pneumonia], finger in glove [Figures 1a–c] pattern [seen in mucus plugging], tramline shadows [airway thickening], and nodules) or permanent changes such as bronchiectasis which is mostly central (inverted wine glass pattern), ring shadows, and pulmonary fibrosis. Central bronchiectasis (Figure 2) is seen because of the larger size of the fungal hyphae/spores which get deposited mainly in central airways and the inciting inflammation causes damage to the cartilage leading to central bronchiectasis. ABPA-S is diagnosed when major and two out of three minor criteria are present in the absence of bronchiectasis. ABPA-CB is the above with central bronchiectasis diagnosed by either chest X-ray or HRCT thorax. There are other supportive criteria: expectoration of brown mucus plugs, positive culture for *A. fumigatus*, patchy fleeting infiltrates, and mucoid-impacted bronchi. In many cases, eosinophilia may be absent, especially if the patient is being treated.

Figures 1a–c show a dilated airway filled with mucus, the classical finger in glove sign seen in ABPA.

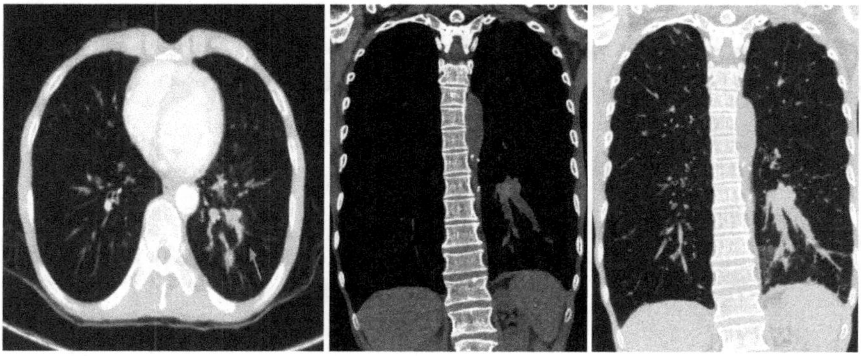

(a) (b) (c)

Figure 1: (a) Finger in glove. (b) Lung window. (c) Soft tissue window.

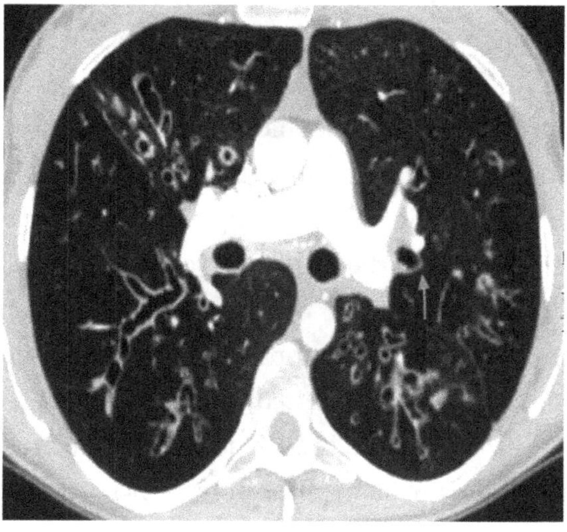

Figure 2: Bilateral bronchiectasis. Blue arrow points to central bronchiectasis, where the airway is larger than the accompanying artery.

Major criteria	Minor criteria (two out of three)
Presence of predisposing condition, either asthma or CF Elevated total IgE >1,000 IU/mL Presence of one of these two criteria: Aspergillus SPT is positive Aspergillus serum specific IgE is positive	Elevated aspergillus-specific IgG antibodies OR Presence of serum precipitins (gel diffusion) Characteristic radiological findings Elevated eosinophil counts (usually the total counts are more than 10,000 cells/cm^3 and AEC > 2,000)

Differential diagnosis

The key differential diagnosis includes other eosinophilic lung diseases.[1] The differentiating features of these eosinophilic lung diseases are listed in the following table. The other differential diagnosis includes pneumonias (bacterial, tubercular, fungal), parasitic infestations (*Ascaris lumbricoides*, *Strongyloides stercoralis*), BOOP, other causes of bronchiectasis, hypersensitivity pneumonitis sarcoidosis, and rheumatoid lung.

Eosinophilic lung diseases	Characteristics
Acute eosinophilic pneumonia	Presentation: acute onset of usually less than 1 month. Common symptoms: fever, cough, dyspnea. Chest X-ray: bilateral diffuse radiological infiltrates. HRCT: ground glass, reticular opacities. May present with acute respiratory failure, severe hypoxia, and needs intensive care unit care initially. Bronchoalveolar lavage (BAL): greater than 25% eosinophils. Associations: some occupational exposures, smoking. Diagnosis: other causes of eosinophilic pneumonia must be ruled out. Treatment: steroids — highly responsive. Relapse: chances are rare.

(*Continued*)

(*Continued*)

Eosinophilic lung diseases	Characteristics
Chronic eosinophilic pneumonia	Presentation: chronic, weeks to months. Common symptoms: fever, productive cough, dyspnea, weight loss, night sweats. Middle aged, female dominant. Chest X-ray: bilateral diffuse radiological infiltrates that is peripherally located (opposite of pulmonary edema is highly suggestive). HRCT: atelectasis, lymph node enlargement, pleural effusions, septal thickening. BAL: greater than 25% eosinophils, all cases have peripheral eosinophilia. Associations: asthma. Diagnosis: BAL is sufficient, rarely lung biopsy (eosinophilic infiltration in interstitium and alveoli). Treatment: steroids — highly responsive. Inhaled steroids and anti-IgE may be added to reduce the dose of steroids. Prognosis is generally good.
Loeffler's syndrome	Associated with helminth infections. Transpulmonary migration of larvae or blood spread. Sometimes seen in other infections and some drugs. Transient pulmonary infiltrates. Peripheral eosinophilia. Mild and self-limited symptoms, cough, breathlessness, and cough. Treatment: antihelminths and antimicrobials.
Tropical pulmonary eosinophilia	Acute onset of fever, cough, dyspnea, bronchospasm. Some cases may present as asthma. Usually in areas endemic to filariasis. Due to microfilaria (*Wuchereria bancrofti* and *Brugia malayi*). Peripheral eosinophilia and high total IgE in the background of total white blood cell count >10,000 cells/mm. Treatment: diethylcarbazine citrate for 21 days. Prognosis: Generally good. If diagnosed and treated late can lead to pulmonary fibrosis with chronic respiratory failure.

(*Continued*)

Eosinophilic lung diseases	Characteristics
Churg–Strauss syndrome	Now known as eosinophilic granulomatosis with polyangiitis. Setting of asthma. Vasculitis of small- and medium-sized vessels that involves both pulmonary and extrapulmonary systems. Presentation: cough, dyspnea, wheezing, fever. Imaging: nodules, consolidation, and patchy infiltrates. Other organ systems: heart, GIT, renal, nervous system, skin. Treatment: steroids, immunosuppressants. Prognosis: poor unless treated aggressively.
Drug reaction with eosinophilia and systemic symptoms (DRESS)	Due to various drugs such as antibiotics, iodine, methotrexate, sulfa drugs, captopril, amiodarone, and bleomycin. Associated with skin eruptions and fever. Imaging: bilateral infiltrates. High degree of suspicion is needed. BAL to exclude infections and other causes. Treatment: avoidance of the drug and steroids.
Hypereosinophilic syndrome	Unexplained cause of peripheral and tissue eosinophilia of >6-month duration. Heart, lungs, GIT, nervous system. Causes organ damage if untreated. Lungs are affected in 25% of these cases. Imaging: consolidation, lymphadenopathy, bilateral infiltrates. Treatment: steroids. Some cases are associated with myeloproliferative diseases (*FIP1L1-PDGFRA* mutations), then treated with imatinib.

Treatment

The key components of the ABPA treatment is discussed in the table below and include systemic corticosteroids, inhaled corticosteroids, bronchodilators, itraconazole, and chest physiotherapy. There is a steady development of evidence for biologicals, such as anti-IgE, benralizumab, mepolizumab, and dupilumab.

Treatment	Key features
OCS	Necessary since the immunopathology includes type I, III, and IV hypersensitivity reactions. Dose: 0.5–1 mg/kg body weight daily for 2 weeks. 0.5 mg/kg on alternate days for 6–8 weeks. Taper by 5 mg every 2 weeks. Many need maintenance dose of 5–7.5 mg/day or alternate days on a long-term basis. Monitor for the reduction in IgE (one-third to half after treatment), serum aspergillus-specific IgG, imaging, eosinophilia.
Inhaled corticosteroids	Of some benefit. In some cases, helps to reduce the dose of OCS.
Inhaled bronchodilators	Symptomatic benefit in the treatment of cough and bronchospasm.
Itraconazole	Other antifungal drugs have not found to help. Voriconazole has the same effect, but very expensive. Dose: 200–400 mg/day for 6–8 weeks. Significant improvements in clinical, imaging, and laboratory parameters. Caution: Drug interactions — interferes with hepatic metabolism of cyclosporine, tacrolimus, and oral hypoglycemic agents. PPIs may decrease itraconazole absorption. Can cause adrenal insufficiency by two mechanisms (direct effect on adrenal steroid production and reduces the clearance of steroids and high levels of serum corticosteroids can lead to adrenal suppression). Some cases of azole-resistant aspergillus are noted, then the subject would not respond to itraconazole. Less effective than OCS.
Anti-IgE[2]	Studies have documented benefit across clinical, exacerbations, imaging, and laboratory parameters. Expensive. Dose: 375 mg every 2 weeks subcutaneously.

(Continued)

Treatment	Key features
Anti-IL-5[3]	Mepolizumab Th2 cascade inhibitor. Indications reported in studies. a. Subjects with ABPA not responding to omalizumab. b. Concurrently used both omalizumab and mepolizumab. Study outcomes: Improvement of clinical symptoms and signs. Radiological improvement.
Anti-IL-4 receptor alpha[4]	Dupilumab Case series. Subjects who did not respond completely to OCS, omalizumab, and mepolizumab were given dupilumab. Reduces OCS use. Reduces exacerbations. Can result in hypereosinophilia.
Anti-IL-5 receptor[5]	Benralizumab Case report. Improvement in peripheral eosinophilia. Resolution of radiological shadow. Resolution of clinical symptoms.

Prognosis

It is important to have a high degree of suspicion and evaluate every difficult asthmatic and CF patient for ABPA. If the diagnosis is made early, without any permanent lung damage, long-term OCS helps to control the disease well and usually further sequelae can be avoided with careful monitoring. Adding antifungal treatment has improved the prognosis in these patients. Subjects who have permanent lung damage at the time of diagnosis generally continue to suffer and the prognosis is worse when there is a persistent reduction in forced expiratory volume in 1 second (FEV_1) of <0.8 L.

References and suggested readings

1. Bains SN, Judson MA. Allergic bronchopulmonary aspergillosis. Clin Chest Med. 2012 Jun;33(2):265–810.
2. Homma T, Kurokawa M, Matsukura S, Yamaguchi M, Adachi M. Anti-IgE therapy for allergic bronchopulmonary aspergillosis. J Microbiol Immunol Infect. 2016 Jun;49(3):459–463.
3. Hirota S, Kobayashi Y, Ishiguro T, Nishida T, Kagiyama N, Shimizu Y, et al. Allergic bronchopulmonary aspergillosis successfully treated with mepolizumab: case report and review of the literature. Respir Med Case Rep. 2019;26:59–62.
4. Ramonell RP, Lee FE-H, Swenson C, Kuruvilla M. Dupilumab treatment for allergic bronchopulmonary aspergillosis: a case series. J Allergy Clin Immunol Pract. 2020 Feb;8(2):742–743.
5. Soeda S, Kono Y, Tsuzuki R, Yamawaki S, Katsube O, To M, et al. Allergic bronchopulmonary aspergillosis successfully treated with benralizumab. J Allergy Clin Immunol Pract. 2019 May;7(5):1633–1635.
6. Ozyigit LP, Pashley CH, Wardlaw AJ. Fungal bronchitis and not allergic bronchopulmonary aspergillosis. Chron Respir Dis. 2021 Jan–Dec;18:14799731211001888. doi: 10.1177/14799731211001888. PMID: 33719619; PMCID: PMC7968014.
7. Sehgal IS, Muthu V, Agarwal R. Fungal bronchitis or allergic bronchopulmonary aspergillosis that is the question. Chron Respir Dis. 2021 Jan–Dec;18:14799731211001887. doi: 10.1177/14799731211001887. PMID: 33719589; PMCID: PMC7968008.
8. Muñoz-Bellido FJ, Moreno E, Dávila I. Dupilumab: a review of present indications and off-label uses. J Investig Allergol Clin Immunol. 2022 Apr 19;32(2):97–115. doi: 10.18176/jiaci.0682. Epub 2021 Mar 3. PMID: 33661102.
9. Muthu V, Agarwal R. Is bronchial thermoplasty safe in allergic bronchopulmonary aspergillosis or severe asthma with fungal sensitization? BMC Pulm Med. 2021 May 18;21(1):169. doi: 10.1186/s12890-021-01535-1. PMID: 34006244; PMCID: PMC8130423.
10. Ali M, Green O. Dupilumab: a new contestant to corticosteroid in allergic bronchopulmonary aspergillosis. Oxf Med Case Rep. 2021 Apr 28;2021(4):omaa029. doi: 10.1093/omcr/omaa029. PMID: 33948179; PMCID: PMC8081018.

11. Grehn C, Eschenhagen P, Temming S, Düesberg U, Neumann K, Schwarz C. Frequent pet contact as risk factor for allergic bronchopulmonary aspergillosis in cystic fibrosis. Front Cell Infect Microbiol. 2021 Jan 11;10:601821. doi: 10.3389/fcimb.2020.601821. PMID: 33585274; PMCID: PMC7873990.
12. Yang Y, Gao Q, Jin Y, Qi M, Lu G, HequanLi. Eosinophils may serve as CEA-secreting cells for allergic bronchopulmonary aspergillosis (ABPA) patients. Sci Rep. 2021 Feb 17;11(1):4025. doi: 10.1038/s41598-021-83470-z. Erratum in: Sci Rep. 2021 May 6;11(1):10126. PMID: 33597608; PMCID: PMC7889926.
13. Kaur K, Sharma K, Girdhar N, Gupta A, Chopra V. Another rare presentation of allergic bronchopulmonary aspergillosis in a high burden tuberculosis country. Monaldi Arch Chest Dis. 2021 Mar 8;91(3). doi: 10.4081/monaldi.2021.1696. PMID: 33691393.
14. Tsubouchi K, Arimura-Omori M, Inoue S, Okamatsu Y, Inoue K, Harada T. A case of allergic bronchopulmonary aspergillosis with marked peripheral blood eosinophilia successfully treated with benralizumab. Respir Med Case Rep. 2021 Jan 5;32:101339. doi: 10.1016/j.rmcr.2021.101339. PMID: 33489747; PMCID: PMC7807250.
15. Yang Y, Qiqi G, Jin Y, Qi M, Lu G, HequanLi. Author correction: eosinophils may serve as CEA-secreting cells for allergic bronchopulmonary aspergillosis (ABPA) patients. Sci Rep. 2021 May 6;11(1):10126. doi: 10.1038/s41598-021-89003-y. Erratum for: Sci Rep. 2021 Feb 17;11(1):4025. PMID: 33958672; PMCID: PMC8102584.
16. Kurihara Y, Tashiro H, Takahashi K, Komiya N, Sadamatsu H, Kimura S, Sueoka-Aragane N. Clinical manifestations of allergic bronchopulmonary aspergillosis without major features of asthma diagnosed by the new criteria in Japan. Intern Med. 2021 Apr 15;60(8):1251–1255. doi: 10.2169/internalmedicine.6072-20. Epub 2020 Nov 9. PMID: 33162484; PMCID: PMC8112978.

https://doi.org/10.1142/9789811271410_0019

19 Cardiopulmonary indications of oxygen therapy

Introduction

Oxygen therapy is indicated in hypoxia of cardiopulmonary origin associated with varying degrees of hypoxemia. And the requirement for oxygen is more and for a short duration in acute illness as compared to chronic cardiorespiratory conditions. Appropriate use of oxygen therapy and for a required duration would receive an optional benefit, avoiding unnecessary oxygen toxicity.

A. Pulmonary indications: Hypoxemia of acute illness and acute on chronic exacerbation is the presentation of acute respiratory failure. Hypercapnia is the usual accompaniment whenever there is hypoventilation. Continuous monitoring of oxygen therapy is aimed at its utilization at the tissue level and on correction of blood PaO_2 level.

1. Chronic obstructive pulmonary disease (COPD): Hypoxia in COPD occurs due to the ventilation–perfusion mismatch and is accompanied by hypercapnia due to airway obstruction, muscle weakness of respiratory muscles, and alveolar and central hypoventilation; reflex pulmonary vasoconstriction due to hypoxemia further aggravates pulmonary hypertension.

   The goal of O_2 therapy is to maintain a PaO_2 of 55–60 mmHg corresponding to SpO_2 of 99%–12%. High-flow delivery in the acute situation has to be shifted to more comfortable nasal prongs as the patient gets stabilized.

Table 1: Indications for oxygen therapy

Intermittent oxygen
During exercise: $PaO_2 > 59$ mmHg or oxygen saturation ≤88% with a low level of exertion.
During sleep: $PaO_2 \leq 55$ mmHg or oxygen saturation ≤88% with associated complications (pulmonary hypertension and cardiac arrhythmias).
Continuous oxygen (more than 12 hours a day)
Resting PaO_2 of ≤55 mmHg or oxygen saturation ≤88%.
Resting PaO_2 of 56–59 mmHg or oxygen saturation of 89% in the presence of the following:
Congestive heart failure and right ventricular failure.
Cor pulmonale on the electrocardiogram (P-wave greater than 3 mm in standard leads II, III, or VF) or echocardiography.
Polycythemia (hematocrit >65%).

2. Bronchial asthma: A mismatch of ventilation to perfusion is observed in asthma. The airway obstruction is diffuse, but CO_2, retention is usually not present despite impaired ventilation. Humidified oxygen with a flow rate of 4–6 L/minute, aiming at F_2O_2 of 35%–40% is to be achieved and adjusted at SaO_2 of at least 92%, and PaO_2 about to mmHg. Along with the usual anti-inflammatory and bronchodilator nebulized therapy, oxygen has a bronchodilatory effect. It also reduces hypoxic pulmonary constriction that directly improves pulmonary hypertension that usually accompanies asthma.
3. ILDS: Hypoxemia occurs because of impaired diffusion as well as ventilation–perfusion mismatch. Hypoxemia which is due to the thickened lung interstitium gets aggravated following a little effort (exercise). In late cases, CO_2 retention may also occur, oxygen therapy is held in correcting hypoxemia and can be given in higher concentration or high flow rates, but continuous research is still on for long-term oxygen therapy in these cases.

4. Bronchiectasis: Extensive lung involvement may be responsible for chronic hypoxemia. Intermittent oxygen for long-term therapy is being investigated.
5. Acute chest infections: Acute upper airway infection in the case of COPD may precipitate respiratory failure, requiring oxygen therapy. Similarly, pneumonia may be a life-threatening condition requiring specific antimicrobials with supportive oxygen therapy which is called for depending on the presence of hypoxemia and not determined by the etiology of pneumonia. Those developing acute respiratory distress syndrome (ARDS) may require intubation and assisted respiratory support also.
6. Pneumothorax/pneumomediastinum: Hypoxemia occurs due to respiratory distress, especially in the presence of diffuse lung disease with compromised lung function. Oxygen therapy treats hypoxemia as well as helps in enhanced absorption of the presence of abnormal air by fourfold (which is normally absorbed from pleural space at the rate of 1.25% per day).
7. Kyphoscoliosis: Ventilation gets diminished and lung expansion is restricted as a result of severe form of spine deformity (kyphoscoliosis). This may get worsened during pregnancy or lower respiratory tract infection. Chronic respiratory failure may occur with the development of pulmonary hypertension and chronic cor pulmonale. NIPPY improves resting arterial PCO_2.
8. Sleep apnea syndrome: Oxygen therapy improves arterial oxygenation during excessive daytime sleep, improves excessive fatigue, and cuts down cardiovascular complications of arterial desaturation, including cardiac arrhythmias.
9. Pulmonary hypertension: Pulmonary hypertension has varied etiology, and alveolar hypoxia in itself is an important cause of pulmonary hypertension. It causes reflex pulmonary vasoconstriction that enhances pulmonary vascular pressure. Oxygen therapy, in

these cases with alveolar hypoxia, corrects hypoxemia and abolishes hypoxic pulmonary vasoconstriction. Supplemental oxygen of 100% acts as a selective primary vasodilator also, irrespective of primary diagnosis, and has a definite role in treating pulmonary hypertension with documented hypoxemia.

10. Pulmonary thromboembolism: Hypoxemia occurs because of V/Q abnormality and the presence of pulmonary edema. Hypocapnia occurs due to hyperventilation, but occasionally hypercapnia may occur in a patient with marked ventilatory insufficiency. Oxygen of 100% and even hyperbaric oxygen is useful in correcting arterial hypoxemia, and therapy prevents pulmonary infarction (seen in 10% of cases) by enriching lung tissue oxygen supply via alveolar air as well as expanded bronchopulmonary vascular anastomoses. Additionally, oxygen therapy helps in absorbing embolism if it is "air embolism."
11. ARDS: ARDS is diagnosed when there is severe hypoxemia, that is, PaO_2/FiO_2 ratio than 200 and is labeled as acute lung injury and if there is less severe hypoxemia, that is, PaO_2/FiO_2 ratio of 300 or less, oxygen therapy aims at adequate tissue oxygenation and not at achieving normal or high PaO_2. An initial FiO_2 of >0.6 is used but soon it is attempted to reduce FiO_2 to achieve satisfactory PaO_2 (and actual arterial oxygen content) These patients may require higher alveolar pressure (achieved with the help of assisted ventilation). But it must be kept in mind that risks of higher alveolar pressure are greater than those of high FiO_2.

B. Cardiovascular indications: Non-pulmonary conditions have a doubtful indication of oxygen therapy. But certain cardiovascular disorders genuinely need oxygen therapy especially when there is demonstrable tissue hypoxemia.

1. IHD: Oxygen therapy is a double-edged sword improving cardiac muscle and tissue oxygenation and relieving dyspnea although there is no arterial hypoxemia. At the same time, excessive administration of oxygen should be avoided since it may cause systemic

vasoconstriction and increase after load. There is not much conclusive evidence that myocardial infarction can be prevented by supplemental oxygen therapy. However, 100% of oxygen improves both myocardial oxygenation and contractility and is indicated in complicated infarctions such as cardiogenic shock or congestive cardiac failure. Definite indications requiring urgent oxygen therapy include left ventricular failure with pulmonary congestion or edema. Oxygen therapy along with drugs and maintenance of blood pressure in heart failure corrects tissue hypoperfusion and hypoxia, although arterial PaO_2 is normal. For acute decompensation of heart failure, oxygen therapy offers basic life care support. Similarly, in chronic heart failure, nocturnal oxygen therapy provides relief of sleep-disturbed breathing and improves left ventricular dysfunction, thus offering a better quality of life.

2. Cerebrovascular disorders: Conflicting reports of transient improvement or prevention of infarction in acute ischemic stroke have appeared, but uncertainty in outcome exists with the use of hyperbaric oxygen treatment. Cluster headache has shown a favorable outcome in three-fourth of cases, attributing to the vasoconstrictive effects of oxygen administration.

C. Operative procedure and oxygen therapy: Preoperative oxygenation has been practiced by a few. Nevertheless, oxygen is routinely administered during anesthesia and surgery. It is routinely given even in endoscopic procedure without anesthesia, especially in patients with a history of respiratory disorder. Obese, smokers, aged, and people with pre-existing lung disease often have postoperative infection, atelectasis, and thromboembolism. Hypoventilation or mismatched ventilation–perfusion often leads to hypoxemia with or without CO_2, retention, underlining the need for oxygen administration, which improves partial pressure in different organs and subcutaneous tissue as well as prevents post-operative emesis and wound infection. Inspired O_2 fraction of 80% is usually considered optimal to give only a small increase in FiO_2 administered with nasal cannula at flow rates of S-6 L/minute.

With significant cardiorespiratory disorder and after cardiothoracic surgery, oxygen administration has to be continued till blood gas analysis shows that it is not required.

Comments: Oxygen therapy plays an important role in the management of cardiopulmonary and other serious illnesses, and these indications are expanding with the increasing understanding regarding physiological and clinical aspects of oxygen. The physiological and pharmacological basis of oxygen therapy remains incompletely understood, and at the same time, erroneous administration in various cardiorespiratory indications is quite prevalent in this part of the country. The cardiopulmonary indications have to be properly assessed; O_2 therapy has to be administered for a proper duration, and delinking has to be done as and when there is no need to supplement oxygen, realizing that oxygen therapy is a "drug" and physician must make optional use of it, avoiding side effects and toxicity of this double-edged sword.

References and suggested readings

1. Josten SA, et al. The effect of oxygen therapy in patients presenting to an emergency department with exacerbation of COPD. Med J Aust. 2007;186:235–238.
2. Bhatia RS. Sleep apnoea syndrome. Curr Med Trends. 2009;9:1769–1774.
3. Bhatia RS, Sidia SS. Management of spontaneous pneumothorax. Med Updates; API. 2004;14:721–726.
4. Helms AK, et al. A review of O_2 therapy in ischemic stroke. Cerebrovas Dis. 2005;20:417–476.
5. Nicholson C. A systemic review of effectiveness of oxygen in reducing acute myocardial ischemia. J Clin Neurol. 2004;13:996–1007.
6. Gulati V. Pulmonary thromboembolism. Med Update. 2009;17:155–162.
7. Tarpy SP, Celli BR. N Engl J Med. 1995;333:710–714.
8. Fletcher DJ, Boller M. Fluid therapy during cardiopulmonary resuscitation. Front Vet Sci. 2021 Jan 28;7:625361. doi: 10.3389/fvets.2020.625361. PMID: 33585610; PMCID: PMC7876065.
9. Niyibizi E, Kembi GE, Lae C, Pignel R, Sologashvili T. Delayed hyperbaric oxygen therapy for air emboli after open heart surgery: case report and review

of a success story. J Cardiothorac Surg. 2016 Dec 5;11(1):167. doi: 10.1186/s13019-016-0553-5. PMID: 27919270; PMCID: PMC5139121.

10. Li J, Tu M, Yang L, Jing G, Fink JB, Burtin C, Andrade AD, Gong L, Xie L, Ehrmann S. Worldwide clinical practice of high-flow nasal cannula and concomitant aerosol therapy in the adult ICU setting. Respir Care. 2021 Sep;66(9):1416–1424. doi: 10.4187/respcare.08996. Epub 2021 Apr 6. PMID: 33824172.
11. Liptzin DR, Abman SH, Giesenhagen A, Ivy DD. An approach to children with pulmonary edema at high altitude. High Alt Med Biol. 2018 Mar;19(1):91–98. doi: 10.1089/ham.2017.0096. Epub 2018 Feb 22. PMID: 29470103; PMCID: PMC5905943.
12. Marcadet DM, Pavy B, Bosser G, Claudot F, Corone S, Douard H, Iliou MC, Vergès-Patois B, Amedro P, Le Tourneau T, Cueff C, Avedian T, Solal AC, Carré F. French Society of Cardiology guidelines on exercise tests (part 1): methods and interpretation. Arch Cardiovasc Dis. 2018 Dec;111(12):782–790. doi: 10.1016/j.acvd.2018.05.005. Epub 2018 Aug 6. PMID: 30093254.
13. Beshai JF, Grimm RA, Nagueh SF, Baker JH 2nd, Beau SL, Greenberg SM, Pires LA, Tchou PJ; RethinQ Study Investigators. Cardiac-resynchronization therapy in heart failure with narrow QRS complexes. N Engl J Med. 2007 Dec 13;357(24):2461–2471. doi: 10.1056/NEJMoa0706695. Epub 2007 Nov 6. PMID: 17986493.
14. Yu M, Li S, Li S, Li J, Xu H, Chen K. Baduanjin exercise for patients with ischemic heart failure on phase-II cardiac rehabilitation (BEAR trial): study protocol for a prospective randomized controlled trial. Trials. 2018 Jul 16;19(1):381. doi: 10.1186/s13063-018-2759-4. PMID: 30012193; PMCID: PMC6048837.
15. Stec SM, Szmit S, Szydłowski L, Dudek K, Zagrodzka M, Futyma M, Opolski G, Kułakowski P. Dyspnoea related to pre-excitation during sinus rhythm as a new indication for catheter ablation. Kardiol Pol. 2014;72(7):646–653. doi: 10.5603/KP.a2014.0047. Epub 2014 Feb 14. PMID: 24526564.

https://doi.org/10.1142/9789811271410_0020

20 Lung cancer

Introduction

Lung cancers are one of the most important causes of cancers in men and women with very high mortality rates and very poor 5-year survival rates of less than 20% in most studies. They are usually diagnosed late in the course of the disease, and most cases are not surgically resectable at the time of the diagnosis. Many patients present in stage III with a short history of a few months, and it is not clear whether it is because the patients are poor perceivers of symptoms or because the malignancy is very aggressive. The incidence of lung cancers is increasing over the last decade and there is an urgent need to reduce the risk factors in the community, identify subjects who are at higher risk of developing lung cancers early in their life course, and research is needed on how to improve tumor immunity and DNA repair in these high-risk subjects. A good number of subjects are women who are nonsmokers and have no environmental tobacco exposure. Further studies are necessary to identify the risks in women. There is also a need to develop effective screening tools that are sensitive and specific and can detect early disease. Liquid biopsies using newer molecular biology can be very useful tools for screening in the future to detect early disease.

Classification

The classification can be dependent on the pathology as well as the TNM staging of lung cancers. Classification based on pathology has not changed much over the years and is mainly divided into two groups: non-small cell lung cancer (NSCLC), which causes 85% of the total lung cancers, and small cell lung cancer (SCLC), which accounts for the remaining 15%. SCLC is kept in a separate group due to its aggressive nature. It is classified into a limited or an extensive group due to its predilection for extensive metastases early in the course of its disease. One of the main reasons is the absence of much inflammation around the tumor, a feature seen in the NSCLC that probably slows down the spread of the disease. SCLC usually has little inflammation and that could be a reason for the easy and extensive spread observed. The details of the pathologic diagnosis given depend on the availability of the tissue. If it is a cytology specimen, then the diagnosis may be limited to NSCLC (squamous and adenocarcinoma) and SCLC. When the specimen appears to be poorly differentiated, immunohistochemistry can help with an appropriate diagnosis. When larger specimens are available, a more prognostic diagnosis can be given for adenocarcinomas; low-grade tumors such as lepidic adenocarcinoma, intermediate grade tumors such as papillary and adenocarcinomas and high-grade tumors such as micropapillary and solid adenocarcinomas. A more detailed World Health Organization (WHO) classification of lung cancer is given in the following table.

Adenocarcinoma	Others
Minimally invasive adenocarcinoma	Squamous cell carcinoma Large cell carcinoma
Lepidic adenocarcinoma	Adenosquamous carcinoma
Acinar adenocarcinoma	Carcinosarcoma
Papillary adenocarcinoma	Giant cell tumors
Micropapillary adenocarcinoma	Spindle cell tumors
Solid adenocarcinoma	Neuroendocrine tumors
Invasive mucinous adenocarcinoma	Carcinoid (typical, atypical) Small cell carcinoma
Colloid adenocarcinoma	Large cell neuroendocrine carcinoma

The TNM staging gives the anatomic extent of the lung cancers and aids in further management of the patient. The current TNM staging is in its eighth edition, and a brief summary is given in the following table.

Tumor	Node (regional lymph nodes)	Metastases
T0 — no primary tumor Tis — carcinoma in situ T1 — tumor <3 cm (further classified as a [<1 cm], b [1–2 cm], and c [2 to <3 cm]) T2 — >3 cm but <5 cm May involve the visceral pleura and main bronchus without involving carina (further classified as a [3–4 cm] and b [>4 but <5 cm]) T3 — >5 cm but <7 cm Involvement of phrenic nerve, chest wall, and pericardium One or more tumor nodules that are separate from the primary tumor in the same lobe T4 — >7 cm Involves carina, esophagus, diaphragm, heart, great vessels, recurrent laryngeal nerve, and ipsilateral another lobe	N0 — no regional lymph nodes N1 — involvement of ipsilateral hilar or pulmonary nodes N2 — involvement of ipsilateral mediastinal or subcarinal nodes N3 — involvement of contralateral hilar or mediastinal or supraclavicular nodes	M0 — no metastases M1a — *pleural or pericardial involvement in the form of effusions or nodules *nodules in the contralateral lung M1b — single extrathoracic metastases M1c — multiple extrathoracic metastases Either in one or more than one organ

Etiology and risk factors

Most of the lung cancers are caused by tobacco consumption which accounts for a total of 75% of all lung cancer cases. Cigarette smoke contains more than 3,000 chemicals of which 60 have been strongly associated with cancers. The most dangerous of these are the polyaromatic hydrocarbons, including benzo(a)pyrene and nitrosamines such as nicotine-derived nitrosoaminoketone. On metabolism by P450 enzymes, these have the potential to bind to the DNA and cause bulky adducts. In the usual course, once these bulky adducts are formed, either they are removed by nucleotide excision repair mechanisms or the cell undergoes apoptosis. In some cases, both do not happen, and there is a chance for mutations in the KRAS or the TP53 genes causing gene instability, an important step in the initiation of lung cancers. The risk contributed by tobacco smoking varies with the type of lung cancer: highest risk is seen for the development of squamous and large cell cancers and lesser risk but still substantial is seen for adenocarcinoma. Ex-smokers have half the risk of developing lung cancer as current active smokers. The other occupational risks are associated with asbestos, arsenic, chromium, nickel, and mustard gas.

More than half of women and nearly 15% of men with lung cancer have never smoked accounting for 25% of lung cancer in subjects who have never smoked. It is important to understand the risk factors to reduce the burden of cancer in these subjects. A list of all the possible risk factors with the quantum of risk is listed in the table below in the order of the associated risk.

Risk factor	Quantum of risk compared to general population
Tobacco smoking	10–20 times
Human papilloma virus	10 times
Asbestos	5 times
Residential radon	An increase of risk by 11% (US population) and 8.4% (European population) for every 100 Bq/m^3 in households
Genetic factors: Mutations of *CYP1A1* Ile462Val polymorphism and *XRCC1* variants	2.99 times

(*Continued*)

Risk factor	Quantum of risk compared to general population
Indoor coal and wood burning	2.66 times
Cooking oil vapors	2.12 times
Environmental tobacco smoke	1.24 times
Various mosquito repellants	Not yet estimated
Agarbathies (incense sticks), dhoop sticks	Not yet estimated

Molecular biology: recent advances in lung cancer

With the advent of next-generation sequencing (NGS), liquid biopsy is likely to be the future of lung cancer care. Many oncogene driver mutations can be studied in a single step by measuring them in the cell-free tumor DNA obtained from the plasma. It helps in monitoring the treatment response and to observe the development of new mutations that may necessitate the modification of the treatment without the need for repeated tissue biopsy from the tumor would be very difficult. Obtaining such information has transformed lung cancer care in the world, though there is a need for this to be cost-effective and accessible to all patients in low-middle-income countries. These oncogenes also determine the drugs that are most effective in a given patient. The most important of these is the epidermal growth factor receptor (EGFR), for which the first-line drug is gefitinib. Over the course of treatment, many subjects can develop resistance to that drug which is identified by the presence of EGFR T790M mutation, which necessitates the modification of the treatment regimen; gefitinib is replaced by a third-generation tyrosine kinase inhibitors (TKIs), such as afatinib and neratinib. There are many other mutations in both adenocarcinoma and squamous cell carcinoma, and further studies are needed to understand the relevance of a combination of these mutations and whether these mutations will guide the development of new targeted treatments. The list of important mutations is given in the table below.

Squamous cell carcinoma	Adenocarcinoma
Common: TP53, CDKN2A, PTEN, PIK3CA, KEAP1, MLL2, HLA-A, NFE2L2, NOTCH1, RB1, and PDYN	Common: *TP53* (46%), *KRAS* (33%), *KEAP1* (17%), *STK11* (17%), *EGFR* (14%), *NF1* (11%), and *BRAF* (10%). Less common: *SETD2, RBM10, MGA, MET, ARID1A, PIK3CA, SMARCA4, RB1, CDKN2A, U2AF1, RIT1, MET* exon 14 skipping, *ERBB2* (or *HER2*) mutation, *ROS1* fusion, *ALK* fusion, *MAP2K1* mutation, *RET* fusion, *NRAS* mutation, and *HRAS* mutation
Mutations that have the potential for being therapeutic targets	
RTK pathway RAS pathway PI(3)K pathway	*ALK, RET, ROS1* *NTRK1, NRG1, ERBB4, BRAF*

There are differences in mutations among smokers and nonsmokers with adenocarcinoma. KRAS mutations are common in smokers, whereas EGFR is more common in nonsmokers. EGFR mutations are also common among Asians as compared to Caucasians.

Clinical features

Many of the clinical features may be innocuous, so a high degree of suspicion is always needed by the clinician. The most common symptom remains cough, but many patients with chronic obstructive pulmonary disease (COPD) or chronic respiratory disease always have cough. In such situations, a change in the nature of the cough, a cough (due to COPD acute exacerbation) that does not respond as usual, and a cough that is associated with a change in the voice (hoarseness) should warrant additional evaluation. The other important sign is hemoptysis, which is usually seen in airway tumors. It usually presents as streaking of the sputum with blood and in a smoker above the age of 40 years needs further evaluation. It is important to remember that airway lesions or in situ mucosal lesions do not cast any shadow in the chest X-ray. Chest discomfort and chest pain that does not respond to analgesics is a very important clue to underlying malignancy. It becomes difficult when the underlying lung is damaged as in a destroyed lung due to old tuberculosis. In a white opaque lobe or lung, it is difficult to differentiate a new lesion and in many cases, even a computed tomography (CT) cannot help in localizing the lesion. We have found that in cases with strong suspicion, a positron emission tomography scan can help to localize the lesion for confirmation by biopsy. In a couple of cases, magnetic resonance imaging had picked up metastases in the rib and vertebral body that were not picked up on CT and a biopsy helped to confirm the diagnosis. The other common symptoms and signs are weight loss, dyspnea, fever, bone pain, clubbing, dysphagia, wheezing, or stridor.

In some cases, the presentation is classical, immediately raising doubts of malignancy, though some of these may not be very common. The important conditions are listed in the table below:

Condition	Clinical features
Horner's syndrome	Involvement of the stellate ganglion and the sympathetic chain. Enophthalmos, absence of sweating in that half of the face, ptosis, pupillary narrowing.
Pancoast tumor (Figure 3)	Superior sulcus tumor. Apex of the upper lobe. Infiltrates C8, T1, and T2 nerve roots. Muscle wasting, pain, and skin temperature change along the involved nerve root.

(*Continued*)

(*Continued*)

Condition	Clinical features
Phrenic nerve palsy	Presents as a raised hemidiaphragm and in patients with already compromised lungs, this may aggravate breathlessness.
SVC obstruction	Most common causes of SVC obstruction are involved by Direct invasion. Pressure from enlarged right paratracheal nodes. Can be at two levels: Supraazygous — drainage will happen through the azygous vein and only the veins over the upper chest wall will be dilated. Infra-azygous — drainage will happen via the inferior vena cava, and the dilated veins will be found over the chest wall and upper abdomen, with a reversal of the direction of flow. Presents with persistent swelling of the face, neck, and eyelids; dyspnea; vertigo; dysphagia in some cases; cough; and blurring of vision.
Recurrent laryngeal nerve involvement	Presents with hoarseness of voice. Usually left nerve is involved as it enters into the thorax, unlike the right whose course is limited only to the neck. Indirect laryngoscopy shows left vocal cord palsy.
Malignant pleural effusion	Usually, hemorrhagic. Large effusion that recurs after pleural tap. May be associated with chest pain and dyspnea. Due to the direct invasion of pleura. Mediastinal lymph node involvement and lymphatic obstruction.

A careful evaluation is needed to understand whether there are any metastases from the primary lung tumor. The common sites are the brain (70% of subjects who present with a central nervous system symptom due to metastases have their primary in the lung; Figure 2), liver (carries a poor prognosis), adrenals (Figure 1; usually asymptomatic and detected only

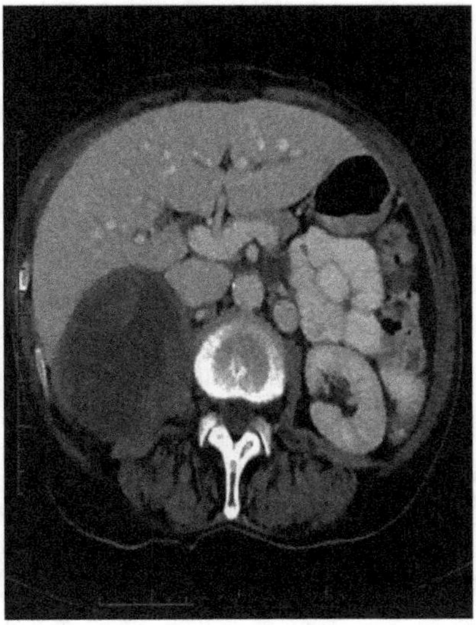

Figure 1: Adrenal metastases.

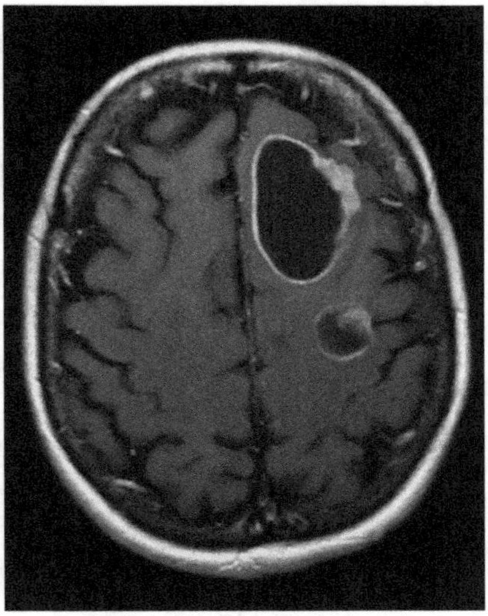

Figure 2: Brain metastases.

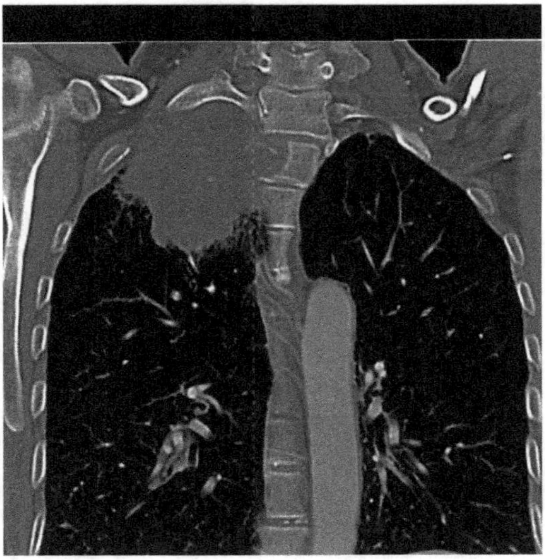

Figure 3: Pancoast tumor — CT.

on screening), spinal cord (usually in subjects who already have cerebral metastases), chest wall (usually presents with chest pain and seen in 50% of subjects at some time), heart and pericardium (mainly spreads from the lymphatic route), and bones (lung cancer can spread to any bone with preference to ribs, long bones, and the axial skeleton).

Paraneoplastic syndromes

Organ system	Paraneoplastic involvement
Neurologic	SCLC (almost exclusively) Mainly due to autoimmune antibodies (anti-Hu antibodies; antineuronal nuclear antibodies) Diagnosis of exclusion (electrolyte imbalance, metastases, treatment toxicity, infections, cerebral vascular disease are ruled out) Eaton–Lambert syndrome (myasthenia-like features, gradual onset of proximal lower and upper limb weakness, worse in the morning and better during the day) Others: Cerebellar degeneration Encephalomyelitis Sensory neuropathy
Skeletal	Squamous and adenocarcinoma Clubbing (most common) (hormonal, neurogenic, and vascular mechanisms) Hypertrophic pulmonary osteoarthropathy (<5%) Painful bilateral symmetric joint pains (wrist, knee, and ankles), periosteal new bone formation of distal long bones Vascular hyperplasia, new osteoblast, and fibroblast formation Due to increased VEGF

(*Continued*)

Organ system	Paraneoplastic involvement
Endocrine	SIADH (5%) elevated ADH secretion from tumor cells or from the hypothalamus leads to hyponatremia and small cell carcinoma (confusion, seizures, coma) Hypercalcemia (2%–6%), parathormone-related protein (PTHrp) Cushing's syndrome (1%–5%) — ectopic production of ACTH or its precursor proopiomelanocortin from tumor cells, small cell carcinoma (weakness, moon face, muscle weakness, hyperglycemia, hypokalemic alkalosis) Gynecomastia — due to ectopic production of beta-HCG Hypercalcitonemia Carcinoid syndrome Hyperthyroidism
Metabolic	Lactic acidosis
Renal	Nephrotic syndrome Glomerulonephritis
Hematologic	Anemia Leukocytosis and leukemoid reactions Thrombocytosis
Coagulopathy	Migratory thrombophlebitis (Trousseau syndrome) Disseminated intravascular coagulation
Systemic	Weight loss (cachexia), fever
Cutaneous	Acanthosis nigricans Erythroderma Urticaria Hypertrichosis Erythema multiforme
Collagen vascular	SLE Dermatomyositis, polymyositis

Diagnosis

A high degree of suspicion is needed to request for investigations to confirm the diagnosis of lung cancer, especially at younger ages. It is not uncommon to find adenocarcinoma in women below the age of 40 years. Many of the cases are classical, above the age of 60 years, male longtime smokers, with a mass lesion either centrally located or at the periphery. Though many of the images may be strongly suggestive, confirmation is only by histopathology. Specimens may be obtained by FNAC of the peripheral lung lesion or from the mediastinal lymph nodes (EBUS) or central lung lesion (routine bronchoscopy), or lymph nodes outside the thorax such as the supraclavicular lymph nodes. If a larger sample is needed from a lung, a tru-cut biopsy can be attempted for a peripheral lesion. Sputum cytology for 5 days or pleural fluid cytology when a malignant pleural effusion is suspected can identify malignant cells but may be difficult to give more details that may be necessary for a precise management. It is important that the cytology is performed within 1 hour since the cells can get lyzed and the examination will return negative for malignant cells.

The common radiological signs of lung cancer are listed in the following table:

Chest X-ray	Contrast-enhanced CT thorax
Mass lesion Solitary pulmonary nodule (Figures 4 and 5) Irregular and spiculated borders Bone erosion Associated with hilar or mediastinal lymphadenopathy Pleural effusion Pleural effusion with ipsilateral shift of the trachea suggesting underlying collapse	Mass lesion is better characterized Solitary pulmonary nodule (Figure 4) CT angiogram sign (in bronchioloalveolar carcinoma, enhancing vessels in a low attenuation mass lesion) Mass lesion with corona radiata Pleural tail/pleural tag sign Lymphangitis carcinomatosa Chest wall involvement Pancoast's tumor

(*Continued*)

Chest X-ray	Contrast-enhanced CT thorax
Noncalcified, usually, some peripheral calcification may be seen when there is a scar carcinoma Increased subcarinal angle suggesting subcarinal lymph node enlargement Postobstructive pneumonia In many cases, pneumonia shadows do not have air bronchograms Hilum overlay sign Golden "S" sign Thick-walled cavity (Figure 7) Collapse of a segment, lobe, or lung Cannon ball metastases Luftsichel sign (left upper lobe collapse)	Central mass with mediastinal involvement Rib and vertebral involvement Mixed solid and ground-glass (sub-solid) lesions Bubbly or cystic lucencies Cavitating lung cancer with thick walls Bronchioloalveolar carcinoma: unilateral or bilateral confluent airspace opacities Mass with pleural effusion Cannon ball metastases (Figure 6)

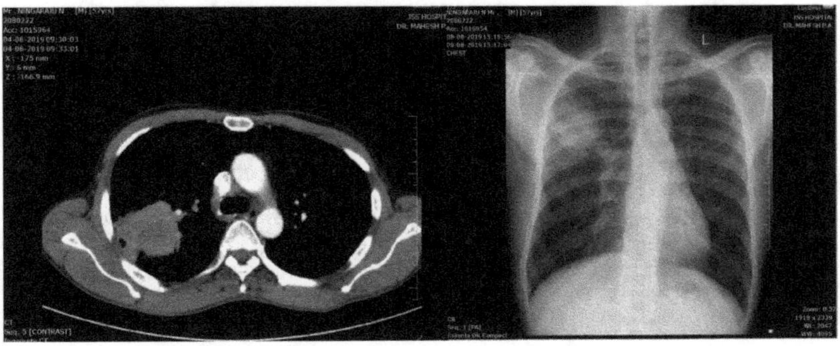

Figure 4: CT scans and chest X-ray of solitary pulmonary nodule.

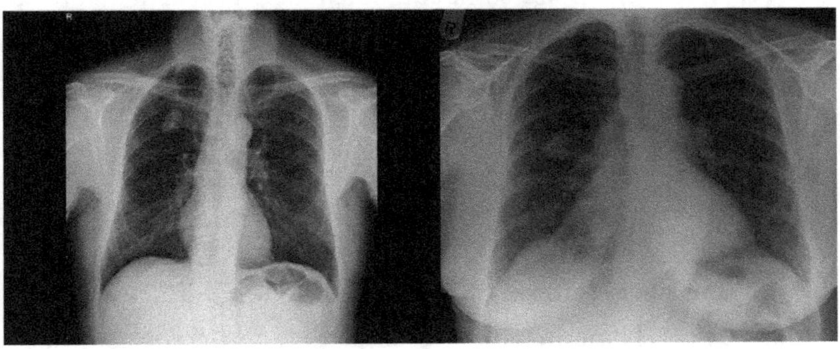

Figure 5: Chest X-ray of solitary pulmonary nodule.

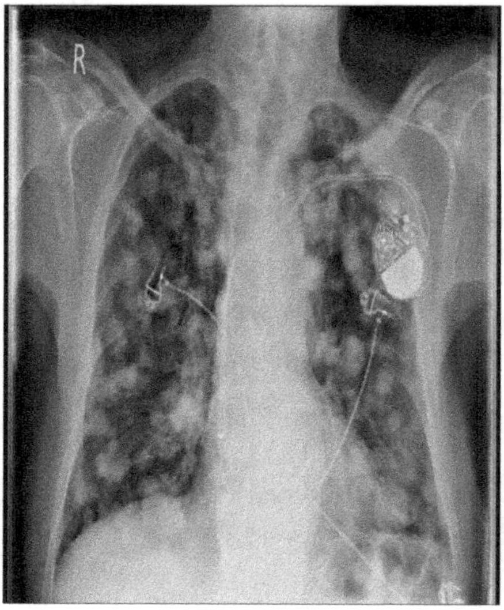

Figure 6: Cannon ball metastases.

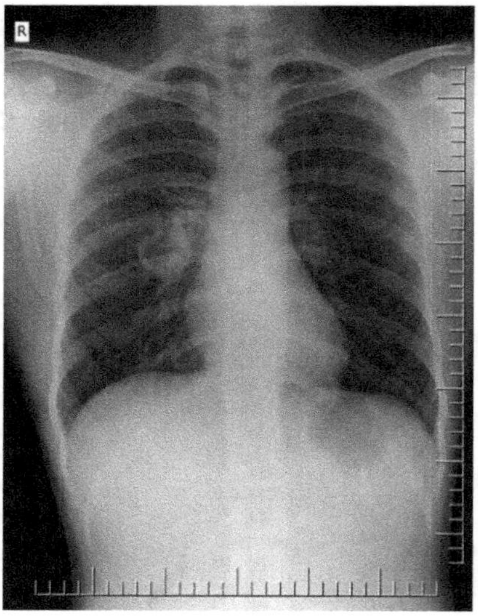

Figure 7: Cavitating lung cancer with thick walls.

Management

Management depends on the stage of the disease. A summary of management is given in the following.

Stage I:

The first choice is surgical resection. It is not clear whether every case needs adjuvant chemotherapy. Large studies have confirmed the role of adjuvant chemotherapy when the size of the mass lesion exceeds 4 cm and is shown to have survival benefits. It may be considered when lesions are between 3.1 and 3.9 cm in size, some additional survival benefit may be seen.

For subjects unwilling or unable to undergo surgical resection, stereotactic radiotherapy may be an option, when there are no lymph node metastases. When lymph node metastases are present, then radiotherapy, chemotherapy, and durvalumab (immune checkpoint inhibitor) are recommended.

Stage II:

If the performance status is good, the preferred choice is surgical resection, followed by chemotherapy, with cisplatin and one of gemcitabine, docetaxel, or pemetrexed. The survival rates are the same with any of the three combinations, but cisplatin and pemetrexed have the least side effects. Routine postoperative radiotherapy can be harmful rather than beneficial in patients undergoing surgery.

For subjects unwilling or unable to undergo surgical resection, stereotactic radiotherapy may be an option, when there are no lymph node metastases. When lymph node metastases are present, then a combination of radiotherapy and chemotherapy is recommended.

Stage IIIA:

For subjects with N0 and N1 disease, consider surgery. Chemotherapy and radiotherapy can be given in various combinations: preoperative chemotherapy, surgery followed by postoperative radiotherapy, or surgery followed by concurrent chemoradiotherapy.

For subjects with N2, no benefits from surgical resection are observed. They have advised chemoradiotherapy with durvalumab recommended for subjects whose disease has not progressed after two to three cycles of chemotherapy.

Stage IIIB:

These are surgically unresectable. Concurrent chemoradiotherapy is the rule. Additional biologic agents such as bevacizumab may be useful in selected cases. The role of TKIs is still being evaluated. Additionally, durvalumab is recommended for subjects whose disease has not progressed after two to three cycles of chemotherapy.

Stage IV:

Not resectable. Treatment depends mainly on the molecular signatures of the tumor. The key drugs based on these signatures are the presence of EGFR mutations (gefitinib, osemeritinib, dacomitinib, erlotinib, and afatinib), ALK rearrangements (crizotinib, ceritinib, alectinib, and brigatinib), BRAF mutations (trametinib, dabrafenib), ROS1 rearrangement (crizotinib, ceritinib), and human immune checkpoint inhibitors programmed death-1 (PD-1) or programmed death-ligand 1 (PD-L1) monoclonal antibodies (pembrolizumab, nivolumab, durvalumab, and atexolizumab). Among the drugs available within each group, the benefits are almost the same and anyone can be chosen.

Pharmacologic management of SCLC

Platinum-based therapy (cisplatin and carboplatin)

On penetrating the cell membrane, cisplatin loses its chlorides in the low-chloride milieu causing the substitution of the chloride ligands for water molecules. On the other hand, the chelating dicarboxylate of carboplatin exchanges for water and is activated by carbonate. These aquated/activated complexes then react with nucleophilic centers on purine bases of DNA, particularly the N7 positions of guanosine and adenosine residues causing cross-linking of guanine bases. These intrastrand and interstrand cross-linking results in distortion to the shape of the DNA preventing effective repair.

Etoposide

It is a semisynthetic derivative of the plant alkaloid, podophyllotoxin. It arrests the cells in the late S to the G2 phase of the cell cycle. Its major target is topoisomerase II that is involved in the resolution of various topological entanglements that occur during various processes like unwinding and rewinding of the double helix, coiling of DNA in higher order structures, and movement of protein along DNA. During this process of resolution, a short-lived enzyme–DNA complex called cleavable or cleavage complex is formed. The drug binds to the enzyme–DNA complex stabilizing the transient form, thereby rendering it susceptible to irreversible double-stranded breaks in the genome that are extremely toxic to the cell.

Irinotecan/topotecan

Irinotecan/topotecan are a semisynthetic derivative of the plant alkaloid camptothecin. It has S-phase–specific cytotoxicity. The major target is topoisomerase I which is involved in relieving torsional strain by inducing reversible single-stranded breaks. Irinotecan, and to a much greater extent its active metabolite SN-38, which is approximately 1,000 times as potent as irinotecan, prevents relegation of these breaks by binding to the topoisomerase I–DNA complex. TopoisomeraseI–drug–DNA complex, though not lethal by itself, collides with the advancing replication forks, forming double-stranded DNA break and irreversible arrest of the replication fork and cell death.

Regimens

First-line CT for limited or concurrent SCLC			
Regimen	**Dose (mg/m^2)**	**Days**	**Repeat cycle**
Etoposide/cisplatin (EP)	80/80, IV	1–3/3	Q 21 days
Etoposide/carboplatin (EP)	100/AUC 6, IV	1–3/3	Q 28 days
Irinotecan/cisplatin (IC)	**60/60, IV**	**1, 8, 15/1**	Q 28 days
Recurrent SCLC			
Topotecan	**1.5, IV**	**1–5**	**Q 21 days**
Recurrence occurs in more than 3 months			
Etoposide	160, PO	1–5	Q 28 days
Etoposide	50, PO	1–21	Repeat as tolerated
Paclitaxel	80–100, IV	Q week for 3 weeks	Q 28 days
Gemcitabine	1,000, PO	1, 8, and 15	Q 28 days
Cyclophosphamide/ doxorubicin/vincristine	1,000/40/1, IV	1/1/1	Q 21 days

Adverse drug reactions (ADRs)

Many adverse reactions have been reported, and most of them are related to the pharmacologic effect of the drugs on normal cells.

System disorders	Cisplatin	Carboplatin	Topotecan	Irinotecan	Etoposide
Infections and infestations	Sepsis	Infections	Infection, sepsis		Infection
Neoplasms					Acute leukemia
Blood and lymphatic system	Bone marrow failure, thrombocytopenia, leukopenia, anemia	Thrombocytopenia, neutropenia, leukopenia, anemia, hemorrhage	Febrile neutropenia, neutropenia, thrombocytopenia, anemia, leukopenia	Neutropenia (reversible and not cumulative) Anemia Thrombocytopenia (in case of combination therapy) Infectious episodes (with monotherapy)	Anemia, leukopenia, myelosuppression, neutropenia, thrombocytopenia, anaphylactic reactions
Immune system		Hypersensitivity, anaphylactoid type reaction	Hypersensitivity reactions including rash		
Metabolism and nutrition	Hyponatremia		Anorexia		
Nervous system		Neuropathy peripheral, paraesthesia, decrease of osteotendinous reflexes, sensory disturbance, dysgeusia			Dizziness
Cardiac system	Arrhythmia, bradycardia, tachycardia	Cardiovascular disorders			Arrhythmia, myocardial infarction

Vascular					Hypertension, transient systolic hypotension following rapid intravenous administration
Respiratory		Respiratory disorder, interstitial lung disease, bronchospasm			
Gastrointestinal		Vomiting, nausea, abdominal pain, diarrhea, constipation, mucous membrane disorder	Nausea, vomiting, and diarrhea (all of which may be severe), constipation, abdominal pain, mucositis	Severe delayed diarrhea Severe nausea and vomiting	Abdominal pain, anorexia, constipation, nausea, and vomiting Diarrhea, mucositis
Hepatobiliary			Hyperbilirubinemia		Increased AST, ALT, ALP, bilirubin, hepatotoxicity
Skin and subcutaneous tissue		Alopecia, skin disorder	Alopecia	Alopecia	Alopecia, pigmentation, pruritis, rash, urticaria
Musculoskeletal and connective tissue		Musculoskeletal disorder			
Renal and urinary		Urogenital disorder			

(*Continued*)

(*Continued*)

System disorders	Cisplatin	Carboplatin	Topotecan	Irinotecan	Etoposide
Reproductive and breast tissue					
General disorder and administration site disorders		Asthenia	Pyrexia, asthenia, fatigue, malaise	Fever in the absence of infection and without concomitant severe neutropenia	Asthenia, malaise, extravasation, phlebitis
Eye		Visual disturbances			
Ear and labyrinth		Ototoxicity			
Investigations		Decreased creatinine renal clearance, decreased blood sodium, potassium, calcium, magnesium, increased blood urea, abnormal liver function test		During combination therapy, transient serum levels (grade 1 and 2) of either ALT, AST, alkaline phosphatase, or bilirubin	

Pharmacologic management of NSCLC

- **Platinum-based therapy (cisplatin and carboplatin)**

  On penetrating the cell membrane, cisplatin loses its chlorides in the low-chloride milieu causing the substitution of the chloride ligands for water molecules. On the other hand, the chelating dicarboxylate of carboplatin exchanges for water and is activated by carbonate. These aquated/activated complexes then react with nucleophilic centers on purine bases of DNA, particularly the N7 positions of guanosine and adenosine residues causing cross-linking of guanine bases. These intrastrand and interstrand cross-linking results in distortion to the shape of the DNA preventing effective repair.
- **Vinca alkaloids**

  Vinorelbine is a mitotic spindle poison that impairs chromosomal segregation during mitosis. They are cell cycle and phase-specific because they block mitosis in metaphase (M-phase). Microtubules derived from polymers of tubulin are the principal target of vinorelbine. By binding to tubulin, they prevent its polymerization and assembly of microtubules, instead forming paracrystalline aggregates of tubulin dimers causing the disruption of mitotic spindle and prevention of chromosomal segregation and cell proliferation.
- **Antimetabolite**

  After entering the cell, gemcitabine is phosphorylated to an active form gemcitabine diphosphate and gemcitabine triphosphate (dFdCTP) by the enzyme deoxycytidine kinase. dFdCTP is incorporated into the DNA followed by one or more deoxynucleotides masking gemcitabine and preventing DNA repair by 3′–5′ exonuclease activity resulting in chain termination.
- **Taxanes**

  In contrast to other microtubule poisons, such as Vinca alkaloids, which inhibit tubulin polymerization, taxanes promote polymerization and stabilization of the polymer leading to the accumulation of microtubules. These overtly stable microtubules formed are nonfunctional resulting in the inhibition of normal dynamic reorganization of the microtubule network that is essential for interphase and mitotic functions.

Between paclitaxel and docetaxel, the latter has a 2-fold higher affinity to the tubulin-binding site and 2.5-fold more potent than paclitaxel as an inhibitor of cell replication. Also, docetaxel acts at the S-phase, whereas paclitaxel acts at the G(2)/M phases of the cell cycle. The slight structural difference between the two drugs makes paclitaxel 25% more aqueous soluble than paclitaxel.

Because of the low aqueous solubility of paclitaxel, a purified polyoxyethylated castor oil has been used as a vehicle that has been implicated in hypersensitivity reactions and may contribute to neuropathy. To overcome this nanoparticle, albumin–bound paclitaxel was developed with the advantage of lesser hypersensitivity reactions and shorter infusion time.

- **Folate analogs**

  Pemetrexed is a multitargeted anticancer antifolate agent that exerts its action by inhibiting thymidylate synthase (TS), dihydrofolate reductase, and glycinamide ribonucleotide formyltransferase (GARFT), which are key folate-dependent enzymes for the de novo biosynthesis of thymidine and purine nucleotides. Pemetrexed enters cells via the reduced folate carrier and binds to folate receptor-α with a very high affinity. Intracellularly, pemetrexed is polyglutamated to the active pentaglutamide, which is over 60-fold more potent than the parent, in the inhibition of TS and GRAFT by a reaction catalyzed by folylpolyglutamate synthase. Inhibition of these enzymes leads to a decrease in thymidine for DNA synthesis and purine synthesis, respectively.

- **Epipodophyllotoxins**

  Etoposide is a semisynthetic derivative of the plant alkaloid, podophyllotoxin. It arrests the cells in the late S to the G2 phase of the cell cycle. Its major target is topoisomerase II that is involved in the resolution of various topological entanglements that occur during various processes like unwinding and rewinding of the double helix, coiling of DNA in higher order structures, and movement of protein along DNA. During this process of resolution, a short-lived enzyme–DNA complex called cleavable or cleavage complex is formed. The drug binds to the enzyme–DNA complex stabilizing the transient form, thereby rendering it susceptible to irreversible double-stranded breaks in the genome that are extremely toxic to the cell.

Regimens

Regimen	Dose (mg/m^2)	Days	Repeat cycle
Adjuvant therapy			
Cisplatin/vinorelbine	50/25, IV	1, 8/weekly for 16 weeks	Q 28 days for 4 cycles
Cisplatin/etoposide	100/100, IV	1/1–3	Q 28 days for 4 cycles
Paclitaxel/carboplatin	175/AUC 6, IV	1/1	Q 21 days for 4 cycles
Cisplatin/pemetrexed	80/500, IV	1/1	Q 21 days for 6 cycles
Metastatic disease			
Cisplatin/gemcitabine	100/1,000, IV	1/1, 8, 15	Q 21 days

Adverse drug reactions

Most of the adverse reactions are due to the pharmacologic effect of the drugs on normal cell metabolism and cell division.

Drugs	Common ADRs
Cisplatin/carboplatin	Neurotoxicity, myelosuppression, N/V, electrolyte wasting, infusion reactions
Vinorelbine	Infections, myelosuppression, neurological disorders, constipation, asthenia, alopecia, transient elevation of LFT

(*Continued*)

(*Continued*)

Drugs	Common ADRs
Gemcitabine	N/V, alopecia, rash, flu-like syndrome
Paclitaxel/docetaxel	Neutropenia, leukopenia, alopecia, hypersensitivity reactions
Pemetrexed	Granulocytopenia, sensory neuropathy, N/V, rash, alopecia, creatinine elevation, fatigue
Etoposide	Myelosuppression, hypotension, alopecia, N/V, arrhythmia, myocardial infarction

- **Tyrosine kinase inhibitors**

  Two classes of tyrosine kinases are distinguished: Receptor tyrosine kinase (RTK) and cellular tyrosine kinase (CTK).

  RTKs consist of an extracellular ligand–binding domain, a transmembrane domain, and an intracellular catalytic domain. Dimerization of two RTKs on ligand binding results in autophosphorylation of tyrosine residues of the intracellular catalytic domains, which leads to an active confirmation and subsequent activation of signal transduction cascade within the cell. In this downstream signaling transduction pathway, CTKs play a primary role. Autophosphorylation of EGFR activates downstream signaling cascades such as the AKT, mitogen-activated protein kinase (MAPK), and JNK (c-Jun N-terminal kinase) pathways, which ultimately leads to DNA synthesis, cell cycle progression, and proliferation.

  ➢ **For the treatment of metastatic disease with EGFR deletions/mutations**

Generation	Name of drug	Blockade	Family members	
First generation	Erlotinib	Reversible	HER 1	19 deletion 21 mutation
	Gefitinib	Reversible	EGFR (HER 1, ErbB1)	19 deletion

(*Continued*)

Generation	Name of drug	Blockade	Family members	
Second generation	Afatinib	Irreversible	EGFR (ErbB1), HER2 (ErbB2), ErbB3 and ErbB4	19 deletion, L858R
	Dacomitinib	Irreversible	ErbB family	Exon 19 deletion, exon 21 1858R substitution
Third generation	Osimertinib	Irreversible	EGFRs	Sensitizing mutations (EGFRm) and TKI-resistance mutation T790M

➢ **For the treatment of anaplastic lymphoma kinase (ALK)–positive metastatic disease**

Alectinib is an ALK and RET TKI leading to the blockage of downstream signaling pathways including STAT3 and PI3K/AKT and induction of apoptosis.

Brigatinib is a TKI that targets ALK, c-ros oncogene 1 (ROS1), and insulin-like growth factor 1 receptor (IGF-1R). Brigatinib inhibits autophosphorylation of ALK and ALK-mediated phosphorylation of the downstream signaling protein STAT3.

Ceritinib and crizotinib are described under the following heading.

Generation	Name	Dose	ADR
Second	Alectinib	600 mg bid	Anemia, increased AST, ALT, ALP, fatigue, hyperbilirubinemia, hyperglycemia, constipation, cough, rash
Second	Brigatinib	90 mg for 7 days and then 180 mg per day	

➤ **For the treatment of ROS1-positive metastatic disease**

ROS1 protein–tyrosine kinase fusion proteins are expressed in 1%–2% of NSCLCs. The ROS1 locus is located on chromosome 6 and encodes for an orphan tyrosine kinase receptor, that is, with no known ligand and biologic function in humans. ROS1 rearrangements/translocations lead to fusions of an intact ROS1 tyrosine kinase domain with partner genes CD74–ROS1 fusion has been reported as the most common rearrangement in NSCLC. These fusion events lead to constitutive activation of the ROS1 kinase that drives cellular transformation and promotes survival and proliferation through downstream signaling via SHP-1/SHP-2, JAK/STAT, PI3K/AKT/mTOR, and MAPK/ERK pathways.

Generation	Name	Dose	ADR
Second	Ceritinib	750 mg/ day PO	Anemia, decreased appetite, vision disorder, bradycardia, diarrhea, nausea, vomiting, abdominal pain, constipation esophageal disorder
First	Crizotinib	250 mg PO bid	plus neutropenia, leukopenia, neuropathy, dysgeusia, dizziness, edema

➤ **For the treatment of BRAF V600E mutation-positive metastatic disease**

Mutations in V-raf murine sarcoma viral oncogene homolog B (BRAF) are identified in 2%–4% of lung adenocarcinomas. BRAF mutation results in the activation of the MAPK pathway that promotes cell growth, proliferation, and survival.

Generation	Name	Dose	ADR
First	Dabrafenib	150 mg/ bid, PO	Papilloma, decreased appetite, headache, cough, nausea, vomiting, diarrhea, hyperkeratosis, alopecia, rash, palmar–plantar erythrodysesthesia syndrome, arthralgia, myalgia, pain in extremity, pyrexia, fatigue, chills, asthenia

(*Continued*)

Generation	Name	Dose	ADR
First	Vemurafenib	960 mg/ bid, PO	* + SCC of the skin, keratoacanthoma, seborrheic keratosis, skin papilloma, headache, dysgeusia, dizziness, constipation, photosensitivity reaction, actinic keratosis, hyperkeratosis, sunburn, pain in extremity, musculoskeletal pain, back pain, edema peripheral
Second	Trametinib	2 mg/ day, PO	* + Folliculitis, paronychia, cellulitis, hypersensitivity, dehydration, blurred vision, periorbital edema, visual impairment, left ventricular dysfunction, ejection fraction decreased, bradycardia, hypertension, hemorrhage, abdominal pain, dry mouth, dermatitis acneiform, dry skin, pruritus, edema peripheral, pyrexia, increased AST

- **Monoclonal antibodies**
  - Immune checkpoint inhibitors against the PD-1/PD-L1 pathway

    PD-1 is an advanced checkpoint molecule and is expressed on the surface of all activated T cells. When a T cell recognizes the antigen expressed by the major histocompatibility complex on the target cell, inflammatory process begins as the cytokines are produced. These cytokines result in PD-L1 expression in the tissue, activating the PD-1 protein on the T cell leading to immune tolerance, a phenomenon where the immune system loses control to mount an inflammatory response, even in the presence of actionable antigens. In certain tumors, this protective mechanism is perverted through overexpression of PD-L1; as a result, it circumvents the generation of an immune response to the tumor. PD-1/PD-L1 inhibitors pharmacologically prevent the PD-1/PD-L1 interaction, thus facilitating a positive immune response to kill the tumor.

Drug	Indication	Dose	ADR
Pembrolizumab	Given as monotherapy or combination	200 mg Q 3 weeks	Fatigue, decreased appetite, dyspnea, cough, pneumonitis, colitis, hypophysitis, thyroid disorders
Nivolumab	Monotherapy in locally advanced or metastatic NSCLC after prior chemotherapy	240 mg every 2 weeks	Upper respiratory tract infection (URTI), neutropenia, hypo/hyperthyroidism, nausea, arthralgia, cough, dyspnea, fatigue, elevated hepatic enzymes
Atezolizumab	In combination with bevacizumab, paclitaxel, and carboplatin is indicated for the first-line treatment for metastatic NSCLC	1,200 mg Q 3 weeks	Urinary tract infection, thrombocytopenia, decreased appetite, arthralgia, rash, pruritis
Durvalumab	Monotherapy is indicated for the treatment of locally advanced, unresectable NSCLC in adults whose tumors express PD-L1 on ≥1% of tumor cells and whose disease has not progressed following platinum-based chemoradiation therapy	10 mg/kg IV Q 2 weeks	URTI, pneumonia, hyperthyroidism, cough, pyrexia

➢ **Antiangiogenesis inhibitors**

Angiogenesis plays an important role in tumor growth, hence the inhibition of angiogenesis is considered an important mechanism.

Bevacizumab binds to vascular endothelial growth factor (VEGF), the key driver of vasculogenesis and angiogenesis, and thereby inhibits the binding of VEGF to its receptors and inhibiting the formation of new tumor vasculature, thereby inhibiting tumor growth. It is given in combination with platinum-based chemotherapy or erlotinib, as indicated for the first-line treatment of adult patients with unresectable advanced, metastatic, or recurrent NSCLC.

Ramucirumab specifically binds VEGF receptor 2 and blocks the binding of VEGF-A, VEGF-C, and VEGF-D. It is given in combination with docetaxel for the treatment of adult patients with locally advanced or metastatic NSCLC with disease progression after platinum-based chemotherapy.

Necitumumab binds with high affinity and specificity to the human EGFR 1 altering malignant progression, induction of angiogenesis, and inhibition of apoptosis. It is administered in addition to gemcitabine and cisplatin-based chemotherapy for up to six cycles of treatment followed as a single agent in patients whose disease has not progressed.

<table>
<tr><th>Drug</th><th>Dose</th><th>ADR</th></tr>
<tr><td>Bevacizumab</td><td>7.5–15 mg/kg Q 3 weeks</td><td rowspan="2">Myelosuppression, anorexia, electrolyte disturbance, dyspnea, epistaxis, increased lacrimation, hypertension</td></tr>
<tr><td>Ramucirumab</td><td>8 mg/kg Q 2 weeks</td></tr>
<tr><td>Necitumumab</td><td>800 mg on day 1, 8 of 3-week cycle</td><td>Hypomagnesemia, hypocalcemia, rash, vomiting</td></tr>
</table>

- **Bisphosphonates**

Bisphosphonates like zoledronic acid, pamidronate, and clodronate have an established role in treating tumor-induced hypercalcemia and decreasing the incidence of skeletal-related events and when added to chemotherapy or radiotherapy, it resulted in better pain control, quality of life, and less progression of bone lesions than the other therapies alone.

- **Denosumab**

  Denosumab is the first example of targeted therapy for bone metastasis. It is a fully human monoclonal antibody directed against the receptor activator of nuclear factor kappa-B ligand inhibiting the maturation of preosteoclasts into osteoclasts. An exploratory analysis showed that denosumab was associated with improved overall survival compared with zoledronate in patients with bone metastases from lung cancer.

Complications

Lung cancer can present with many complications due to the primary tumor, metastases, or due to treatment. The adverse events associated with the chemotherapeutic agents are listed separately.

Primary tumor	Metastases	Treatment
Pulmonary hemorrhage Superior venacaval obstruction Venous thromboembolism Central airway obstruction with stridor, respiratory failure, and death Postobstructive pneumonia	Liver: anorexia, nausea, vomiting, liver failure Brain: asymptomatic, hemorrhage, stroke, focal neurologic deficit, seizures, personality changes, headaches Bone: severe pain not responding to analgesics Pathologic fractures Vertebrospinal involvement	Febrile neutropenia secondary to chemotherapy Radiation pneumonitis and later on fibrosis Postoperative complications including pneumonia Skin rashes, acneiform, lichenoid eruptions

Survival

Five-year survival rates are still dismal in lung cancer in spite of advances in radiotherapy and chemotherapy. The survival rates in one of the large series of patients were as follows: Stage I A (49%), Stage IB (45%), Stage II A, B (around 30%), Stage III A (14%) and III B (5%), Stage IV (0%–1%). The key factors that determine survival are not only the TNM staging of the disease but also the functional status of the patient as assessed by the Karnofsky score or the Eastern Cooperative Oncology Group WHO score, the presence of other comorbidities, and whether they are able to tolerate and complete the recommended treatment. The untreated mean survival for NSCLC is about 7.5 months.

References and suggested readings

1. Zheng M. Classification and pathology of lung cancer. Surg Oncol Clin N Am. 2016;25:447–468.
2. Heinemann S, Zabel P, Hauber H-P. Paraneoplastic syndromes in lung cancer. Cancer Ther. 2008;6:687–698.
3. Sun S, Schiller JH, Gazdar AF. Lung cancer in never smokers — a different disease. Nat Rev Cancer. 2007;7:778–790.
4. Inamura K. Lung cancer: understanding its molecular pathology and the 2015 WHO classification. Front Oncol. 2017;7:193.
5. Kanaji N, Watanabe N, Kita N, Bandoh S, Tadokoro A, Ishii T, Dobashi H, Matsunaga T. Paraneoplastic syndromes associated with lung cancer. World J Clin Oncol. 2014 Aug 10;5(3):197–223.
6. Initial evaluation of the patient with lung cancer: symptoms, signs, laboratory tests, and paraneoplastic syndromes. Chest. 2003;123:97S–104S.
7. Darnell RB, Posner JB. Paraneoplastic syndromes involving the nervous system. N Engl J Med. 2003;349:1543–1554.
8. Graus F, Delattre JY, Antoine JC, Dalmau J, Giometto B, Grisold W, Honnorat J, Sillevis Smitt P, Vedeler Ch, Verschuuren JJGM, Vincent A, Voltz R. Recommended diagnostic criteria for paraneoplastic neurological syndromes. J Neurol Neurosurg Psychiatry. 2004;75:1135–1140.
9. Rudin CM, Brambilla E, Faivre-Finn C, Sage J. Small-cell lung cancer. Nat Rev Dis Primers. 2021 Jan 14;7(1):3. doi: 10.1038/s41572-020-00235-0. PMID: 33446664; PMCID: PMC8177722.
10. Chaft JE, Rimner A, Weder W, Azzoli CG, Kris MG, Cascone T. Evolution of systemic therapy for stages I–III non-metastatic non-small-cell lung cancer.

Nat Rev Clin Oncol. 2021 Sep;18(9):547–557. doi: 10.1038/s41571-021-00501-4. Epub 2021 Apr 28. PMID: 33911215; PMCID: PMC9447511.

11. Zhao Y, Liu Y, Li S, Peng Z, Liu X, Chen J, Zheng X. Role of lung and gut microbiota on lung cancer pathogenesis. J Cancer Res Clin Oncol. 2021 Aug;147(8):2177–2186. doi: 10.1007/s00432-021-03644-0. Epub 2021 May 20. PMID: 34018055; PMCID: PMC8236441.
12. Xu K, Zhang C, Du T, Gabriel ANA, Wang X, Li X, Sun L, Wang N, Jiang X, Zhang Y. Progress of exosomes in the diagnosis and treatment of lung cancer. Biomed Pharmacother. 2021 Feb;134:111111. doi: 10.1016/j.biopha.2020.111111. Epub 2020 Dec 24. PMID: 33352449.
13. Fan Y, Liu B, Chen F, Song Z, Han B, Meng Y, Hou J, Cao P, Chang Y, Tan K. Hepcidin upregulation in lung cancer: a potential therapeutic target associated with immune infiltration. Front Immunol. 2021 Apr 1;12:612144. doi: 10.3389/fimmu.2021.612144. PMID: 33868231; PMCID: PMC8047218.
14. Li Z, Feiyue Z, Gaofeng L. Traditional Chinese medicine and lung cancer: from theory to practice. Biomed Pharmacother. 2021 May;137:111381. doi: 10.1016/j.biopha.2021.111381. Epub 2021 Feb 15. PMID: 33601147.
15. Fois SS, Paliogiannis P, Zinellu A, Fois AG, Cossu A, Palmieri G. Molecular epidemiology of the main druggable genetic alterations in non-small cell lung cancer. Int J Mol Sci. 2021 Jan 9;22(2):612. doi: 10.3390/ijms22020612. PMID: 33435440; PMCID: PMC7827915.

https://doi.org/10.1142/9789811271410_0021

21 Chest imaging in pulmonary tuberculosis

Introduction

As blood is to life, conventional radiology is to tuberculosis (TB). TB affects different organs, giving different radiological pictures which along with clinical and other pathological investigations help in diagnosing TB. Interventional radiology is utilized in inoperable cases with massive hemoptysis in TB using bronchial artery embolization. The common signs of TB are enumerated in Table 1.

Table 1:

Radiologic features in tuberculosis-active TB	
Infiltrate or consolidation	Opacification of airspaces within the lung parenchyma. It can be dense or patchy and might have irregular, ill-defined borders.
Cavity	Dark areas within the lung parenchyma, with or without irregular margins that might be surrounded by an area of airspace consolidation or infiltrates, by nodular or fibrotic densities, or both. The walls surrounding the lucent area can be thick or thin. Calcification can exist.
Pleural effusion	Presence of a significant amount of fluid within the pleural space (Figures 15 and 16). This finding can be seen in active pulmonary TB, and empyema is also common in TB. Pneumothorax including tension pneumothorax is also a common presentation of TB. Hydropneumothorax and pyopneumothorax with or without tension are also common presentations in TB (Figures 8 and 9).
Nodule	Round density within the lung parenchyma also called a tuberculoma. Nodules included in this category are those with margins that are indistinct or poorly defined.
Hilar or mediastinal lymphadenopathy	Enlargement of lymph nodes in one or both hila or within the mediastinum, with or without associated atelectasis or consolidation.

(*Continued*)

Table 1: (*Continued*)

Radiologic features in tuberculosis-inactive TB	
Airways and parenchyma	Fibrosis (unilateral or bilateral), loss of lung volume (Figures 25 and 26), bronchiectasis, persisting cavity, aspergilloma, calcification (Figures 5 and 6).
Pleura	Pleural thickening, pleural calcification (Figure 7), loss of lung volume (Figures 23 and 24).

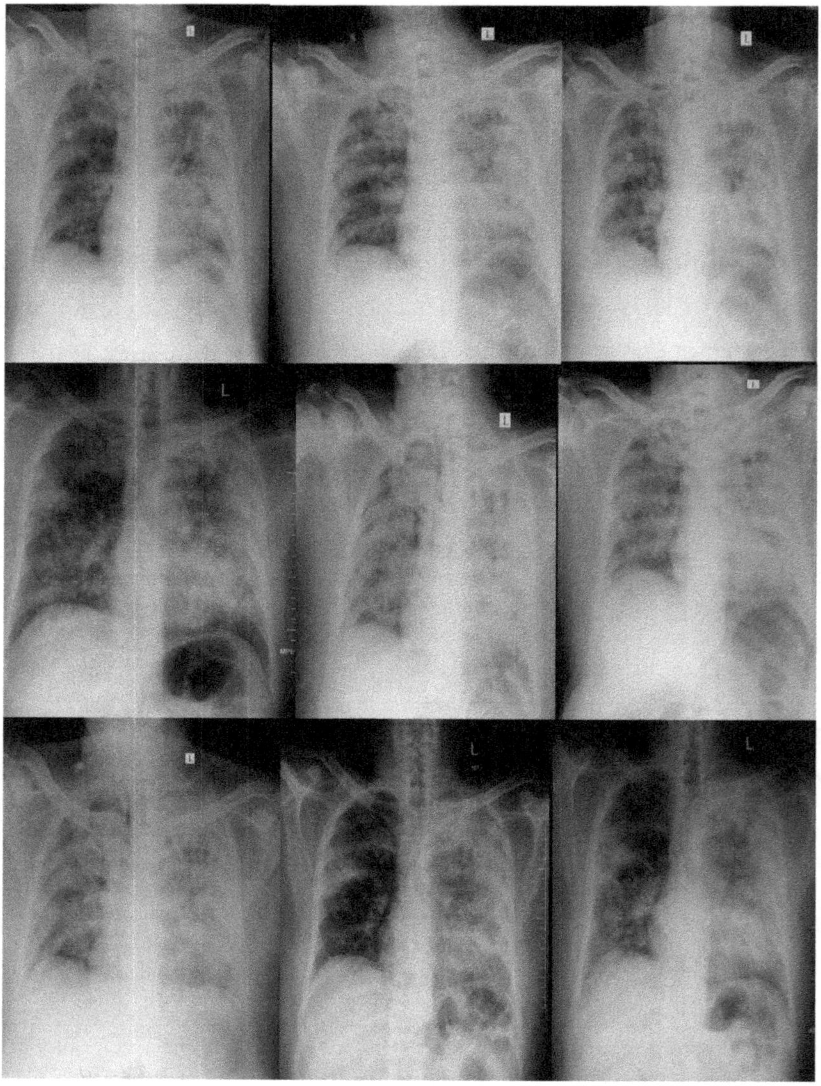

Figure 1: Series of X-ray in sputum-positive patient with TB admitted in intensive care unit with bilateral extensive opacities and respiratory failure.

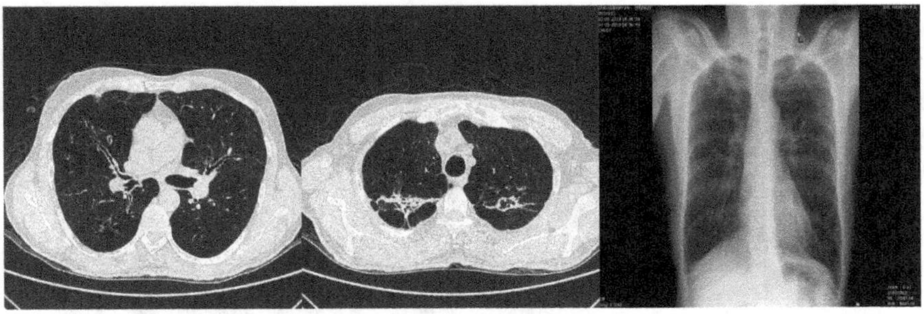

Figure 2: Computed tomography (CT) and X-rays of chronic obstructive pulmonary disease TB cavity with fibrosis.

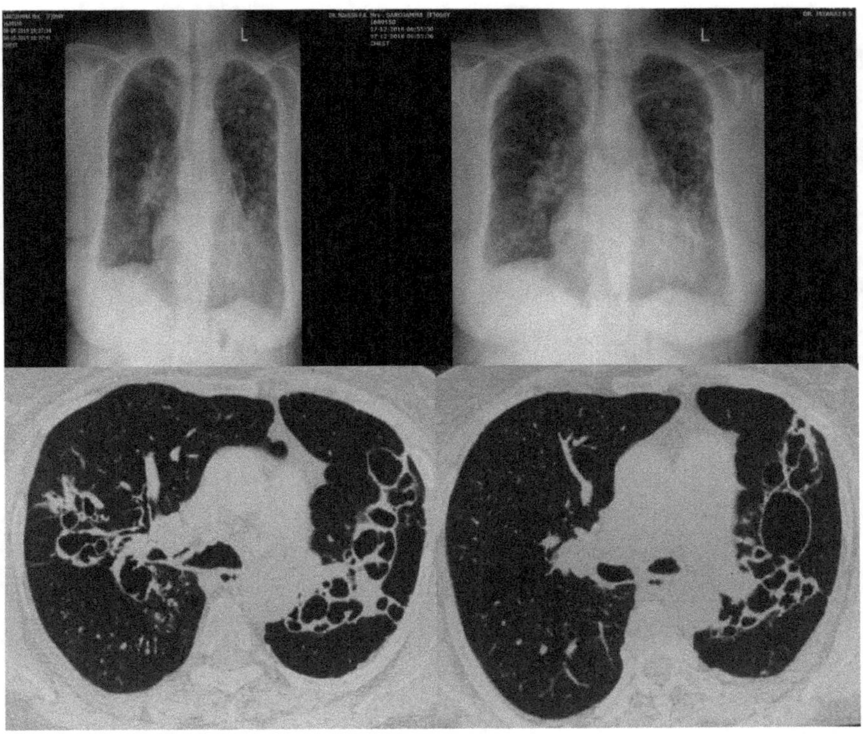

Figure 3: X-ray and CT scans of extensive bronchiectasis post-TB sequelae.

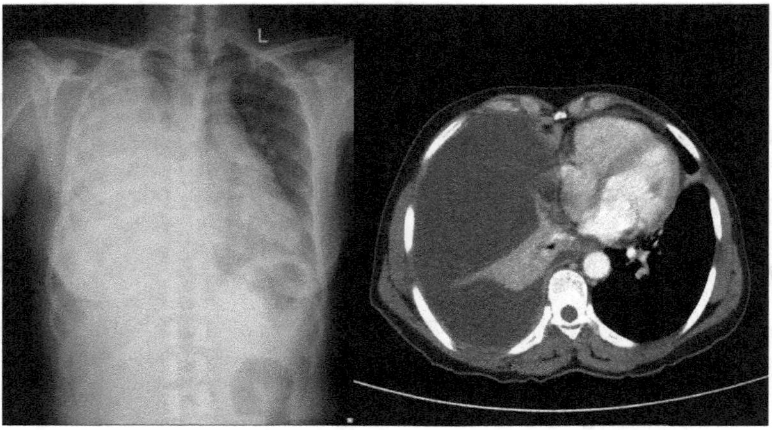

Figure 4: Massive pleural effusion TB.

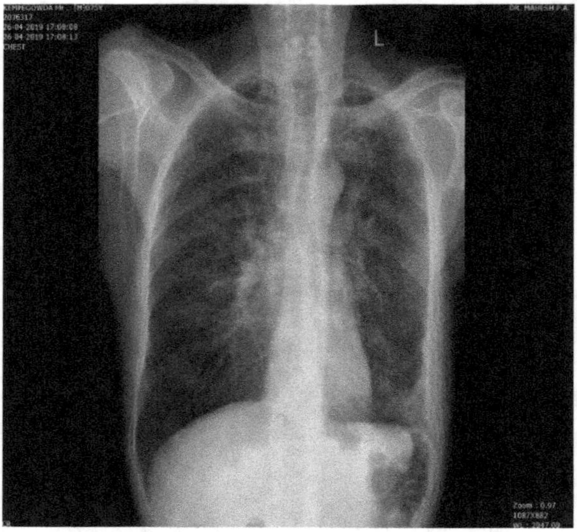

Figure 5: Left pleural calcification.

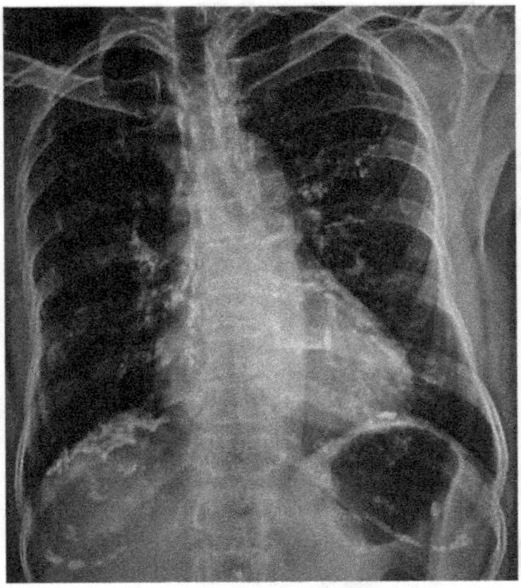

Figure 6: Pleural and pulmonary calcification — improperly drained PLEF overexposed film, no nipple shadow.

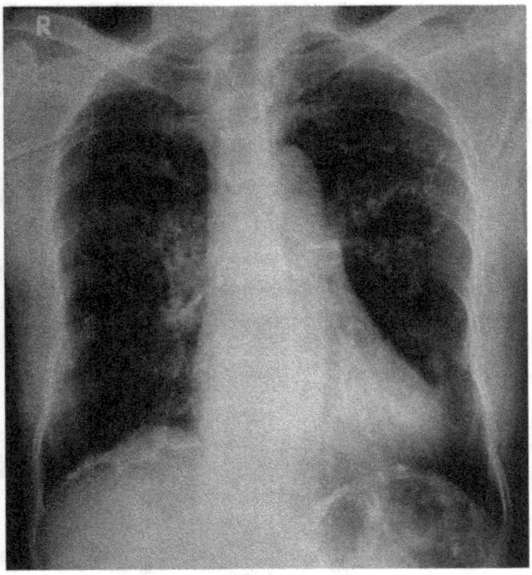

Figure 7: Pleural and pulmonary calcification — normal exposure, nipple shadow left, not a nodule.

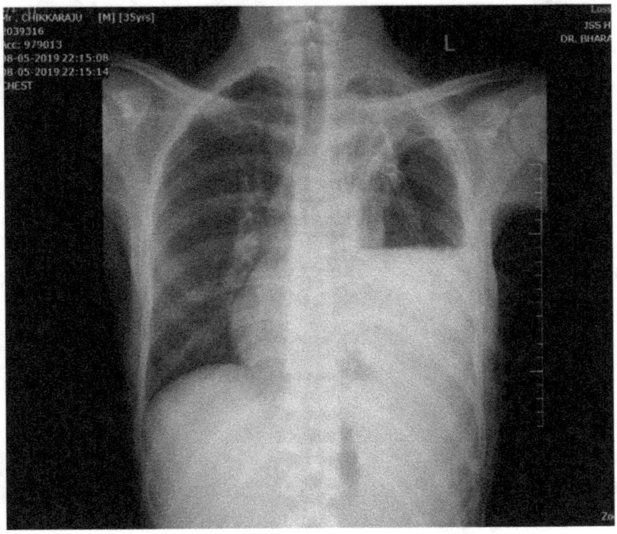

Figure 8: Tension pyopneumothorax.

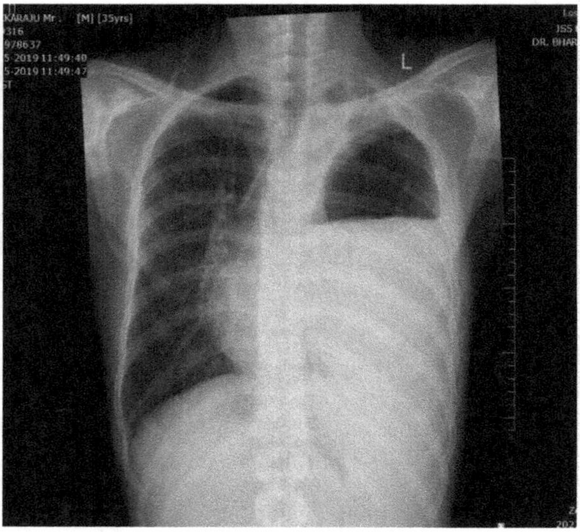

Figure 9: Tension pyopneumothorax with ICD TB.

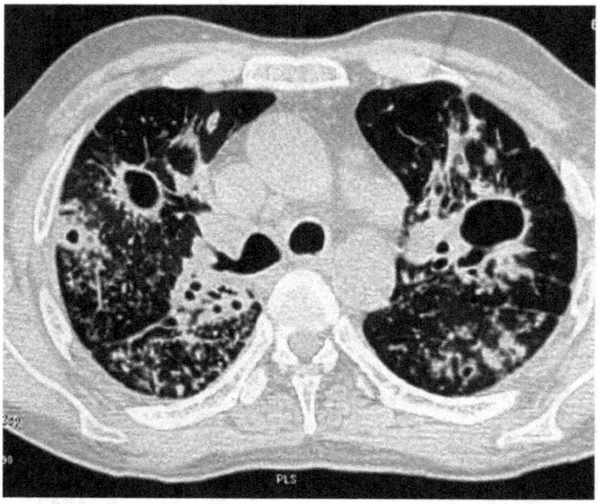

Figure 10: Bilateral extensive sputum-positive cavitary TB.

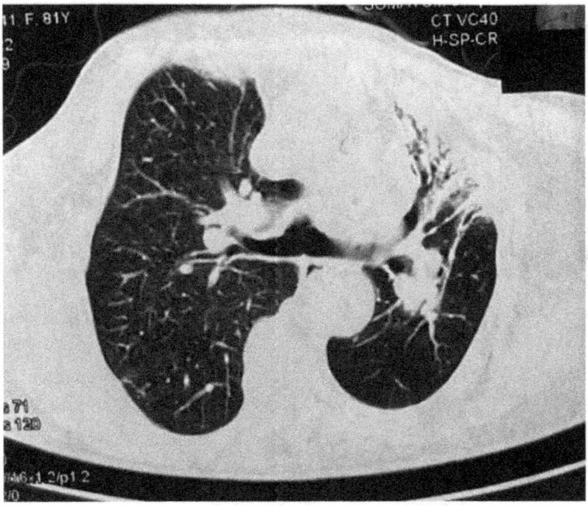

Figure 11: Lingular pneumonia TB.

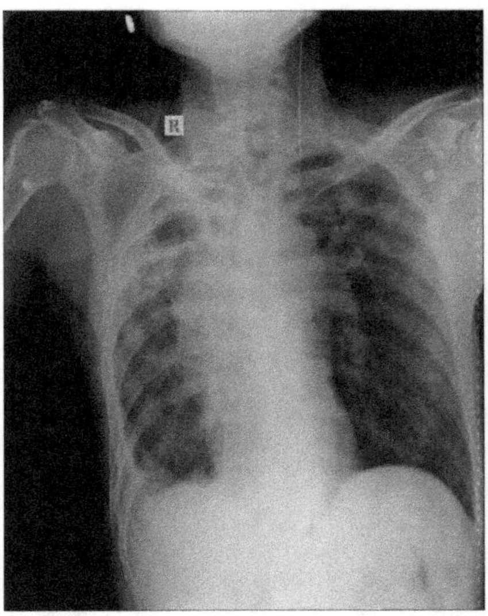

Figure 12: Lobectomy for massive hemoptysis.

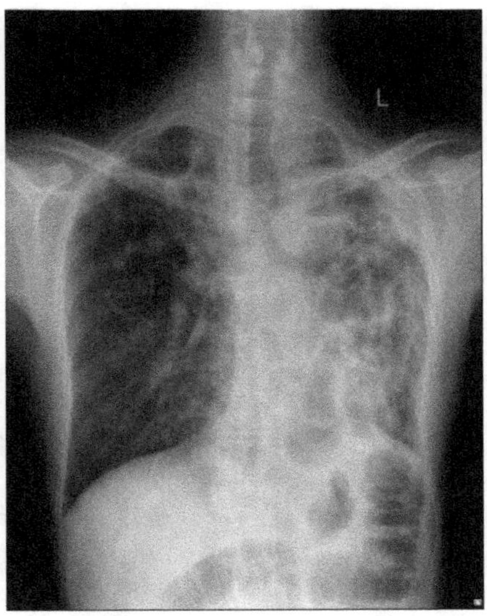

Figure 13: Partially destroyed lung left post-TB.

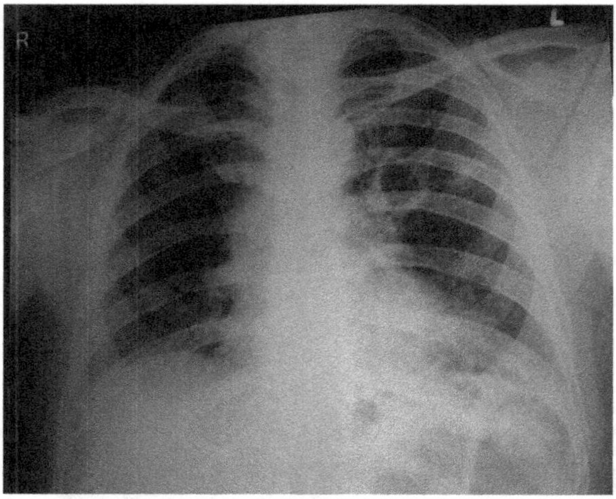

Figure 14: Sputum-positive cavitary lesion left upper lobe and infiltrates left lower lobe.

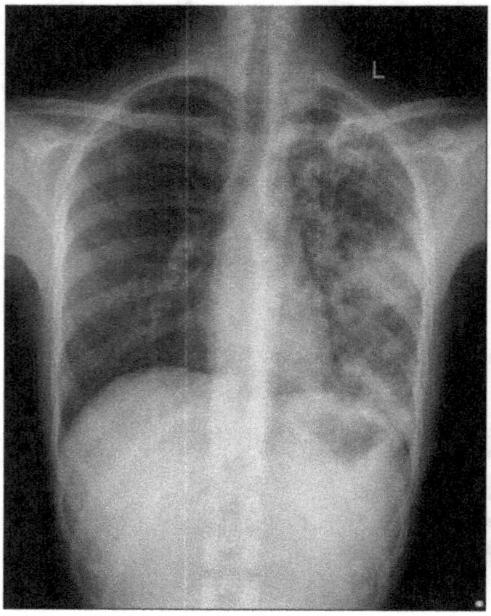

Figure 15: Sputum-positive PTB cavity with fluid level.

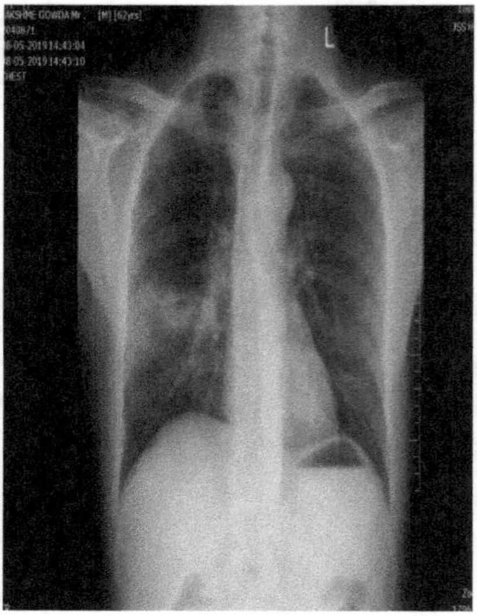

Figure 16: Sputum-positive PTB cavity without fluid level.

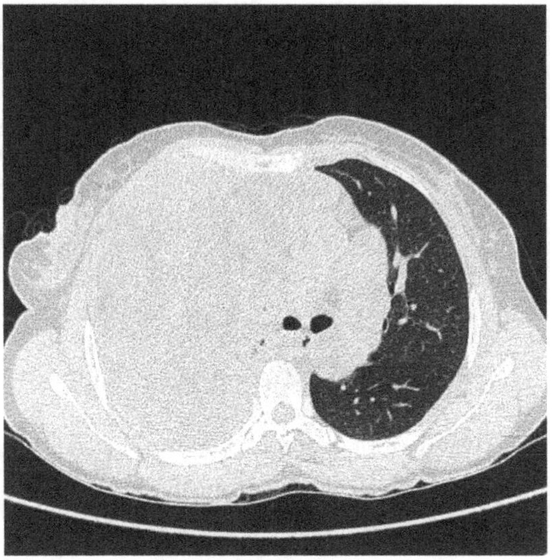

Figure 17: Pleural effusion massive lung window.

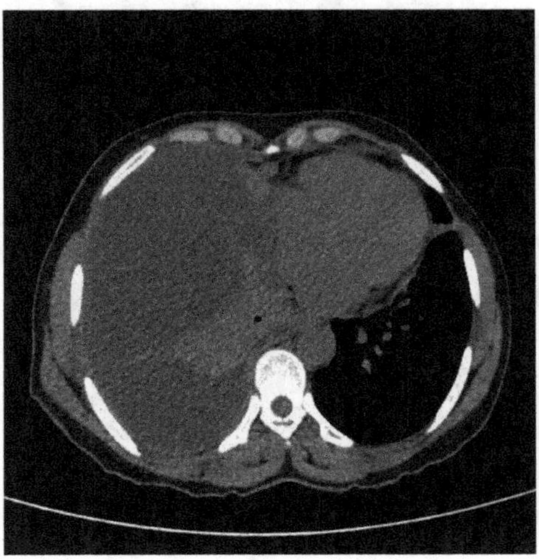

Figure 18: Pleural effusion massive mediastinal window.

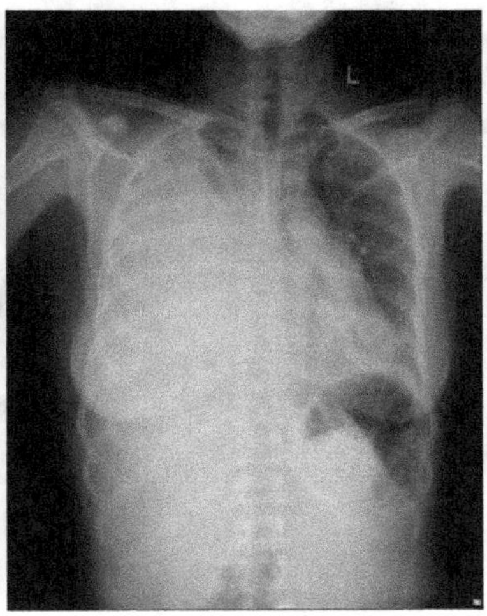

Figure 19: Pleural effusion — plain CT massive tubercular.

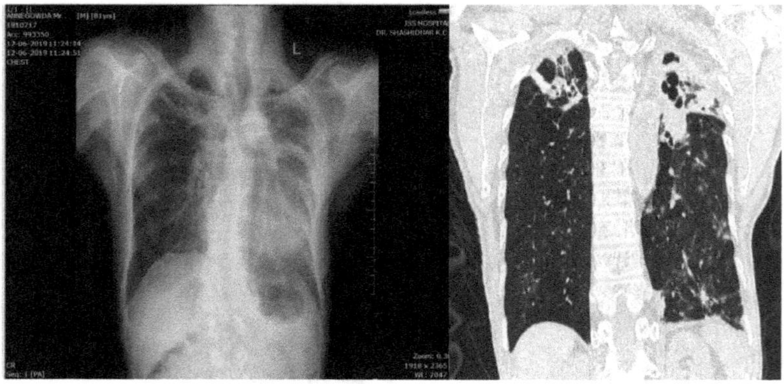

Figure 20: X-ray and CT scans of post-TB sequelae (bilateral upper lobe fibrosis, nodules in the left upper lobe, and tenting of the left hemidiaphragm).

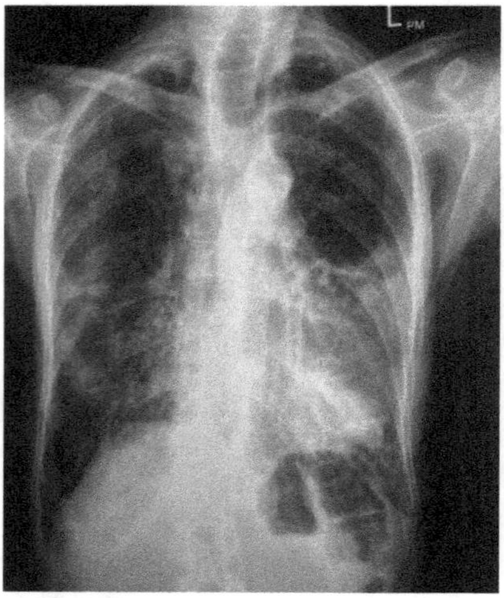

Figure 21: Post-TB sequelae.

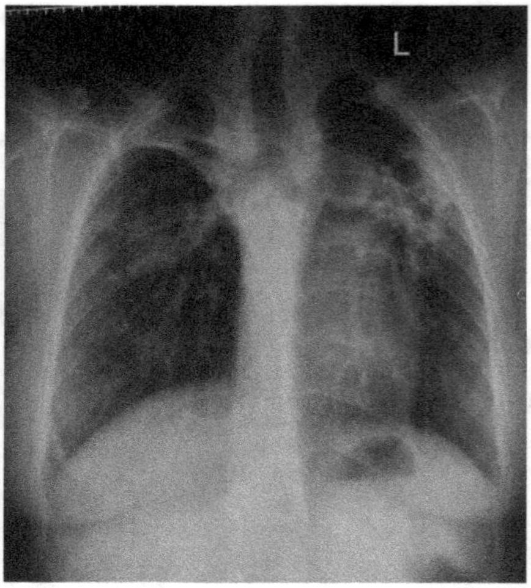

Figure 22: Post-TB sequelae with persistent cavity left upper lobe.

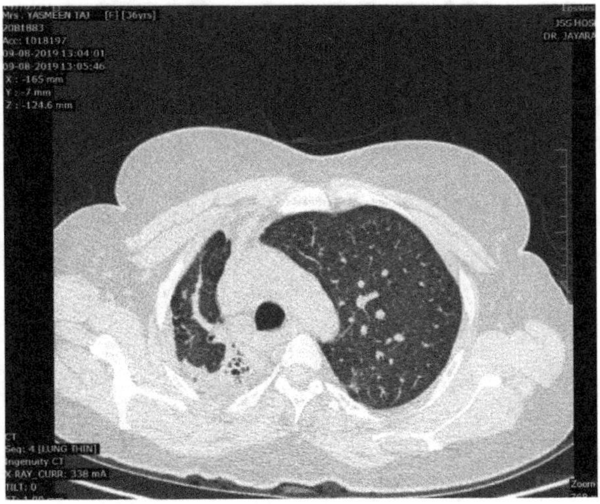

Figure 23: Loss of lung volume lung herniation.

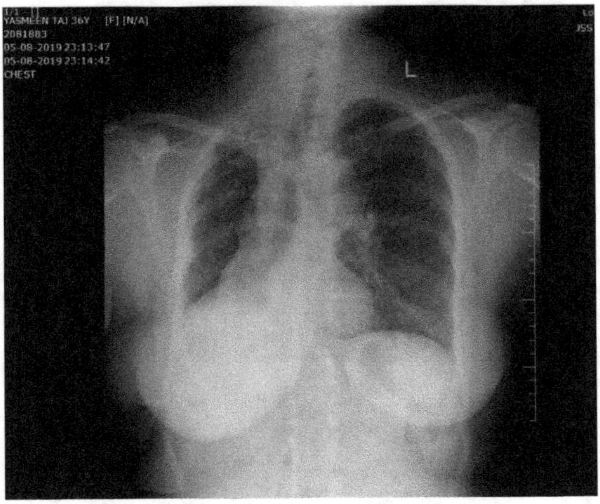

Figure 24: Loss of lung volume right left lung herniation right.

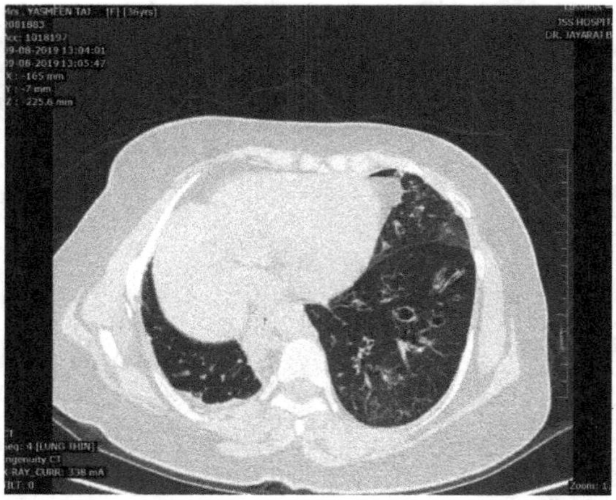

Figure 25: Loss of lung volume post-TB — bronchiectasis left lung.

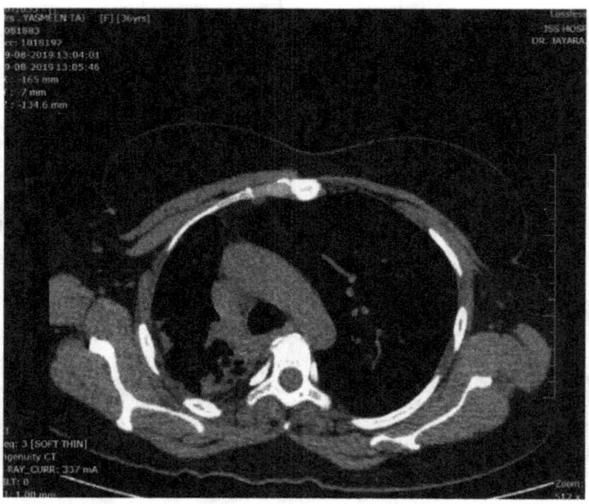

Figure 26: Post-TB sequelae loss of lung volume right.

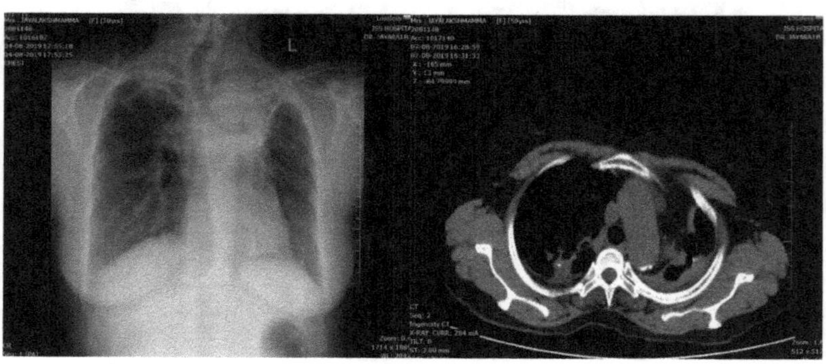

Figure 27: X-ray and CT scans of post-TB sequelae bilateral upper lobe.

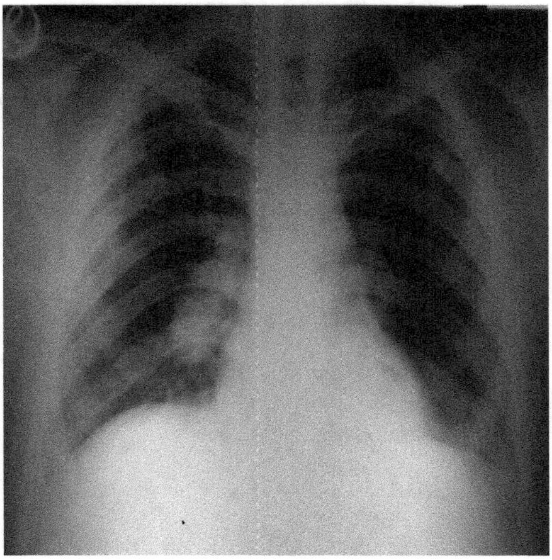

Figure 28: Hilar lymph node TB.

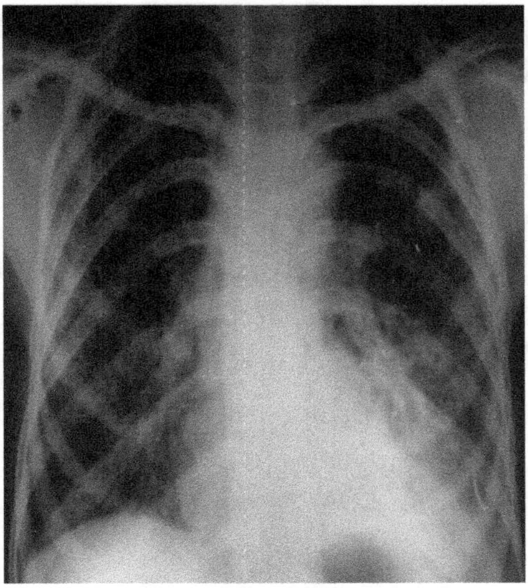

Figure 29: Miliary TB.

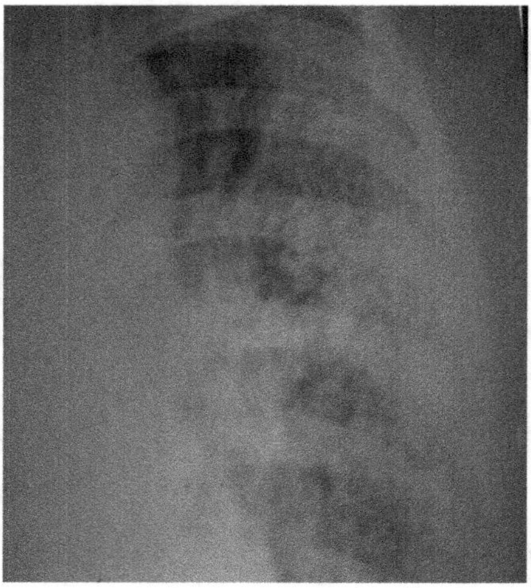

Figure 30: Miliary post-TB.

Chest wall TB

Rib erosion along with localized swelling on the chest wall makes one suspect TB of chest wall. Soft tissue mass in the chest wall with or without bony destruction is the radiographic finding of rib TB. Juxtacostal soft tissue mass with central low attenuation and peripheral rim enhancement seen are CT findings of rib TB. Bony destruction, osteolytic expansile lesions with cortical disruption, or mild cortical irregularity may be associated. In addition, soft tissue mass with calcification and rim enhancement of soft tissue mass following intravenous contrast medium administration can be demonstrated on CT. Magnetic resonance imaging (MRI) is occasionally helpful in evaluating the complications of TB.

Pleural TB

Pleural effusion is present in about 10% of all new TB infections. The frequency is higher in adult patients with AIDS.[1] Tubercular pleural effusion on plain radiograph appears either as free fluid along the chest wall or loculated in lateral or mediastinal pleura. Sometimes nodularity can be appreciated on a pleural surface on the radiograph.[2] In early tuberculous effusion, ultrasonography may show simple anechoic pleural fluid.[57] In acute tuberculous effusion, CT scan may show parenchymal cavitation, including small subpleural cavity, the site of communication between the cavity and the pleural space, parenchymal infiltrates, and hilar adenopathy as well as fluid collection in the pleural cavity. This regular pleural thickening can be shown on CT scans.

In chronic tuberculous empyema, CT scan shows focal fluid collection in association with pleural thickening and calcification. In these cases, the presence of residual pleural fluid signifies active infection.[3] Contrast-enhanced CT scans demonstrate emphysema with the enhancement of the parietal and visceral pleurae. The enhancing septa are seen within the pleural fluid collections. The pleural fluid collections are characterized by low attenuation. The so-called split pleura sign, consisting of the pleural fluid collection tracking between the abnormally enhancing parietal and visceral pleura, is observed in empyema.

Primary TB

Primary TB radiologically usually appears as lobar pneumonia along with recognizable enlarged lymph nodes in the hilum or the mediastinum.[4] The consolidation is usually homogeneous, dense, and well-defined. In patients who are immunocompromised, diabetics, or on corticosteroids, lobar or segmental pneumonia breaks down into a cavity. Primary TB appears as a solitary cavity lesion in about 10% of patients.[4]

Postprimary TB

Postprimary TB radiologically appears with local exudative lesions, local fibronodular lesions, cavitation, and bronchogenic involvement. Approximately 40% of adults with TB have some form of cavitation, usually in combination with pulmonary infiltration. High-resolution CT (HRCT) findings of active pulmonary TB are centrilobular lesions appearing as a nodule or branching linear structure (95%), bronchial wall thickening (73%), tree-in-bud appearance (71%), poorly defined nodule (61%), cavity (51%), and lobular consolidation (41%).[5]

In postprimary TB, the pattern, distribution, and extension of parenchymal lesions can be accurately demonstrated by CT. Cavities, the most important radiological evidence of activity, can be also well depicted on CT. The nature of pulmonary damage, including bronchiectasis, cicatrization, atelectasis, and scarring, can be characterized, even when extensive disease makes radiological interpretation difficult.

Tuberculoma

Primary TB in adults may appear as solitary or multiple macronodular lesions (tuberculomas). Postprimary TB also presents large nodular masses or densities that are considered neoplastic. On CT scan, these are usually regular and smooth but may have a rough edge. Cavitation in the lesion or surrounding satellite nodule(s), sometimes differentiates from lung cancer on CT scans. Calcification is found in 20%–30% of the lesions and is usually nodular and diffuse.[6] Rarely tuberculoma appears with CT-halo sign (halo of round-glass attenuation surrounding the nodule in a patient with hemoptysis).

Miliary TB

In the early stage of miliary TB, chest radiograph may be normal. Follow-up usually shows a poorly defined haze through both lungs. Typical nodules of 1–2 mm become recognizable even as late as 2–3 months. As the infection progresses, the miliary nodules coalesce. Cavitation may occasionally occur in the nodules.

HRCT scans show well-defined, marginated nodules of 1–2 mm in size widely disseminated throughout the lungs in association with diffuse reticulation. Other features signifying nodular presence include nodular interlobular septae, nodular irregularity of vessels, subpleural dots, and studded fissures. Diffuse intra- and interlobular septal thickening is not uncommon.[7]

Airway TB

Usually, airway TB radiologically presents with persistent infiltration, atelectasis, cavitating lesion as mass-like lesion or rarely miliary mottling. CT scans of the involved bronchi demonstrate stenosis with wall thickening, obstruction with peribronchial cuff of soft tissue, stenosis, or obstruction with adjacent tuberculous lymphadenitis or intraluminal polypoid mass of low attenuation with bronchial narrowing.[8]

Bronchiectasis is commonly seen in the upper lobes, often manifesting as traction bronchiectasis on the basis of fibrotic disease with subsequent traction on the airways. Minimal and uniform thickening of the bronchial wall in tuberculous bronchitis may mimic radiologically an early bronchogenic carcinoma. The presence of enlarged lymph nodes lying close to the stenotic bronchus with low attenuation, on enhanced CT scans, when combined with peripheral parenchymal atelectasis or consolidation, may simulate the findings of lung cancer. Bronchoscopy can differentiate and confirm the diagnosis.

Mediastinal TB

Tuberculous lymphadenitis often accompanying a pulmonary lesion (the primary compel) is a frequent manifestation of primary TB in children. The lesion is also seen in adults. On enhanced CT scans, nodes larger than 2 cm in diameter invariably show central areas of low attenuation and peripheral rim enhancement. Enhanced walls are usually irregular in thickness. In few patients, solid or calcified type of nodes can be seen. On MRI, tuberculous lymphadenitis with central areas of low attenuation and peripheral rim enhancement at CT scans show homogeneous nodes with hyperintensity both on T1- and T2-weighted images. The lymphadenitis with solid type at CT scans similarly show homogeneous nodes with hyperintensity on both T1 and T2 weighted images but with less marked T2 prolongation than that with central areas of low attenuation and peripheral rim enhancement. The presence of calcification along with lymphadenitis shows inhomogeneous nodes with hypointensity both on T1 and T2-weighted images.[9]

Pericardial TB

Calcification related to prior tuberculous pericarditis is more readily apparent on CT images.[10,11]

Ultrasonography may be used for thoracentesis guidance or to evaluate the pericardium for secondary tuberculous involvement, especially as a bedside non-invasive modality.

Comments

Chest X-ray is considered very important from patient's point of view for the diagnosis of TB, but TB is never diagnosed only with a solitary radiological picture of the chest by the physician since no radiographic pattern is pathognomonic of TB, although the classical hallmarks of the disease are cavitation, apical distribution, pulmonary fibrosis, shrinkage, and calcification. Human immunodeficiency virus–infected persons with a well preserved immunity will show these typical features. However, with immune suppression, chest X-ray more often shows typical findings such as pulmonary infiltrates affecting the lower lobes, intrathoracic lymphadenopathy, miliary TB, and rarely a normal chest radiograph.[12,13]

Diseases other than TB can cause both classical and atypical chest X-ray findings, and if sputum smears are negative, differential diagnosis becomes difficult, requiring other investigations.

CT is a very useful mode of examination for the visualization of the features of pulmonary changes and localized lesions in pulmonary TB. Interventional radiology may be the choice procedure in inoperable cases of massive hemoptysis in TB by bronchial artery embolization.[14] MRI is of less importance; it possibly plays a role in the examination of the mediastinal lesions. Ultrasonic examination is another simple non-invasive bedside investigation, which is useful for very sick patients.

Nuclear medicine has no diagnostic value in TB.

References and suggested readings

1. Tanaka A, Komiya K, Yamasue M, Ando Y, Takeno Y, Takikawa S, Hiramatsu K, Kadota JI. Quantitative assessment of the association between erector spinae muscle and in-hospital mortality in elderly patients with pulmonary tuberculosis. BMC Res Notes. 2021 Apr 13;14(1):134. doi: 10.1186/s13104-021-05546-3. PMID: 33849637; PMCID: PMC8042463.
2. Akhan O, Demirkazik FB, Ozmen MN, et al. Tuberculous pleural effusion: ultrasonic diagnosis. Clin Ultrasound. 1992;20:461–465.
3. Hulnick DH, Niaidch DP, McCauley DI. Pleural tuberculosis evaluated by computed tomography. Radiology. 1983;149:759–765.
4. Afessa B. Pleural effusions and pneumothoraces in AIDS. Curr Opin Pulm Med. 2001;7:20.
5. Im J-G, Roll H. Shim Y-S, et al. Pulmonary tuberculosis: CT findings-early active disease and sequential change with antituberculous therapy. Radiology. 1993;186:653–660.
6. Lee S, Kim HT, Cho WS, Kin PN, Bae WK, Kim W. Active solitary tuberculoma of the lung: CT and clinical findings. J Kor Rad Soc. 1993;29:1200–1207 (Korean).
7. McGuiness G, Naidich DP, Jagirdari J, Leitmen B, McCauley DI. High resolution CT finding in miliary lung disease. J Comput Assist Tomogr. 1992;16:384–390.
8. Lee KS, Kim YH, Kim WS, Hwang SH, Kim PN, Lee BH. Endobronchial tuberculosis: CT features. J Comput Assist Tomogr. 1991;15:414–428.
9. Moon WK, Im J-G, Han MC. CT and MR imaging of mediastinal tuberculous lymphadenitis. Radiology. 1993;189:437.
10. Prakash SC. Calcified constrictive pericarditis. Curr Med Trends. 2005;9:1783–1786.
11. Bhatia RS. TB of serous membranes. IN: RS Bhatia, ed. Tuberculosis. Pee Pee Publ. 2007;7:47–51.
12. Bhatia RS. TB and AIDS. JAPI. 2000;48:613–616.
13. Bhatia RS. Pulmonary opportunistic infections in AIDS. Med Update. 1997;7:1088–1090.
14. Mahalakshmi H, et al. Bronchial artery embolisation to control massive haemoptysis in tuberculosis. Lung India. 2000;18:27–28.

15. Lee G, Im J-G, Kim JS, Kang HS, Han MC. Tuberculosis of the ribs: CT appearance. J Comput Assist Tomogr. 1993;17:363–366.
16. Bhattacharya A. Pleural effusions in AIDS. Lung India. 2005;22:101–110.
17. Mathur RB, et al. Ultrasonic evaluating of pleural opacities. Ind J Chest Dr Allied Sci. 1994;36:21–25.
18. Narang P, Bhargava SK. Ultrasonic features of tuberculous pleural effusion. Ind J Radiol Imaging. 1993;2:217–220.
19. Singh S, et al. Role of sonography in diagnosis of pleural and lung diseases. Lung India. 2005;22:97–98.
20. Huang C, Huang L, Wang Y, Li X, Ren L, Gu X, Kang L, Guo L, Liu M, Zhou X, Luo J, Huang Z, Tu S, Zhao Y, Chen L, Xu D, Li Y, Li C, Peng L, Li Y, Xie W, Cui D, Shang L, Fan G, Xu J, Wang G, Wang Y, Zhong J, Wang C, Wang J, Zhang D, Cao B. 6-Month consequences of COVID-19 in patients discharged from hospital: a cohort study. Lancet. 2021 Jan 16;397(10270):220–232. doi: 10.1016/S0140-6736(20)32656-8. Epub 2021 Jan 8. PMID: 33428867; PMCID: PMC7833295.
21. Cao XF, Li Y, Xin HN, Zhang HR, Pai M, Gao L. Application of artificial intelligence in digital chest radiography reading for pulmonary tuberculosis screening. Chronic Dis Transl Med. 2021 Mar 3;7(1):35–40. doi: 10.1016/j.cdtm.2021.02.001. PMID: 34013178; PMCID: PMC8110935.
22. Le Roux CE, Vlok SSC. The silent pandemic in South Africa: extra-pulmonary tuberculosis from head to heel. SA J Radiol. 2021 Apr 16;25(1):2026. doi: 10.4102/sajr.v25i1.2026. PMID: 33936795; PMCID: PMC8063767.
23. Nagu TJ, Mboka MA, Nkrumbih ZF, Shayo G, Mizinduko MM, Komba EV, Maeurer M, Zumla A, Mugusi F. Clinical and imaging features of adults with recurrent pulmonary tuberculosis — a prospective case-controlled study. Int J Infect Dis. 2021 Dec;113(Suppl 1):S33–S39. doi: 10.1016/j.ijid.2021.01.071. Epub 2021 Mar 11. PMID: 33716197.

https://doi.org/10.1142/9789811271410_0022

22 Extrapulmonary tuberculosis

Summary: Diagnosis of non-pulmonary tuberculosis (NIP) is important, and any delay would have diverse consequences leading to fatality. It assumes further importance as being commonest infection in human immunodeficiency virus (HIV) patients. Four-drug medical regimen is effective, obviating the need for surgery in the majority of cases. The outcome is favorable if diagnosed early and short-course regular chemotherapy is instituted. The duration of chemotherapy should be 12 months in case of joint and brain tuberculosis (TB).

Introduction: The incidence of NIP (other than lungs) in India is 10%–15% of all forms of TB; higher incidence is expected due to the rising trend of HIV disease and here TB is the most common opportunistic infection. Organs such as lymph nodes, kidneys, meninges, growing ends of bones, and the spine which have higher vascularity are mostly involved. In the absence of classical clinical presentation, noncontributory chest X-ray and sputum analysis reports, insignificant contributory utility of Mantoux test in patients aged 3 years or so, and variable specificity and sensitivity of immunological tests, the diagnosis of NIP becomes difficult many a times. A Mantoux test may be negative for malnutrition, severe anemia, immunosuppression, acquired immunodeficiency syndrome (AIDS), sarcoidosis, and Hodgkin's disease. Treatment with short-course chemotherapy remains the mainstay of management; an equal efficacy of intermittent regimen has also been documented. To achieve a nearly 99% of cure rate, the duration can be increased up to 12 months, especially in the case of joint and brain TB. Excellent patient compliance yields a total cure and helps in the prevention of MDR-TB.

Common sites	Uncommon sites
1. Serous membranes ❖ Pleura ❖ Peritoneum	1. Serous membranes ❖ Pericardium
2. Gastrointestinal system ❖ Duodenum ❖ Esophagus ❖ Liver ❖ Colon and rectum	2. Gastrointestinal system ❖ Spleen ❖ Pancreas
3. Central nervous system ❖ Brain ❖ Meninges	3. Breast
4. Urogenital tract	4. Kidney
5. Endometrium	5. Thyroid glands
	6. Bone marrow
	7. Tongue
	8. Kidney
	9. Eye
	10. Sino nasal
	11. Parotid gland

TB of serous membranes

Introduction

Serosal involvement in TB is not uncommon. Fluid collection is quite commonly seen in routine practice, and the number of cases involved is increasing because of the increasing number of HIV coexisting with TB. Drug management with the present-day anti-TB chemotherapy is sufficient to treat these cases. Surgery is rarely indicated when complicated.

Tuberculous pleural effusion

Pleural affection and effusion in TB are the most common afflictions in high TB prevalence regions. Incidence is increased with coexisting HIV disease.[1,2] Pleural involvement may occur as a part of primary TB in children, and young adults with pyrexia and pleurisy or as a part of disseminated TB in AIDS patients. The coexistence of lung cancer with a malignant and tuberculous pleural effusion can also rarely occur. The immunosuppression and defective cell-mediated immunity (due to age, poor nutrition, alcohol intake of almost, lung neoplasm) may reactivate endogenous TB or predispose it to exogenous reinfection. The malignant parenchymal extension to pleura might erode the subpleural focus of mycobacteria into pleural space, setting the chain of events leading to the development of tuberculous pleural effusion.[3]

Pathogenesis of pleural effusion involves a delayed type of hypersensitivity, which occurs due to the release of tuberculous protein into the pleural space following the rupture of subpleural caseous focus into the pleural space. Local inflammatory reaction occurs because of the release of cytokines such as interleukin (IL)-2, 11.1, tumor necrosis factor α (TNF-α), IL-6, IL-10, IL-11, IL-12, and interferon-γ (IFN-γ) by the activated lymphocytes and macrophages. Lymphocytes in the pleural fluid are in a ratio of CDA4:CD8::3:4. Pleural fluid culture for *Mycobacterium tuberculosis* is most of the time noncontributory (negative). PPD skin test may be negative in one-third of the cases, possibly due to the circulating adherent cell, which suppresses the specifically sensitized circulatory T lymphocytes in the peripheral blood, or due to the sequestration of PPD reaction T lymphocytes in the pleural space.

Clinical manifestations include fever, chest pain, and nonproductive cough in almost three-fourths of the cases, and these patients, generally one-third, reach the family physician within a week's time. Those with chronic infection, generally two-thirds of cases, present with malaise, dyspnea, and weight loss within a month's period. Rarely, patients may present in a critically sick situation with polyserositis, afflicting multiple serosal involvement. TB pleural effusion is generally unilateral and is of a moderate degree. In primary TB, effusion may be present without any evidence of lung parenchymal disease, while lung parenchyma may be accompanying the effusion in postprimary (reactivation) TB.[1]

Negative TB test initially in one-third of cases generally becomes positive after 6–8 weeks. Therefore, a negative test does not rule out tuberculous pleuritis. Plain X-ray chest may show tubercular parenchymal infiltration accompanying pleural effusion in one-third of cases. Aspirated fluid is never bloody, mostly serosanguinous, testing proteins >5 g/dL, and glucose <60 mg/dL. Cellular analysis may show polymorphs in the early phase (with 7–10 days) but later on, predominantly small lymphocytes are seen. Eosinophils rarely exceed 10% and mesothelial cells are rare, and if more than 5%, this disfavors the diagnosis of TB. ADA levels of >70 IU/L have 98% and 96% of sensitivity and specificity, respectively. However, ADA levels may go down to <40 IU/L in immunocompromised patients. Pleural fluid interferon level >200 pg/mL favors the diagnosis of TB. Sensitivity and specificity of 81% and 78%, respectively, using polymerase chain reaction (PCR) is diagnosing TB etiology. Demonstration of *M. tuberculosis* in the fluid from pleural cavity is possible in less than 10% of cases. Three different pleural biopsy specimens may increase the diagnostic yield from 60% to 100%.[4] The presence of granuloma in parietal pleura, without the demonstration of caseous necrosis and acid fast bacilli (AFB), is suggestive of diagnosis although granuloma may be present in other diseases, such as fungal, RA, and tularemia. The use of lysozyme, IFN-γ, and immunodiagnostic studies (enzyme-linked immunosorbent assay [ELISA]) help in differentiating tuberculous from nontuberculous pleural fluids. Short-course anti-TB treatment is sufficient to treat these patients. Corticosteroids are only indicated for acute symptoms and should be rapidly tapered off as soon as the patient responds.

Therapeutic thoracentesis has not been indicated, and decortication is only considered when there is empyema; extrapleural pneumonectomy and thoracoplasty are also recommended. Complete resolution occurs otherwise, with a short course of ATT given for a complete duration.[5]

Tubercular peritonitis

Peritoneal involvement in TB can occur secondary to abdominal TB, but it is more commonly affected by hematogenous spread from foci in the lungs. The most common variety is exudative peritonitis leading to ascites, and other varieties include encysted or loculated type, fibrous or plastic type, and rarely the purulent type of TB peritonitis.[6]

The onset is insidious in almost three-fourths of cases, taking 3–4 months, presenting with fever, anorexia, weight loss, abdominal pain, and a mass in fibroadhesive variety. Abdominal examination gives a tender and doughy feel.[7] Shifting dullness in ascites is present except when the fluid is loculated. Ascitic fluid tap may demonstrate total proteins >3.0 g/dL. SAAG is <1.1. Lymphocytes and AFB are rarely demonstrable, and fluid culture is positive for AFB in <20% of cases. ADA is highly specific for tuberculous ascites. Mantoux test is usually positive. Computed tomography (CT) abdomen may reveal local pathology of thickened blood, lymphadenopathy, and genital affection in females, and CT-guided biopsy of the lesion may reveal caseating granuloma in >90% of cases. Chest X-ray may be positive for tuberculous pathology in case of hemotogenous spread from foci in the lungs.[1] Short-course antituberculous treatment is effective.

Tuberculous pericarditis

A rising trend from 0.4% to the highest trend of 11% in acute pericarditis has been observed in tuberculous pericarditis in the last five decades all over the world, the effect may be due to the resurgence of tuberculosis due to AIDS in the past two decades. Indian tuberculous pericarditis has been reported to have a prevalance rate of 3.3% in cases of chronic pericardial effusions. Tuberculous pericarditis occurs in 1%–2% of cases of pulmonary TB. Disease mostly spreads from local tracheobronchial, mediastinal, or hilar nodal lesions; hematogenous spread from lungs and other organs can also occur. Initial deposit of pericardial fibrin is associated with serosanguinous or even blood-stained effusion that occurs because of the hypersensitive reaction to tubercular protein. In the subacute stage, granulomatous pericardial inflammation is followed by the infiltration of epithelioid histiocytes and Langhans giant cells with caseating necrosis. In the chronic (adhesive) phase, there is pericardial (both visceral and parietal) thickening with fibroblastic proliferation, which assumes a pattern of effusion constrictive pericarditis if there is a persistent effusion. In the later stage, obliteration of the pericardial cavity without effusion may occur, eventually with pericardial calcification in developing frank constrictive pericarditis. Involvement of myocardium by *Mycobacterium* (as myocarditis) and developing cardiac tamponade are future-associated complications.

Clinical presentation with a typical slow onset and accidental finding of large pericardial effusion is not uncommon, mostly seen in third to fifth decades of life. Children and immunocompromised persons may present with acute pericarditis, cough, dyspnea, fever, weight loss, chest pain, ankle edema (especially in cardiac tamponade or constrictive pericarditis resulting in raised systemic venous pressure), and pain in right upper quadrant due to hepatic congestion. Clinically silent disease with ascites and hepatic congestion may mimic cirrhosis (Pick's disease). Eight different syndromes have been described, such as acute painful pericarditis, silent large effusion, cardiac tamponade, acute pericardial constriction, subacute constriction, chronic constriction, pericardial calcification, and undiagnosed pyrexia with weight loss and malaise. Pericardial pain and rub are seen in few patients. Exertional dyspnea may be present in a patient with large effusion or associated pleural effusion (polyserosal affection). Symptoms of cardiac tamponade or constrictive pericarditis are similar to those caused by other diseases. The patient is febrile, has tachycardia, hepatomegaly, and cardiomegaly, with pulsus paradoxus. A respiratory swelling of the neck veins (Kussmaul's sign) may be seen in patients with constrictive pericarditis. A pericardial knock can also be heard. Raised jugular venous pressure, pulsus paradoxus, and hypotension are present in a patient with cardiac tamponade, which is attended as a medical emergency.[1]

Chest X-ray reveals pulmonary infiltrates in one-third to three-fourths of patients. Pericardial or effusive constrictive pericarditis is seen in almost 95% of cases as an enlarged cardiac silhouette. Accompanying pleural effusion may be present in three-fourths of cases. Pericardial calcification, though very rare, always points towards tubercular etiology. Electrocardiogram shows low-voltage tracings. Electrical alternans may suggest cardiac tamponade. Atrial fibrillation may occasionally be present. Pericardial fluid is serosanguinous or thickly bloody and has high protein content and increased leukocyte contents, mainly lymphocytes. However, polymorphs may predgmiriatelh early phase (first 1–2 weeks). AFB smear positivity is up to 40%, culture positivity is up to 60%, and guinea pig inoculation may yield 80% APB positivity. Echocardiogram is noncontributory, and CT scan and magnetic resonance imaging (MRI) give information about effusion and thickening of the pericardium. PPD skin test is positive in 75%–100% of cases; a negative PPD skin test is observed in 60% of cases with AIDS.[8] False positivity of test is seen in one-third of cases of idiopathic pericarditis, whereas false negative test is observed in one-fourth of cases of TB pericarditis. The value of adenosine deaminase activity of >45 IU/L has been 100% sensitive and 97% specific for tuberculous pleural fluid and has not been found applicable to tuberculous pericardial fluid.

Anti-Koch's treatment with four drugs regimen is sufficient to treat tuberculous pericarditis; corticosteroids when added, reduce the mortality and the need for pericardiocentesis but do not lessen the need for operation for constrictive pericarditis. Pericardiectomy is recommended only in selected cases of tuberculous pericarditis.

A. **Tubercular lymphadenitis**: This is the commonest type of TB, mainly affecting the cervical region.

Younger age group, immunostatus, race (more in blacks, and female sex (female>male, 2:1) are considered risk factors. Regional nodes are involved from the primary focus, followed by spread via lymphatic to other lymph nodes and hematogenous spread occurs if not contained.

M. tuberculosis is the commonest infection in India, followed by *Mycobacterium bovis* and African and non-TB mycobacteria such as MAC and *Mycobacterium scrofulaceum* should be suspected in HIV disease.

Necrotizing granulomatous lymph node biopsy, patient mostly a young girl not responding to ATT should be suspected of Kikuchi disease.

Clinically patients present with no specific symptoms and a painless swelling, generally of multiple matted nodes of variable consistency, with or without discharging sinus or scar. Generalized lymphadenopathy, dysphagia, abnormal pain, and jaundice may rarely be seen. FNAC is a simple and safe method for easy and early diagnosis. Histology reveals epitheloid cells, modified histiocytes, and Langhans giant cells surrounded by dense infiltrate of lymphocytes, with or without the presence of caseation. CT scan of the chest and abdomen may rarely be required to distinguish between *M. tuberculosis* and MAC where local visceral lesions with low attenuation in lymph node favors *M. tuberculosis*, and accompanying hepatosplenomegaly with enlarged soft dense (density > muscle) nodes are suggestive of MAC infection.

B. TB of bones and joints: It is common in old age; children and young people are also more affected, the incidence being 30%. Involvement of skeletal tissue may accompany 3% of patients. Single joint is involved, usually secondary to primary lung lesion or ountagious nodes. Usually, constitutional symptoms are favored for localizing signs depending on the site of involvement. Histopathologically, two types of microscopic lesions are seen, one with predominant necrosis and cold abscess called caseating exudation type 4 and another with predominant proliferation with minimal or no caseation called proliferative type, the extreme form involving the shoulder as tuberculous granuloma called caries sicca.

B1. TB of spine: Because of the excessive weight bearing at thoraco lumbar level, the spine is involved at the paradise region, central body, anterior type, appendiceal lesion, or articular region. TB spine, also called Pott's spine, affects 50%–65% of the total incidence of skeletal TB. The destruction of intervertebral disc and adjacent vertebral body leads to the collapse and obliteration of intervertebral space, leading to angular kyphosis called gibbus. Cold abscess is formed owing to spreading caseation and osteolysis. Clinically, a patient presents with localized or referred pain and rigidity due to paraspinal muscle spasm. Gibbus may show density in the thoracic area and a cold abscess in the paravertebral region. In 10% of patients, paraplegia may occur, especially when the disease is in active stage: late-onset paraplegia is due to deformity or sequelae. Rarely, a gradual onset type of paraplegia, due to ingrown granulation tissue pressing the spinal cord may occur as spinal cord tumor syndrome. Narrowing of intervertebral space due to erosion is the earlier radiological sign followed by obliteration of intervertebral spine due to destruction and collapse. CT spine may show caries spine and associated paravertebral cold abscess. Even cervical spine involvement from retropharyngeal tubercular abscess has been documented. Anti-Koch's chemotherapy from 9 to 12 months is effective and rarely requires surgery when signs of recovery on chemotherapy are insignificant or paraplegia is worsening or spastic paraplegia is appearing.

Hip joint involvement is another important affection found mostly in 5–15 years of age groups. Joint may be kept flexed, abducted, and externally rotated in case there is exudation in the joint cavity or the next stage of adduction, flexion, and internal rotation and if not treated, the destroyed joint ends up with real shortening of the limb. Cold abscess sinus may appear, pouring out pus. Plain X-ray may show a widening of joint space due to effusion or narrowing of joint space due to erosion of articular surface or destroyed femur with dislocated acetabulum called traveling acetabulum. Short-course chemotherapy with complete rest for a minimum of 3 months, followed by supported weight bearing can be uneventful.

B2. Tuberculous osteomyelitis: This occurs in children; phalanges and shafts are involved in tuberculous infection. Short bones become spindle shaped called spina ventosa due to subperiosteal new bone formation and thickening of bone. Benign type of osteomyelitis may be seen as a rare complication of Bacillus Calmette–Guérin (BCG) vaccination, which is completely cured by instituting anti-tuberculous therapy. Polyarthritis resembling rheumatoid arthritis may occur during the treatment with chemotherapy and is called Poncet's osteomyelitis. This requires symptomatic treatment only.

C. **Abdominal TB**: Intestinal TB constitutes 5% of NIP, which occurs by ingesting infected sputum or by hematogenous spread. It can affect the gastrointestinal tract, right from the mouth to the anus, ileocecal junction being the commonest, possibly due to minimal digestion activity, more physiological stasis, increased rate of absorption, and preponderance of lymphoid tissue at this site. Esophagus, pancreas, and appendix are more affected by TB bacilli in HIV disease.

Clinically, nonspecific symptomology with off and on diarrhea, constipation, abdominal distension are observed, and occasionally bleeding may occur. Due to the extensive inflammation and fibrous adhesions, abdominal examination may give a doughy feel. Pathologically, intestinal TB has an ulcerative variety, having multiple coalescing ulcers. Healing with extensive fibrosis-forming napkin-ring appearance strictures, hypertrophic variety where submucosal inflammation and fibrosis may mimic neoplasm, mixed variety with pseudopolyps giving cobblestone appearance, and lastly diffuse variety resembling ulcerative colitis have been described. Caseation is commonly seen in the granulomas in the bowel and it's draining lymph nodes. Lumina narrowing and strictures of the bowel may complicate subsequent obstruction. Fistula formation due to infection may occur, and malabsorption syndrome due to bacterial overgrowth may cause stagnant loop syndrome.

Peritoneal involvement occurs in 5%–10% of cases of NIP, mostly by hematogenous spread. Ascites is common, mostly due to exudation, in exudation-type hyperplastic type affecting the greater omentum and fibrotic type with focal, fibroblastic peritoneal adhesions.

Clinically, distended abdomen is presented, mostly in females and a doughy feel of abdomen called a cotton wool sign is observed. A lump may be found in hyperplastic form, while signs of obstruction may be observed in the fibrotic type. Glandular TB infection affecting mesenteric nodes is called tabes mesenterica and is often seen in children, clinically mimicking appendicitis, presenting with fever and pain in the right iliac fossa. CT scan shows high-density ascites and abdominal lymphadenopathy. Classical straw-colored, high-protein fluid may be seen on paracentesis, with increased adrenaline deaminase activity, 1%–3% of AFB positivity, and 10%–20% of culture positivity, and the sensitivity of these tests is further decreased in cases of association with HIV disease. Stool tests for AFB culture have better diagnostic positivity index. CT-guided biopsy has a 60%–75% of diagnostic yield.

D. **Hepatobiliary TB**: Almost two-thirds of cases of primary TB have the evidence of liver involvement. In hepatic granuloma and miliary affection of the liver, 80% and 90% of patients may be affected. The incidence of liver involvement by TB in AIDS cases is almost seen in two-thirds of cases. Specific lesions include granuloma, granulomatous hepatitis, tuberculoma, caseous necrosis, tubercular abscess, fulminant hepatic failure, cholangitis, and cholecystitis. Nonspecific hepatic lesions include Kupffer cell hyperplasia, sinusoidal dilatation, fatty change, focal necrosis, periportal fibrosis, amyloidosis, siderosis, acidophilic bodies, and glycogen nuclei.

Clinically hepatic TB may be asymptomatic or with nonspecific symptoms such as fever, fatigue, night sweats, loss of appetite, and loss of weight. Abdominal pain, jaundice, or without ascites in a few patients may be seen. Serum transaminases are raised in three-fourths of patients, serum bilirubin is elevated in 20% of cases, and serum proteins are lowered in 80% of cases. Chest X-ray may reveal pulmonary TB in 10% of cases. Liver calcification is highly suggestive of hepatobiliary TB, seen in 50% of cases. Ultrasonography shows diffuse small nodules in the miliary TB of the liver. Larger nodules may mimic neoplasm. ERCP and PTCA may be required in cases of jaundiced patients. Choledoscopic biopsy from a common hepatic duct structure may reveal TB in the biliary epithelium.

Congenital TB may involve liver in 80% of cases, presenting with hepatomegaly and jaundice. Primary hepatic TB may have local lymph node affection and splenic involvement.

Biliary TB may present with obstructive jaundice. Tuberculous cholangitis is rare. Gallbladder involvement by TB is also rare and may be localized to the gallbladder or in association with other peritoneal organs. The majority of patients are women above 30 years of age. In children, miliary form with ulcerating tubercles may be present. Hepatic TB is seen in >50% of cases in AIDS patients, suggestive of extrapulmonary involvement. *Mycobacterium avium* intracellular complex infection is commonly found in AIDS patients and is suggestive of marked immunosuppression if the infection is disseminated.

TB in liver transplant patients is also reported. Isoniazid-associated hepatitis may affect the liver. Treatment with first-line four-drug regimen is effective. In AIDS and TB dual affection, rifabutin may be used along with antiretroviral therapy. Mortality rate is 12% and may increase to 75% in jaundiced patients. Prognosis is poor in patients with *M. avium* intracellular complex infection.

E. **Cutaneous TB**: 1.5% of cases of extrapulmonary TB suffer from cutaneous TB. Rising incidence is expected as 20% and a rise in NIP has been observed due to impaired cellular immunity as a consequence of HIV infection. Mostly, *M. tuberculosis* and *M. bovis* have been implicated as causative organisms, depending on factors such as sensitization status of host, immune reactivity of the host, route of infection, and pathogenicity of the infection strain. Cutaneous TB can be primary as TB chancre and acute miliary TB or secondary infection such as lupus vulgaris, tuberculosis verrucosa cutis, scrofuloderma, and tuberculosis cutis orificialis. An overlap may be seen in secondary varieties due to the continuous immunologic spectrum.

E1. Tuberculous primary complex or tuberculous chancre: This occurs following the inoculation of *Mycobacterium* into the skin of an individual who is not previously infected. The tuberculous chancre and the affected regional lymph nodes constitute the tuberculous primary complex of the skin. Clinically, a painless ulcer, granulating with an inflammatory reaction and regional node involvement may have 3–6 weeks to acquire a tuberculoid appearance. Depending on the host immunity, the reaction heals with scarring, yielding satisfactory host immunity but develops lupus vulgaris at the healed tuberculous chance site. Post-host resistance may allow primary inoculation of TB to progress to acute miliary disease with a fatal outcome.

E2. Tuberculous verrucosa cutis: It is an indolent, warty form of TB that occurs following the inoculation of organism into the skin of a previously infected person with a moderate degree of immunity. This is seen in the inoculation of PPD. In certain cattle butchers, such an infection is mostly due to *M. bovis*. Following accidental inoculation, the lesion starts as a small, indurated, warty papule with irregular purplish margins. Histology reveals pseudoepitheliomatous hyperplasia with marked hyperkeratosis and dense inflammatory infiltrates. Epitheloid and giant cells are present in the middle position of the dermis. Mycobacteria are occasionally demonstrated. Extension is slow and lesions remain inactive for months and years. Response to anti-TB treatment is good.

E3. Lupus vulgaris: This cutaneous TB is seen in patients with a moderate degree of immunity. A plaque lesion of nodules of apple jelly color is seen, which is potentially destructive in nature. Infection starts from the hematogeneous or lymphatic route, mostly from cervical lymph nodes or pulmonary TB, and rarely following BCG vaccination. About 40% of lupus vulgaris patients have TB lymphadenitis, and 20% of these are having primary TB or bone TB. Lupus vulgaris is asymptomatic. Early lesions may progress as elevated deep brown lesions, followed by a plaque with gyrate outline, having ulcerating and scarring course, exhibiting diverse manifestations, such as plaque form, ulcerating and mutilating form, vegetating form, tumor-like form, papular and nodular form, and lupus of mucus membrane. A chronic form called lupus exanthematicus may linger on for many years without treatment.

E4. **Scrofuloderma**: It is a subcutaneous TB leading to cold abscess formation, usually over a focus on the lymph node, lacrimal duct, or bone. Histopathology reveals tuberculous granulation with caseation in the deeper dermis, and tubercle bacilli are usually demonstrable in the pus. Clinically a bluish-red nodule, over an infected gland, having multiple intercommunicating fistulae beneath the irregular, inflammatory, ulcerating lesion, may be seen, and excessive granulation may give rise to a fundating tumor-like appearance. Scarring at the site may take years, and lupus vulgaris may appear in the vicinity of the scrofuloderma.

E5. **Metastatic tuberculous abscess**: Develops by hemotogenous spread from the primary focus due to decreased host immunity, in the form of solitary or multiple cutaneous lesions. These subcutaneous abscesses are non-tender, and histopathology may reveal massive necrosis with a large number of demonstrable AFB. It is also called tuberculous gumma.

E6. **Orificial TB**: This is the TB of mucous membranes and the skin, where mouth, tongue, and soft palate are mainly affected. A yellowish-pinkish mucosal lesion of soft consistency showing yellowish tubercular nodules beneath an inflamed and swollen mucus. Lesions are often painful causing difficulty in eating. Histopathology shows nonspecific inflammatory infiltration with necrosis. Caseation is seen in the deeper part of the tubercles in the dermis. Mycobacteria are demonstrable.

E7. **Acute miliary TB of skin**: It is a rare skin manifestation of fulminant variety, seen in children. Spreading via hematogenous route, from pulmonary or meningeal foci, especially where the host resistance is reduced due to measles or HIV disease. The lesions are seen in the body, as maculopapular pruritic rash, sometimes converting into umbilicated vesicles. Histopathology shows initial nonspecific inflammatory infiltrates and vasculitis, with mycobacteria mostly present in and around the blood vessels. Lymphocytic cuffing of vessels and tubercles appear later on. The prognosis is poor.

E8. **Tuberculids**: These are symmetrically disseminated varieties of skin eruptions associated with the internal focus of TB. They respond well to anti-TB treatment. Spread is hematogenous and patients do retain their immunity.

Lichen scrofulosorum is a lichenoid papular eruption seen in children and adolescents with TB. It is often present on the trunk and is asymptomatic. The yellowish pinkish small, firm, tubercular papule around the hair follicle is a superficial tuberculoid granuloma that does not contain mycobacteria.

Papulonecrotic tuberculid is a symmetrical necrotizing papular rash that comes in a crop and heals with scarring, mostly appearing on the lower trunk and buttocks. In case of deeper lesions, spontaneous healing occurs with pitted scars. Histopathology shows wedge spread necrosis surrounded with nonspecific infiltrates, usually tuberculoid. Granulomatous vasculitis is a feature, sometimes causing thrombosis and complete luminal occlusion.

Erythema induratum of the skin is yet another chronic recurring noduloulcerative disorder of the lower legs, mostly seen in females. Diagnostic features include characteristic histopathology with the recovery of AFB in the lesion, confirmed by follow-up positive culture of *M. tuberculosis* on U medium after 4–6 weeks of inoculation. Response to anti-Koch's four-drug regimen chemotherapy is good.

F. **Renal TB**: NIP has a rising trend in HIV-infected patients. TB of the genitourinary tract has most of the cases with renal involvement that accounts for 15%–33% of all extrapulmonary TB; *M. tuberculosis* is the main causative agent, and *Mycobacterium kansasii* is a very rare culprit. Right-sided kidney is more commonly affected. Spread is mainly hematogenous from primary pulmonary focus, leading to seeding of cortex that gradually spreads towards renal papillae, destroying calyces and forming characteristic ulcerocavernous lesions in the medulla. This is followed by ureteric and bladder involvement. Healing by fibrosis often leads to multiple ureteric structures. Total destruction of kidney may occur if the infection is severe, leading to autonephrectomy and formation of nonfunctional calcified cement kidney. An asymptomatic patient may rapidly progress into chronic renal failure. Apart from the constitutional symptoms, patients may experience painless hematuria, renal colic, isolated sterile dysuria, cystitis, and acute or chronic renal failure, which may be detected incidentally or as a part of an infertility investigation.

Routine urine examination included red blood cells, urine culture for AFB (recovery of AFB is low), plain X-ray KUB showing cumulus cloud or cement kidney, cystoscopy showing golf hole orifice (characteristic) of tubercular bladder, renal function tests and other supportive investigations such as plain X-ray chest (showing primary focus), serological and molecular diagnosis by ELISA and PCR, and tuberculin test for suspecting TB (although it does not differentiate primary and secondary infections or active and inactive diseases). Short-course anti-TB treatment is effective; streptomycin has to be avoided. Corticosteroids are only coadministered in preserving renal functions if there is tubercular interstitial nephritis. Conservative surgery is done to preserve the functional renal tissue. Total nephrectomy is only indicated when there is autonephrectomized kidney, gross and persistent hematuria, or malignant hypertension.

G. **TB of brain:** In India, 50%–55% of bacterial meningitis are due to tuberculosis, where 20%–60% of dying children with active tuberculosis have brain or meningeal affection. TB brain occurs in 5%–10% of adult cases of clinical tuberculosis. *M. tuberculosis* is the main culprit; non-tubercular mycobacteria and bovine variety are responsible for less than 5% of cases.

G1. **Tubercular meningitis**: It has a continuously changing profile due to mass BCG vaccination, HIV/AIDS, malnutrition, and late onset of primary infection. The early stage has nonspecific symptomology in a conscious, alert child, followed by the second stage of meningism, drowsiness, lassitude, cranial nerve palsy (sixth, followed by second, fourth, seventh), and hydrocephalus. Stupor, systemic toxicity, paralysis, seizures, choreoathetosis, and coma are seen in the advanced stage. Ophthalmic signs such as choroidal tubercles, papilledema, and internuclear ophthalmoplegia are seen. Chest X-ray may reveal healed or active pulmonary lesion. CT scan may reveal enhancing exudates. MRI may give a better visualization of hydrocephalus, infarcts, tuberculoma, or miliary nodules. Antitubercular chemotherapy is effective. Corticosteroids are indicated in the second or third stage only when there is significant cerebral edema, spinal cord disease, or drug reaction. Surgery is indicated to release hydrocephalus if raised intracranial tension is life-threatening, and vision is being compromised, or increase in ventricle size despite adequate anti-TB therapy. The outcome much depends on the adequate treatment, stage of the disease, BCG (priority given or not), raised intracranial tension, encephalopathy, and drug resistance.

G2. Tuberculoma is another manifestation of TB brain where an aggregated lesion of small granulomatous lesion is seen in the brain parenchyma, without rupturing into subarachnoid space. This may produce a paradoxical reaction at times with anti-TB therapy, resulting in an enlargement due to an inflammatory response arising out of released antigens. Clinical presentation is due to signs and symptoms of raised intracranial tension, focal signs may occur in 85% of supratentorial type with seizures, and focal motor deficit. Fever and systemic symptoms, unlike meningitis, are absent. CT brain reveals a thick ring of enhancement surrounded by punctuate central clearing (representing central caseous lesions). It may have three varieties: tuberculous plaque, cystic tuberculoma, and tuberculous abscess. Short-course chemotherapy is effective.

G3. TB and HIV — dual effect: TB enhances HIV replication by secreting TNF-α, by destroying CD4 cells, and by enhancing the release of virions from infected cells and increasing apoptosis. At the same time, HIV promotes TB by decreasing the macrophage-activating lymphocytes, by decreasing CD4 cells, and by enhancing tissue destruction. Individual contribution of *M. tuberculosis* to immunosuppression is well documented. TB remains the most common opportunistic infection in HIV disease in India. The degree of this immunosuppression directly affects the clinicoradiological features when both of these infections coexist. Non-pulmonary involvement by TB, other than lungs, in AIDS patients may go as high as 70%. And this higher tendency of non-pulmonary affection as well as more of disseminated TB increases as the immunity further decreases. Anti-TB treatment is started first and course completed if CD4 cell count is more than 200 cells/mm to avoid enhanced drug adverse effects that occur mostly in the first 2 months. But it is not wise to wait in starting antiretroviral treatment if the CD4 cells count goes lesser than 50 cells/mm^3. Modified antiretroviral treatment can be given in case of interaction between rifampicin and nevirapine and rifampicin and other protease inhibitors. Often there is radiological worsening in the form of aggravation of symptoms and flaring up of institution of antiretroviral therapy, usually in 1–4 weeks. Such a paradoxical reaction or immunoreconstruction inflammatory syndrome is often observed with anti-TB treatment of tuberculoma of the brain and lymph nodes. Corticosteroids may help in tiding over the situation without stopping any therapies against TB or HIV disease.

References for further readings

1. McGrath EE, Anderson PB. Diagnosis of pleural effusion — a systemic approach. Am J Crit Care. 2011;20:119–127.
2. Bhatia RS. TB and AIDS. JAPI. 2000;48:613–616.
3. Sahoo RC, Acharya PR. Pleural effusion of a dual etiology. JAPI. 2007;55:76–77.
4. Bhatia RS, Nigam P. Pulmonary TB — an update. Curr Med J. 1997;3(5):19–24.
5. Vora A, Suigh N. Algorithmic approach for the management of pleural effusion. Med Update; API. 2016;26:1031–1037.
6. Baal R, et al. Site specific incidence of abdominal TB. Ind J Gastroenterol. 2000;19(Supp. 2):A44.
7. Amrapurkar, D. Abdominal TB in India. IN: S. Das, ed. Med Update; API. 2003;13:108–111.
8. Patel KA, Patel KK. HIV and TB. IN: SB Gupta, ed. Med Update. Mumbai: API. 2005;15:726–730.
9. Bhatia RS. Diagnostic value of EUSA and ADA in TB. JAPI. 1998;46:574.
10. Ferriro L, et al. Systemic diseases and the pleura. Arch Bronchoneurol. 2011;47:361–370.
11. Henry M, Holzman R. TB of brain, meninges and spinal cord. IN: W Rom, S Gary, ed. TB. New York: Lippincott Williams and Wilkins. 2004;445–464.
12. Dipti Gothi., et al. "Lymph Node Tuberculosis". EC Pulmonology and Respiratory Medicine (2016): 194-211.
13. Andola SK, et al. K-Fs disease-clinical pathological correlation. JAPI. 2016;64:83–84.
14. Ekka M, Sinha S. Retropharyngeal abscess a rare presentation of TB. Lung India. 2015;32:262–264.
15. Khas AS, Hague SF. Renal TB in India. IN: S Das, ed. Med Update; API. 2003;13:119–122.
16. Jain P, Puwar P. Primary TB of tongue. JAPI. 2016;64:78–79.
17. Bandyopadhyay S, Mainty PK. Hepatobiliary TB. JAPI. 2013;61:404.
18. Manoharan G. IRIS. Med Update; API. 2015;25:962–969.
19. Rathi P, Gambhir P. Abdominal TB. JAPI. 2016;64:38–47.

https://doi.org/10.1142/9789811271410_0023

23 Tuberculosis of female genitalia

Introduction

Tuberculosis (TB) of female genital organs is the main cause of infertility in developing countries. The prevalence can be up to 10% in patients attending gynecology clinics. The true incidence is not known; however, it is almost 1% in those attending hospital gynecology outpatient departments. Mostly it occurs secondary to tubercular disease elsewhere in the body, at least in 80% of cases.

Pathogenesis

The common mode of spread is by hematogenous route. Lymphohematogenous spread may occur from the primary complex in the lungs. Lung lesions heal while infection remains dormant for a variable period, manifesting at a later stage. Lymphatic spread may occur from peritoneal TB, intestine, and kidneys. However, a reverse spread more commonly occurs from spill-over infection from fallopian tubes in the peritoneum. External female genitalia, that is, vagina and cervix gets infected through sexual contact regional lymph nodes are involved. Female genitalia may also be involved as a part of miliary TB.

Pathology

Vaginal involvement may occur in up to 10% of cases, cervix may be involved in up to 15% of cases, ovaries in one-fourth of cases, uterus in half of the cases, and fallopian tubes in almost all the cases in genitalia involvement in females.

Vulvovaginal involvement, a nodular involvement, followed by ulceration and discharging caseous material are seen. Similar changes are seen in the cervix. Hyperplastic mucosa with caseation and abscess formation is also seen. Direct -spread often leads to perioophoritis. Uterine involvement may be seen in up to three-fourths of cases where endometrium has granular, fungative, and ulcerative lesions. Granulomas can best be seen within 24 hours of year onset of menstruation. Total destruction of endometrium leads to amenorrhea. Pyometra may occur due to the release of caseous material into the uterine cavity.

Acute tubercular infection of fallopian tubes often causes bilateral salpingitis in less than 5% of cases. Destruction of muscle often replaces with fibrous tissue, leading to thickening of tube and calcification, which causes occlusion in three-fourths of cases, leading to infertility or ectopic pregnancies.

Clinical presentation

Genital TB can occur in 5%–10% of cases, where the previous history of pulmonary TB in a childbearing female is often positive. Genital TB in an unmarried girl can be suspected if present with pelvic infection. Up to 10% of patients may remain asymptomatic, and in three-fourths of cases, genital TB may present within the lower abdomen. Nearly half of the patients had amenorrhea. TB must be suspected in case of ectopic pregnancy. Clinical examination may be noncontributory in more than half of the cases, while adnexal mass may be palpable in nearly one-fourth of cases and nearly half the number of cases may present with peritonitis. Painful ulcerative lesions may be seen in renal infection, and painless nodules with ulcerative lesions may be seen in vaginal tubercular involvement.

Investigations and diagnosis

Culture positivity from the menstrual flow is hardly 10%; AAFB positivity from culture samples is observed in 25% of cases; granulomatous histological lesions are demonstrable only in 50% of cases; chest X-ray may show old lung lesions in 20%–30% of cases; and calcified lymph nodes may be seen in very few cases on plain X-ray abdomen. Adnexal solid mass can also be demonstrated by ultrasonography. Hysterosalpingography is a contra-indication in a proven case of genital TB for the fear of reactivation of the lesion. Renal involvement can be seen in 10% of cases. Laparoscopy may be helpful in a few cases.

Management

A short course of four drugs-anti-TB therapy is sufficient to treat cases of female genital TB. Surgical treatment such as bilateral salpingo-oophorectomy or hysterectomy is only indicated if the disease persists despite adequate treatment, the persistence of pain amenorrhea, coexistence of neoplasm, non-heaking fistulae or suspasim of MDR-TB.

Complications like sterility may persist in a few number of cases and ectopic pregnancy (more so in those who are treated for TB).

<table>
<tr><th colspan="3">Female genital tract TB</th></tr>
<tr><td>Incidence</td><td>13%–19% in India.</td><td>Infertility, the incidence of genital TB is 17.4%.</td></tr>
<tr><td>Pathogenesis</td><td>Almost always secondary to TB elsewhere in the body — usually pulmonary.</td><td>The mode of spread is usually hematogenous or lymphatic or by way of direct contiguity with an intra-abdominal or peritoneal focus.</td></tr>
<tr><td></td><td><table>
<tr><th>Organ</th><th>Frequency (%)</th></tr>
<tr><td>Fallopian tubes</td><td>90–100</td></tr>
<tr><td>Endometrium</td><td>50–60</td></tr>
<tr><td>Ovaries</td><td>20–30</td></tr>
<tr><td>Cervix</td><td>5–15</td></tr>
<tr><td>Vulva and vagina</td><td>1</td></tr>
</table></td><td></td></tr>
</table>

(*Continued*)

Female genital tract TB		
Microscopy	Microscopically, granulomatous and a chronic inflammatory infiltrate may involve the full thickness of the tubal wall, and caseation necrosis is common.	
Clinical features	Weight loss, undue fatigue, low-grade fever, or vague lower abdominal discomfort is often elicited in patients with genital TB. Menstrual disturbances Amenorrhea Menorrhagia Metrorrhagia Oligomenorrhea Abdominal swelling Postcoital bleeding Vaginal discharge Dyspareunia Infertility	
Signs	Normal Abdominal mass Pelvic mass Adnexal mass Abdominal tenderness Pelvic/adnexal tenderness Ascites Excessive vaginal discharge Ulcer in the vulva, vagina, and cervix Pyometra Fistula	

(*Continued*)

Female genital tract TB		
Differential diagnosis	Crohn's disease Actinomycosis Leprosy Granuloma inguinale Lymphogranuloma venereum Syphilis	

Hematological manifestations of bone marrow TB — anemia		
Demography	Gender	Male > female
	Peak age:	30–39 years
Pathology: peripheral blood smear	Anemia of chronic disease — most common	Red cell volume distribution width is decreased
	Microcytic anemia	Malnutrition, iron deficiency
	Macrocytic anemia	Secondary to anorexia, increased utilization and ileal involvement
	Autoimmune hemolytic anemia	Most commonly seen in disseminated TB due to the proliferation of reticuloendothelial tissues
Biochemistry	Serum iron and total iron-binding capacity decreased	
	Serum ferritin increased	
	Bone marrow erythropoietin response reduced	Due to elevated tumor necrosis factor-alpha, bone marrow fibrosis, aplasia, and amyloid infiltration of bone marrow

Hematological manifestations of bone marrow TB — leukocytes		
Leukocytes	Leukocytosis	Due to the inflammatory response
	Leukemoid reaction	
	Leukopenia	TB infection, folate deficiency, anorexia, bone marrow fibrosis, aplasia, and amyloid infiltration of bone marrow
Lymphocytes	Lymphopenia	TB infection
	Lymphocytosis	Inflammatory response

Manifestations in bone marrow due to TB — platelets		
Platelets	Thrombocytosis	Acute-phase reactant
	Thrombocytopenia	Immunologic mechanisms
		Hypersplenism
		DIC
		Bone marrow fibrosis, aplasia, and amyloid infiltration

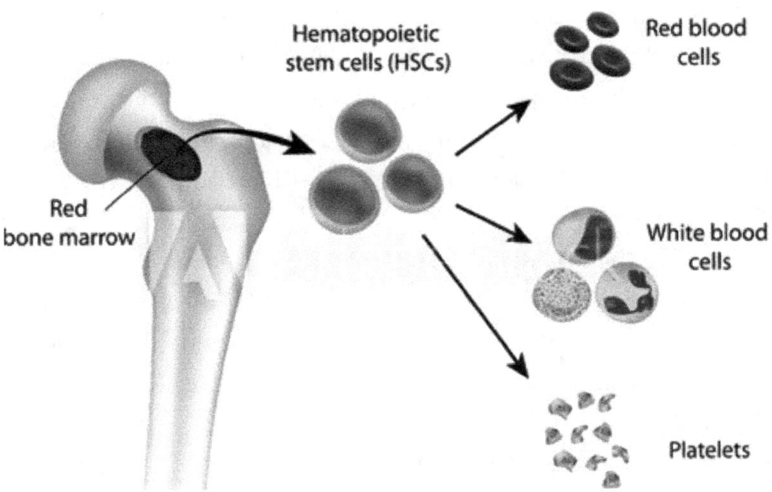

References for further readings

1. Varma TR. Genital tuberculosis and subsequent fertility. Int J Gypaec Obstet. 1991;35:1–11.
2. Dara Coglu OF, et al. Pelvic tuberculosis. Int J Gynaec Obstet. 1992;37:115–120.
3. Sinha P, et al. Pelvic TB-an uncommon gynaecological problem presenting as ovarian mass. Brit Obstet Gynaec. 2000;107:139–140.
4. Bhatia RS. TB — present approach in management. Curr Med Pract. 1992;36:168–170.
5. Bhatia RS, Bhardwaj BL. Pulmonary TB: tuberculosis of renal, urinary tract and genitourinary system. Lucknow: Aditya Med. Publ. 2005;11:87–89.
6. Bhatia RS. HIV and TB — where we stand? IN: S8 Gupta, ed. Med Update; API. 2002;12:1180–1183.
7. Bhatia RS. TB and AIDS — update article. JAPI. 2000;48:613–616.
8. Aulakh BS, Bhatia RS. Genitourinary TB. IN: RS Bhatia, ed. Tuberculosis. New Delhi: Pee Pee Publ. 2007;8:52–54.
9. Dogra Y, Singh N, Vanamail P. Autologous platelet-rich plasma optimizes endometrial thickness and pregnancy outcomes in women with refractory thin endometrium of varied aetiology during fresh and frozen-thawed embryo transfer cycles. JBRA Assist Reprod. 2022 Jan 17;26(1):13–21. doi: 10.5935/1518-0557.20210037. PMID: 34296832; PMCID: PMC8769175.
10. Abdissa S, Abebe T, Ameni G, Teklu S, Bekuretsion Y, Abebe M, Mihret A. Endometrial tuberculosis among patients undergoing endometrial biopsy at Tikur Anbesa specialized hospital, Addis Ababa, Ethiopia. BMC Infect Dis. 2018 Jul 5;18(1):304. doi: 10.1186/s12879-018-3202-x. PMID: 29976147; PMCID: PMC6034314.
11. Polepole P, Kabwe M, Kasonde M, Tembo J, Shibemba A, O'Grady J, Kapata N, Zumla A, Bates M. Performance of the Xpert MTB/RIF assay in the diagnosis of tuberculosis in formalin-fixed, paraffin-embedded tissues. Int J Mycobacteriol. 2017 Jan–Mar;6(1):87–93. doi: 10.4103/2212-5531.201892. PMID: 28317811.
12. Subramani E, Rameshbabu AP, Jothiramajayam M, Subramanian B, Chakravorty D, Bose G, Joshi M, Ray CD, Lodh I, Chattopadhyay R, Saha S, Mukherjee A, Dhara S, Chakravarty B, Chaudhury K. Mycobacterial heat shock protein 65 mediated metabolic shift in decidualization of human

endometrial stromal cells. Sci Rep. 2017 Jun 21;7(1):3942. doi: 10.1038/s41598-017-04024-w. PMID: 28638075; PMCID: PMC5479817.

13. Nibamureke UMC, Wagenaar GM. Histopathological changes in Oreochromis mossambicus (Peters, 1852) ovaries after a chronic exposure to a mixture of the HIV drug nevirapine and the antibiotics sulfamethoxazole and trimethoprim. Chemosphere. 2021 Jul;274:129900. doi: 10.1016/j.chemosphere.2021.129900. Epub 2021 Feb 9. PMID: 33979944; PMCID: PMC8049986.
14. Tulsyan S, Tripathi M, Das K, Yadav D, Shamim SA, Damle N, Bal C. Tc-99m sulfur colloid lymphoscintigraphy with single-photon emission computed tomography/computed tomography in a case of acquired vulval lymphangiomas. Indian J Nucl Med. 2017 Jan–Mar;32(1):73–74. doi: 10.4103/0972-3919.198495. PMID: 28242996; PMCID: PMC5317082.
15. Gilbert NM, O'Brien VP, Lewis AL. Transient microbiota exposures activate dormant Escherichia coli infection in the bladder and drive severe outcomes of recurrent disease. PLoS Pathog. 2017 Mar 30;13(3):e1006238. doi: 10.1371/journal.ppat.1006238. PMID: 28358889; PMCID: PMC5373645.
16. Igiraneza G, Hategekimana T, Manzi OM, Ogbuagu O. Obstructive uropathy as initial presentation of genitourinary tuberculosis and masquerading as a postsurgical complication. BMJ Case Rep. 2017 Oct 15;2017:bcr2017221270. doi: 10.1136/bcr-2017-221270. PMID: 29038191; PMCID: PMC5652372.
17. Assefa S, Desta K, Lema T. Group B streptococci vaginal colonization and drug susceptibility pattern among pregnant women attending in selected public antenatal care centers in Addis Ababa, Ethiopia. BMC Pregnancy Childbirth. 2018 May 4;18(1):135. doi: 10.1186/s12884-018-1791-4. PMID: 29728084; PMCID: PMC5935928.

https://doi.org/10.1142/9789811271410_0024

24 Multidrug-resistant tuberculosis

Epidemiology

Mycobacterium tuberculosis is the bacterium that causes the contagious disease tuberculosis (TB) which spreads through the air and once a person is infected the symptoms can appear immediately or the bacteria can live in a dormant condition called latent TB infection. More than 2 billion people which is about one-third of the global population are infected, many asymptomatically, with the TB bacilli. Globally tuberculosis (TB) remains one of the leading causes of morbidity and mortality from an infectious disease. According to WHO 1.5 million people have died from TB in 2020 worldwide and every year more than 10 million are infected and fell ill with tuberculosis which consists of 5.6 million men, 3.3 million women, and 1.1 million children despite it being a preventable and curable disease[1] because one of the main reasons is that mycobacterium continuous to gain drug resistances and evolve rapidly. The incidence rate of TB had declined over the past 20 years in most region of the world, however, the emergence of strains resistant to antituberculotic drugs have threatened the future world. The subjects with the drug-susceptible TB are treatable with the standard potent drugs isoniazid and rifampicin resulting in an excellent cure. The subjects who are infected with the strains resistant to antituberculotic drugs i.e., isoniazid and rifampicin are called Multi-Drug Resistant TB (MDR-TB), Rifampicin-resistant TB causes illness in more than half a million people every year and an increase in this resistance can be seen in countries like Russia, Myanmar, China, and South Africa.[1,2]

First-line therapy is not able to cure the subject thus they need to switch to the second-line therapy. In the same way, Extensively Drug-Resistant TB (EDR-TB) is a type of MDR — TB, resistant to fluoroquinolones and second-line therapy. Technically drug susceptibility testing is challenging and it requires a specialized person and also the laboratory facilities, these are not commonly available in the affected countries. Henceforth the World Health Organisation WHO and the International Union Against Tuberculosis and Lung Disease (IUATLD) launched a global surveillance program in 1994 that helps to estimate the global burden of MDR tuberculosis over time. Globally, MDR-TB is present in 3.8% of new TB patients and 20% of patients who have a history of previous treatment. Recent studies had estimated that about a half-million new cases of rifampicin-resistant TB (RR-TB) occurred in 2019 with 78% of them having confirmed MDR-TB. The incidence rate of MDR-TB is highest in the South — African general population, about 50% of MDR-TB cases account for India, China, and Russia the total pulmonary diseases worldwide. In India, a total of 96 913 patients were put on a shorter MDR-TB regimen with injectable second-line drugs (SLD) till December 2020. From 2014 to 2017 average success rate of the conventional regimen of MDR-TB was 49%. From 2016 to 2018 the average success rate of conventional XDR — TB patients on treatment is 29% and in 2017 it increased to 34%. In 2019, the success rate of mono or poly DR — TB regimen registered was 78%. One and five tuberculosis subjects were resistant to at least one major first-line therapy drug or second-line therapy drug. India and China have the second-highest number of MDR-TB cases in the world. Worldwide it is estimated that 9.6% of MDR-TB cases have XDR-TB (WHO 2013a) because in poor countries the access to second-line drug susceptibility tests is low, in most cases XDR-TB goes unrecognized.

Pathogenesis

Types of drug-resistant TB

1. **Monoresistance:** Resistance to one first-line anti-TB drug only.
2. **Polydrug resistance:** Resistance to more than one first-line anti-TB drug, other than both isoniazid and rifampicin.

3. **Multidrug resistance (MDR):** Resistance to at least both isoniazid and rifampicin.
4. **Rifampicin resistance (RR):** Resistance to rifampicin detected using phenotypic or genotypic methods, with or without resistance to other anti-TB drugs. It includes any resistance to rifampicin, whether monoresistance, multidrug resistance, polydrug resistance, or extensive drug resistance.
5. **Pre-Extensively drug resistance (pre-XDR):** Resistance to isoniazid, rifampicin, and a fluoroquinolone or resistant to isoniazid, rifampicin, and a second-line injectable (amikacin, capreomycin, and kanamycin).
6. **Extensive drug resistance (XDR):** Resistance to any fluoroquinolone, and at least one of three second-line injectable drugs (capreomycin, kanamycin, and amikacin), in addition to multidrug resistance.

Causes of drug resistance

- **Community transmission:** patients infected directly with MDR-TB strain rather than the strain acquiring drug resistance after infecting the patients
- **Nosocomial transmission:** crowded hospitals and health centers are likely one of the major drivers of the epidemic, especially in high HIV prevalence settings. This can result in the spread of drug-resistant strains among patients receiving therapy for drug-susceptible TB as well as among the health workers
- **Other causes:** misuse or mismanagement of drugs used to treat TB. Other causes leading to drug-resistant TB are incomplete TB treatment, prescribing wrong treatment (the wrong dose or length of time) by the health care workers, availability of drugs for treatment, and poor-quality drugs.

Common mutations and compensatory mutations

Risk factors of MDR — TB

- Failure to respond to a first-line DOTS regimen (WHO Category I or II)
- Relapse after a full course of treatment with a first-line regimen

Table 1: Common target mutations and compensatory mutations in drug-resistant Mycobacterium tuberculosis isolates

Common target mutations		Compensatory mutations
Rifampicin: inhibition of transcriptional activity		
rpoB	Asp516Val or Asp516Tyr, His526Arg or His526Asp or His526Tyr, Ser531Leu	rpoA mutations: Arg186Cys, Thr187Pro/Ala, Glu319Lys; rpoC mutations: Val483Ala, Asp485Asn, Gly594Glu, Asn689Ser, Asn826Lys
Isoniazid: inhibition of cell wall mycolic acid synthesis		
katG	Thr275Pro, Trp300Gly, Ser315Thr or Ser315Asn, Gln434X, Ala478del	Intergenic region between oxyR' and ahpC: –9G→A, −15C→T
Rv1910c-furA intergenic region	−12G→A, −10A→C, −7G→A	Unknown
furA-katG intergenic region	Truncation of 134-bp fragment (2156592–2156726)*	Unknown
mabA (fabG)-inhA	−17G→T, −15C→T, −8t→A, Ser94Ala	Unknown
Fluoroquinolones: inhibition of DNA replication, transcription, and recombination		
gyrA	Ala74Ser, Gly88Ala or Gly88Cys, Ala90Val, Ser91Pro, Asp94Gly or Asp94His or Asp94Ala	gyrA mutations: Thr80Ala, Ala90Gly
gyrB	Asp461His or Asp461Asn or Asp461Ala, Gly470Ala, Asp494Ala, Asn499Asp, Glu501Val	Unknown

Table 1: (*Continued*)

Common target mutations		Compensatory mutations
Ethambutol: inhibition of biosynthesis of cell wall arabinogalactan		
embB	Met306Val or Met306Ile, Gly406Ser or Gly406Ala or Gly406Asp or Gly406Cys, Gln497Arg	Unknown
ubiA	Val188Ala, Ala237Val, Arg240Cys, Ala249Gly	Unknown
Linezolid: inhibition of protein synthesis		
rrl	2061G→T, 2270G→C or 2270G→T, 2576G→T, 2746G→A	Unknown
rplC	Cys154Asn, His155Asp	Unknown
Bedaquiline: inhibition of mycobacterial ATP synthase		
atpE	Asp28Val, Glu61Asp, Ala63Pro	Unknown
Rv0678	Ser68Gly, Arg94Gln, Glu138Gly, Trp92_Phe93insGly, Arg38_Leu39insAla¶	Unknown
Ethionamide: inhibition of cell wall mycolic acid synthesis		
ethA	Diverse mutations scattered along entire gene	Unknown
ethR	Ala95Thr, Phe110Leu	Unknown
mabA (fabG)-inhA	−17G→T, −15C→T, −8T→A, Ser94Ala	Unknown
Para-aminosalicylic acid: inhibitor of folic acid and thymine nucleotide metabolism		
ribD	−11 G→A	Unknown
thyA	Gln111X, Leu143Pro, Ala182Pro, Thr202Ala, Tyr251X, Val261Gly X264Arg	Unknown

(*Continued*)

Table 1: (*Continued*)

Common target mutations		Compensatory mutations
dfrA	Val54Ala, Ser66Cys, Cys110Arg	Unknown
folC	Glu40Ala or Glu40Gly, Ile43Ala or Ile43Thr	Unknown
Kanamycin and amikacin: inhibition of protein synthesis		
rrs	1401A→G, 1484G→T	1409C→A, 1491G→T
eis‡	−10G→A, −14C→T, −37G→T	Unknown
whiB7	86del C, 124del C, 128del G, 133del C, 133_134insC, 179del G§	Unknown
Streptomycin: inhibition of protein synthesis		
rpsL	Lys43Arg, Lys88Arg	Unknown
rrs	462C→T, 492C→T, 514A→C, 517C→T	Unknown
gidB	n/a†	Unknown
Capreomycin: inhibition of protein synthesis		
rrs	1401A→G, 1484G→T	Unknown
tlyA	Asn236Lys	Unknown
Pyrazinamide: interference with membrane energy transduction, inhibition of trans-translation, inhibition of pantothenate and inhibition of CoA biosynthesis		
pncA	Diverse mutations scattered along entire gene	Unknown
rpsA	Thr5Ser, Asp123Ala, Ala438del	Unknown
panD	Met117Ile, Pro134Ser	Unknown
D-cycloserine: inhibition of cell wall peptidoglycan synthesis		
alr	−26 G→T‖	Unknown
ddl	None identified	Unknown
cycA	Gly122Ser**	Unknown

- Treatment after defaulting from treatment with a first-line regimen
- Exposure to a known case of MDR-TB
- Exposure to TB in institutions with a high prevalence of MDR-TB, such as a prison or hospital
- Living in areas or countries with a high prevalence of MDR-TB
- HIV coinfection

Transmission

A person with pulmonary or laryngeal TB disease when sneezes, coughs, shouts or sings the M. tuberculosis bacteria transmit as airborne particles, called droplet nuclei (1-5 microns in diameter) which can remain suspended in the air for several hours depending on the environment. When a normal healthy person inhales these droplets containing M. tuberculosis, they traverse the mouth or nasal passages, upper respiratory tract, and bronchi to reach the alveoli of the lungs. The risk of infection is dependent on several factors such as susceptibility, infectiousness, environment, and exposure (Table 2).

Table 2: Factors involved in the transmission of Mycobacterium tuberculosis

Factors		Description
Susceptibility		Immune status of the exposed individual
Infectiousness of the person with TB disease is directly related to the number of tubercle bacilli that he or she expels into the air.	Clinical	Presence of cough, especially lasting 3 weeks or longer

Table 2: (*Continued*)

Factors		Description
		Respiratory tract disease, especially with the involvement of the larynx (highly infectious)
		Failure to cover the mouth and nose when coughing
		Inappropriate or inadequate treatment (drugs, duration)
	Procedure	Undergoing cough-inducing or aerosol-generating procedures (e.g., bronchoscopy, sputum induction, administration of aerosolized medications)
	Radiographic and laboratory	Cavitation on chest radiograph
		A positive culture for M. tuberculosis
		Positive AFB sputum smear result
Environment: Environmental factors that affect the concentration of M. tuberculosis organisms	The concentration of infectious droplet nuclei	The more droplet nuclei in the air, the more probable that M. tuberculosis will be transmitted
	Space	Exposure in small, enclosed spaces
	Ventilation	Inadequate local or general ventilation that results in insufficient dilution or removal of infectious droplet nuclei
	Air circulation	Recirculation of air containing infectious droplet nuclei
	Specimen handling	Improper specimen handling procedures that generate infectious droplet nuclei
	Air Pressure	Positive air pressure in infectious patient's room that causes M. tuberculosis organisms to flow to other areas

(*Continued*)

Table 2: (*Continued*)

Factors		Description
Exposure: Proximity, frequency and duration of exposure	Duration of exposure to a person with infectious TB	The longer the duration of exposure, the higher the risk for transmission
	Frequency of exposure to an infectious person	The more frequent the exposure, the higher the risk for transmission
	Physical proximity to an infectious person	The closer the proximity, the higher the risk for transmission

Pathogenesis

Upon inhalation of the droplet nuclei by a healthy person majority of the droplet nuclei containing MTB from infectious patients are trapped in upper airway and expelled by ciliated mucosal cells: only a fraction reaches alveoli which avoids the defenses of the bronchi due to their small size and penetrate into the terminal alveoli where they are infect the phagocytic immune cells (macrophages and dendritic cells) or nonphagocytic cells in the alveolar space including M cells, alveolar endothelial, and type 1 and type 2 epithelial cells (pneumocytes) where they replicate, usually majority of infected patients the pathogens multiplication is stopped by cell-mediated immune response which develops after 2-8 weeks upon infection but in some individuals the pathogen is not completely eradicated as it has evolved effective strategies to evade the immune response resulting in survival and persistence of some bacilli in a nonreplicating state in the host which can be referred to as Latent TB infection (LTBI). More than 90% of the individuals infected with M. tuberculosis have asymptomatic LTBI, with only a 10% lifetime chance of LTBI progressing to active TB disease.

The pathogen binds to the cell surface of alveolar macrophages through complement receptors, mannose receptors, or type A scavenger receptors and the cells undergo phagocytosis, and the M. tuberculosis reduces acidity in the phagosome and a cell wall component (i.e., lipoarabinomannan) impairs Ca+/calmodulin pathway thus inhibiting phagosome-lysosome fusion which in turn stops the phagosome maturation and once this happens the bacteria multiplies and eventually kills the immune cell by multiplying in it and rupturing it to release the multiplied bacteria's which again are taken up by healthy macrophages and again the same infection cycle repeats.

The primary site of infection in the lungs is known as the Ghon focus, during primary infection, M. tuberculosis undergoes hematogenous and lymphatic dissemination involving hilar and mediastinal lymph nodes forming primary Ghon's complex. Eventually, bacteria enter the bloodstream and reach various organs. This lympho-hematogenous dissemination results in extrapulmonary tuberculosis (EPTB) during primary infection or later in life during reactivation of the disease. EPTB can spread the infection to more distant site's lymph nodes, kidneys, brain, and bones. When the infection worsens tissue destruction and necrosis are often balanced by healing and fibrosis which replace the affected tissues with scarring and cavities filled with caseous necrotic material.

Regimen for rifampicin-susceptible, isoniazid-resistant tuberculosis

Once the patient is found to be rifampicin sensitive, the second specimen available must be sent immediately FL-LPA test and the patient is initiated on standard regimen for DS-TB. If H resistance is not detected, the patient will be continued on DS TB regimen and monitored for response to treatment. If H resistance is detected on FL-LPA, the LPA deposit must be subjected to SL-LPA and LC&DST to Mfx, Z, Lzd, Cfz. Appropriate clinical evaluation is conducted and H mono/poly DR-TB regimen is initiated while waiting for the results of SL-LPA and LC&DST.

The treating doctor may need to modify the regimen using the replacement sequence in the event of additional resistance or intolerance or non-availability of any drug in use or emergence of exclusion criteria.

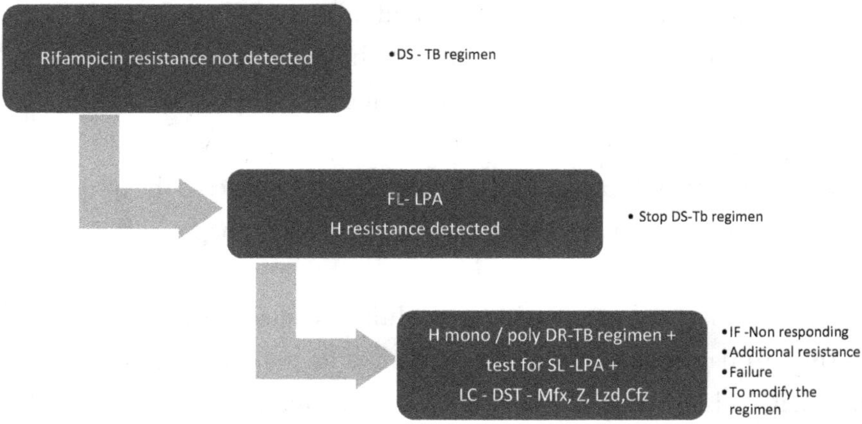

Figure 1: Steps considered while designing rifampicin-susceptible, isoniazid-resistant tuberculosis regimen

At any time during the treatment with DS-TB or H mono/poly DR-TB regimen with or without modifications, if there are signs of non-response, the patient must be subjected to NAAT again to rule out amplification of rifampicin resistance and further LPA and DST at specific time points as detailed in the follow-up monitoring.

H mono/poly DR-TB regimen is of 6 or 9 months with no separate IP/CP. In exceptional situations of unavailability of loose drug R or E or Z, the use of 4 FDC (HREZ) with Lfx loose tablets may be considered as an option rather than not starting the H mono/poly DR-TB patients on treatment.

In patients with H mono/poly DR-TB, treatment success rates were higher when fluoroquinolones were added to (H)REZ regimens than when patients were treated with 6(H)REZ or >6(H)REZ without the addition of fluoroquinolones. With the addition of fluoroquinolones in patients receiving (H)REZ, the number of deaths was reduced. Acquisition of additional resistance with progression to MDR-TB was also reduced when fluoroquinolones were added to a ≥6(H)REZ regimen, albeit with small absolute numbers.

Replacement sequence in H Mono/Poly regimen

Table 3: Situations to be considered while replacing H Mono/Poly regimen

Situation	Sequence of using replacement drugs
If Lfx can't be used	Replace with Mfxh if SL LPA pattern suggests. Do LC DST for detection of resistance to Mfxh, Z, Lzd & Cfz*
If Mfxh or Z can't be used	Replace with Lzd. If Lzd also cannot be given, replace with Cfz* + Cs
If both Mfxh and Z can't be used	Add 2 drugs of the 3 – Lzd, Cfz*, Cs in order of preference based on resistance, tolerability & availability
If R resistance	Switch to appropriate shorter or longer regimen

Table 4: Adverse effects and drugs given for the MDR-TB regimen

Adverse Drug Events	Drugs
Hepatitis	R, Z
QT prolongation	FQ, Cfz
Rash, allergic reaction and anaphylaxis	Any drug
Gastrointestinal symptoms	Z, E, Cfz, FQs
Giddiness	FQ, Z
Arthralgia	Z, FQ
Peripheral neuropathy	FQ, E
Depression, Psychotic symptoms, Seizures, Tendonitis and tendon rupture, Vestibular toxicity (tinnitus and dizziness), Metallic Taste, Superficial fungal infection and thrush	FQ
Optic neuritis	E, Lzd, Cfz

Treatment algorithm of M/XDR-TB

Rifampicin resistance (RR) is primarily being diagnosed in the field using NAAT among all the presumptive TB patients in areas that have transitioned to rapid molecular tests for TB diagnosis and in areas yet to transition, among key populations (PLHIV, children, EPTB, smear negative or

NA with X-ray suggestive of TB, contact of DR-TB patient, other vulnerable groups) or in all TB patients or among the non-responders of DS-TB or H mono/poly DR-TB patients.

MDR-TB patients get diagnosed among the H mono/poly DR-TB patients or among RR-TB patients which are subjected to FL-LPA during their treatment or if the specimen is directly tested for UDST on FL-LPA occasionally. Refer to integrated diagnostic and treatment algorithm in Chapter 3 for more details.

Shorter oral Bedaquiline-containing MDR/RR-TB regimen

Inclusion criteria

1. DST based inclusion criteria
   Rifampicin resistance detected/inferred
   MDR/RR-TB with H resistance detected/inferred based on InhA mutation only or based on KatG mutation only (not both)
   MDR/RR-TB with FQ resistance not detected
2. Other inclusion criteria
   Children, aged 5 years to less than 18 years of age and weighing at least 15 kg, given their special needs, in consultation with the pediatrician
   No history of exposure to previous treatment with second-line medicines in the regimen (Bdq, Lfx, Eto or Cfz) for more than 1 month (unless susceptibility to these medicines is confirmed)
   No extensive TB disease
   No severe extra-pulmonary TB
   Women who are not pregnant or lactating

Exclusion criteria

1. DST based exclusion criteria
   MDR/RR-TB patients with H resistance detected with both KatG and InhA mutation; and
   MDR/RR-TB patients with FQ resistance detected.

2. Other exclusion criteria

   If result for FL-LPA, SL-LPA and DST to Z, BDQ* & Cfz* is not available after pre-treatment evaluation is completed and it is a time to initiate the first dose of the regimen, then, exclude those with history of exposure for > 1 month to Bdq, Lfx, Eto or Cfz;

   Intolerance to any drug or risk of toxicity from a drug in shorter oral Bedaquiline-containing MDR/RR-TB regimen (e.g. drug–drug interactions);

   Extensive TB disease found in presence of bilateral cavitary disease or extensive parenchymal damage on chest radiography. In children aged under 15 years, presence of cavities or bilateral disease on chest radiography;

   Severe EP-TB disease where there is a presence of miliary TB or TB meningitis or central nervous system (CNS) TB. In children aged under 15 years, extrapulmonary forms of disease other than lymphadenopathy (peripheral nodes or isolated mediastinal mass without compression);

   Pregnant and lactating women (as ethionamide has eratogenic effects in animal models) and

   Children below 5 years

Investigations before starting short oral regimen

A shorter oral Bedaquiline-containing MDR/RR-TB regimen of 9–11 months duration is recommended in eligible patients with confirmed

Table 5: Clinical investigations before stating shot of oral regimen

Clinical Evaluation
Symptoms, history
Height, weight, BMI
clinical examination
ECG
Psychiatric evaluation when needed

Table 6: Laboratory based investigations to be considered before starting the oral regimen

Laboratory tests
Chest X Ray
RBS, Evaluation for Diabetes Mellitus
Complete blood counts (Hb, WBC count, Differential count, Platelets
ICTC Referral for counselling and HIV Testing
Serum Electrolytes (Na, K, Cl, Mg, Ca)
Liver Function Test (Bilirubin, proteins and enzymes)
TSH Levels
Urine routine and microscopy
Urine pregnancy test for the women in reproductive age group

MDR/RR-TB who have not been exposed to treatment with second-line TB medicines used in this regimen for more than 1 month, and in whom resistance to fluoroquinolones has been excluded.

The regimen consists of an initial phase of 4 months that may be extended up to 6 months and a continuation phase of 5 months, giving a total duration of 9–11 months. Bdq is used for a duration of 6 months.

- From start to end of 4th month – Bdq, Lfx, Cfz, Z, E, Hh, Eto
- From start of 5th month to end of 6th month – (If IP not extended) – Bdq, Lfx, Cfz, Z, E
- From start of 7th month to end of 9th month – Lfx, Cfz, Z, E
- If the IP is extended up to 6 months then all 3 drugs Bdq, Hh and Eto are stopped together

Need for stopping/replacing any drug in the shorter oral Bedaquiline-containing MDR/RR-TB regimen warrants stopping the regimen and evaluating the patient to switch to longer oral M/XDR-TB regimen.

Bedaquiline (Bdq) is a diarylquinoline that specifically targets mycobacterial ATP synthase, an enzyme essential for the supply of energy to Mycobacterium TB. Strong bactericidal and sterilizing activities against

Mtb have been shown in pre-clinical, laboratory and animal experiments. The drug has a high volume of distribution, with extensive tissue distribution, highly bound to plasma proteins and is hepatically metabolized. The drug has an extended half-life, which means that it is still present in the plasma up to 5.5 months post stopping Bdq. Bdq has shown significant benefits in improving the time to culture conversion in MDR-TB patients.

Delamanid (Dlm) is the first approved drug in the class of nitro-dihydro-imidazo-oxazoles for the treatment of MDR-TB. It is bactericidal drug with 36 hours of half-life and act with two different mechanism of action. It blocks the synthesis of mycolic acids (i.e., stopping the bacteria from creating building blocks important for their cell walls) as well as poison the bacilli with nitric oxide, which the drugs release when metabolized.

Longer oral M/XDR-TB regimen

Eligibility criteria:

- Longer oral M/XDR-TB regimen is recommended for MDR/RR-TB patients who are excluded from shorter oral Bedaquiline-containing MDR/RR-TB regimen including for the XDR-TB patients.
- In case of additional resistance or intolerance or non-availability of any drug in use or emergence of exclusion criteria to shorter oral Bedaquiline-containing MDR/RR-TB regimen or any longer regimen, the patient would be re-evaluated and initiated on longer oral M/XDR-TB regimen at N/DDR-TBC with any modifications, if additional resistance to any second-line drugs especially Lfx, Mfx, Bdq*, Lzd, Cfz*, Dlm* and Z (*whenever available). The regimen modification would be done using replacement sequence from group C detailed in the later section.

In MDR/RR-TB patients on longer oral M/XDR-TB regimen, all three Group A agents and at least one Group B agent should be included to

Table 7: Adverse drug events and suitable drugs given for the MDR-TB patients

Adverse Drug Events	Drugs	Adverse Drug Events	Drugs
QT prolongation	Bdq, FQ, Cfz	Psychotic symptoms	H, FQ,
Rash, allergic reaction and anaphylaxis	Any drug	Suicidal ideation	H, Eto
Gastrointestinal symptoms	Eto, Z, E, Bdq, Cfz, FQs, H	Seizures	H, FQ
Diarrhoea and/ or flatulence	Eto	Tendonitis and tendon rupture	FQ
Hepatitis	Z, H, Eto, Bdq	Vestibular toxicity (tinnitus and dizziness)	FQs, H, Eto
Giddiness	Eto, FQ, Z	Optic neuritis	E, Lzd, Eto, Cfz, H
Hypothyroidism	Eto	Metallic taste	Eto, FQs
Arthralgia	Z, FQ, Bdq	Gynaecomastia	Eto
Peripheral neuropathy	H, FQ, rarely Eto, E	Alopecia	H, Eto
Headache	Bdq	Superficial fungal Infection and thrush	FQ
Depression	FQ H, Eto	Dysglycaemia and hyperglycaemia	Eto

ensure that treatment starts with at least four TB agents likely to be effective and that at least three agents are included for rest of the treatment if Bdq is stopped. If only one or two Group A agents are used, both Group B agents are to be included. If the regimen cannot be composed with agents from Groups A and B alone, Group C agents are added to complete it as recommended by WHO. In India the experts concurred to start with all 5 drugs of Group A and B and continue with 4 drugs in the latter part of the regimen (beyond 6–8 months) if the patient can tolerate the drugs

Table 8: Group of drugs and steps to be followed while designing the Longer oral M/XDR-TB regimen

Groups & steps	Medicine	Abbreviation
Group A Include all three medicines	Levofloxacin or Moxifloxacin	Lfx Mfx
	Bedaquiline	Bdq
	Linezolid	Lzd
Group B Add one or both medicines	Clofazimine	Cfz
	Cycloserine or Terizidone	Cs Trd
Group C Add to complete the regimen and when medicines from Group A and B cannot be used	Ethambutol	E
	Delamanid	Dlm
	Pyrazinamide	Z
	Imipenem-cilastatin or Meropenem	Ipm-Cln Mpm
	Amikacin (OR Streptomycin)	Am (S)
	Ethionamide or Prothionamide	Eto Pto
	p-aminosalicylic acid	PAS

and for operational ease in the field. Longer oral M/XDR-TB regimen is of 18–20 months with no separate IP or CP. Although standardization in the design of longer regimens is possible, in many cases, the modification of the composition and duration of a regimen to make it individualized could enhance regimen effectiveness or safety. Once a patient is placed on a longer oral M/XDR-TB regimen for at least 4 weeks, normally that patient can no longer be switched to the shorter oral Bedaquiline-containing MDR/RR-TB regimen because this 4-weeks treatment would represent an exposure to second-line medicines. dose of Lzd will be tapered to 300 mg after the initial 6–8 months of treatment.

Bdq will be given for 6 months & extended beyond 6 months as an exception Pyridoxine to be given to all DR-TB patients as per weight band. For Pre-XDR-TB and XDR-TB patients the duration of longer oral XDR-TB regimen would be for 20 months with appropriate modifications. Total duration of longer oral M/XDR-TB regimen is 18–20 months. After month 6 of treatment, the patient must be reviewed based on month 5 culture results. If month 5 culture result is not available at the end of month 6, decision to taper the dose of Lzd to 300 mg will be based on month 4 culture result. If the month 5 or 4 culture result (whichever applicable) remains positive, the dose of Lzd (600 mg) and the regimen is extended by 1 month to month 7 and for a maximum till month 8 based on monthly culture results of month 6 and 7 respectively and clinical/radiographic response. If the month 8 culture is also positive, subject the culture isolate to FL-LPA, SL-LPA and C&DST. If any additional resistant to Group A, B or C drugs in use is detected, the patient needs to be reassessed at N/DDR-TBC for modification of longer oral M/XDR-TB regimen immediately on receiving the report. The duration of Bedaquiline is limited to 6 months. Extension beyond 6 months is to be considered in patients in whom an effective regimen cannot otherwise be designed if only 2 of 5 drugs are available from Groups A & B and adequate number of Group C drugs are not available due to high background resistance, non-availability or unreliability of DST. Maximum duration of treatment is not more than 20 months. A treatment duration of 15–17 months after culture conversion is suggested for most patients. The duration may be modified according to the patient's response to treatment.

Replacement sequence

In case of the need for replacement of any of the component(s) in the longer oral M/XDR-TB regimen, the following broad principles apply:

No drugs to be replaced

- 3group A + 2 Group B drugs to be included
- Lfx, Bdq, Lzd, Cfz, Cs

To replace 1 Group A drug

- 2 Group A + 2 Group B + 1 Group C drugs
- To replace the 1 group A drug which cannot be used with Delamanid

To replace 2 group A drugs

- 1 Group A + 2 Group B + 2 Group C
- To replace the Group A drugs which cannot be used with Delamanid and Amikacin

To replace 1 group A and 1 Group B drug

- 2 Group A + 1 Group B + 2 Group C
- To replace with delamanid and Amikacin

To replace 1 Group B drug

- 3 Group A + 1 group B + 1 Group C
- To replace the group B drug whiich cannot be used with Delamanid

To replace 2 Group B drug

- 3 Group A + 2 group C
- To replace Group B drugs with Delamanid and Amikacin

To replace 3 or more drugs from Group A and Group B

- To use the remaining Group A and B drugs + 3 or more Group C drugs
- To make a regime with at least 5–6 drugs

- The drugs are replaced according to their efficacy, no demonstrable resistance, prior use, side-effects profile and background resistance to the replacement drug in the country as per the NDRS report (4).
- The regimen should preferably be fully oral. However, in certain circumstances, injectables may have to be used for the need of efficacy and side-effect profile.
- At least 4–5 drugs are to be used in the initial 6 to 8 months. In situations where no replacement of any drug is required in the first 6 or 8 months of treatment in MDR-TB or XDR-TB patients, continue with

at least 3 drugs after this depending upon resistance, tolerability, availability, contraindication etc. of any one of Group A or B drugs.

- Replacement sequence of Group C drugs for longer oral M/XDR-TB regimen was recommended in the order of - delamanid, amikacin, pyrazinamide, ethionamide, PAS, ethambutol, penems.
- Combined use of Bdq and Dlm in the regimen is recommended for those M/XDR-TB patients in whom an appropriate regimen cannot be designed using all 5 drugs from Group A and B.
- In the final 12 months, at least 3–4 drugs are to be used from Group A & B. In situations where this cannot be done, the remaining drugs from Group C may be added as per the replacement sequence to complete 4 drugs (except Dlm and Am).
- Dlm and Am will not be started in the final 12 months of treatment.
- The duration of new drugs (Bdq or Dlm) is limited to 6 months. Extension beyond 6 months to be considered in patients in whom an effective regimen cannot be otherwise designed if only 2 of 5 drugs are available from Groups A & B and adequate number of Group C drugs are not available due to high background resistance, non-availability or unreliability of DST.
- Though Imp-Cln is 4th in the sequence of drugs of group C in WHO guidelines (15), it will only be used as the last resort for designing the regimens, operational issues of a Peripherally Inserted Central Catheter (PICC) placement for the entire duration of its use, need for admission.
- In individual patients for whom the design of an effective regimen is not possible as per recommendations, BPaL can be considered as a last resort under prevailing ethical standards, if Bdq and Lzd are available for use.
- To modify the longer oral M/XDR-TB regimen, the physician must look for the resistance pattern, tolerability history, contraindications and availability of first and second-line drugs to identify the number of drugs from Group A and Group B that need to be replaced.

Shorter injectable containing regimen

In the unavailability of bedaquiline, shorter injectable containing regimen to be considered for MDR/RR TB.

The regimen consists of

IP phase (4months, extendable to 6 months) – Mfx^{h}, Km / Am, Eto, Cfz, Z, H^{h}, E

CP phase (5 months) – Mfx^{h}, Cfz, Z, E

- If IP phase is extended, injectable agent to be given 3 times in a week during the extended IP phase.
- The regimen cannot be extended beyond 11 months
- No replacement of drug (except for Am instead of Km) is permitted.
- Baseline audiometry evaluation and every 2 months till the completion of injectable course is recommended.
- Baseline Serum Creatinine level and monthly evaluation till the completion of Injectable course.

Exclusion criteria:

DST based –

MDR/RR TB with H resistance detected for both KatG and InhA mutation

MDR/RR TB patients with Flouroquinolone or SLI resistance detected.

Other Criteria-

Unavailability of FL, SL LPA and DST to Z and Cfz.

Intolerance to any drug in the regimen

Severe EP-TB disease in the presence of miliary TB or TB meningitis.

Extensive Tb with bilateral cavitary disease or extensive parenchymal destruction on CXR.

Pregnant and lactating women.

References and suggested readings

1. Conradie F, Diacon AH, Ngubane N, Howell P, Everitt D, Crook AM, Mendel CM, Egizi E, Moreira J, Timm J, McHugh TD, Wills GH, Bateson A, Hunt R, Van Niekerk C, Li M, Olugbosi M, Spigelman M; Nix-TB Trial Team. Treatment of highly drug-resistant pulmonary tuberculosis. N Engl

J Med. 2020 Mar 5;382(10):893–902. doi: 10.1056/NEJMoa1901814. PMID: 32130813; PMCID: PMC6955640.

2. Sultana ZZ, Hoque FU, Beyene J, Akhlak-Ul-Islam M, Khan MHR, Ahmed S, Hawlader DH, Hossain A. HIV infection and multidrug resistant tuberculosis: a systematic review and meta-analysis. BMC Infect Dis. 2021 Jan 11;21(1):51. doi: 10.1186/s12879-020-05749-2. Erratum in: BMC Infect Dis. 2021 Jan 20;21(1):86. PMID: 33430786; PMCID: PMC7802168.
3. Rao Muvva J, Ahmed S, Rekha RS, Kalsum S, Groenheit R, Schön T, Agerberth B, Bergman P, Brighenti S. Immunomodulatory agents combat multidrug-resistant tuberculosis by improving antimicrobial immunity. J Infect Dis. 2021 Jul 15;224(2):332–344. doi: 10.1093/infdis/jiab100. PMID: 33606878; PMCID: PMC8280489.
4. Diel R, Sotgiu G, Andres S, Hillemann D, Maurer FP. Cost of multidrug resistant tuberculosis in Germany-An update. Int J Infect Dis. 2021 Feb;103:102–109. doi: 10.1016/j.ijid.2020.10.084. Epub 2020 Nov 3. PMID: 33157286.
5. Grobbel HP, Merker M, Köhler N, Andres S, Hoffmann H, Heyckendorf J, Reimann M, Barilar I, Dreyer V, Hillemann D, Kalsdorf B, Kohl TA, Sanchez Carballo P, Schaub D, Todt K, Utpatel C, Maurer FP, Lange C, Niemann S. Design of multidrug-resistant tuberculosis treatment regimens based on DNA sequencing. Clin Infect Dis. 2021 Oct 5;73(7):1194–1202. doi: 10.1093/cid/ciab359. PMID: 33900387; PMCID: PMC8492214.
6. Santos FLD, et al. Patients' perceptions regarding multidrug-resistant tuberculosis and barriers to seeking care in a priority city in Brazil during COVID-19 pandemic: a qualitative study. PloS One. 2021 Apr 9; 16(4):e0249822. doi: 10.1371/journal.pone.0249822.
7. Du L, et al. Prevalence of multidrug-resistant tuberculosis in Dalian, China: a retrospective study. Infect Drug Resist. 2021 Mar 16;14:1037–1047. doi: 10.2147/IDR.S294611.
8. Katrak S, et al. Bedaquiline for multidrug-resistant tuberculosis and QTc prolongation in California. J Clin Tuberc Other Mycobact Dis. 2021 Jan 10;23:100216. doi: 10.1016/j.jctube.2021.100216.
9. Ernest JP, et al. Development of new tuberculosis drugs: translation to regimen composition for drug-sensitive and multidrug-resistant tuberculosis. Ann Rev Pharmacol Toxicol. 2021;61:495–516. doi: 10.1146/annurev-pharmtox-030920-011143.

10. Biswas SS, et al. In silico approach for phytocompound-based drug designing to fight efflux pump-mediated multidrug-resistant mycobacterium tuberculosis. Appl Biochemis Biotechnol. 2021;193(6):1757–1779. doi: 10.1007/s12010-021-03557-1.
11. Dooley KE, et al. QT effects of bedaquiline, delamanid, or both in patients with rifampicin-resistant tuberculosis: a phase 2, open-label, randomised, controlled trial. Lancet Infect Dis. 2021;21(7):975–983. doi: 10.1016/S1473-3099(20)30770-2.
12. Guglielmetti L, et al. Evaluating newly approved drugs for multidrug-resistant tuberculosis (endTB): study protocol for an adaptive, multi-country randomized controlled trial. Trials. 2021 Sep 25;22(1):651. doi: 10.1186/s13063-021-05491-3.
13. Usmanova R, et al. Treatment compliance of multidrug resistant tuberculosis in Uzbekistan: does practice follow policy? Int J Environ Res Public Health. 2021 Apr 12;18(8):4071. doi: 10.3390/ijerph18084071.
14. Singh AV, et al. Genetic variability in multidrug-resistant mycobacterium tuberculosis isolates from patients with pulmonary tuberculosis in North India. BMC Microbiol. 2021 Apr 21;21(1):123. doi: 10.1186/s12866-021-02174-6.
15. Edwards BD, et al. Rifampin-resistant/multidrug-resistant tuberculosis in Alberta, Canada: epidemiology and treatment outcomes in a low-incidence setting. PloS One. 2021 Feb 16;16(2):e0246993. doi: 10.1371/journal.pone.0246993.

https://doi.org/10.1142/9789811271410_0025

25 Tuberculosis and diabetes mellitus

Hyperglycemia or uncontrolled diabetes predisposes to tuberculosis (TB) and is also considered a risk factor for its activation. Centuries-old association has seen diabetes in less than 10% of cases of TB hospital admissions, which is increased to 10% in TB patients over the age of 40 years who are having diabetes at present in India.

Radiological diagnosis of TB among diabetic patients in Korea varied from 9.6% to 12.8%, whereas 2002 Imphal study revealed the prevalence of pulmonary TB is 100 diabetic patients with 27% of radiologic diagnosis and 60% of sputum positivity. The risk of TB in diabetes increases by 3.4 times, which is directly related to uncontrolled hyperglycemia of a longer duration. Relative risk is higher among younger age groups, that is, 9.88% (30–39 years), 4.72% (40–49 years), and 1.76%–2.3% (above 49 years). TB among male diabetics is 2.2 times more than among female diabetics. Both bronchial and pleuropulmonary involvements are known to occur. Multiple lobe involvement can occur, and lower lung fields are commonly affected in diabetes mellitus. Duration of diabetes does not correlate with the occurrence of TB, but the risk of developing multidrug-resistant TB is more, and various types of lesions of TB in diabetes mellitus are listed in Table 1.

A higher prevalence of pulmonary TB in diabetes is attributed to existing inadequate substrate for immunity formation due to disturbed protein metabolism. At the same time, higher chances of infection are due to low opsonic index, reduced antibacterial activity, poor tissue resistance, reduced collagen synthesis, impaired defensive function of RE cells, and increased

Table 1: Tubercular disease and variety of tubercular lesions in diabetes mellitus

1. Minimal
2. Moderate
3. Advanced
1. Cavitary
2. Homogeneous opacities
3. Hetergeneous opacities
4. Pleural effusion
5. Consolidation
6. Fibrosis

availability of tissue glycerol as a substrate that enhances the growth of TB bacilli. Prognosis is not favorable, and doctors must be vigilant to suspect infection in cases with uncontrolled hyperglycemia. Keeping blood sugar fasting level at 100 mg/dL is the prudent target. Diagnosis and management with anti-TB drugs for an appropriate duration with the maintenance of glucose status is rewarding and is not dependent on the type of hypoglycemic therapy (insulin or OHA) used. Bacterial chest infections are increased in the presence of hyperglycemia, and this is attributed to reduced availability of NABPH, producing decreased production of superoxide anion along with depressed respiratory burst, which would contribute to impaired chemotaxis, phagocytosis, and intracellular killing of microorganisms by granulocytes and mononuclear cells in diabetes mellitus. Similarly, an impaired ability of alveolar macrophages in inhibiting fungal spore germination would enhance zygomycosis.

Comorbidities and altered pulmonary functions in two-third of diabetic cases and the influence of obesity, muscle weakness, and congestive heart failure add to the agony. Reduced lung columns (in insulin-dependent diabetes), pulmonary elastic recoil and impaired pulmonary diffusion, and pulmonary epithelial permeability along with the abnormal ventilatory response to hypoxia can cause unexpected cardiorespiratory arrest in diabetic patients, possibly due to an increased sleep-related breathing disorder produced as a result of autonomic neuropathy.

Reduced gradient between pulmonary wedge pressure and serum colloid oncotic pressure may produce cerebral edema, which may cause neurogenic pulmonary edema due to increased permeability during acidosis. Acute respiratory distress syndrome can also occur because of cardiogenic pulmonary edema while treating diabetic ketoacidosis, which may produce alveolar hypoventilation due to hypokalemia and hypophosphatemia because of severe muscular weakness.

Bronchial asthma may rarely be coexisting with diabetes mellitus. Nevertheless, exacerbation of bronchospasm may occur in bronchial asthma during hypoglycemia. Diabetic autonomic neuropathy, on the other hand, reduces bronchial hyperreactivity possibly because of depressed cholinergic bronchomotor tone. Diabetic neuropathy and persistent transudatic pleural effusion due to left ventricular dysfunction may produce transient vocal cord paralysis. Pulmonary thromboembolism may get precipitated due to dehydration in the case of diabetic ketoacidosis.

Metabolic disorders and lung involvement require elaborated diagnostic procedures to establish the diagnosis. And at the same time, these facilities may not be available at all centers or may not be affordable for all patients. Hence, the clinical acumen used is rewarding.

Comments

Diabetes and chest infections including TB are directly related in the case of uncontrolled hyperglycemia due to higher susceptibility sustenance and reduced bactericidal activity and tissue resistance because of the inability of granulocytes, mononuclear cells, and even alveolar macrophages to contain the infection. Comorbidities and diabetic ketoacidosis would add agony to the existing problem. Maintenance of fasting blood glucose as/around 100 mg/dL would prevent as well as help in the early recovery of accompanying chest disorders in diabetes mellitus.

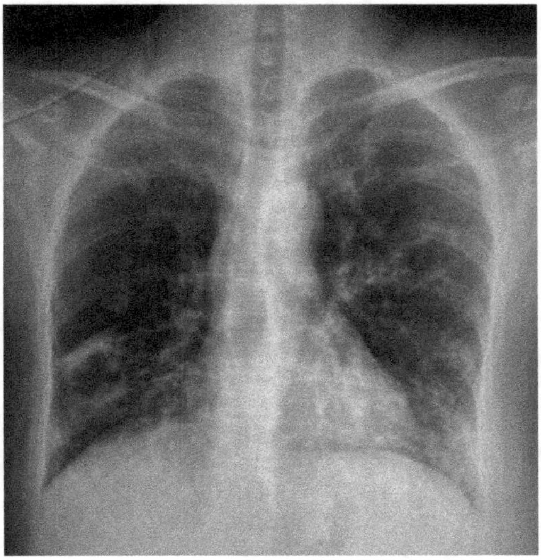

Figure 1: Lower zone TB diabetic.

References and suggested readings

1. Ezung T, et al. Pulmonary TB and diabetes. J Ind Med Assn. 2002;100:376–379.
2. Bhatia RS, Singh H. Cardio pulmonary complications in diabetes. IN: Cardiopulmonary topic. Pee Pee Publ. 2008;15:123–129.
3. Maj D. Endocrine emergencies. IN: M Panja, ed. Med Update; API. 2001;11:463–471.
4. Vigg A, et al. Sleep in type 2 diabetes. JAPI. 2003;51:797–781.
5. Bhatia RS. Metabolic disorders and lungs. IN: BB Thakur, ed. PG Med; API. 2002;16:125–129.
6. Antonio-Arques V, Franch-Nadal J, Caylà JA. Diabetes and tuberculosis: a syndemic complicated by COVID-19. Med Clin (Barc). 2021 Sep 24;157(6):288–293. English, Spanish. doi: 10.1016/j.medcli.2021.04.004. Epub 2021 May 6. PMID: 34049681; PMCID: PMC8101986.
7. Mave V, Gaikwad S, Barthwal M, Chandanwale A, Lokhande R, Kadam D, Dharmshale S, Bharadwaj R, Kagal A, Pradhan N, Deshmukh S, Atre S, Sahasrabudhe T, Meshram S, Kakrani A, Kulkarni V, Raskar S, Suryavanshi N, Kornfeld H, Dooley KE, Chon S, Gupte A, Gupta A, Gupte N, Golub JE. Diabetes mellitus and tuberculosis treatment outcomes in Pune, India.

Open Forum Infect Dis. 2021 Mar 4;8(4):ofab097. doi: 10.1093/ofid/ofab097. PMID: 33884278; PMCID: PMC8047862.

8. Gibbons C, Blundell J, Tetens Hoff S, Dahl K, Bauer R, Baekdal T. Effects of oral semaglutide on energy intake, food preference, appetite, control of eating and body weight in subjects with type 2 diabetes. Diabetes Obes Metab. 2021 Feb;23(2):581–588. doi: 10.1111/dom.14255. Epub 2020 Nov 27. PMID: 33184979; PMCID: PMC7839771.
9. Phillip M, Bergenstal RM, Close KL, Danne T, Garg SK, Heinemann L, Hirsch IB, Kovatchev BP, Laffel LM, Mohan V, Parkin CG, Battelino T. The digital/virtual diabetes clinic: the future is now-recommendations from an international panel on diabetes digital technologies introduction. Diabetes Technol Ther. 2021 Feb;23(2):146–154. doi: 10.1089/dia.2020.0375. Epub 2020 Sep 28. PMID: 32905711; PMCID: PMC8098767.
10. Araia ZZ, Mesfin AB, Mebrahtu AH, Tewelde AG, Osman R, Tuumzghi HA. Diabetes mellitus and its associated factors in tuberculosis patients in Maekel region, eritrea: analytical cross-sectional study. Diabetes Metab Syndr Obes. 2021 Feb 4;14:515–523. doi: 10.2147/DMSO.S293557. PMID: 33568928; PMCID: PMC7869713.
11. Tamuhla T, Dave JA, Raubenheimer P, Tiffin N. Diabetes in a TB and HIV-endemic South African population: analysis of a virtual cohort using routine health data. PLoS One. 2021 May 7;16(5):e0251303. doi: 10.1371/journal.pone.0251303. PMID: 33961671; PMCID: PMC8104376.
12. van Crevel R, Critchley JA. The interaction of diabetes and tuberculosis: translating research to policy and practice. Trop Med Infect Dis. 2021 Jan 8;6(1):8. doi: 10.3390/tropicalmed6010008. PMID: 33435609; PMCID: PMC7838867.
13. Fu CP, Lee CL, Li YH, Lin SY. Metformin as a potential protective therapy against tuberculosis in patients with diabetes mellitus: a retrospective cohort study in a single teaching hospital. J Diabetes Investig. 2021 Sep;12(9):1603–1609. doi: 10.1111/jdi.13523. Epub 2021 Mar 3. PMID: 33550691; PMCID: PMC8409838.
14. Xiao W, Huang D, Li S, Zhou S, Wei X, Chen B, Zou G. Delayed diagnosis of tuberculosis in patients with diabetes mellitus co-morbidity and its associated factors in Zhejiang Province, China. BMC Infect Dis. 2021 Mar 18;21(1):272. doi: 10.1186/s12879-021-05929-8. PMID: 33736610; PMCID: PMC7977257.

https://doi.org/10.1142/9789811271410_0026

26 Pharmacotherapy of tuberculosis

First-line agents

- Isoniazid
- Rifampicin
- Ethambutol
- Pyrazinamide
- Streptomycin

Second-line agents

- Ethionamide
- Cycloserine
- Kanamycin
- Amikacin
- Capreomycin
- Ciprofloxacin
- Ofloxacin
- Clarithromycin
- Azithromycin
- Rifabutin

Recommended dose in adults

Drugs	Recommended daily dose (mg/kg)	Maximum daily dose (mg)	Recommended 3 times/week (mg/kg)	Maximum dose (mg)
Isoniazid	5 (4–6)	300	10 (8–12)	900
Rifampicin	10 (8–12)	600	10 (8–12)	600
Pyrazinamide	25 (20–30)	—	35 (30–40)	—
Ethambutol	15 (15–20)	—	30 (25–35)	—
Streptomycin	15 (12–18)	—	15 (12–18)	1,000

Recommended dose in children

Drug	Dose in mg/kg/day
Isoniazid	10–15
Rifampicin	10
Pyrazinamide	35
Ethambutol	30
Streptomycin	15

Mechanism of actions

Isoniazid

Isoniazid is a prodrug and is activated by bacterial catalase. Activation is associated with reduction of the mycobacterial ferric KatG catalase-peroxidase by hydrazine and reaction with oxygen to form an oxyferrous enzyme complex. Once activated, isoniazid inhibits the synthesis of mycolic acids, an essential component of the bacterial cell wall. At therapeutic levels, isoniazid is bactericidal against actively growing intracellular and extracellular *Mycobacterium tuberculosis* organisms. Specifically, isoniazid inhibits InhA, the enoyl reductase from *M. tuberculosis*, by forming a covalent bond with the NAD cofactor. It is the INH–NAD complex that acts as a slow, tight-binding competitive inhibitor of InhA.

Rifampicin

Rifampicin acts via the inhibition of DNA-dependent RNA polymerase, leading to the suppression of RNA synthesis and cell death.

Pyrazinamide

Pyrazinamide diffuses into *M. tuberculosis*, where the enzyme pyrazinamidase converts pyrazinamide to the active form pyrazinoic acid. Under acidic conditions, the pyrazinoic acid converts to the protonated conjugate acid, which diffuses easily back into the bacilli and accumulates. The net effect is that more pyrazinoic acid accumulates inside the bacillus at acid pH than at neutral pH. Pyrazinoic acid inhibits the enzyme fatty acid synthase (FAS) I, which is required by the bacterium to synthesize fatty acids. The accumulation of pyrazinoic acid disrupts membrane potential and interferes with energy production, necessary for the survival of *M. tuberculosis* at an acidic site of infection.

Ethambutol

Ethambutol inhibits RNA synthesis and decreases tubercle bacilli replication. Nearly all strains of *M. tuberculosis* and *M. kansasii* as well as a number of strains of MAC are sensitive to ethambutol. Ethambutol inhibits arabinosyltransferases which is involved in cell wall biosynthesis. By inhibiting this enzyme, the bacterial cell wall complex production is inhibited. This leads to an increase in cell wall permeability.

Streptomycin

Streptomycin is an aminoglycoside antibiotic produced by the soil actinomycete *Streptomyces griseus*. It acts by binding to the 30S ribosomal subunit of susceptible organisms and disrupting the initiation and elongation steps in protein synthesis.

Common side effects of essential anti-TB drugs

Drugs	Common effects	Rare effects
Isoniazid	Peripheral neuropathy, hepatitis, skin rash, sleepiness, lethargy	Convulsions, psychosis, arthralgia, anemia
Rifampicin	Abdominal pain, nausea, vomiting, hepatitis, generalized cutaneous reactions, thrombocytopenic purpura	Osteomalacia, pseudomembranous colitis, pseudo adrenal crisis, acute renal failure, hemolytic anemia
Pyrazinamide	Arthralgia, hepatitis, abdominal pain, nausea, and vomiting	Cutaneous reactions, sideroblastic anemia
Ethambutol	Retrobulbar neuritis	Generalized cutaneous reactions, arthralgia, peripheral neuropathy, hepatitis (very rare)

Adverse effects of reserve anti-TB drugs

Drugs	Common effects	Rare effects
Aminoglycosides	Vestibular and auditory nerve damage, nephrotoxicity	Cutaneous hypersensitivity, clinical renal failure
Ethionamide	Anorexia, nausea, diarrhea, abdominal pain, hepatotoxicity	Convulsions, mental symptoms, impotence, gynecomastia
Fluoroquinolones	Anorexia, nausea, vomiting	Dizziness, headache, convulsions, rupture of Achilles tendon
Cycloserine	Dizziness, headache, depression, hepatitis, psychosis, convulsion	Suicide, generalized hypersensitivity, hepatitis

Newer classification of anti-TB drugs

Group name	Anti-tuberculosis drugs
Group 1	First-line oral drugs: HRZE
Group 2	Quinolones: high-dose levofloxacin, moxifloxacin
Group 3	Linezolid, bedaquiline, delamanid
Group 4	Injectable second-line drugs: kanamycin, amikacin, capreomycin
Group 5	Ethionamide/prothionamide, clofazimine, carbapenems
Group 6	Cycloserine, PASA, amoxicillin/clavulanate

WHO guidelines (2019) for drug-resistant tuberculosis

<table>
<tr><th>Groups and steps</th><th>Drugs</th></tr>
<tr><td rowspan="3">Group A:
Include all three medicines</td><td>Levofloxacin
Moxifloxacin</td></tr>
<tr><td>Bedaquiline</td></tr>
<tr><td>Linezolid</td></tr>
<tr><td rowspan="2">Group B:
Add one or both medicines</td><td>Clofazimine</td></tr>
<tr><td>Cycloserine or terizidone</td></tr>
<tr><td rowspan="7">Group C:
Add to complete the regimen and when medicines from Groups A and B cannot be used</td><td>Ethambutol</td></tr>
<tr><td>Delamanid</td></tr>
<tr><td>Pyrazinamide</td></tr>
<tr><td>Imipenem–cilastatin or meropenem</td></tr>
<tr><td>Amikacin</td></tr>
<tr><td>Ethionamide</td></tr>
<tr><td>p-Aminosalicylic acid</td></tr>
</table>

Mechanism of Bedaquiline (Sirturo) — Janssen Therapeutics

Approval: Dec. 2012

Indication: as part of combination therapy in adults (≥18 years) to treat MDR-TB when other alternatives are not available

MoA: inhibits mycobacterial ATP (adenosine 5'-triphosphate) synthase, an enzyme that is essential for the generation of energy in *M. tuberculosis*

Dose: 400 mg once daily for the first 2 weeks and 200 mg three times per week for the following 22 weeks

Mechanism of delamanid

Delamanid is a dihydro-nitroimidazole oxazole derivative. Delamanid is a prodrug that gets activated by the enzyme deazaflavin-dependent nitroreductase. It acts by inhibiting the synthesis of mycobacterial cell wall components, methoxy mycolic acid, and keto mycolic acid. A reactive intermediate metabolite, formed between delamanid and des-nitroimidazole oxazole derivative, is considered to play a vital role in the inhibition of mycolic acid production.

Dose: 100 mg once daily orally

Side effects: QT prolongation, syncope, arrhythmia

Clinical trials

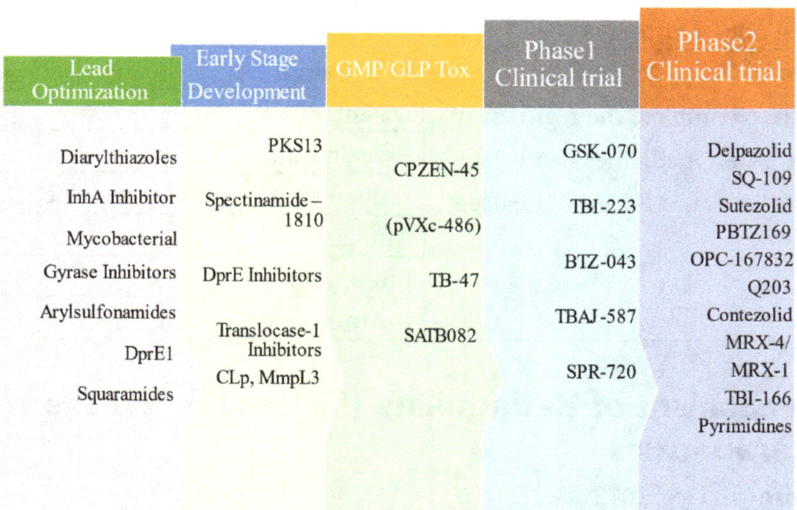

Two new drugs (bedaquiline and delamanid) are in confirmatory phase 3 trials, having received accelerated approvals for MDR tuberculosis based on phase 2 data in 2012 and 2014, respectively.

The FDA and European medicines agency both gave conditional approval to both bedaquiline and delamanid to be used individually as a component of an optimized background regimen for pulmonary MDR-TB up to 24 weeks; they are not recommended for extrapulmonary TB, and efficacy in meningitis is currently lacking.

Both bedaquiline and delamanid are not currently recommended in pregnancy. Both delamanid and bedaquiline may have to be used for more than 24 weeks in many pre-XDR and XDR-TB patients with few options, as removing these drugs may then compromise therapy.

Two formalized clinical trials assessing the safety and efficacy of the combination have recently started enrolling: The US National Institutes of Health's AIDS Clinical Trials Group protocol ACTG5343, which will evaluate the safety, tolerability, and pharmacokinetics of bedaquiline and delamanid alone and in combination; and the endTB trial, which is a randomized, controlled, open-label, Phase III trial evaluating the efficacy of several regimens for the treatment of MDR-TB, including the one combining bedaquiline and delamanid. The results of these trials, however, are expected only in three to five years.

Study name	Description	Aim	Experimental arm	Phase and number of patients	Status
MDR-END NCT02619994 Seoul National University Hospital	Open-label randomized control phase 2 study Assessment of standard treatment regimen of anti-tuberculosis drugs for patients with RR but FQ-susceptible TB	Comparison of a standard MDR/XDR TB regimen (containing an injectable) and 9–12 month (all oral) delamanid-containing regimen	Dld + Lzd + Lfx + Z	Phase 2 238 patients Duration 9–12 months according to treatment response	Recruitment ongoing. Results expected 2019
NeXT NCT02454205, PACTR201409000848428 University of Cape Town Bedaquiline	Open-label phase 3 randomized control trial Investigating a new treatment regimen for patients with MDR tuberculosis: a prospective open-label randomized controlled trial	Open-label RCT of a 6–9-month injection-free regimen containing bedaquiline, linezolid, levofloxacin, ethionamide or high-dose isoniazid, and pyrazinamide	Lzd + Bdq + Lfx + Z + (Eto or hH or Tzd, according to genotype)	Phase 3 300 patients Duration 6–9 months according to treatment response	Recruitment ongoing. Results expected 2019
STAND NCT02342886 Global alliance for TB Drug Development Pretomanid	A phase 3 open-label, partially randomized trial to assess the efficacy, safety, and tolerability of the combination of moxifloxacin plus PA-824 plus pyrazinamide after 4	Efficacy, safety, and tolerability of a combination of moxifloxacin, PA-824, and pyrazinamide treatments after 6 months of treatment in patients with MDR	Mfx + Pa + Z	Phase 3 1,500 cases Duration 26 weeks	Suspended recruitment due to episodes of severe liver toxicity

	and 6 months of treatment in adults with smear-positive pulmonary drug-sensitive tuberculosis, and after 6 months of treatment in adults with smear-positive pulmonary MDR tuberculosis	tuberculosis compared with a combination of moxifloxacin, PA-824, and pyrazinamide treatments in drug-sensitive tuberculosis subjects; there will be a comparator arm for MDR tuberculosis			
STREAM Stage 2 NCT02409290 IUATLD Bedaquiline	STREAM Stage 2 NCT02409290 IUATLD Bedaquiline	Comparison of a 6-month (containing an injectable) and 9-month (all oral) bedaquiline-containing regimen versus the WHO and Bangladesh regimen	Bdq + Lfx + Cfz + E + Z for 40 weeks; hH + Pro for 16 weeks Bdq + Lfx + Cfz + Z for 28 weeks; hH + Km for 8 weeks	Phase 3 1,155 patients 6 or 9 months	Recruitment ongoing. Expected completion 2021
NiX-TB NCT02333799 Global alliance for TB Drug Development Bedaquiline, pretomanid, linezolid	Phase 3 open-label trial assessing the safety and efficacy of bedaquiline plus PA-824 plus linezolid in subjects with pulmonary infection of either XDR tuberculosis, treatment-intolerant tuberculosis, or pre-XDR nonresponsive MDR tuberculosis	Study of bedaquiline, pretomanid, and linezolid in patients with XDR tuberculosis and MDR tuberculosis for 6 months with an option of 9 months' treatment	Bdq + Pa + Led	Phase 3 200 patients Duration 6–9 months according to treatment response	Recruitment ongoing. Results expected 2021

Diet in tuberculosis

Introduction

Contents and consistency of diet in a tuberculosis patient depend upon the severity of pathologic condition and acute or chronic status of the disease. The initial infection is found to be benign, mostly kept in check by the body's immune system. However, the acute phase is more exhaustive, having lesser wasting, with features of cough, high-grade fever, and increased cardiorespiratory activities as compared to the chronic illness, with low-grade fever, lower metabolic rate, and considerable wasting.

Dietary care

To have desirable weight gain, patients with chronic illness often require increased energy. Energy needs in the acute phase are also increased at least by 50% because of high temperature, tissue destruction, and higher requirement of calories due to restlessness.

Liberal intake of carbohydrates should be allowed. Simple sugars are assimilated into blood without any need of enzymes. Sweet preparations, potato, rice, wheat preparations, banana, grapes, dates, and chiku should be generously taken.

Protein intake replenishes and regenerates serum albumins; generally, nonvegetarian foods are high in protein, but legumes, ground nuts, leafy vegetables, and sprouted whole grain and moong are also useful.

Fats may be permitted but judiciously used, keeping in view the digestion capability of the individual. Iron supplement is necessary for hemoglobin levels. Calcium promotes healing of tuberculosis lesions. Milk, cheese, jaggery, and nuts are useful. Vitamin A, D, and E supplements are very useful.

Fluid intake is most important in TB patients for renal excretion of toxins of infection as well as eliminating the increased metabolic wastes resulting from high intake of protein. Fluids act as an essential carrier of other dietary constituents, are easy to take, and help in digestion and assimilation of nutrients with minimal mechanical activity in the body. The protective effect of fluids on the urinary tract from irritative, toxic, and inflammatory products being excreted cannot be underrated. Regular intake of fluids assumes further importance in clearing the daily intake of drugs, to enable to receive the next-day dose, since the treatment with multi-drug-dosage has to be given for a longer duration. Thus, fluids help in giving continuous dietary, energic, and necessary nutrients even in most debilitated and difficult patients who are unable to eat.

Comments

High proteins, high calorie, heavy fluids, and frequent diets are always good in the acute phase. Gradually, appetite and disturbed psyche needs personal touch in providing sour and salty mid-meals in between sweet meals. Fluid intake in the form of sweet and tasty drinks is very important.

References and suggested readings

1. López-López JP, Posada-Martínez EL, Saldarriaga C, Wyss F, Ponte-Negretti CI, Alexander B, Miranda-Arboleda AF, Martínez-Sellés M, Baranchuk A. Neglected Tropical Diseases, Other Infectious Diseases Affecting the Heart (the NET-Heart Project). Tuberculosis and the heart. J Am Heart Assoc. 2021 Apr 6;10(7):e019435. doi: 10.1161/JAHA.120.019435. Epub 2021 Mar 18. PMID: 33733808; PMCID: PMC8174360.
2. Antonio-Arques V, Franch-Nadal J, Caylà JA. Diabetes and tuberculosis: a syndemic complicated by COVID-19. Med Clin (Barc). 2021 Sep 24;157(6):288–293. English, Spanish. doi: 10.1016/j.medcli.2021.04.004. Epub 2021 May 6. PMID: 34049681; PMCID: PMC8101986.
3. Boom WH, Schaible UE, Achkar JM. The knowns and unknowns of latent mycobacterium tuberculosis infection. J Clin Invest. 2021 Feb 1;131(3): e136222. doi: 10.1172/JCI136222. PMID: 33529162; PMCID: PMC7843221.
4. Koegelenberg CFN, Schoch OD, Lange C. Tuberculosis: the past, the present and the future. Respiration. 2021;100(7):553–556. doi: 10.1159/000516509. Epub 2021 May 25. PMID: 34034257.

5. The Lancet Infectious Diseases. Tuberculosis and malaria in the age of COVID-19. Lancet Infect Dis. 2021 Jan;21(1):1. doi: 10.1016/S1473-3099(20)30946-4. PMID: 33357386; PMCID: PMC7758173.
6. Visca D, Ong CWM, Tiberi S, Centis R, D'Ambrosio L, Chen B, Mueller J, Mueller P, Duarte R, Dalcolmo M, Sotgiu G, Migliori GB, Goletti D. Tuberculosis and COVID-19 interaction: a review of biological, clinical and public health effects. Pulmonology. 2021 Mar–Apr;27(2):151–165. doi: 10.1016/j.pulmoe.2020.12.012. Epub 2021 Jan 22. PMID: 33547029; PMCID: PMC7825946.
7. Zhou J, Lv J, Carlson C, Liu H, Wang H, Xu T, Wu F, Song C, Wang X, Wang T, Qian Z. Trained immunity contributes to the prevention of *Mycobacterium tuberculosis* infection, a novel role of autophagy. Emerg Microbes Infect. 2021 Dec;10(1):578–588. doi: 10.1080/22221751.2021.1899771. PMID: 33666534; PMCID: PMC8018485.
8. Kanabalan RD, Lee LJ, Lee TY, Chong PP, Hassan L, Ismail R, Chin VK. Human tuberculosis and Mycobacterium tuberculosis complex: a review on genetic diversity, pathogenesis and omics approaches in host biomarkers discovery. Microbiol Res. 2021 May;246:126674. doi: 10.1016/j.micres.2020.126674. Epub 2021 Jan 29. PMID: 33549960.
9. Dian S, Ganiem AR, van Laarhoven A. Central nervous system tuberculosis. Curr Opin Neurol. 2021 Jun 1;34(3):396–402. doi: 10.1097/WCO.0000000000000920. PMID: 33661159; PMCID: PMC8283909.
10. Hamada Y, Getahun H, Tadesse BT, Ford N. HIV-associated tuberculosis. Int J STD AIDS. 2021 Aug;32(9):780–790. doi: 10.1177/0956462421992257. Epub 2021 Feb 20. PMID: 33612015; PMCID: PMC8236666.
11. Mpande CAM, Musvosvi M, Rozot V, Mosito B, Reid TD, Schreuder C, Lloyd T, Bilek N, Huang H, Obermoser G, Davis MM, Ruhwald M, Hatherill M, Scriba TJ, Nemes E; ACS Study Team. Antigen-specific T-cell activation distinguishes between recent and remote tuberculosis infection. Am J Respir Crit Care Med. 2021 Jun 15;203(12):1556–1565. doi: 10.1164/rccm.202007-2686OC. PMID: 33406011; PMCID: PMC8483229.
12. Kohli M, Schiller I, Dendukuri N, Yao M, Dheda K, Denkinger CM, Schumacher SG, Steingart KR. Xpert MTB/RIF Ultra and Xpert MTB/RIF assays for extrapulmonary tuberculosis and rifampicin resistance

in adults. Cochrane Database Syst Rev. 2021 Jan 15;1(1):CD012768. doi: 10.1002/14651858.CD012768.pub3. PMID: 33448348; PMCID: PMC8078545.

13. Fatima S, Bhaskar A, Dwivedi VP. Repurposing immunomodulatory drugs to combat tuberculosis. Front Immunol. 2021 Apr 13;12:645485. doi: 10.3389/fimmu.2021.645485. PMID: 33927718; PMCID: PMC8076598.
14. Sinha P, Lönnroth K, Bhargava A, Heysell SK, Sarkar S, Salgame P, Rudgard W, Boccia D, Van Aartsen D, Hochberg NS. Food for thought: addressing undernutrition to end tuberculosis. Lancet Infect Dis. 2021 Oct;21(10):e318–e325. doi: 10.1016/S1473-3099(20)30792-1. Epub 2021 Mar 23. PMID: 33770535; PMCID: PMC8458477.
15. Ordonez AA, Tucker EW, Anderson CJ, Carter CL, Ganatra S, Kaushal D, Kramnik I, Lin PL, Madigan CA, Mendez S, Rao J, Savic RM, Tobin DM, Walzl G, Wilkinson RJ, Lacourciere KA, Via LE, Jain SK. Visualizing the dynamics of tuberculosis pathology using molecular imaging. J Clin Invest. 2021 Mar 1;131(5):e145107. doi: 10.1172/JCI145107. PMID: 33645551; PMCID: PMC7919721.
16. Allué-Guardia A, Saranathan R, Chan J, Torrelles JB. Mycobacteriophages as potential therapeutic agents against drug-resistant tuberculosis. Int J Mol Sci. 2021 Jan 13;22(2):735. doi: 10.3390/ijms22020735. PMID: 33450990; PMCID: PMC7828454.

https://doi.org/10.1142/9789811271410_0027

27 Lungs in HIV

Introduction

The lung is a very common organ involved in HIV infections due to the fact that it is continuously exposed to ambient air replete with a large number of organisms capable of causing infection in humans. A reduced ability to combat these infections will lead to infection and disease with a large number of opportunistic infections, cancers and other lung diseases, which is the focus of this chapter. HIV infection can affect any part of the lung, including parenchyma, interstitium, pulmonary blood vessels, airways, and even pleura. The common diseases are infections (*Pneumocystis jirovecii, Mycobacterium tuberculosis, Mycobacterium avium*, various bacterial infections, various viral infections, fungal infections, and parasitic infections), cancers, and other lung diseases such as the lymphocytic interstitial pneumonia.

The burden of HIV-associated lung disorder has changed in the past few decades. This is because of the introduction of co-trimoxazole prophylaxis therapy and highly effective antiretroviral therapy (like HAART). The total number of people living with HIV (PLHIV) in India was estimated at 23.19 lakh (18.33–29.78 lakh) in 2020.

Pneumocystis carinii pneumonia/*P. jirovecii* pneumonia

The first report of infection with *P. carinii* was reported in humans in 1942, and they have significantly increased after the onset of HIV infection. The terminology has been modified, and *P. carinii* is now termed as *P. jirovecii.*

This was changed to differentiate the organism *Pneumocystis* that infects rats (*P. carinii*) from that infecting humans (*P. jirovecii*). *Pneumocystis carinii* pneumonia (PCP) is an opportunistic infection, and studies have shown that a significant reduction or altered function of the T helper lymphocytes leads to the disease. Though the most common cause of PCP in humans is HIV, individuals with defective T helper cells that are acquired secondary to cancers (e.g., Hodgkin's lymphoma) or medications such as immunosuppressant drugs (steroids and anticancer drugs) are at risk of PCP. Clinical studies suggest that PCP is mostly due to the reactivation of an asymptomatic infection. Similar to tuberculosis in high-endemic countries, *Pneumocystis* is acquired during childhood. The classical clinical features include an increasing shortness of breath, which is usually exertional to begin with and progresses to severe dyspnea at rest. This is usually accompanied by a nonproductive cough, which can be severe in some cases. Dyspnea is usually accompanied with hypoxia. These classical symptoms are usually preceded by several days or weeks of fever, malaise, tiredness, and even weight loss.

The gold standard for the diagnosis is the identification of the organism by either a bronchoalveolar lavage or a lung biopsy. Immunofluorescent staining of induced sputum could be used. When facilities are not available, then one could attempt empirical therapy on clinical diagnosis which is a 4% drop in oxygen saturation on exertion in a patient with HIV or immunosuppressive conditions. This suggest interstitial involvement and can be seen also in other conditions such as cytomegalovirus (CMV) pneumonia in HIV patients. If the clinical diagnosis is correct, with appropriate treatment, subjects usually start improving by the third to fifth day. Treatment should be started at the earliest when PCP is suspected. The drug of choice is trimethoprim–sulfamethoxazole (trimethoprim 5 mg–sulfamethoxazole 25 mg/kg/day every 6 hours). The second drug of choice is intravenous pentamidine (4 mg/kg/day). In moderate to severe cases, there is a role for adjunctive steroid therapy, which has been shown to improve survival. The presence of severe hypoxia, respiratory failure, and pneumothorax worsens the prognosis. The usual duration of the treatment is 21 days and is generally effective. The infection, however, remains and can recur. Therefore, every subject treated for PCP should continue prophylaxis with one double strength tablet daily. This has been shown to reduce recurrence of PCP by more than 85%. Prophylaxis can also be given by using aerosolized pentamidine, which increases the risk of pneumothorax as well as extrapulmonary infection.

M. avium and other nontuberculous mycobacteria

These infections have gained prominence in the past couple of decades due to their occurrence in not only HIV patients but also other immunosuppressed conditions such as cystic fibrosis, malignancies, chemotherapy, and transplant recipients. Clinical presentation usually involves lymphatic involvement, pulmonary involvement, or both and is rarely disseminated or have systemic symptoms. The disease progresses insidiously and is rarely acute. Lymph nodes involvement is usually in the head and neck region and rarely mediastinal, is unilateral (in around 95%) and nontender, and have the potential to enlarge rapidly. Rupture of these lymph nodes when left untreated is a risk and leads to sinus tracts that takes a long time to heal. The symptoms of nontuberculous mycobacteria (NTM) involving the lungs are nonspecific and similar to pulmonary tuberculosis and other indolent infections. Chronic cough is the most common symptom along with expectoration, tiredness, malaise, shortness of breath, fever, chest pain, hemoptysis, chest pain, and loss of weight, especially more than 20%; systemic symptoms can progressively become more distressing with extensive disease. Clinical findings include rhonchi and crepitations and bronchial breathing when there is a consolidation or a cavity. The classic radiologic features of the NTM lung disease include fibro-cavitary lesions (usually thin-walled cavities), or small nodules (<5 mm) and bronchiectasis and pleural involvement can be observed. Sometimes, a dense consolidation or even a solitary pulmonary nodule can be observed. Pleural effusion is uncommon, and the pulmonary involvement is usually in the mid and lower lung zones unlike the usual pulmonary tuberculosis.

The diagnosis of MAC and other NTM involves a combination of clinical and microbiologic investigations. The clinical criteria include the presence of respiratory symptoms such as cough sputum, dyspnea, and hemoptysis; presence of nodular or cavitary opacities on chest X-ray or CT scan; and presence of multifocal bronchiectasis on HRCT along with multiple small nodules. It is important to exclude other possible diagnosis including *M. tuberculosis* hominis infection. The microbiologic criteria include a positive culture from two separate sputum samples or a positive culture result from bronchial lavage specimen or a transbronchial or lung biopsy with a positive culture for NTM and presence of histopathologic features suggestive of a mycobacterial infection such as a granulomatous inflammation or presence of AFB.

Bacterial infections

The most common pulmonary infection in an HIV patient is a bacterial infection, with more than 10 times increased incidence as compared to a non-HIV patient. Other than the HIV infection, these subjects have other risk factors, which may further accentuate the risk; smoking increases the risk of bacterial pneumonia fivefold; older age, IV drug use, and previous pneumonia are other risk factors. The most common organism is the *Streptococcus pneumoniae*, followed by *Haemophilus influenzae*, *Staphylococcus aureus*, and Gram-negative bacteria. Greater risk is observed in HIV patients with lower CD4 counts. Most bacterial pneumonia cases are seen in subjects with a CD4 count less than 400 cells/mm^3. It is observed that the bacterial pneumonia risk is increased with a greater viral load and reduction of the viral load with treatment (HAART) reduces the risk of bacterial pneumonia. Even in patients with CD4 counts above 500 cells/mm^3, antiretroviral treatment reduced the risk of pneumonia. Compared to non-HIV patients, the incidence of pneumococcal bacteremia is high in HIV patients, with some studies observing greater than 50% of their study subjects. The role of pneumococcal vaccination in preventing bacterial pneumonia still needs to be resolved; while majority of studies reported benefit, some studies reported an increase in incidence of pneumonia after vaccination. *Haemophilus* pneumonia is the second most common cause of bacterial pneumonia among HIV patients, and the course can be atypical, with 30% reporting sub-acute clinical presentation, and more than 50% of patients have bilateral pneumonia. It is seen in HIV patients with advanced disease. *S. aureus* and *Pseudomonas aeruginosa* are seen as community-acquired pneumonia in HIV patients and are associated with high risk of mortality. Staph is the third most common bacterial pneumonia in HIV patients, and *Pseudomonas* infections is usually seen in subjects with very low CD4 counts. *Legionella* infections are uncommon but are reported in greater frequency among HIV patients than non-HIV patients. Rarely *Rhodococcus equi* and *Nocardia* are reported as causes of pneumonia as are *Mycoplasma pneumoniae* and *Chlamydia pneumoniae.* The clinical course of bacterial pneumonia is similar in HIV patients to non-HIV patients with greater risk of bacteremia and bilateral lung lesions. Staph and *Pseudomonas* may present with cavitary lung lesions.

Viral infections

Seasonal viral infections are common among patients with HIV infection, and the most common virus is the *Influenza* virus, and the patients are at a higher risk of complications, especially if they are not on HAART. Subjects who are treated well have similar risks of complications to influenza (even with infections with the pandemic H1N1 virus) as compared to non-HIV patients. Annual influenza vaccines are recommended according to the CDC guidelines. Systematic reviews have observed that it is useful to give vaccinations to HIV patients in spite of variable antibody responses. Parainfluenza virus and metapneumovirus are also the important causes of virus infections along with respiratory syncytial virus and adenoviruses similar to the normal population. CMV is an important cause of morbidity and mortality in HIV patients especially in those with very low CD4 counts. CMV has retinitis and gastroenteritis as common manifestations, but also pneumonitis, usually seen when the CD4 counts are below 50 cells/mm^3. The problem is accentuated when there is a coinfection with both *P. jirovecii* and CMV. Diagnosis of CMV infection as a cause of pneumonitis is difficult and would need isolation of CMV from BAL fluid, characteristic cytopathic changes in the lungs that is associated with CMV and identification of CMV inclusion bodies.

Fungal infections

The most common fungal infections causing pneumonia in HIV patients are *Histoplasma*, *Coccidioides*, and *Blastomyces*, and the most common route of reaching the lung is by inhalation. Pneumonia can be either due to the reactivation of a latent infection, which can occur years after moving away from an endemic region, or due to a new infection. The disseminated forms of these fungal infections occur in HIV patients with CD4 counts <100 cells/mm^3, while the localized forms can be seen in HIV patients with CD4 counts even above 250 cells/mm^3. Blastomycosis is rarer than histoplasmosis and coccidioidomycosis, but it is associated with poor prognosis. The main treatment of all these infections are amphotericin B followed by triazoles such as itraconazole for a long-term such as 1 year or more. *Penicillium marneffei* is endemic in countries such as China and India, but it is not seen in western countries. Cryptococcal pneumonia presents as bilateral interstitial infiltrates similar to the picture seen in PCP patients. Rarely, the lesions can be unilateral, associated with nodules, cavitation, and hilar lymphadenopathy. Culture can be positive in sputum or in BAL. CSF testing for cryptococcal antigen and culture must be done in suspected cases, along with blood cultures, which are positive in nearly three-fourths of subjects. Treatment is with amphotericin B along with flucytosine, followed by fluconazole. Invasive aspergillosis can be seen in severely immunosuppressed HIV patients (<100 CD4 cells/mm^3) but is reduced after the advent of HAART.

Parasitic infections

These are important causes of mortality and morbidity among HIV patients, and the most common organisms implicated are *Cryptosporidium*, *Microsporidium*, *Strongyloides stercoralis*, and *Toxoplasma gondii*. The most common cause of pneumonia due to parasitic infection is *T. gondii* and is usually seen in HIV patients with CD4 counts less than 100 cells/mm^3 and is usually due to the reactivation of a latent infection. The clinical presentation is similar to many other pulmonary infections in HIV patients such as tuberculosis, nontuberculous mycobacteria, PCP, and fungal infections such as histoplasmosis and cryptococcosis. The radiologic features include bilateral lung infiltrates, which can be either fine or coarse nodular pattern. Diagnosis is confirmed by a positive IgG antibody to *T. gondii*, and a high degree of suspicion is needed. Sometimes, bronchoscopy and BAL may be needed to confirm the diagnosis. Other parasitic infections such as *Strongyloides*, *Cryptosporidium*, and *Microsporidium* usually present as disseminated infections.

Table 1: Prevalence of opportunistic infections affecting the lung in patients with HIV

Organism	Brief clinical presentation	CD4 counts below which the infection is likely to occur
Mycobacterium tuberculosis	Productive cough for more than 2 weeks, continuous fever, night sweats	250–500
Pneumocystis carnii/ Pneumocystis jiroveci	Progressive dyspnea Weight loss Fever Chills Nonproductive cough	75–125. 100–200 cells/μL = risk; 100–200 cells/μL + ART = lower risk. Rarely occurs when CD4 counts more than 250/μL

Table 1: (*Continued*)

Organism	Brief clinical presentation	CD4 counts below which the infection is likely to occur
Mycobacterium avium intracellulare (disseminated)	High-grade fever, night sweats, chills, body pain, diarrhea	75–125
Streptococcus pneumoniae	Pneumonia: breathlessness, woody dullness upon percussion, fever	If <200 cells/μL, then 4 times risk as compared to >500 cells/μL
Staphylococcus aureus	Symptoms of pneumonia	<185/μL
Haemophilus influenzae	Pneumonia	200–250/μL
Pseudomonas aeruginosa	Pneumonia, history of indwelling central venous catheters and/or chronic steroid use, cavitary lesions on radiograph	<50/μL
Influenza virus	Cough with green/yellow sputum, fever, chills, fatigue, sweating, cyanosis	No data
Cytomegalovirus	Fever, progressive dyspnea, hypoxemia	No data
Adenovirus	Fever, shortness of breath, myalgia, chills, sore throat, chest pain, pneumonia	No data

(*Continued*)

Table 1: (*Continued*)

Organism	Brief clinical presentation	CD4 counts below which the infection is likely to occur
Toxoplasma gondii	Febrile illness associated with unspecific respiratory involvement like cough and dyspnea. Cough is nonproductive unless there is a coinfection with other microbes. Lymphadenopathy may also provide nonspecific clues to diagnosis.	<100 cells/μL
Strongyloides stercoralis	Progressive dyspnea, dry cough, epigastric pain, diarrhea, weight loss, dry bibasilar end inspiratory crackles	GI infection can be expected at CD4 counts of <250/μL. Therefore, pulmonary manifestations can also be expected below this count.
Cryptococcus neoformans	Cough, shortness of breath, chest pain, fever	<200/μL
Histoplasma capsulatum	Fever, chills, dry cough, headache, muscle soreness, chest discomfort	<50/μL

Table 1: (*Continued*)

Organism	Brief clinical presentation	CD4 counts below which the infection is likely to occur
Penicillium marneffei	Cough, fever, dyspnea, chest pain, symptoms of reticuloendothelial system infection like generalized lymphadenopathy, hepatosplenomegaly	<200/μL
Nocardia		<200/μL

Table 2: First-line and alternative treatment strategies for the common lung infections seen in HIV patients

Organism	First-line drugs	Alternative drugs
Mycobacterium Tuberculosis	Multidrug therapy as per national programme. Isoniazid, Rifampicin, pyrazinamide, ethambutol (NTEP guidelines)	Streptomycin, levofloxacin, ethionamide, PAS
Pneumocystis carnii/ Pneumocystis jiroveci	Trimethoprim–sulfamethoxazole (TMP–SMZ)	Pentamidine, dapsone with trimethoprim, clindamycin with primaquine, and atovaquone
Mycobacterium avium intracellulare (disseminated)	Multidrug therapy, clarithromycin, ethambutol, levofloxacin (+rifabutin)	

(*Continued*)

Table 2: (*Continued*)

Organism	First-line drugs	Alternative drugs
Streptococcus pneumonia	Oral beta-lactam plus (high-dose amoxicillin or amoxicillin-clavulanate) an oral macrolide (azithromycin or clarithromycin) IV therapy if pneumonia is severe	Respiratory fluoroquinolone if TB is not suspected (moxifloxacin or levofloxacin) Doxycycline + beta-lactam when there is macrolide resistance
Staphylococcus aureus	Vancomycin or linezolid should be added to the antibiotic regimen	
Hemophilus influenza	Oral beta-lactam plus (high-dose amoxicillin or amoxicillin-clavulanate) and oral macrolide (azithromycin or clarithromycin) IV therapy if pneumonia is severe	Respiratory fluoroquinolone if TB is not suspected (moxifloxacin or levofloxacin) Doxycycline + beta-lactam when there is macrolide resistance.
Pseudomonas aeruginosa	Antipneumococcal, antipseudomonal beta-lactam plus either ciprofloxacin or levofloxacin (750-mg dose) should be used. Preferred beta-lactams are piperacillin-tazobactam, cefepime, imipenem, or meropenem	Antipneumococcal, antipseudomonal beta-lactam plus an aminoglycoside and azithromycin Antipneumococcal, antipseudomonal beta-lactam plus an aminoglycoside and an antipneumococcal fluoroquinolone

Table 2: (*Continued*)

Organism	First-line drugs	Alternative drugs
		In patients who are allergic to penicillin, aztreonam is recommended to be used in place of the beta-lactam
Influenza virus	Oseltamivir	
Cytomegalovirus	Oral valganciclovir or intravenous ganciclovir	IV foscarnet and IV cidofovir
Adenovirus	Supportive and symptomatic therapy	
Toxoplasma gondii	Pyrimethamine + sulfadiazine + leucovorin	Pyrimethamine + clindamycin + leucovorin TMP-SMX atovaquone
Strongyloides stercoralis	Ivermectin	Albendazole
Cryptococcus neoformans	Induction therapy: IV amphotericin B + oral flucytosine Consolidation and maintenance therapy: fluconazole	Fluconazole + flucytosine Mild to moderate symptoms with focal pulmonary involvement: fluconazole
Histoplasma capsulatum	Intravenous (IV) liposomal amphotericin B/standard IV amphotericin B	Oral itraconazole
Penicillium marneffei	Amphotericin B	Itraconazole, voriconazole
Nocardia		

Table 3: Effect of HIV on the lung

Pathology	Mechanism
1. Recurrent pneumonia	Low $CD4^+$ count
2. Emphysema	Recurrent bacterial infection, ART use (1)
3. Pleural effusion	Parapneumonic effusion
4. Asthma	RANTES and macrophage inflammatory protein-1α and –1β release during inflammation (2)
5. Lung cancer	Recurrent pneumonia
6. Pulmonary hypertension	Endothelial dysfunction by HIV Nef protein (3)

Table 4: Radiologic manifestations of different opportunistic infections affecting the lung in HIV patients

Organism	Typical, chest X-ray, CT thorax	Atypical, chest X-ray, CT thorax
1. *Pneumocystis jiroveci*	Normal X-ray, diffuse interstitial infiltrates, cavities, lung cysts, pneumothorax	Pleural effusion, focal infiltrates, lymphadenopathy, nodular lesions
2. *Mycobacterium tuberculosis*	Cavities, hilar lymphadenopathy, diffuse infiltrates, military nodules	
3. *Aspergillus*	Invasion, halo sign, cavities, air crescent sign, finger in glove sign	Nodular lesions, pleural effusion
4. *Toxoplasma gondii*	Diffuse infiltrates	Pleural effusion, lymphadenopathy
5. *Streptococcus pneumoniae*	Consolidation	
6. *Candida*	Focal or diffuse infiltrates, nodular infiltrates	Pleural effusion
7. SARS COV-2	Peripheral ground glass opacities with consolidation	Pneumothorax, pleural effusion
8. Nontubercular mycobacterium	Normal X-ray, cavities, diffuse infiltrates	Pleural effusion
9. *Cryptococcus*	Reticulonodular opacities, nodules	Lymphadenopathy, pleural effusion, miliary nodules

Table 5: Cancers in the lung due to HIV, clinical and radiologic presentations

Cancers in the lung	Clinical presentations (including at what CD4 counts)	Radiologic presentations
Kaposi's sarcoma		Plain radiograph reveals peribronchovascular thickening, extending from the hila to the periphery as the disease progresses. Then, this thickening becomes nodular. Findings also include areas of consolidation, developing from coalescence of nodules. Middle and lower lobes are most commonly involved. CT features are bronchial wall thickening, speculated nodules 1–2 cm in diameter, thickening of the interlobular septae, which may be smooth or nodular, unilateral or bilateral pleural effusion (35%–50%), and hilar and mediastinal lymphadenopathy (16%), as an advanced manifestation of the disease
Lymphoma	Non-Hodgkin's lymphoma: this is the most common (70%); it occurs with CD4 count <100 cells/mm^3, and it has a high degree of malignancy.	Well-defined nodules greater than 1 cm in diameter, which are often peripheral and predominantly present in the lung bases

(Continued)

Table 5: (*Continued*)

	Hodgkin's lymphoma: it is less common and of early onset; it occurs with CD4 >200 cells/mm^3, and it has a high degree of malignancy and aggressive behavior.	
Carcinoma		Central or peripheral pulmonary mass associated with mediastinal adenopathy, atelectasis, and pleural effusion

Table 6: Noninfectious and noncancerous manifestation of the lung in patients with HIV

Noninfectious and noncancerous manifestation	Clinical features	Radiologic features
Lymphocytic interstitial pneumonitis	Gradually progressive dyspnea and cough. There will be diffuse infiltration of pulmonary lymphatics. There can be infiltration of parotid glands, liver, and bone marrow	CXR: reticular or reticulonodular infiltrates, predominantly in the lower zones, and consolidation CT: bilateral ground-glass opacity, poorly defined centrilobular nodules, subpleural and peribronchovascular nodules, air space consolidation, bronchiectasis, pleural thickening, and lymphadenopathy

Table 6: (*Continued*)

Noninfectious and noncancerous manifestation	Clinical features	Radiologic features
Bronchiolitis obliterans		Bilateral areas of parenchymal consolidation or ground-glass infiltrate in a geographical distribution Poorly defined nodular infiltrates, subtle diffuse reticular infiltrates, or scattered centrilobular nodules may be less commonly observed
Nonspecific interstitial pneumonitis	Diagnosis of NSIP should be considered when the patient fails to respond to treatment for infectious conditions	Diffuse interstitial infiltrate or bronchiectasis and less commonly alveolar infiltrate

HIV disease and pleural effusion

Introduction

Pleural effusion in HIV disease is not uncommon; association of pleural effusion is more with the advanced stages of HIV disease. Although the etiology may remain obscure in a few cases, diagnosis can be made in most of these patients, pinpointing infective or noninfective etiology in almost one-third and two-thirds of cases, respectively.

Infective etiology of pleural effusion

Pleural effusion is present in association with AIDS, in infections causing pulmonary infiltration. Pleural effusion is present in almost one-third of cases of bacterial pneumonia in HIV disease. In 50% of cases, *S. pneumoniae* is responsible for pneumonitis; *H. influenzae*, *M. pneumoniae*, *Legionella*, and *Nocardia asteroides* have also been implicated. Right-sided endocarditis may also lead to septic pulmonary embolization that may result in small pleural effusion; the effusions are small, ipsilateral, and exudative in nature with low nucleated cell count and rarely become empyematous, especially in parapneumonic effusions in AIDS. *S. aureus* may be responsible for life-threatening community-acquired pneumonia with parapneumonic effusion in association with HIV disease, with a history of intravenous drug users.

Precisely, 2%–11% of pleural effusion is observed in cases of *P. carinii* pneumoniae, more so in patients receiving aerosolized pentamidine therapy and is often accompanied with pleural masses or pneumothorax. The effusions are usually small, unilateral or bilateral, serous or bloody in nature, with raised LDH levels, having a fluid-to-serum ratio of more than 1.0 (i.e., exudate in nature) and without any acidosis or alteration in fluid amylase and glucose levels. Total nucleated cell count in the fluid is low with predominant mononuclear cells. Trophozoites of *P. carinii* in the fluid can be demonstrated by Grocott silver staining; however, examination of an air-dried Diff-Quick-stained cytospin preparation is ideal. Pleural fluid demonstrates numerous vacuolated macrophages, granular eosinophilic aggregates, and scattered benign mesothelial cell clusters. Occurrence of pleural effusion does not alter the prognosis of the PCP, although the occurrence of pneumothorax often means prolonged drainage of the indwelling chest tube.

Tuberculous pleural effusion accounts for 10% of cases with AIDS, and the effusion is usually a larger one. Accompanying miliary or pulmonary parenchymal infiltration may be present. This exudative fluid has neither fluid acidosis nor low glucose levels. Nucleated cell count is low in the fluid with predominance of lymphocytes: AFB positivity in the fluid is less than 15%. Pleural biopsy reveals granulomatous lesion in almost 90% of cases. Tuberculin positivity is varying from 20% to 64%.

In cryptococcal neoformans in HIV disease, pleural effusion in an isolated finding, but often it represents disseminated cryptococcal disease in AIDS patients. Fluid is exudative with low count of nucleated cells.

Cryptococcal antigen determination in the fluid is a rapid and specific test

Pleural effusion with *Histoplasma capsulatum* in AIDS patients is rare, and occurs with disseminated disease, contiguous spread, hypersensitivity pleuritis, or active pericarditis. Effusion is serosanguinous with low number of nucleated cells. Wright–Giemsa staining demonstrates intracellular yeast, typical of *H. capsulatum.*

Unilateral or bilateral pleural effusion may rarely be seen in *T. gondii* infection in late stages of AIDS. *T. gondii* trophozoites within the neutrophils can be demonstrated by Giemsa staining in the centrifuged pleural fluid.

Noninfective pleural etiology

Hypoalbuminemic pleural effusion may occur in progressive HIV disease. These are moderate-sized transudates that occur bilaterally. Nucleated cells are low in the fluid, with predominant mononuclear cells.

Isolated pleural effusion is a sole presentation of AIDS-related lymphoma, occurring in 5%–10% of cases. Thoracic involvement in AIDS-related lymphoma is uncommon with the absence of mediastinal and hilar involvement of lymph nodes. Such an effusion is unilateral and larger one, serosanguinous exudate with normal glucose contents and lymphocytic predominance.

Pleural pulmonary involvement is seen in one-fifth of cases of AIDS with Kaposi's sarcoma, and 60% of these cases have pleural effusion. Cutaneous and thoracic involvement may not correlate, and pleuritic pain may be absent because of the involvement of the visceral pleura and sparing of the parietal pleura. Unilateral or bilateral alveolar or interstitial involvement is present along with hilar or mediastinal lymphadenopathy in 25%–60% of cases. Effusions are large and predominantly bilateral. Autopsy findings reveal bilateral hemorrhagic pleural effusions, visceral pleural purplish lesions of Kaposi's sarcoma, and infiltration of lung parenchymal lymphatics and mediastinal lymph nodes. Bleeding from highly vascular visceral pleural lesions make the fluid serosanguinous that gets complicated because of impaired drainage, secondary to the obstruction of lymphatics. Nucleated cell count in the fluid is low, with predominance of mononuclear cells. The fluid is exudative, pH being more than 7.4, with higher glucose contents and LDH levels varying from 111 to 3,301 U/L. Percutaneous pleural biopsy is noncontributory (because of the absence of a lesion on the parietal pleura). Open lung biopsy is diagnostic in more than three-fourths of cases but not recommended for being highly risky. Bronchoscopy demonstrates diagnostic cherry-red endobronchial lesions in a patient with bilateral hemorrhagic pleural effusion in cases of Kaposi's sarcoma.

Pleural effusion due to congestive cardiac failure may occur in AIDS patients, due to cardiomyopathy, usually caused by infectious myocarditis with toxoplasmosis, CMV, and human immunodeficiency virus. These are small transudates, unilateral or bilateral, and usually resolve following the treatment of cardiac failure.

Management: Infection is empirically treated in intravenous drug abusers in bacterial pneumonia. PCP is managed with intravenous pentamidine, supplemented with aerosolized pentamidine. TB is treated with full-dose, four-drug regimen for 9–12 months. Amphotericin B is useful in treating *C. neoformans* infection in HIV disease. *H. capsulatum* pleural effusion resolves spontaneously. Effusion with lymphoma in HIV disease responds to chemotherapy. Treatment of pleural effusion with Kaposi's sarcoma is symptomatic; radiation may offer palliative management. Tetracycline pleurodesis is effective. Alpha interferon or combined chemotherapy gives partial relief. Transudate effusion resolves by itself when heart failure is treated.

Tuberculosis and HIV disease

TB is the most common opportunistic infection amongst HIV-infected individuals. HIV-infected persons have eight times greater risk of TB. Two million people are living with HIV in India. The adult HIV prevalence in India is of 0.27%. The dual infection adds morbidity, where HIV infection helps in spreading the tuberculosis, and the interaction between the two has lethal implications. Tuberculosis in HIV disease brings forth many issues such as atypical presentations posing diagnostic difficulties, drug–drug interaction, and paradoxical reactions posing treatment difficulties and emerging MDR-TB and occurrence of polymicrobial infections such as *P. carinii* pneumonia, CMV, and other bacterial infections posing management difficulties, especially in the advanced disease. Tuberculosis assumes particular importance for its contagious spread by inhalation and as it is readily treatable with the current effective drugs that are required to be used effectively in full dose and for appropriate duration.

Introduction

Poor and (over) populated societies have high prevalence of tuberculosis, even up to 80% of adults carrying TB germ in overcrowded cities of some developing countries.[1] In addition, 9% of the total 8.3 million new TB adult cases are attributable to HIV infection; the risk of developing active TB is increased by 25–30 times than those with *Mycobacterium* infection alone.[2] Again, out of 1.8 million deaths this from TB, 12% are attributable to HIV, where TB remains the immediate cause of adult deaths in AIDS.[3] Out of 52,000 deaths due to TB every week, more than 40% occur in Southeast Asia. Tuberculosis is a major health problem in Southeast Asia,[4] infecting 40%–50% of nearly 6 million adults living with HIV disease in this region. Due to the interaction of HIV and TB, prevalence of extrapulmonary TB may increase from 15% to up to 70%, especially when CD cell count is decreased to 100 cells/mm.[4–6] Diagnostic difficulties of TB in HIV disease occur because of the following features such as extrapulmonary

Table 7: Chest X-ray finding in pulmonary TB in association with HIV infection

Hilar lymphadenopathy	42%
Pleural effusion	29%
Liner lobe infiltrates	25%
Miliary pattern	13%
Cavitation	0.6%

presentation, AFB negativity, tuberculin test negativity or weak response, and lower and middle zone involvement. There is an increased risk to community along with concomitant emergence of MDR-TB.[7]

Due to constraints of laboratory facilities in India, a highly sensitive tuberculin test can be used positively with a cut-off criterion of 2 mm induration[8] for the early detection of mycobacterial infection amongst HIV-positive individuals, especially when the CD cell count is not possible.[9] The positive tuberculin test when stratified by induration measured reveals positivity of the test (**2 mm induration**) in HIV-positive cases in 80% as compared to 24% in HIV-negative cases. Clinical features are most atypical, where lungs are less affected and the disease is more disseminated to other organs. Chest X-ray findings are given in Table 7.

Sputum smear and stool smear are positive for AFB hardly in 40% of cases. This necessitates the need for more sensitive and rapid diagnostic tests. The dual infection has pulmonary involvement, in 74%–100% of cases, and physical findings are indistinguishable between those with and those without HIV infection, posing a lot of difficulty in differential diagnosis. Extrapulmonary involvement in the form of lymphadenitis, miliary or disseminated tuberculosis, has been included as AIDS indicator of disease in the Indian context HIV disease with tuberculosis can present as chronic meningitis with headache and altered sensorium. Fever and signs of meningeal irritation are less common.

	CD4 cell count	*>200 cells/mm*^{3}	*<200 cells/mm*^{3}
Clinical pattern of TB in HIV disease			
• **Involvement of CNS, testis, BM, liver, and soft tissue is also seen (tuberculomas)**			
• **Pleural effusion is more common** • **TB lymphadenopathy may be acute and resemble acute pyogenic lymphadenitis**			
• **Miliary TB**			
• **Diffuse pulmonary disease without cavitation involving lower lobes**			
• **Prominent mediastinal or Paratracheal adenopathy**			

Diagnosis

Diagnosis is difficult in AIDS since TB has unusual presentation and lacks simultaneous histologic reaction in some cases due to depressed cell-mediated immunity. Tuberculin test is no longer recommended for routine use in TB screening program of HIV-infected persons. The results of anergy testing using a panel of antigens give inconsistent and ambiguous observations. The test positivity of 5 mm^3 induration in HIV and TB coinfection with CD_4 count >500 cells/mm^3 as 50%–90% may fall to 0%–20% with CD cell count falling to less than 200 cells/mm^3. Those with relatively well-preserved cell immunity (manifested by a positive tuberculin test and lack of other HIV-associated infections) have chest findings that are similar to those of reactivation TB in immunocompetent patients, including cavitation and upper lobe infiltration. In contrast, those with immunosuppression due to HIV infection have chest findings that are typical of primary TB in immunocompetent patients such as hilar lymphadenopathy, miliary TB, and pleural effusion. Diseases other than TB can give both classical and atypical findings on chest X-ray, and in cases with sputum smear negativity, other differentials, especially the HIV-related pulmonary diseases such as bacterial pneumonia, *P. carinii* pneumonia, Kaposi's sarcoma, fungal infections, and nocardiosis have to be considered.

Sputum positivity for AFB may vary from 31% to 82%. The positivity of AR falls to 5% in HIV-infected patients with pulmonary tuberculosis, although it forms the cornerstone of diagnosis of TB even in high HIV prevalence areas. Additional growth from sputum on U medium and venous blood subjected to glutaraldehyde test which offers sensitivity of 85% and specificity of 95% for fresh TB cases. Both for pulmonary and extrapulmonary TB, auramine phenol (fluorescent staining) offers 87.5% sensitivity and 87% specificity as compared to simultaneous ZN staining showing 48% sensitivity and 94% specificity. All types of pleural involvement may occur. Those with isolated unilateral involvement may have better prognosis. Multi-drug-resistant TB (MDR-TB) is caused by a strain of *M. tuberculosis* that is resistant to two or more antitubercular drugs, usually isoniazid and rifampicin. It is a serious problem, and case fatality in HIV with MDR-TB is 70% in 4–6 weeks as compared to non-HIV with MDR-TB where it is 25%. MDR-TB associated with HIV infection is being labeled as the third epidemic' that is one of the most malignant of opportunistic infections.

Primary resistance in developing countries like India is 15%. Acquired resistance from initial response is constantly increasing, and this problems shall further worsen with HIV endemicity. In MDR-TB, risk factors include inadequate treatment, noncompliance, especially in lower socio-economic patients, presence of cavitary lesions, HIV infection, IV drug use, following anticancer therapy, and after organ transplant.

Mechanism of development of resistance includes:

(a) Natural resistance due to spontaneous mutation.
(b) Primary resistance through infection with resistant tubercle bacilli.
(c) Acquired resistance in those having inadequate therapy, this being the strongest predictor for MDR-TB.
(d) Initially, resistance may be seen in those who have taken the chemotherapy intentionally or unintentionally. Extrapulmonary disease are unintentional. Extrapulmonary diseases are up to 70% in HIV-related TB if the CD cell count is less than $100/mm^3$. Diagnosis of extrapulmonary TB is often difficult. Variety of diagnostic tests have to be indicated depending on the site of infection.

Pathogenesis

In an immunocompetent person on infection with tuberculosis, the organism is presented in the macrophage through ingestion; thereafter, the processed mycobacterial antigens are presented to T cells. The CD4 cells secrete lymphokines that enhance the capacity of macrophage to ingest and kill the mycobacteria. In majority of the people, the infection is contained, and TB does not develop, although a number of dormant bacilli remain in the body. Only 10% of cases develop clinical TB, soon after the primary infection or years later as reactivation TB. The consequences in the HIV-positive background are possibly due to defects in T cells and/or macrophages functions."

Progressive depletion and dysfunction of CD4 cells, coupled with defects in macrophage and monocyte function, form the hallmark of HIV infection. An epidemiological evidence favors that HIV infection increases the risk of late reactivation of TB and also the risk of progressive disease from a new infection.

Treatment

Treatment of TB aims at curing the patient along with minimizing the transmission of *M. tuberculosis* to the community. The recommendations for the treatment remain the same for TB in HIV-infected or uninfected patients.

Intermittent regimens are contraindicated, adherence strategies including DOTS are given importance, and drug–drug interaction is strictly observed for better compliance and results. Hepatotoxicity always looked for being a serious obstacle. Effective treatment with four drugs (rifampicin, isoniazid, ethambutol, and pyrazinamide) for 2 months, followed by three drugs for 7 months without pyrazinamide, gives 80% conversion after 3 months of treatment. However, relapses have been reported, but mortality, if occurs, is due to other opportunistic infections. Adverse reactions to drugs are more frequent in these cases; 90% of these occur in the 2 months. Anti-TB drugs are to be given first at least the 2 months intensive therapy, if not complete 9 months treatment, provided the CD4 cell count is more than 200/mm^3. But if the count is below 60/mm^3, ART has to be initiated. The attending physician must be watchful for paradoxical reaction or immune reconstitution inflammatory syndrome (IRIS). IRIS: incidence being 4%–45%, it is mainly studied in HIV-TB coinfection in India and occurs 15.2% annually. Mostly develop within 2 months of HAART initiation but can take up tp2 years. Classified as infectious, autoimmune, and sarcoid IRIS.

Major criteria

1. Reduction of plasma HIV RNA bylog
2. Tumors or atypical opportunistic infections such as (a) localised disease in lymph nodes, spleen, or liver, (b) high fever with painful lesions, (c) atypical inflammatory tissue response such as granuloma, suppuration/necrosis, or perivascular lymphocytic infiltration, and (d) progressive organ dysfunction, such as (1) development of SOL following the treatment of cerebral toxoplasmosis or cryptococcosis, (2) progressive or organizing pneumonia following the treatment of PCP or TB, (3) worsening of uveitis after resolution of CMV retinitis, (4) fever and cytopenia following MAC treatment, and (5) enlargement/spontaneous resolution (without treatment) of Kaposi's sarcoma.

Minor criteria

1. Increased CD cell count increase
2. Enhanced immune response specific to reactive antigen such as DTH or mycobacterial agent
3. Spontaneous resolution of the disease

Risk factors for IRIS

CD cell count <50 cells/mm

Presence of an opportunistic infection

Early initiation of HAART

Rapid HIV-RNA level suppression during the first 3 months of therapy

Clinical presentation of IRIS

• Fever
• Increase in size or development of lymphadenopathy
• Respiratory failure
• Appearance of new lesions or worsening of existing pulmonary infiltrates
• Worsening of pleuritic
• Pericarditis or ascites
• Disseminated skin lesions
• Hepatosplenomegaly

Cotrimoxazole prophylaxis therapy (CPT) for HIV-TB pts

1. **CPT reduces mortality and morbidity**
2. **Dosage: 160 mg TMP + 800 mg SMX daily**
3. **CPT is provided to patients in monthly pouches**
4. **Can be taken along with ATT and ART**

WHO policy — 3 I's

- **ICF = Intensified case finding**
- **IPT = Isoniazid prevention therapy**
- **IC = Infection control at all clinical encounters**

Unanswered question

Why improvement in immunity interacts with pathogens and that too, why only some people develop IRIS. Better understanding of pathogenesis will open newer preventive, modifying and therapeutic options to tackle IRIS. One NMRTI two NRTI has been suggested for Indian patients.[10] HAART is started only as soon as anti-TB therapy is tolerated.[11] Patients with CD4 cells count more than 200/mm^3 have a low risk. ZDV/dd1/3TC combination triple therapy is less potent, more complicating hepatotoxicity. ZD (or dMT) 3TC/EF2 is another option for patients being coadministered rifampicin. Another option for PI-containing combinations of ZDV/3TC/SQV/r or d4T/3TC/SQV/r with the concomitant use of rifampicin is in offering where the dose of ritonavir should be 400 mg twice a day. In treating MDR-TB, a five-drug regimen has been suggested, while treating MDR-TB in HIV patients, even six drugs have been suggested to be used. There is a need to add two new drugs instead of one.

A case–control study in a large New York City Hospital that included MDR-TB cases with and without HIV revealed that five- or six-drug combination that was used included either of the following additional drugs:

1. Capreomycin plus ciprofloxacin
2. Capreomycin plus cycloserine
3. Ciprofloxacin + cycloserine + capreomycin

In meningeal tuberculosis in HIV disease, in areas where initial resistance is less than 4%, three- to four-drug combination for a minimum of 12 months is necessary, but 50% of patients may need longer treatment which is essential because of concurrent HIV disease. In case of infection with MDR-TB, more than five drugs including ciprofloxacin, clofazimine, clarithromycin, or cyclosporine should be dispensed. It has to be differentiated from *M. avium* complex infection, typically presenting as mass lesions such as tuberculoma and cerebral or spinal cord abscess. Prevention of these infections, both TB and AIDS — the ancient and modern plagues which dare to raise their ugly heads — can only be done through public awareness and education regarding correct behavior and code of conduct in human sexual needs. While treating the patients with HIV disease, the aim is maximal suppression of HIV replication for as long as possible. Three-drug combination of two nucleoside analogues with a protease inhibitor (PI), initiated early in the course of HIV infection, forms the current standard care of HIV patients.

Combination of one NNRTI + two NRTI has been suggested for Indian patients 15b. HAART is started only when (as soon as) ATT is tolerated." Patients with CD cell count 200/mm^3 have a low risk.

Drug interaction is less pronounced with some PIs with rifabutin, but it is available only in resource limited setting. Paradoxical reaction/immune reconstitution inflammatory syndrome (IRIS) appears to occur more commonly on initiation of HAART and not because of anti-TB treatment, generally within 15 days (median) and mostly in patients with advanced HIV infection." This happens in 36% of patients receiving antiretroviral therapy along with anti-TB drugs as compared to 7%in patients receiving anti-TB drugs alone, in the form of worsening of pleuropulmonary lesions, cutaneous and psoas abscess, effusions in pleura, peritoneum and pericardium, tuberculoma, and lymphadenopathy. Life-threatening IRIS such as meningitis, raised intracranial tension, and pulmonary opacities leading to ARDS require urgent corticosteroids.

Chemoprophylaxis

Public education regarding correct sexual behavior forms the cornerstone in presenting this dual infection. Chemoprophylaxis of healthy contacts is highly important. Chemoprophylaxis with isoniazid alone may not look to be a prudent step. The criterion for a positive tuberculin test should be taken as 5-mm induration instead of 10 mm. So, the criteria for isoniazid chemoprophylaxis has been suggested to be either tuberculin test of more than 5-mm induration with 5 IU or CD cell count below 200/cu mm, and prophylaxis is recommended for 12 months for any person of any age. However, efficiency of rifampicin in combination with pyrazinamide for 2 months shows better compliance than that of rifampicin and isoniazid combination for 6 months chemoprophylaxis in preventing active TB in HIV seropositive.

Nosocomial infection of tuberculosis in indoor patients and in health care workers adds gravity to hospitalized morbidity and burden on health care agencies, respectively. These infections especially MDR-TB have been recorded even as an outbreak by CDC in the health department of Florida and New York City. That is why CDC and American Thoracic Society have recommended preventive therapy, especially in patients exposed to MDR-TB to decrease the risk of active disease. This includes the use of ciprofloxacin 750 mg BD or ofloxacin 400 mg or pyrazinamide 35 mg/kg/day for contacts deemed likely to be newly infected with MDR-TB and at high risk for active disease.

BCG is beneficial in HIV infection in preventing the TB infection and putting aside the theoretical fear of disseminating TB infection in HIV-infected infants. BCG vaccination should be given to all infants even when the mother is a known suspected case of HIV infection; however, BCG should be without from patients with symptomatic HIV infection.

AIDS vaccine trials and their evaluation have been entrusted to NARI of ICMR. There are certain difficulties such as maintenance of high-level immune response and variability of virus. Ideal HIV vaccine would be that which works against all the major five subtypes of the virus.[12,13] Trials have been started recently. We have to wait for their results.

India scenario

- **TB is the most common opportunistic infection amongst HIV-infected individuals**
- **HIV-infected persons have eight times greater risk of TB**
- **2.1 million people are living with HIV in India**
- **Adult HIV prevalence is of 0.27% in India**
- **TB accounts for 25% of deaths among PLHIV in India**
- **5% cases of incident TB have HIV**
- **HIV is not a predisposing factor for the development of MDR-TB**
- **MDR-TB is not more common in HIV infected**

HIV/TB policy 2013 salient features

- **All patients screened with four symptom-complex:**
  1. **Current cough of any duration**

2. Fever of any duration
3. Significant weight loss
4. Drenching night sweats

- Integrated HIV and TB services (e.g., HIV screening at RNTCP DMC)
- Focus on early detection and early care (all ICTC's and ART centers will do ICF for TB)
- Targeted intervention projects for high-risk groups like IV drug users
- CBNAAT use among PLHIV
- One-stop service — diagnostic facility for TB and HIV to be offered at same premises
- Single-window delivery services where all HIV/TB patients get TB medications from the ART center itself
- Travel support for patients going to ART centers via RNTCP
- Strengthening HIV testing in presumptive DR-TB cases
- Implementation of IPT for all PLHIV (on ART + pre-ART)
- Strengthening implementation of airborne infection control strategies
- PLHIV having DRTB are managed by DRTB center in consultation with ART center
- ART supply to all HIV-infected TB cases irrespective of CD4 count
- Prompt ART initiation — within the first eight weeks of starting ATT

Comments

Deficient-cell mediated immunity is the common denominator, both for tuberculosis and HIV disease. More than 50% of AIDS cases suffer from tuberculosis in India. HIV infection and tuberculosis relationship is exhibited in Table 8. Reactivation of tuberculosis is common in early HIV disease. Clinical presentation and response to antitubercular therapy is similar to non-HIV tubercular disease. Progressive HIV disease with severe immunodeficiency leads to extrapulmonary and disseminated tuberculosis requiring aggressive and prolonged treatment." Incidence of multi-drug-resistant tuberculosis has increased.

Table 8: Features of TB in HIV

More frequency of EPTB, especially lymph node
Involvement of CNS, testis, BM, liver, and soft tissue is also seen (tuberculomas)
Tb pleural effusion is more common
Cavitation involving lower lobes
Prominent mediastinal or paratracheal adenopathy
Tuberculin skin test negative
Sputum AFB maybe negative
MTB may be isolated from blood or feces

MAC infection is often a late opportunistic infection. HIV is not a predisposing factor for the development of MDR-TB. MDR-TB is not more common in HIV infected. A combination of six or even more drugs, including fluroquinolones, is recommended for combating MDR-tuberculosis." Although sparfloxacin has shown dose-related activity both in vivo and in vitro, a caution has been given to use in MDR-TB" only after extended human studies are undertaken. Many novel approaches are being explored, but prevention of MDR-TB is more important than treating the same.[14,15]

References and suggested readings

1. McCarthy GA, Mercey D. The changing clinical features of HIV-1 infection in the United Kingdom. Commun Dis Rep CDR Rev. 1994 Apr 29;4(5):R53–R58.
2. Wingfield T, Wilkins E. Opportunistic infections in HIV disease. Br J Nurs. 2010 Jun 27;19(10):621–627.
3. Poh KC, Zheng S. A rare case of CMV pneumonia in HIV-infection. Respir Med Case Rep. 2019;28:100945.
4. Velásquez JN, Ledesma BA, Nigro MG, Vittar N, Rueda N, De Carolis L, et al. Pulmonary toxoplasmosis in human immunodeficiency virus-infected patients in the era of antiretroviral therapy. Lung India. 2016 Feb;33(1):88–91.
5. Pomeroy C, Filice GA. Pulmonary toxoplasmosis: a review. Clin Infect Dis. 1992 Apr;14(4):863–870.

6. Capocci S, Lipman M. Respiratory infections in HIV-infected adults: epidemiology, clinical features, diagnosis and treatment. Curr Opin Pulm Med. 2013 May;19(3):238–243.
7. Everett CK, Subramanian A, Jarisberg LG, Fei M, Huang L. Characteristics of drug-susceptible and drug-resistant staphylococcus aureus pneumonia in patients with HIV. Epidemiology (Sunnyvale). 2013 May 6;3(1).
8. Jung AC, Paauw DS. Diagnosing HIV-related disease: using the CD4 count as a guide. J Gen Intern Med. 1998 Feb;13(2):131.
9. Mokhlesi B, Shulzhenko O, Garimella PS, Kuma L, Monti C. Pulmonary strongyloidiasis: the varied clinical presentations. Clin Pulm Med. 2004 Jan;11(1):6–13.
10. Almodovar S, Knight R, Allshouse AA, Roemer S, Lozupone C, McDonald D, Widmann J, Voelkel NF, Shelton RJ, Suarez EB, Hammer KW. Human immunodeficiency virus nef signature sequences are associated with pulmonary hypertension. AIDS Res Hum Retrovir. 2012 Jun 1;28(6):607–618.
11. Franquet T, Müller NL, Lee KS, Oikonomou A, Flint JD. Pulmonary candidiasis after hematopoietic stem cell transplantation: thin-section CT findings. Radiology. 2005 Jul;236(1):332–337.
12. Afione C, Sala AD, Frank L. Pulmonary manifestations in patients with AIDS. RAR. 2011;75(4).
13. Bhatia RS, Deivanygam CN. HIV disease-the great waster upon us (editorial). Lung India. 1992;10:91–93.
14. Mehta AA, et al. Diagnostic utility of ADA in exudative pleural effusion. Lung India. 2014;31:142–144.
15. How do TB and HIV infect in individuals. AIDS Update. 1996;2(2):1.
16. Vazquez Guillamet LJ, Saul Z, Miljkovich G, Vilchez GA, Mendonca N, Gourineni V, et al. Strongyloides stercoralis infection among human immunodeficiency virus (HIV)-infected patients in the United States of America: a case report and review of literature. Am J Case Rep. 2017 Apr 3;18:339–346.
17. Guidelines for the prevention and treatment of opportunistic infections in adults and adolescents with HIV. Available at: https://clinicalinfo.hiv.gov/en/guidelines/adult-and-adolescent-opportunistic-infection/.
18. Gingo MR, George MP, Kessinger CJ, Lucht L, Rissler B, Weinman R, Slivka WA, McMahon DK, Wenzel SE, Sciurba FC, Morris A. Pulmonary function

abnormalities in HIV-infected patients during the current antiretroviral therapy era. Am J Respir Crit. Care Med. 2010 Sep 15;182(6):790–796.
19. Kuhlman JE, Kavuru M, Fishman EK, Siegelman SS. Pneumocystis carinii pneumonia: spectrum of parenchymal CT findings. Radiology. 1990 Jun;175(3):711–714.
20. Cocchi F, DeVico AL, Garzino-Demo A, Arya SK, Gallo RC, Lusso P. Identification of RANTES, MIP-1α, and MIP-1β as the major HIV-suppressive factors produced by CD8+ T cells. Science. 1995 Dec 15;270(5243):1811–1815.
21. McGuinness G. Changing trends in the pulmonary manifestations of AIDS. Radiol Clin North Am. 1997 Sep 1;35(5):1029–1082.
22. Bhatia RS. Common pulmonary opportunistic infections in AIDS. Med Update. 1999;7:1088–1090.
23. Bhatia RS. TB and AIDS. JAPI. 2000;48:613–616.
24. Bhattacharya AK. Pleural effusion in AIDS. Lung India. 2005;22:101–104.
25. Prabhu VG, Narsimhan R. Role of pleuroscopy in undiagnosed exudative pleural effusion. Lung India. 2012;29:128–130. UNAIDS. TB and AIDS, UNAIDSA point of view. UNAIDS best practive collections. 1997 Oct.
26. Banarjee K. HIV/AIDS-criteria of diagnosis: an overview. IN: YP Munjal, ed. Med Update; API. 1997;7:497–503.
27. Rau NR. Serosal tuberculosis. IN: S Das, ed. Med Update; API. 2003;13:112–119.
28. Bhatia RS. TB of serous membranes. IN: RS Bhatia, ed. Tuberculosis. New Delhi: Pee Publ. 2007;17:47–51.
29. Bhatia RS, Khan GQ. TB and AIDS. Pulmoary Medicine. Pee Pee Publ. 2007;12:110–119.
30. Johnson JL, et al. Duration of efficiency of treatment of latent TB infection is HIV-infected adults. AIDS. 2001;15:2137–2147.
31. Bhatia RS, Parkash S. AIDS/HIV disease. New Delhi: Pee Pee Publ. 2007;103–104. 15a. Vajpayee M, Dar L. Anti retroviral drugs in HIV infection. Ind J Pharm. 1999;31(2):96–103. 15b. Gupta SB, et al. API-ARI guidelines. JAPI. 2006;54:57–74.
32. Dean GI, et al. Treatment of TB in HI infected persons in the era of highly active anti-retroviral therapy. AIDS. 2002;16:75–83.
33. Pozniak A. BHIVA treatment guidelines for TB/HIV infection. HIV Med. 2003(Suppl. 1):1–41.

34. Prasad BNBM. A study on comparative efficiency of anti TB prophylaxis with two different regimens in HIV infected tuberculosis reactors. Lung India. 2006;23:64. Jayasingh FtS. Vacine update. IN: YP Munjal, ed. Med Update; API. 1997;7:856–862.
35. Bhatia RS. HIV and TB: the ominous connection. IN: PC Manoria, ed. PG Med; API. Mumabi. 1998;12(110):104–107.
36. Bhatia RS, Singh H. Cardio pulmonary manifestation in HIV disease/AIDS. Pee Pee Publ. 2008;17:137–164.
37. Alanzaden GJ, Lerner SA. The clinical use of fluoroquinolones for the treatment of mycobacterial diseases. Clin Inf Dis. 1997;25:1213–1221.
38. Bhatia RS, Sibia SS. Treatment of tuberculosis: role of sparfloxacin? JAPI. 1999;47:750.
39. Prakash P, Agarwal P. Current concepts in treatment of TB. RNTCP, WHO and Indian guidelines. Med Update; API. 2016;26:944–952.
40. Bhardwaj BL, Bhatia RS. MDR-TB. IN: RS Bhatia, ed. Tuberculosised. Pee Publ. 2007;19:110–121.
41. Thandra KC, Barsouk A, Saginala K, Aluru JS, Barsouk A. Epidemiology of lung cancer. Contemp Oncol (Pozn). 2021;25(1):45–52. doi: 10.5114/wo.2021.103829. Epub 2021 Feb 23. PMID: 33911981; PMCID: PMC8063897.
42. Breijyeh Z, Jubeh B, Bufo SA, Karaman R, Scrano L. Cannabis: a toxin-producing plant with potential therapeutic uses. Toxins (Basel). 2021 Feb 5;13(2):117. doi: 10.3390/toxins13020117. PMID: 33562446; PMCID: PMC7915118.
43. Wahl A, Gralinski LE, Johnson CE, Yao W, Kovarova M, Dinnon KH 3rd, Liu H, Madden VJ, Krzystek HM, De C, White KK, Gully K. SARS-CoV-2 infection is effectively treated and prevented by EIDD-2801. Nature. 2021 Mar;591(7850):451–457. doi: 10.1038/s41586-021-03312-w. Epub 2021 Feb 9. PMID: 33561864; PMCID: PMC7979515.
44. Devadoss D, Singh SP, Acharya A, Do KC, Periyasamy P, Manevski M, Mishra N, Tellez CS, Ramakrishnan S, Belinsky SA, Byrareddy SN, Buch S, Chand HS, Sopori M. HIV-1 productively infects and integrates in bronchial epithelial cells. Front Cell Infect Microbiol. 2021 Feb 4;10:612360. doi: 10.3389/fcimb.2020.612360. PMID: 33614527; PMCID: PMC7890076.

https://doi.org/10.1142/9789811271410_0028

28 Surgery in tuberculosis

Introduction

Less than 2% of cases, out of 2 million of *new* cases of active tuberculosis occurring every year in India, require surgical consideration. Most of these cases belong to multidrug-resistant tuberculosis (MDR-TB) infection. The role of surgery also lies in the management of pulmonary complications such as severe hemoptysis, chronic emphysema, bronchiectasis, scar carcinoma, and so on.[1,2] Surgical treatment of pulmonary tuberculosis is based mainly on three principles:

1. Collapse therapy (artificial pneumothorax, pneumoperitoneum, thoracoplasty).
2. Excisional surgery (pulmonary resection).
3. Drainage procedures (Cavernostomy Monaldi).

Collapse therapy

This is required to restrict the lung movements, to reduce the lung cavities, to close down the lung cavities, or to reduce the thoracic space volume, especially in post-resection cases. This can be compared to a splint or a crutch for protection of an injured extremity. Collapse therapy may be of temporary or permanent type. Temporary methods include artificial pneumothorax, pneumoperitoneum, and phrenic nerve crushing for paralyzing the diaphragm. This method is now being used sporadically in patients with pulmonary tuberculosis. Pneumoperitoneum is the procedure of choice for the purpose of relaxing a diseased lower lobe. There is no permanent loss of lung function. Thoracoplasty is a permanent method to relax or compress the tuberculous lung. The majority of the patients requiring surgical care are successfully treated by resection, but thoracoplasty is still justified in certain "Salvage Cases," in which resection is not possible because of bilateral extensive, disease with highly productive drug-resistant organisms, and poor cardiorespiratory reserve. Thoracoplasty is done in chemotherapy failure drug resistance cases, cases with persistently positive sputum for acid fast bacilli with hemoptysis, and cavities in the lung apex which are nor too medial, too big, too thin or under tension. The combined thoracoplasty with intercostal myoplasty has been used for treating chronic empyema with or without bronchopleural fistula where resectional surgery is not possible.[3]

Resection (excision) therapy[4,5]

This method offers a curative treatment of pulmonary tuberculosis in association with adequate chemotherapy. The surgery is done to assist in the healing, to remove the destructive residuals that offer hurdle or cause failure of the medical treatment and in a way reactivate the disease process. The indications include the following:

A. Removal of residual caseous necrotic foci.
B. A persisting open cavity *even* after 6 months of continuous chemotherapy.
C. Persistent positive sputum cultures even after 6 months of chemotherapy, without any demonstrable cavitation but with a destroyed lobe of the lung, localized bronchiectasis, or bronchial stenosis with resultant atelectasis.
D. Sputum-negative patients with a residual destroyed segment or lobe of the lung to avoid any threat of reactivation of tuberculosis and troublesome hemoptysis.
E. The presence of a localized infection with atypical group III (Battery) organisms requiring resection because of the organism's primary resistance to drugs.
F. Poorly drained tubercular bronchiectasis of the middle and lower lobes requiring resection.

G. A concomitant neoplasm within a tuberculous lesion suspected.
H. Recurrent or persistent life-threatening hemoptysis.
I. Pleural empyema with spontaneous bronchopleural fistula or any postoperative bronchopleural fistula requiring resection and decortication.
J. Lung tuberculoma.
K. MDR tuberculosis.

Surgical resection is contraindicated in patients with inadequate cardiopulmonary reserve, ventilatory insufficiency, coexisting debilitating disease with a poor prognosis, generalized or extrapulmonary tuberculosis that is progressive despite adequate chemotherapy, and the presence of an active arteriosclerotic heart disease. Active endobronchial tuberculosis and associated lung carcinoma, which cannot be controlled by operation, may also obviate surgical intervention.

Patient selection and preoperative measures

As compared to elderly, younger patients tolerate resection better. Young women and adolescent girls are prone to recurrence of arrested tuberculosis and hence require "Curative" resectional surgery. Thoracoplasty at the same time should not be planned in growing children and young adults. Resection may be recommended in patients with thick-walled cavities, patients who have responded slowly as determined by sputum conversion and by lack of radiographic improvement, and patients who are likely to be unreliable in taking medicine or obtaining follow-up examination, such as alcoholics and drug addicts. Occupational and the economic status of the patients, particularly in men, should always be kept in mind. Those with poor socioeconomic and poor educational resources who must perform strenuous labor for their livelihood require a more definitive treatment.

All patients need preoperative evaluation and measures to improve bronchial hygiene by using bronchodilators, nebulized mists, and appropriate antibiotic therapy. Pulmonary function studies and arterial blood gas levels are helpful, particularly in the borderline cases. In elected cases, bronchograms and CT scans are useful in demonstrating unsuspected bronchiectasis and in delineating the diseased segments. Fiberoptic bronchoscopy reveals the unsuspected presence of endobronchial tuberculosis, bronchostenosis, or other non-tuberculosis endobronchial lesions. Anemia can be improved by adding a high-protein, high-calorie diet along with Vitamin C and iron preparations.

Management of complications of surgery

Appropriate timing of the operative procedure, meticulous surgical technique, and rapid physiotherapy for re-expansion of the remaining lung tissue minimize the complications of surgery. The usual complications of thoracotomy can be prevented by postoperative care, use of proper antibiotics, and maintenance of the fluid balance. The most distressing postoperative complications include bronchopleural fistula and empyema. In 3%–7% of cases of pulmonary tuberculosis following surgery, bronchopleural fistula usually occurs at the end of the first week following surgery. Patients may complain of fever and blood-tinged sputum. Chest X-ray shows the presence of air or air–fluid level in the pleural cavity, or there may be continuous air leak via the intercostal catheter for more than 2 weeks. Tension pneumothorax may develop in some cases if the stump is poorly closed, infection of the stump by tubercular mycobacteria or non-tubercular organism, or sometimes due to poor healing as in old age, marked debility and after radiation therapy.

The cardinal rule in the management of bronchopleural fistula is the establishment of pleural drainage. If fistula becomes apparent within 3–4 days of the initial resection, an immediate operative reclosure is justified. Unfortunately, most fistulas do not become apparent until several weeks following resection, and in such cases, consideration is given to the appropriate timing of a tailoring thoracoplasty to obliterate the pleural space. If this fails in closing the fistula, a myoplasty utilizing a lap based on the intercostal muscles or pectoral muscles has been rewarding.

Comments

Pulmonary tuberculosis, a global threat, threatening further with a rising number of patients with MDR-TB, will require resectional surgery along with second-line antituberculosis chemotherapy.[6,7] The role of thoracoplasty still exists in treating a localized cavitary disease with persistent positive sputum. Nevertheless, strict implementation of DOTS can help in the eradication of the disease,[8] as well as in minimizing the role of surgery in tuberculosis.

References and suggested readings

1. Harrison LH. Current aspects of the surgical management of tuberculosis. Surg Clin North Am. 1980;60:88395.
2. Weissbery D, Ready Y. The place of surgery in the treatment of *ree*merging pulmonary tuberculosis. Ann Ital Chir. 2001;71:649–652.
3. Sarkar SK, Sharma TN, Singh H, Singh A, Purohit SD, Sharma VK. Thoracoplasty with intercostal myoplasty for closure of an empyma cavity and bronchopleural fistula. Int Surg. 1985;70:219–221.
4. Das PB, David JG. Excisional surgery in the treatment of pulmonary tuberculosis. 1977;69:217.
5. Hankins JR, Miller JE, Attat S, et al. Bronchopleural fistula. J Thorac Cardiovasc Surg. 1978;76:755.
6. Shiraishi Y, Nakejema Y, Katsuragi N, Kurai M, Takashasti M. Resectionalsurgry combined with chemotherapy remains the treatment of choice for multidrug-resistant tuberculosis. J Thorac Cardivasc Surg. 2004;128:523–528.
7. Chan ED, Laurel V, Strand MJ, Chan J, Huynh MN, Goble M, et al. Treatment and outcome analysis of 205 patients with multidrug-resistant tuberculosis. Am J Respir Crit Care Med. 2004;169:1103.
8. Bhatia RS, Bhardwaj BL. MDR-TB. IN: Pulmonary tuberculosis. Lukcows: Aditya Publ. 2006;139.
9. Sarkar SK. Current aspects in the surgical management of TB. IN: RS Bhatia, ed. Tuberculosis. N Delhi: Pee PeePubl. 2007;17:96–101.
10. Pairolero PC, Arnold PG, Piehler JM. Intrathoracic transposition of extrathoracic skeletal muscle. J Thorac Cardiovasc Surg. 1983;86:809–817.

11. Lin L, Ke Z, Cheng S. Efficacy and safety of short-term chemotherapy for patients with spinal tuberculosis undergoing surgery in Chinese population: a meta-analysis. J Orthop Surg Res. 2021 Mar 29;16(1):229. doi: 10.1186/s13018-021-02375-9. PMID: 33781290; PMCID: PMC8006363.
12. Bao YC, Yu M, Tang L, Ning HY, Zhang WL. Changes in serum prealbumin and incision complications following spinal tuberculosis surgery: a preliminary study. Orthop Surg. 2021 Apr;13(2):501–505. doi: 10.1111/os.12896. Epub 2021 Feb 11. PMID: 33570256; PMCID: PMC7957422.
13. Sun YF, Pi J, Xu JF. Emerging role of exosomes in tuberculosis: from immunity regulations to vaccine and immunotherapy. Front Immunol. 2021 Apr 1;12:628973. doi: 10.3389/fimmu.2021.628973. PMID: 33868247; PMCID: PMC8047325.
14. Mousa H, Abdel-Kader S, Abu-Zidan FM. Management of abdominal tuberculosis in a community-based hospital in a high-income developing country. World J Emerg Surg. 2021 May 26;16(1):25. doi: 10.1186/s13017-021-00370-3. PMID: 34039395; PMCID: PMC8153524.
15. Pérez-López LM, Subirá-Álvarez T, Martínez-Ruíz A, Noguera-Julian A, Moreno-Romo D, Torner-Rubies F, Fontecha CG. Non-axial osteoarticular tuberculosis in the paediatric age. Rev Esp Cir OrtopTraumatol (Engl Ed). 2021 May–Jun;65(3):186–194. English, Spanish. doi: 10.1016/j.recot.2020.09.004. Epub 2021 Jan 23. PMID: 33495138.
16. Wang JL, Yin QY, Han C, Liu FL, Wang MS. Risk factors for death in tuberculosis patients requiring ICU care. Epidemiol Infect. 2021 Jan 5;149:e22. doi: 10.1017/S0950268820003106. PMID: 33397522; PMCID: PMC8057484.
17. Meinerz G, Silva CKD, Dorsdt DMB, Adames JB, Andrade JP, Ventura PE, Monteiro AA, Pasqualotto AC, Garcia VD, Keitel E. Latent tuberculosis screening before kidney transplantation in the South of Brazil. J Bras Nefrol. 2021 Oct–Dec;43(4):520–529. doi: 10.1590/2175-8239-JBN-2020-0189. PMID: 33999988; PMCID: PMC8940112.

https://doi.org/10.1142/9789811271410_0029

29 Organisms and antibiotics in respiratory diseases

Infections of the respiratory tract are grouped according to their symptomatology and anatomic involvement. Acute upper respiratory infections (URIs) include the common cold, pharyngitis, epiglottitis, and laryngotracheitis. These infections are usually benign, transitory, and self-limited, although epiglottitis and laryngotracheitis can be serious diseases in children and young infants. Etiologic agents associated with URI include viruses, bacteria, mycoplasma, and fungi.

Gram-positive bacteria	Gram-negative bacteria	Atypical organisms	Viruses	Fungi
Streptococcus pneumoniae, Staphylococcus aureus, *Streptococcus pyogenes*, *Corynebacterium diphtheriae*, *Mycobacterium tuberculosis*, *Enterococcus*, *Nocardia*, MRSA	*Pseudomonas aeruginosa*, *Haemophilus influenzae*, *Klebsiella pneumoniae*, *Escherichia coli*, *Bordetella pertussis*, *Legionella pneumophila*, *Enterobacter*, *Moraxella catarrhalis*, *Acinetobacter*, *Campylobacter*, *Bartonella*	*Mycoplasma pneumoniae*, *Coxiella burnetii*, *Chlamydia psittaci*	Rhinovirus, coronavirus, parainfluenza virus, adenovirus, respiratory syncytial virus, Epstein–Barr virus, cytomegalovirus, herpes simplex virus, varicella zoster virus, hantavirus	*Candida albicans*, *Histoplasma capsulatum*, *Blastomyces dermatitidis*, *Paracoccidioides brasiliensis*, *Coccidioides*, *Cryptococcus*, *Aspergillus*, *Pneumocystis carinii*

Antibiotics for Gram-positive organisms

Most infections due to Gram-positive organisms can be treated with quite a small number of antibiotics. Penicillin, cloxacillin, and erythromycin should be enough to cover 90% of Gram-positive infections. The relatively narrow spectrum of these drugs should be the incentive to prescribers to use them selectively, together with adequate bacteriological investigation, in order to achieve effective treatment with a minimum of disturbance to the patient's normal bacterial flora and without any other harmful side effects.

Antibiotics	Dose	ADR
Penicillin G	1.2 million units IM	Nausea, vomiting, diarrhea, hypersensitivity reactions, epigastric distress, swelling, itching, redness, insomnia, constipation, headache
Amoxicillin	250 mg, 500 mg, 875 mg PO	
Piperacillin–tazobactam	2.25 g, 3.375 g, 4.5 g IV	
Cephalosporins		
Cephalexin	250 mg, 500 mg PO	Nausea, vomiting, diarrhea, rashes, itching, angioedema, urticarial, disulfiram-like interaction with alcohol
Cefazolin Cefuroxime	500 mg, 1 g IV 250 mg, 500 mg, 750 mg PO/IV	
Ceftriaxone Cefpodoxime	250 mg, 500 mg, 1 g, 2 g IV	
Cefixime	200 mg, 400 mg, 500 mg PO	
Cefepime	1 g, 2 g, IV	
Cefotaxime	500 mg, 1 g, 2 g IV/IM	
Fluoroquinolones		
Ciprofloxacin	400 mg, 500 mg, 750 mg PO/IV	Nausea, vomiting, anorexia, anxiety, insomnia, headache, tremors, pruritis, rash, urticarial, tendinitis, tendon rupture
Ofloxacin Levofloxacin Moxifloxacin Gemifloxacin	400 mg PO 500 mg, 750 mg PO/IV 400 mg PO/IV 320 mg PO	
Lincosamide		
Clindamycin Lincomycin	150 mg, 300 mg, 450 mg, 600 mg, 900 mg PO/IV	Rashes, urticarial, abdominal pain, diarrhea

(*Continued*)

(*Continued*)

Antibiotics	Dose	ADR
Glycopeptides		
Vancomycin Teicoplanin	500 mg, 1 g, 2 g IV	Hypotension, chills, fever, urticarial, flushing, red man syndrome
Lipoglycopeptides		
Dalbavancin	500 mg IV	Nausea, headache, vomiting, rash, pruritis, hepatotoxicity
Oritavancin	1,200 mg IV	
Sulfonamides		
Co-trimoxazole	80/400 mg, 40/800 mg PO	Nausea, vomiting, epigastric pain, hepatitis, neutropenia, SJS, exfoliative dermatitis, renal failure
Macrolides		
Erythromycin Azithromycin	200 mg, 400 mg, 800 mg, 1,000 mg PO 250 mg, 500 mg, 600 mg PO	Epigastric pain, hypersensitivity, hepatitis, headache, dizziness
Clarithromycin	250 mg, 500 mg, 100 mg PO	
Oxazolidinone		
Linezolid	600 mg PO	Abdominal pain, nausea, taste disturbance, diarrhea, headache, pruritis, optic neuropathy
Tetracyclines		
Minocycline Tigecycline	100 mg PO 100 mg IV	Nausea, vomiting, diarrhea, odynophagia, hepatotoxicity, phototoxicity, hypersensitivity reactions
Doxycycline	100 mg, 200 mg PO	
Carbapenems		
Imipenem	500 mg, 750 mg IV	Vomiting, diarrhea, skin rashes, seizures
Meropenem	500 mg, 1 g IV	
Faropenem Doripenem	 500 mg IV	
Aminoglycosides		
Streptomycin	15 mg/kg IM	Ototoxicity, nephrotoxicity, neuromuscular blockade, rashes, eosinophilia
Amikacin	20 mg/kg IV	
Gentamicin	3 mg/kg IM/IV	
Chloramphenicol	50 mg/kg IV	Bone marrow suppression, hypersensitivity reactions, Gray baby syndrome

Antibiotics for Gram-negative organisms

Antibiotics	Dose	ADR
Penicillins		
Ampicillin	250 mg, 500 mg PO/ IV/IM	Nausea, vomiting, diarrhea, hypersensitivity reactions, epigastric distress, swelling, itching, redness, insomnia, constipation, headache
Piperacillin–tazobactam	2.25 g, 3.375 g, 4.5 g IV	
Cephalosporins		
Cefuroxime	250 mg, 500 mg, 750 mg PO/IV	Nausea, vomiting, diarrhea, rashes, itching, angioedema, urticarial, disulfiram-like interaction with alcohol
Cefaclor	250 mg, 500 mg PO	
Cefotaxime	1 g IV	
Ceftazidime	30–50 mg/kg, 1 g, 2 g IV	
Cefoperazone	1 g, 1.5 g IV/PO	
Cefixime	200 mg, 400 mg, 500 mg PO	
Cefepime	1 g, 2 g, IV	
Fluroquinolones		
Norfloxacin		Nausea, vomiting, anorexia, anxiety, insomnia, headache, tremors, pruritis, rash, urticarial, tendinitis, tendon rupture
Levofloxacin	500 mg, 750 mg PO/IV	
Ofloxacin	400 mg PO	
Sulfonamides		
Co-trimoxazole	80/400 mg, 40/800 mg PO	Nausea, vomiting, epigastric pain, hepatitis, neutropenia, SJS, exfoliative dermatitis, renal failure
Tetracyclines		
Minocycline Tigecycline	100 mg PO 100 mg IV	Nausea, vomiting, diarrhea, odynophagia, hepatotoxicity, phototoxicity, hypersensitivity reactions
Doxycycline	100 mg, 200 mg PO	

(*Continued*)

(*Continued*)

Antibiotics	Dose	ADR
Aminoglycosides		
Streptomycin	15 mg/kg IM	Ototoxicity, nephrotoxicity, neuromuscular blockade, rashes, eosinophilia
Amikacin	20 mg/kg IV	
Gentamicin	3 mg/kg IM/IV	
Macrolides		
Erythromycin Azithromycin Roxithromycin	200 mg, 400 mg, 800 mg, 1,000 mg PO 250 mg, 500 mg, 600 mg PO	Epigastric pain, hypersensitivity, hepatitis, headache, dizziness.
Clarithromycin	250 mg, 500 mg, 100 mg PO	
Lincosamide		
Clindamycin Lincomycin	150 mg, 300 mg, 450 mg, 600 mg, 900 mg PO/IV	Rashes, urticarial, abdominal pain, diarrhea
Glycopeptides		
Vancomycin Teicoplanin	500 mg, 1 g, 2 g IV	Hypotension, chills, fever, urticarial, flushing, red man syndrome
Polypeptide antibiotics		
Polymyxin B	15,000–25,000 units/kg/day IV	Bacitracin nausea, vomiting, diarrhea, flushing, paresthesias, marked kidney damage, neurological disturbances
Colistin	2.5–5 mg/kg/day	
Carbapenems		
Imipenem	500 mg, 750 mg IV	Vomiting, diarrhea, skin rashes, seizures
Meropenem	500 mg, 1 g IV	
Faropenem Doripenem	500 mg IV	
Monobactams		
Aztreonam	1 g, 2 g IV	Skin rashes, rise in transaminase levels

Mechanism of actions

Penicillin antibiotics

Penicillin G is a broad-spectrum, beta-lactam naturally occurring penicillin antibiotic with antibacterial activity. Penicillin G binds to and inactivates the penicillin-binding proteins (PBPs) located inside the bacterial cell wall. Inactivation of PBPs interferes with the cross-linkage of peptidoglycan chains necessary for bacterial cell wall strength and rigidity. This interrupts bacterial cell wall synthesis and results in the weakening of the bacterial cell wall and eventually causes cell lysis.

Amoxicillin is a moderate-spectrum antibiotic active against a wide range of Gram-positive, and a limited range of Gram-negative organisms.

Piperacillin is an extended-spectrum penicillin antibiotic, but it can be destroyed by an enzyme produced by bacteria called beta-lactamase. Tazobactam inhibits beta-lactamase and prevents the destruction of piperacillin. Therefore, tazobactam is given with piperacillin to enhance the activity of piperacillin in eradicating bacterial infections.

Cephalosporins

Cephalosporin is a beta-lactam antibiotic to target the integrity of the cell wall synthesis. By disrupting the cell wall synthesis, cephalosporins also disrupt the osmotic gradient necessary to retain the structural integrity of the microbe. As the osmotic gradient goes into decline, the microbe begins to swell and, in the end, burst or lyse. More specifically, cephalosporins work by inhibiting the enzymes needed for peptidoglycan cross-linking in the bacterial cell wall. The final step of peptidoglycan synthesis involves cross-linking at the D-Ala-D-Ala site. Cephalosporins mirror this site forbidding PBPs from binding to the D-Ala-D-Ala site.

First-generation cephalosporins have broad spectrum of activity and low toxicity and are very active against Gram-positive cocci such as pneumococci, viridans streptococci, β-hemolytic streptococci, and staphylococci. They are effective against Gram-negative rods such as *Escherichia coli*, *Klebsiella pneumoniae*, and *Proteus mirabilis* but have very little activity against *Pseudomonas aeruginosa*, *P. vulgaris*, *Enterobacter*, *Citrobacter*, *Serratia*, and *Acinetobacter*.

Second-generation cephalosporins have extended Gram-negative coverage than that of first-generation cephalosporins. They are heterogeneous groups of antibiotics with different antimicrobial activities. They are active against *Enterobacter*, *P. vulgaris*, *Klebsiella*, and *Haemophilus influenzae*.

Third-generation cephalosporins have extended spectrum of activities, and they have extended Gram-negative coverage including *Citrobacter*, *Enterobacter*, *Providencia*, *P. aeruginosa*, β-lactamase-producing meningococci, and *H. influenzae*. The third-generation cephalosporins are usually used in the treatment of sepsis of unknown origin, especially in immunocompromised patients and in those individuals where cephalosporin possess least toxicity. Fourth-generation cephalosporins have extended Gram-negative coverage, and they have increased activity against streptococci and methicillin-resistant *Staphylococcus aureus* (MRSA). The activity of fourth-generation cephalosporins can be comparable to ceftazidime against *Pseudomonas*. They are extended-spectrum cephalosporins with extended spectrum of activities against MRSA.

Quinolone antibiotics

Quinolones act by the rapid inhibition of bacterial DNA synthesis, leading to cell death. The primary targets are DNA gyrase and topoisomerase IV which are involved in the maintenance of the superhelical structure of DNA. Both enzymes are composed of two subunits that are homologous: DNA gyrase subunits encoded by gyrA and gyrB; topoisomerase IV encoded by parC (grlA in *S. aureus*) and parE (grlB in *S. aureus*). The relative affinity of a quinolone antibiotic to either the topoisomerase or the gyrase depends both on the structure of fluoroquinolone and the organism in question and may vary from one agent to the next even within a single species. Some organisms (e.g., *Mycobacterium* spp. and *Campylobacter* spp.) do not have topoisomerase IV, such that the only target to quinolones is DNA gyrase in these organisms.

All quinolones are bactericidal against the majority of Gram-negative bacteria. Most are active against the principal varieties of enterococci and staphylococci, but not against streptococci.

Sulfonamides

Sulfonamides are structural analogs of para-aminobenzoic acid (PABA) and thus act as competitive antagonists in microbial cells. Microbes need PABA to form dihydrofolic acid, a precursor of folic acid. Folic acid is required for purine and pyrimidine synthesis and hence nucleic acid synthesis. Sulfonamides not only block the formation of folic acid — they are incorporated into the precursors, forming a pseudometabolite that is reactive and antibacterial. Mammalian cells are not susceptible to sulfonamides as they absorb and use preformed folic acid, resulting in a wide therapeutic index. The combination of sulfonamides with trimethoprim or other diaminopyrimidines potentiates their activity.

Trimethoprim enters bacteria and inhibits bacterial dihydrofolic acid reductase, thus acting on the same metabolic pathway as sulfonamides. Therefore, the combination has a synergistic activity. The binding affinity of trimethoprim is very much greater for the bacterial enzyme than for mammalian enzyme, and hence, selective bacterial toxicity occurs.

Tetracycline antibiotics

Tetracycline is a broad-spectrum polyketide antibiotic produced by the *Streptomyces* genus of *Actinobacteria*. It exerts a bacteriostatic effect on bacteria by binding reversible to the bacterial 30S ribosomal subunit and blocking the incoming aminoacyl tRNA from binding to the ribosome acceptor site. It also binds to some extent to the bacterial 50S ribosomal subunit and may alter the cytoplasmic membrane causing intracellular components to leak from bacterial cells.

Aminoglycosides

Aminoglycosides antibiotics are used to treat serious infections caused by Gram-negative bacteria. Aminoglycosides bind to the bacterial 30S ribosomal subunit. Ribosomes are the protein factories of cells. They are composed of two subunits in bacteria, a 30S and a larger 50S. By binding to the ribosome, aminoglycosides inhibit the translocation of tRNA during translation and leave the bacterium unable to synthesize proteins necessary for growth.

Although the eukaryotic cells of humans also have ribosomes, these cellular protein factories differ in size and structure from the ribosomes of prokaryotes. That is why aminoglycosides do not interfere with protein synthesis in human cells.

Bacterial cell wall damage

It may not be the inhibition of protein synthesis that produces the bactericidal (bacteria killing) effect. Aminoglycosides also appear to displace cations in the bacterial cell biofilm that are responsible for linking the lipopolysaccharide (LPS) molecules characteristic of Gram-negative bacterial cell walls. This creates holes in the cell wall that may kill the bacteria before the aminoglycoside even reaches the ribosome. Because our cells do not have cell walls (some of the chemical structural components of the bacterial cell wall are found only bacteria), human cells are not susceptible to these destructive actions.

Carbapenems

Carbapenems are beta-lactam antibiotics which have a broad spectrum of activity against many Gram-positive and Gram-negative aerobic and anaerobic organisms and are used for treating life-threatening serious infections not responding to standard antibiotic therapy. Carbapenems bind PBPs disrupting the integrity of the bacterial cell wall, thus causing cell death. The mechanism of action is similar to beta-lactam antibiotics and cephalosporins, but carbapenems have a fused beta-lactam ring structure which is resistant to most beta-lactamases produced by bacteria to inactivate penicillin-like antibiotics. Carbapenems are very effective in treating infections caused by streptococci, enterococci, staphylococci, *Listeria*, Enterobacteriaceae, and many *Pseudomonas*, *Bacteroides*, and *Acinetobacter* species. MRSA are resistant to carbapenems. Carbapenems are also very effective against cephalosporin-resistant bacteria which are ESBL producers.

Linezolid

Linezolid is a synthetic antibiotic, the first of the oxazolidinone class, used for the treatment of infections caused by multi-resistant bacteria including *Streptococcus* and MRSA. The drug works by inhibiting the initiation of bacterial protein synthesis.

It has in vitro activity against aerobic Gram-positive bacteria, certain Gram-negative bacteria, and anaerobic microorganisms. It selectively inhibits bacterial protein synthesis through binding to sites on the bacterial ribosome and prevents the formation of a functional 70S-initiation complex. Specifically, linezolid binds to a site on the bacterial 23S ribosomal RNA of the 50S subunit and prevents the formation of a functional 70S initiation complex, which is an essential component of the bacterial translation process. For streptococci, linezolid was found to be bactericidal for the majority of strains. Linezolid is also a reversible, nonselective inhibitor of monoamine oxidase.

Macrolides

The macrolide antibiotics have the common structure of a macrocyclic lactone ring to which are attached one or more deoxy sugars. The macrolide antibiotics are bacteriostatic agents that inhibit bacterial protein synthesis by binding reversibly to 50S ribosomal subunits of sensitive microorganisms.

The antimicrobial spectra of the macrolide agents are similar to those of penicillin.[1,19] These agents are active against Gram-positive cocci, including streptococci, staphylococci, and spirochetes, but are not active against enterococci, penicillin-resistant staphylococci, and most Gram-negative bacteria with the notable exception of *Neisseria gonorrhoeae.* Erythromycin has weak activity against *H. influenzae*, but clarithromycin and azithromycin exhibit considerably better activity against this microorganism. Consequently, macrolides are often used in the treatment of infections caused by Gram-positive bacteria as alternatives for patients who are allergic to penicillin.

The macrolide antibiotics are generally active against strict anaerobes. They are also effective against *Chlamydia*, *Legionella pneumophila*, and *Mycoplasma*, against which many types of antibiotics, including β-lactams, are ineffective.

Lincosamides

The lincosamides are naturally occurring compounds derived from *Streptomyces* spp. The lincosamide antibiotics bind to the 50S subunit at a site that overlaps both the A and P sites on the ribosome, preventing the docking of charged tRNAs and their movement through the peptidyl transferase center, thus inhibiting the formation of protein. The P-site attachment of clindamycin occurs at the same ribosomal-RNA structural bases as the macrolide binding sites, explaining the competitive inhibition between binding of the two classes of antibiotics for the ribosome, as well the resistance that occurs to both antibiotics by altering a single base. Clindamycin has significant activity against many Gram-positive and Gram-negative anaerobic and facultative/aerobic microorganisms.

Glycopeptides

Glycopeptide antibiotics, including vancomycin and teicoplanin, are large, rigid molecules that inhibit a late stage in bacterial cell wall peptidoglycan synthesis. The three-dimensional structure contains a cleft into which peptides of highly specific configuration (L-aa-D-aa-D-aa) can fit: such sequences are found only in bacterial cell walls; hence, glycopeptides are selectively toxic. Glycopeptides interact with peptides of this conformation by hydrogen bonding, forming stable complexes. As a result of binding to L-aa-D-Ala-D-Ala groups in wall intermediates, glycopeptides inhibit, apparently by steric hindrance, the formation of the backbone glycan chains (catalyzed by peptidoglycan polymerase) from the simple wall subunits as they are extruded through the cytoplasmic membrane. The subsequent transpeptidation reaction that imparts rigidity to the cell wall is also thus inhibited. Vancomycin is the foundational member of the class, showing both clinical longevity and a still preferential role in the therapy of MRSA and of susceptible *Enterococcus* spp. Newer lipoglycopeptide derivatives (telavancin, dalbavancin, and oritavancin) were designed in a targeted fashion to increase the antibacterial activity, in some cases through secondary mechanisms of action.

Polypeptides

Bacitracin is a polypeptide antibiotic that inhibits the cell wall synthesis and is active against Gram-positive bacteria.

Colistin (polymyxin E) and polymyxin B are cationic polypeptide antibiotics that disrupt the outer bacterial cell membrane by binding to the anionic outer membrane and thereby neutralizing the bacteria's toxicity and causing bacterial cell death.

Colistin methanesulfonate (colistimethate sodium [CMS]) is a parenteral preparation of a prodrug that is transformed in blood and urine to colistin. CMS is less toxic than colistin.

Monobactams

Monobactams are monocyclic β-lactam agents characterized by the presence of a 2-oxoazetidine-1-sulfonic acid moiety. Aztreonam is the only monobactam currently approved by the FDA. Aztreonam is a synthetic monocyclic β-lactam, the core structure of which was originally isolated from *Chromobacterium violaceum*. It has high affinity for PBP3 of Gram-negative bacteria, causing their filamentation, bacterial lysis, and death. It does not bind to the PBPs of Gram-positive or anaerobic microorganisms; its spectrum is limited to aerobic Gram-negative species.

It has a broad spectrum of activity against Gram-negative bacteria but has no activity against Gram-positive or anaerobic bacteria. Aztreonam readily penetrates the outer membrane of Gram-negative bacteria.

Antivirals

Antivirals are a class of medication which are used to treat viral infections. Most viral infections resolve spontaneously in immunocompetent individuals. The aim of antiviral therapy is to minimize the symptoms and infectivity as well as to shorten the duration of illness. These drugs act by arresting the viral replication cycle at various stages. Currently, antiviral therapy is available only for a limited number of infections.

Agents	Mechanism	Adverse effect	Areas of application
Amantadine — PO 100 mg, 200 mg Rimantadine — PO 100 mg	**Ion channel blocker** Protons flow into the interior of the virus via the M2 ion channel, which leads to viral uncoating. Amantadine blocks these channels and thereby inhibits the release of the viral genome.	• Gastrointestinal (GI) effects • Neurological: • Anxiety • Lightheadedness • Rare: seizures • Amantadine: cardiovascular adverse effects: Orthostatic dysregulation, QT prolongation	Influenza A

(*Continued*)

Agents	Mechanism	Adverse effect	Areas of application
Oseltamivir — PO 75 mg Zanamivir — inhalation powder 5 mg, 10 mg	Neuraminidase inhibitor	• GI disturbances, headache, upper respiratory infections	Influenza A and B
Acyclovir — IV 50 mg/mL PO — 200 mg, 400 mg, 800 mg Valacyclovir — 500 mg PO Famciclovir — 250 mg, 500 mg PO	**Guanosine analogs** Valacyclovir is a prodrug of acyclovir with greater oral bioavailability. Famciclovir is a prodrug of penciclovir with greater oral bioavailability. Acyclovir and penciclovir are monophosphorylated by herpes simplex virus (HSV)-coded thymidine kinase to an active intermediate, which is then phosphorylated, and the phosphorylated drug is incorporated into the replicating viral DNA strand. Termination of viral DNA synthesis by the inhibition of viral DNA polymerase. Selective action in the infected cells only affect the host cell's DNA replication. **Mechanism of resistance**: mutated viral thymidine kinase	Crystal-induced acute kidney injury, increased transaminases, GI disturbances, thrombotic thrombocytopenic purpura	Herpes simplex, varicella zoster

(*Continued*)

Agents	Mechanism	Adverse effect	Areas of application
Ganciclovir — 5 mg/kg IV Valganciclovir — 450 mg PO, 50 mg/mL IV	**Guanosine analogs** Valganciclovir is a prodrug of ganciclovir and has better oral bioavailability.	Pancytopenia, nephrotoxicity, GI disturbances, headache, confusion, paresthesia	Severe cytomegalovirus infection
	Ganciclovir is monophosphorylated by CMV-coded UL97 kinase to an active intermediate, which is then phosphorylated by cellular kinases; the phosphorylated drug is incorporated into the replicating viral DNA strand. Termination of viral DNA synthesis by the inhibition of viral DNA polymerase. Lower selectivity than acyclovir and penciclovir — can affect the host cell's DNA replication. **Mechanism of resistance**: mutated viral UL97 kinase		
Foscarnet — 40–60 mg/kg IV	Directly inhibits the viral DNA polymerases (pyrophosphate analog), Does not require activation by viral kinase. **Mechanism of resistance**: mutated DNA polymerase	Nephrotoxicity, GI disturbances, headache, confusion, paresthesias, seizures due to electrolyte abnormalities (hypocalcemia), leukopenia, neutropenia	CMV retinitis (when ganciclovir fails), acyclovir-resistant HSV

(Continued)

Agents	Mechanism	Adverse effect	Areas of application
Cidofovir — 5 mg/kg IV	Directly inhibits viral DNA polymerases. Does not require activation by viral kinase. **Mechanism of resistance:** mutated DNA polymerase	Nephrotoxicity	CMV retinitis, acyclovir-resistant HSV

Antifungals

Drugs	Dose	Mechanism	Adverse effects
Azoles Fluconazole Itraconazole Voriconazole	100 mg, 150 mg, 200 mg PO 2 mg/mL IV 100 mg, 200 mg PO 50 mg, 200 mg 6 mg/kg IV	The inhibition of 14α-lanosterol demethylase, a key enzyme in ergosterol biosynthesis, resulting in the depletion of ergosterol and accumulation of toxic 14α-methylated sterols in membranes of susceptible yeast species. For some azoles, their antifungal mode of action is not only characterized by the inhibition of ergosterol biosynthesis.	Hepatotoxicity, neurologic toxicities, skin rash, and photosensitivity, abdominal cramps, headache
Polyenes Amphotericin B Nystatin Terbinafine	1 mg/kg IV 5–10 lakh units available as powder, tablet, and capsule 250 mg PO	Acts by binding to ergosterol in the fungal cell membrane, altering the cell permeability with subsequent depolarization and leakage of cytoplasmic contents, eventually leading to cell death.	Malaise, hypotension, tachypnea, nausea, vomiting, diarrhea, dyspepsia, anemia, hypokalemia, thrombophlebitis, azotemia, renal failure

(*Continued*)

Drugs	Dose	Mechanism	Adverse effects
Beta glucan inhibitors Aculeacins, Echinocandins, Papulacandins		β-Glucan inhibitors act as specific noncompetitive inhibitors of β-(1,3)-glucan synthase, a large (210-kDa) integral membrane heterodimeric protein. Inhibitors of glucan synthesis also have secondary effects on other components of intact cells including a reduction in the ergosterol and lanosterol content and an increase in the chitin content of the cell wall. Inhibition of β-(1,3)-glucan synthetase results in cytological and ultrastructural changes in fungi characterized by growth as pseudohyphae, thickened cell wall, and buds failing to separate from the mother cells. Cells also become osmotically sensitive, with lysis being restricted largely to the growing tips of budding cells.	Nausea, vomiting, abdominal pain, diarrhea, dyspnea, flushing, fever, headache, rashes, hypokalemia, hypomagnesemia, hepatobiliary disturbance
5-Fluorocytosine	250 mg, 500 mg PO	5FC is a fluorinated pyrimidine with an inhibitory activity against many yeasts, including *Candida* and *Cryptococcus neoformans*. 5FC is used in combination with other antifungals, such as amphotericin B and fluconazole, but only rarely as a single agent. 5FC enters the	Skin rash, itching, sore throat, fever, headache, abdominal pain, diarrhea, nausea, vomiting, bruising, confusion, hallucination, photosensitivity

(*Continued*)

Drugs	Dose	Mechanism	Adverse effects
		fungal cells aided by a permease enzyme. Once inside, it is converted to 5-fluorouracil (5FU) by the enzyme cytosine deaminase. Subsequently, 5FU is converted by UMP pyrophosphorylase into 5-fluorouridylic acid (FUMP), which is phosphorylated further and incorporated into RNA, resulting in disruption of protein synthesis. 5FU also is converted to 5-fluorodeoxyuridine monophosphate, a potent inhibitor of thymidylate synthase, an enzyme involved in DNA synthesis and nuclear division. Thus, 5FC acts by interfering with pyrimidine metabolism, as well as RNA, DNA, and protein synthesis in the fungal cell.	

Mechanism of resistance of azoles

The following are the mechanisms by which microbial cells might develop resistance: (1) The target enzyme is overproduced so that the drug does not inhibit the biochemical reaction completely. (2) The drug target is altered so that the drug cannot bind to the target. (3) The drug is pumped out by an efflux pump. (4) The entry of the drug is prevented at the cell membrane. (5) The cell has a bypass pathway that compensates for the loss of function inhibition due to the drug activity. (6) Enzymes that convert an inactive drug to its active form are inhibited. (7) The cells secrete some enzymes to the extracellular medium, which degrade the drug.

Mechanism of resistance of polyenes

The development of resistance occurs by the selection of naturally occurring resistant cells, present in small numbers in the population. These naturally resistant cells produce modified sterols that bind nystatin with lower affinity. The growth rate in the presence of nystatin is therefore dependent upon the normal growth rate (in the absence of nystatin) and the rate at which nystatin causes cell membrane damage. This latter rate is presumed to be a function of the affinity of nystatin for the membrane sterols: the greater the nystatin-sterol affinity, the greater the rate of membrane damage. As a corollary, each resistant strain exhibits slower growth than its more susceptible parent. A difference between resistant and susceptible strains was in fact observed. The fact that resistance to polyenes is gradually lost after serial passage on media devoid of nystatin presumably represents repopulation of the culture by cells producing sterols with a higher affinity for nystatin. The molecular genetics underlying these shifts in sterol content are not well worked out.

Mechanism of resistance to allylamines

Although clinical failure has been observed in patients treated with terbinafine, allylamine resistance in association with the clinical use of terbinafine and naftifine has not been found in human pathogenic fungi. However, with the increased use of this agent, resistance may be expected, that a *C. glabrata* strain that became resistant to fluconazole and expressed cross-resistance to terbinafine. Other investigators report that CDR1 can use terbinafine as a substrate. The machinery to develop resistance to allylamines is therefore already present in some fungal species.

Mechanism of resistance of glucan synthesis inhibitors

Inhibitors of glucan synthesis also have secondary effects on other components of intact cells including a reduction in the ergosterol and lanosterol content and an increase in the chitin content of the cell wall. Inhibition of β-(1,3)-glucan synthetase results in cytological and ultrastructural changes in fungi characterized by growth as pseudohyphae, thickened cell wall, and buds failing to separate from the mother cells. Cells also become osmotically sensitive, with lysis being restricted largely to the growing tips of budding cells.

Mechanism of resistance to 5FC

Resistance to 5FC may result from the decreased uptake (loss of permease activity) or loss of enzymatic activity responsible for conversion to FUMP. Blocking the formation of FUMP by the loss of cytosine deaminase activity or by the loss of uracil phosphoribosyltransferase (UPRTase) activity is sufficient to confer 5FC resistance. Decreased UPRTase activity was associated with resistance in a gene dosage-dependent manner in *C. albicans.* FCY/FCY homozygotes possessed high UPRTase specific activity (approximately 3 U), whereas FCY/FCY heterozygotes possessed less activity (approximately 1.5 U), and FCY/FCY homozygotes possessed barely detectable activity.

Newer antimicrobials

Telavancin lipoglycopeptide (approved)

Telavancin is a vancomycin-derived lipoglycopeptide which is characterized by a broad spectrum of microbiologic activity against Gram-positive bacteria, such as *S. pneumoniae* independent of penicillin susceptibility and staphylococci (including MRSA, *hetero-resistant vancomycin-intermediate S. aureus* [hVISA] and VISA strains). Its antibacterial effects are proposed to be achieved through a dual mechanism of action, that is, inhibition of cell wall peptidoglycan synthesis and depolarization of the cell membrane, resulting in disruption of the functional integrity.

ADR: Gastrointestinal discomfort and taste disturbance, nausea, headache, vomiting, insomnia and foamy urine

Ceftaroline cephalosporin — approved by FDA and EMA

Ceftaroline fosamil is a new, bactericidal, parental, extended-spectrum cephalosporin (Table 2) with activity against Gram-positive organisms, including *S. pneumoniae*, *S. pyogenes*, *S. aureus* (including MRSA and *vancomycin-resistant S. aureus* (VRSA) and hVISA), as well as many common Gram-negative organisms, such as *H. influenzae* and *Moraxella catarrhalis.* Like other b-lactam antibiotics, it prevents the cell wall formation by binding to the PBP, especially to PBP e 2a, which confers the methicillin resistance in *S. aureus.*

ADR: Hypersensitivity reactions. The most common adverse effects were rash, diarrhea, headache, hypokalemia, insomnia and phlebitis.

Ceftobiprole cephalosporin HAP, excluded VAP approved in Europe

Ceftobiprole is a new member of the pyrrolidone-3-ylidenemethyl cephem series of cephalosporins. It is active against pneumococci, *S. aureus*, including MRSA and VISA, *Enterococcus faecalis,* and Gram-negative bacilli, especially has anti-pseudomonal activity similar to cefepime and some anaerobes.

Like ceftaroline, it has strong binding affinity to PBP-2x and PBP-2a, resulting in bactericidal activity against resistant *S. pneumoniae* and Ca-MRSA.

ADR: Nausea, vomiting, taste disturbance

Antimicrobials under development

Cethromycin ketolide CAP phase III

Cethromycin is a new fluoroketolide with a reported high potency against Gram-positive, Gram-negative bacteria, and atypicals including *Mycoplasma* and *Ureaplasma.* It also has in vitro activity against penicillin- and macrolide-resistant Gram-positive organisms, possibly due to a higher affinity for the target site on the ribosomal unit.

ADR: Diarrhea, dysgeusia, headache

Omadacycline tetracycline cSSSIs, CAP phase III cSSTI completed

Omadacycline, an aminomethylcycline, is a semisynthetic derivative of minocycline that has in vitro potency against Gram-positive and Gram-negative bacteria and atypicals (*L. pneumophila*) causing ASSSIs and CAP.

ADR: Nausea, elevation of ALT levels, diarrhea, dysgeusia, headache

Solithromycin ketolide CAP phase III

Solithromycin is a novel fluoroketolide with high potency against Gram-positive and Gram-negative bacteria commonly associated with community LRTIs. Against strains with defined susceptibilities to erythromycin, clindamycin, and telithromycin, solithromycin showed potent inhibition against all combinations.

ADR: Diarrhea, headache and nausea

Tedizolid oxazolidinone cSSSIs and HAP phase III cSSTI and HAP

Tedizolid and radezolid are two new oxazolidinones that are currently under development; both retain activity against MRSA strains that are resistant to linezolid. Tedizolid phosphate is a new oxazolidinone prodrug that is transformed in the serum into the active drug torezolid. Tedizolid acts by inhibiting protein synthesis and has broad activity against Gram (þ) pathogens. The methyl tetrazole D-ring system pick up additional binding site interactions with the ribosome and thus confers increased potency, relative to that of linezolid.

ADR: Nausea, diarrhea, headache, vomiting

Nemonoxacin quinolone CAP phase III clinical trial in CAP

Nemonoxacin is a novel non-fluorinated quinolone that is a broad-spectrum, once daily oral therapy for cSSSI and CAP. Nemonoxacin displayed greater activity than the fluoroquinolones (levofloxacin) against MSSA, MSSE, MRSE, *S. pneumoniae*, and *E. faecalis*. Interestingly, nemonoxacin maintained better activity against CA-MRSA than against HA-MRSA. It has also demonstrated a potent antibacterial activity against ciprofloxacin-resistant MRSA, methicillin- and levofloxacin-resistant *S. capitis*, penicillin- and levofloxacin-resistant *S. pneumoniae*, and VRE.

ADR: Headache, contact dermatitis, pruritus, rash

Drugs in trials

Plazomicin

The drug belongs to the aminoglycoside group of antibiotics commonly referred to as next-generation aminoglycoside and was developed from sisomicin. Its structure possesses two substitutions at position 1 (hydroxyl-aminobutyric acid) and 6 (hydroxyethyl), which makes it resistant to inactivation by aminoglycoside-modifying enzymes. However, it is not active against those bacteria that have ribosomal methyltransferases as a mechanism of drug resistance. It acts by inhibiting protein synthesis and has activity against both Gram-negative and Gram-positive bacteria. Synergistic activity of this drug has been demonstrated against *P. aeruginosa* when combined with cefepime, imipenem, doripenem, and piperacillin–tazobactam and against MRSA, VISA, and VRSA when combined with daptomycin or ceftobiprole. This drug is currently in phase III trial, which is aimed to demonstrate its superiority to colistin including a factor of mortality at 28 days for treating bloodstream infections or nosocomial pneumonia caused by CRE.

Newer fluroquinolones

The newer fluoroquinolones under development for the treatment of infections caused by Gram-negative bacteria include avarofloxacin and nemonoxacin. The activity of nemonoxacin against Gram-positive bacteria (including MRSA and multidrug-resistant [MDR] *S. pneumoniae*) is better than ciprofloxacin, levofloxacin, or moxifloxacin. Other newer agents with intracellular activity against Gram-negative bacteria include delafloxacin (phase III trial) and finafloxacin (phase II trial). Another similar compound, DS-8587 (phase II trial), has activity against both Gram-negative (including *Acinetobacter baumannii*) and Gram-positive bacteria. An oxoquinolizine compound, GC-072 (preclinical phase), possesses good efficacy against *A. baumannii* and *Burkholderia pseudomallei.* A pyrrolopyrimidine inhibitor that acts on GyrB and ParE and other compounds have been developed, which have broad-spectrum activity against *P. aeruginosa, A. baumannii, and E. coli,* which have the advantage of lack of cross-resistance.

References and suggested readings

1. Cheng LL, Guan WJ, Duan CY, Zhang NF. Effect of recombinant human granulocyte colony-stimulating factor for patients with coronavirus disease 2019 (COVID-19) and lymphopenia: a randomized clinical trial. JAMA Intern Med. 2021 Jan 1;181(1):71–78. doi: 10.1001/jamainternmed.2020.5503. PMID: 32910179; PMCID: PMC7489414.
2. MacLeod M, Papi A, Contoli M, Beghé B, Celli BR, Wedzicha JA, Fabbri LM. Chronic obstructive pulmonary disease exacerbation fundamentals: diagnosis, treatment, prevention and disease impact. Respirology. 2021 Jun;26(6):532–551. doi: 10.1111/resp.14041. Epub 2021 Apr 24. PMID: 33893708.
3. Pernica JM, Harman S, Kam AJ, Carciumaru R, Vanniyasingam T, Crawford T, Dalgleish D, Khan S, Slinger RS, Fulford M, Main C, Smieja M, Thabane L, Loeb M. Short-course antimicrobial therapy for pediatric community-acquired pneumonia: the SAFER randomized clinical trial. JAMA Pediatr. 2021 May 1;175(5):475–482. doi: 10.1001/jamapediatrics.2020.6735. PMID: 33683325; PMCID: PMC7941245.

4. Westblade LF, Simon MS, Satlin MJ. Bacterial coinfections in coronavirus disease 2019. Trends Microbiol. 2021 Oct;29(10):930–941. doi: 10.1016/j.tim.2021.03.018. Epub 2021 Apr 8. PMID: 33934980; PMCID: PMC8026275.
5. Harper A, Vijayakumar V, Ouwehand AC, Ter Haar J, Obis D, Espadaler J, Binda S, Desiraju S, Day R. Viral infections, the microbiome, and probiotics. Front Cell Infect Microbiol. 2021 Feb 12;10:596166. doi: 10.3389/fcimb.2020.596166. PMID: 33643929; PMCID: PMC7907522.
6. Chong WH, Saha BK, Ramani A, Chopra A. State-of-the-art review of secondary pulmonary infections in patients with COVID-19 pneumonia. Infection. 2021 Aug;49(4):591–605. doi: 10.1007/s15010-021-01602-z. Epub 2021 Mar 11. PMID: 33709380; PMCID: PMC7951131.
7. Khezri MR, Zolbanin NM, Ghasemnejad-Berenji M, Jafari R. Azithromycin: immunomodulatory and antiviral properties for SARS-CoV-2 infection. Eur J Pharmacol. 2021 Aug 15;905:174191. doi: 10.1016/j.ejphar.2021.174191. Epub 2021 May 17. PMID: 34015317; PMCID: PMC8127529.
8. Robichaud A, Fereydoonzad L, Collins SL, Loube JM, Ishii Y, Horton MR, Martin JG, Mitzner W. Airway compliance measurements in mouse models of respiratory diseases. Am J Physiol Lung Cell Mol Physiol. 2021 Jul 1;321(1):L204–L212. doi: 10.1152/ajplung.00470.2020. Epub 2021 May 19. PMID: 34009049; PMCID: PMC8321862.
9. Marin-Corral J, Pascual-Guardia S, Amati F, Aliberti S, Masclans JR, Soni N, Rodriguez A, Sibila O, Sanz F, Sotgiu G, Anzueto A, Dimakou K, Petrino R, van de Garde E, Restrepo MI; GLIMP Investigators. Aspiration risk factors, microbiology, and empiric antibiotics for patients hospitalized with community-acquired pneumonia. Chest. 2021 Jan;159(1):58–72. doi: 10.1016/j.chest.2020.06.079. Epub 2020 Jul 17. PMID: 32687909.
10. Zhong H, Wang Y, Shi Z, Zhang L, Ren H. Characterization of respiratory microbial dysbiosis in hospitalized COVID-19 patients. Cell Discov. 2021 Apr 13;7(1):23. doi: 10.1038/s41421-021-00257-2. PMID: 33850111; PMCID: PMC8043102.

https://doi.org/10.1142/9789811271410_0030

30 Community-acquired pneumonia

Epidemiology

Community-acquired pneumonia (CAP) affects 2 to 3 million people worldwide, leading to 1 million hospitalizations as per CDC data. Mortality is low in nonhospitalized patients, whereas up to 30% of mortality has been reported in hospitalized patients. It is the leading cause of death due to infectious disease and the sixth leading cause of death in patients aged more than 65 years. It has been aptly called the "captain of men of death." It is defined as pneumonia developing in an outpatient setting or a hospitalized patient within 48 hours of hospitalization.

Etiology

The most common etiologies for CAP are bacterial and/or viral. The commonest organisms are *Streptococcus pneumoniae*, *Haemophilus influenzae*, *Mycoplasma pneumoniae*, *Staphylococcus aureus*, *Moraxella catarrhalis*, *Legionella* species, and *Chlamydia pneumoniae*. Additional causes of pneumonia in tropical countries include tuberculosis, leptospirosis, and Q fever. In the United States, an increased incidence of community-acquired methicillin-resistant *Staphylococcus aureus* (MRSA) has also been reported. In severe CAP, the etiological factors also include Enterobacteriaceae species like *Klebsiella*, *Pseudomonas* (more common in those with structural lung disease), and *Escherichia coli*.

The etiology of CAP keeps changing due to the introduction of vaccines (especially pneumococcal), indiscriminate use of antibiotics, and the recent Covid pandemic. Many times, bacterial pathogens coexist with

Table 1:

Clinical setting/geography	Causative organism
Southeast Asia	*Pseudomonas*
Sub-Saharan Africa	Tuberculosis
Scandinavian countries	Legionellosis
South and Central Asia	Tuberculosis
Northern Australia	Q fever
Prison environment	*Mycobacterium* sp. (tuberculosis)
Poor dental hygiene	Anaerobes
Environmental contact Birds, bats	*Chlamydophila psittaci, Cryptococcus neoformans, Histoplasma capsulatum*
Bird droppings	*C. psittaci, H. capsulatum*
Ungulate animals	*Coxiella burnetii* (Q fever)
Hunting (animal and insect bites)	*Yersinia pestis* (plague), *Francisella tularensis* (tularemia)

viruses, and it is difficult to establish a microbiological diagnosis. Up to 20% of severe CAP is caused by polymicrobial organisms.

The common viruses causing CAP include influenza virus (commonest), parainfluenza virus, rhinovirus, respiratory syncytial virus, human metapneumovirus, and adenovirus. In certain parts of the world, Covid-19 has become endemic and now is the most common cause of CAP. Fungal pathogens are seen in patients with chronic illness with immunocompromised status and exposure to bird droppings (*Cryptococcus*) or soil (*Sporothrix schenckii*). Table 1 depicts the common pathogens based on the clinical setting and geography, whereas Table 2 depicts the common pathogens of CAP.

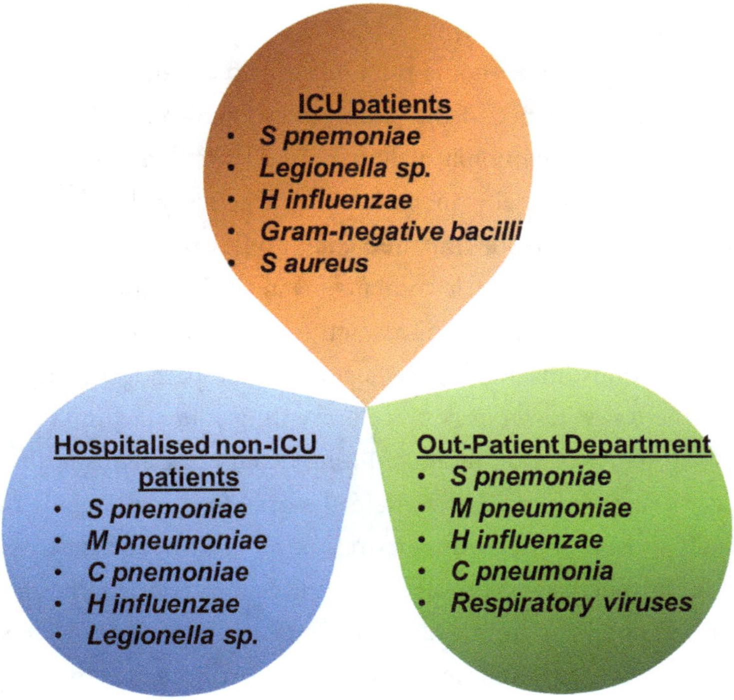

Figure 1:

Table 2:

Gram-positive bacteria	Gram-negative bacteria	Atypical organisms	Viruses	Fungi
S. pneumonia, ***S. aureus***, ***Streptococcus pyogenes***, ***Mycobacterium tuberculosis***, Enterococcus, ***Nocardia***, MRSA	*Pseudomonas aeruginosa*, *H. influenza*, *Klebsiella pneumoniae*, *E. coli*, *Enterobacter*, *M. catarrhalis*, *Campylobacter*, *Bartonella*	*M. pneumoniae*, *Coxiella burnetii*, *Chlamydophila psittaci*, *Legionella pneumophila*	Rhinovirus, coronavirus, parainfluenza virus, adenovirus, respiratory syncytial virus, Epstein–Barr virus, cytomegalovirus, herpes simplex virus, varicella-zoster virus	*Histoplasma capsulatum*, *Blastomyces*, *Paracoccidioides*, *Coccidioides*, *Cryptococcus*, *Aspergillus*, *Pneumocystis jirovecii*

Pathogenesis

The pathogenesis of pneumonia is mainly due to the altered lung defense mechanism and virulence of the pathogenic organism. The endogenous factors leading to pneumonia include chronic bacterial colonization of the oropharynx (especially in chronic obstructive pulmonary disease [COPD] patients), poor or impaired cough reflex (e.g., stroke patients), and microaspiration of gastric contents (as in GERD patients) leading to the seeding of pathogenic organisms in the lower respiratory tract. Under normal conditions, macrophages phagocytize the pathogenic organisms reaching the lower respiratory tract preventing a further inflammatory reaction. In patients with an altered lung defense mechanism, the alveolar macrophage is unable to contain the growth of pathogenic organisms leading to a local inflammatory response. The alveolar macrophages release tumor necrosis factor-alpha, interleukin 6, interleukin 10, interleukin 12, granulocyte colony-stimulating factor, and monocyte chemotactic protein. These cytokines lead to the recruitment of neutrophils, lymphocytes, and monocytes from blood into the alveoli propagating the

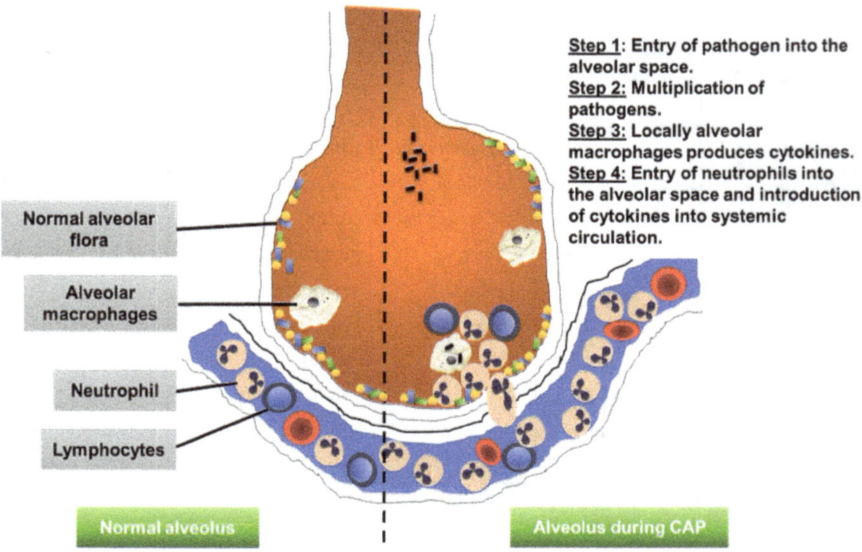

Figure 2: Pathogenesis of community-acquired pneumonia.

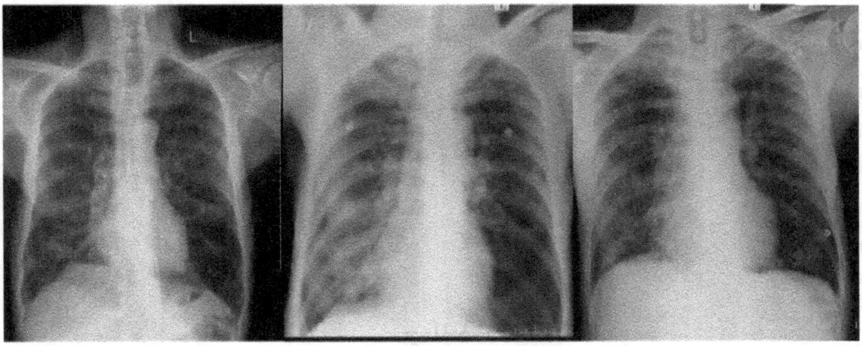

Figure 3: Chest X-ray showing pneumonia COPD.

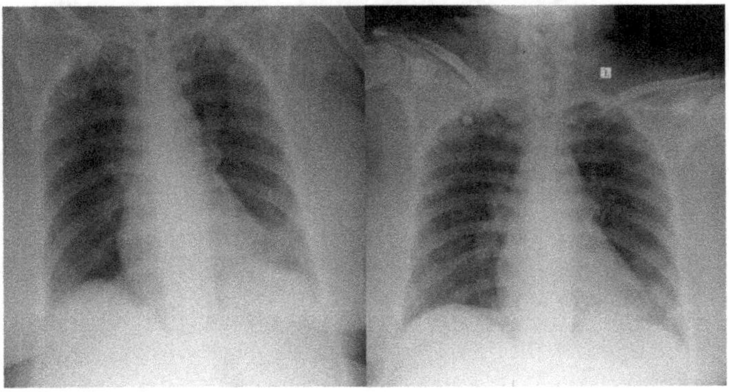

Figure 4: Chest X-ray showing community-acquired pneumonia lingula.

inflammatory process. The above cytokines also enter the systemic circulation leading to a local and systemic inflammatory response. The presence of this local and systemic inflammation leads to classical symptoms, signs, and laboratory manifestations of CAP. The pathogenesis of CAP is summarized in Figure 2.

Risk factors

Clinical conditions associated with an increased risk of development of CAP include a previous history of pneumonia, diabetes, cerebrovascular diseases like stroke or dementia, psychiatric conditions, chronic respiratory

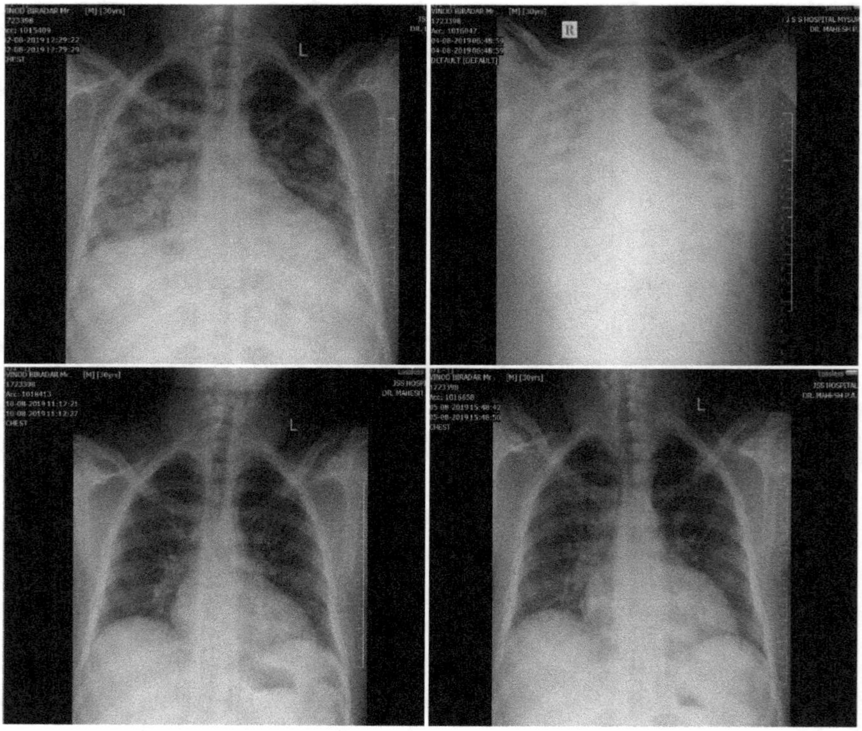

Figure 5: Chest X-ray showing H1N1 pneumonia images.

illnesses like COPD, bronchitis or asthma, chronic liver disease for renal disease, and chronic cardiovascular diseases. Immunocompromised patients, especially those with solid organ malignancy and chemotherapy, are also at an increased risk of development of CAP. Alcohol abuse, malnutrition, and continued smoking status are a few lifestyle factors associated with an increased risk of acquiring pneumonia.

Clinical manifestations

The common presenting symptoms and signs in a patient with CAP are summarized in Table 3.

Clinical presentation of CAP is varied from mild symptoms of fever and cough to severe sepsis and respiratory failure with multiorgan dysfunction syndrome. This is dependent on the host–pathogen interaction which in turn is decided by the patient's immune response, functional status of various organs, and virulence of the pathogen. Diagnosis can be challenging in certain populations like the elderly, immunocompromised patients, or those with atypical presentations. Organisms like *Legionella*, *Mycoplasma*, and *Chlamydia* are known for atypical presentation (hence the name atypical pneumonia), especially in the elderly. Patients with *Legionella* pneumonia can present with headache, confusion, and agitation due to hyponatremia and diarrhea, whereas *M. pneumoniae* is associated with hemolytic anemia, upper respiratory tract symptoms, and skin manifestations (Steven–Johnson syndrome). Table 4 summarizes the

Table 3:

Symptoms	Signs
Fever	Tachycardia
Cough with productive sputum	Crepitations
Shortness of breath	Tachypnea
Pleuritic chest pain	Pleural rub
Mental confusion (atypical presentation in older patients and those with shock)	Hypotension
Nausea, vomiting, or diarrhea (atypical pneumonia)	Hypoxemia

Table 4:

Extrapulmonary manifestation	Possible etiological agent
Skin nodules	*Aspergillus* species, *Nocardia*, *Coccidioides immitis*, *Blastomyces* species
Erythema nodosum	Tuberculosis, *C. immitis*
Pharyngitis	*Mycoplasma pneumoniae*
Herpes labialis	*Streptococcus pneumoniae*
Splenomegaly	*Francisella tularensis*, *C. psittaci*, *C. burnetii*
Erythema multiforme	*M. pneumoniae*, *C. psittaci*
Ecthyma gangrenosum	*Pseudomonas*
Lymphadenopathy	Tularemia

extrapulmonary manifestations and possible etiological agents in CAP. The predictive value of these signs has not been validated rigorously.

Imaging

Diagnosis of CAP requires radiological evidence in the form of infiltrates on the chest X-ray, lung ultrasonography, or CT chest in the background of clinical syndrome compatible with CAP. Diffuse infiltrates on chest X-rays suggest *Pneumocystis jirovecii* pneumonia and viral pneumonia, whereas focal infiltrates suggest Gram-negative bacilli, *S. pneumoniae*, *S. aureus*, and *Legionella* species. Cavitation on the chest X-ray should arouse the suspicion of fungal etiology (*Aspergillus*, *Nocardia*,), necrotizing pneumonia (*S. aureus*, Gram-negative bacilli), tuberculosis, malignancy, and Wegener's granulomatosis.

A chest CT is indicated when there is any inconsistency between the clinical suspicion of pneumonia and a negative chest X-ray if complications are suspected (e.g., lung abscess, empyema), or in the presence of comorbidities (e.g., pulmonary embolism or cancer). Bedsides, lung ultrasonography has shown promise as it is quick, easy to perform, and has a sensitivity of 94% and a specificity of 96% for the diagnosis of pneumonia.

Other diagnostic and microbiological investigations

The suspicion of CAP is clinical, based on the signs or symptoms suggestive of a lower respiratory tract infection which are acute in onset (e.g., cough, fever, sputum production, difficulty in breathing, and pleuritic chest pain), the sensitivity of which is only 60%. Hence, the definitive diagnosis of CAP requires radiological evidence in the form of new infiltrates on a chest X-ray or chest CT, or lung ultrasonography.

The initial investigations required in a patient with CAP can be grouped into two subgroups.

a. Tests to evaluate the disease severity

These include the chest X-ray, CT chest or lung ultrasound, complete blood count, C-reactive protein, and procalcitonin. Procalcitonin is commonly used in the past decade to discriminate between the fungal, viral, and bacterial causes of pneumonia. However, controversies exist due to studies showing the inability of procalcitonin to discriminate between bacterial and viral causes. Also, it is seen to be more of an inflammatory marker than a marker of infection as a rise in procalcitonin is seen in trauma and post-surgical cases also. However, it correlates well with the Pneumonia Severity Index (PSI) score and the development of complications like the need for invasive mechanical ventilation, empyema, and septic shock. Other tests like liver function tests, coagulation tests, and renal function tests should be done to look for multiorgan dysfunction syndrome, especially in cases of severe CAP.

b. Tests to establish the etiological diagnosis

These tests should be tailored to each patient's history and laboratory parameters along with the geographic location and local antibiotic stewardship process. For example, routine testing for tuberculosis is not recommended as per European guidelines, whereas in countries like India, tuberculosis testing has a high yield. Testing is also based on the severity of the disease and the immune status of the patient. For example, routine testing of sputum for Gram stain and cultures are not recommended by all societies in an outpatient setup, whereas it should be done for all ICU patients.

Sputum testing and cultures

Sample for sputum testing should be obtained before the start of an antibiotic therapy, rapidly transported, and should be of good quality (minimal oral contamination, i.e., at least 25 polymorphonuclear cells and less than 10 epithelial cells). Sputum Gram stain may be negative in 50% of patients and should not be used for de-escalation of therapy. Sputum cultures are difficult to interpret due to the inability to differentiate between colonization and infection. Hence, most guidelines do not recommend sputum cultures in nonhospitalized patients, whereas it should be done in those hospitalized patients with a high risk of Multi-Drug-Resistant (MDR) pathogens. Bronchoscopy and sampling should be considered in critically ill, immunocompromised, and mechanically ventilated patients.

The blood culture positivity rate in pneumonia is approximately 15%, and hence, it should not be done routinely. However, it is recommended in all critically ill patients, those at risk of MDR pathogens, and immunocompromised patients.

Serology and urinary antigen testing

Serological testing can be done for atypical organisms like *Mycoplasma*, *Chlamydophila*, and *Legionella*. However, these tests have very low sensitivity and specificity, and the delayed result has led to questioning the clinical utility of these tests. Hence, these tests are not recommended in routine clinical practice. Urinary antigen testing can be done for *S. pneumoniae* and *Legionella*. These are rapid and readily available with high specificity, but limitations include a low sensitivity. These are recommended in severe CAP and cases of outbreaks of CAP (especially *Legionella*).

Multiplex RT-PCR assay

The use of Real-Time multiplex panel Polymerase Chain Reaction techniques of sputum evaluation (e.g., BioFire) aids in the rapid and accurate identification of an array of etiological pathogens including bacteria and viruses within a few hours. However, the routine use of these tests is limited due to prohibitory costs, especially in low- and middle-income countries.

Table 5: Summarizes guidelines for testing by different societies for establishing the etiological diagnosis in CAP

	European Respiratory Society 2011	ATS and IDSA 2019	British Thoracic Society	Comments
Outpatient				
Sputum for Gram stain and culture	No	No	No	May be done if the patient is at risk of MRSA/pseudomonas infection
Blood culture	No	No	No	May be done if the patient is previously infected with MRSA or *P. aeruginosa*
Legionella urinary antigen	No	No	No	The test has high specificity, especially for serogroup-I but low sensitivity. Should be done in case of outbreaks
Pneumococcal antigen	No	No	May be done	The test has high specificity but low sensitivity
Serology for ***Chlamydophila***, ***Mycoplasma***, and ***Legionella***	No	No	No	Test positivity is usually after 7 days of illness, and delayed results may not help in patient care
Tuberculosis and HIV	No	No	May be done	

(*Continued*)

Table 5: (*Continued*)

	European Respiratory Society 2011	ATS and IDSA 2019	British Thoracic Society	Comments
Virus (PCR for influenza, Covid, parainfluenza)	No	No	No	Rapid and accurate results but cannot differentiate between colonization and infection. Useful in outbreaks
Inpatient				
Sputum for Gram stain and culture	Yes	May be done	Yes	May be done if the patient is at risk of MRSA/pseudomonas infection
Blood culture	Yes	May be done	Yes	May be done if the patient is previously infected with MRSA or *P. aeruginosa*
Legionella urinary antigen	May be done	May be done	May be done	The test has high specificity, especially for serogroup-I but low sensitivity. Should be done in case of outbreaks
Pneumococcal antigen	May be done	No	Yes	The test has high specificity but low sensitivity
Serology for ***Chlamydophila***, ***Mycoplasma***, and ***Legionella***	May be done	No	May be done	Test positivity is usually after 7 days of illness, and delayed results may not help in patient care

Table 5: (*Continued*)

	European Respiratory Society 2011	ATS and IDSA 2019	British Thoracic Society	Comments
Tuberculosis and HIV	May be done	No	May be done	
Virus (PCR for influenza, Covid, parainfluenza)	May be done	May be done	May be done	Rapid and accurate results but cannot differentiate between colonization and infection. Useful in outbreaks
ICU				
Sputum for Gram stain and culture	Yes	Yes	Yes	May be done if the patient is at risk of MRSA/pseudomonas infection
Blood culture	Yes	Yes	Yes	May be done if the patient is previously infected with MRSA or *P. aeruginosa*
Legionella urinary antigen	Yes	Yes	Yes	The test has high specificity, especially for serogroup-I but low sensitivity. Should be done in case of outbreaks
Pneumococcal antigen	Yes	Yes	Yes	The test has high specificity but low sensitivity

(*Continued*)

Table 5: (*Continued*)

	European Respiratory Society 2011	ATS and IDSA 2019	British Thoracic Society	Comments
Serology for ***Chlamydophila***, ***Mycoplasma***, and ***Legionella***	May be done	No	May be done	Test positivity is usually after 7 days of illness and delayed results may not help inpatient care
Tuberculosis and HIV	No	No	May be done	
Virus (PCR for influenza, Covid, parainfluenza)	May be done	May be done	May be done	Rapid and accurate results but cannot differentiate between colonization and infection. Useful in outbreaks

Decision on site of care of a patient with CAP

The decision on where to admit a patient with CAP depends on the patient's risk for mortality and the risk of developing a complicated course during the hospital stay. Many scoring systems help clinicians decide on the site of care of a patient with CAP. They are summarized in Table 6.

Table 6:

Scoring system	Determinants of the scoring system	Criteria for admission
CURB-65 (British Thoracic Society scoring system)	**C**onfusion — 1 point **U**rea > 20 mg/dL — 1 point **R**espiratory rate > 30 — 1 point **B**P systolic < 90, diastolic < 60 — 1 point Age > **65** years — 1 point	0/1 point — outpatient care 2/3 — inpatient care 4/5 — ICU admission
Pneumonia Severity Index (recommended by ATS and IDSA)	More than 20 acute health and chronic health parameters classify patients into 5 classes	Predicts mortality risk with lower mortality in classes I–III
SMART-COP	**S**ystolic BP less than 90 mmHg, **M**ultilobar infiltrates, **A**lbumin < 3.5 mg/dL, **R**espiratory rate elevation (> 25 for those younger than 50 years, and > 30 for those older than 50 years), **T**achycardia (> 125/minute), **C**onfusion, low **O**xygen (< 70 mmHg if younger than 50 years or < 60 mmHg if older than 50 years), arterial **p**H less than 7.35	92% sensitive for predicting the need for invasive mechanical ventilation and vasopressors
CURSO-80 (Spanish scoring system)	Two major criteria arterial pH < 7.39 systolic BP < 90 mmHg, or the presence of two of six minor criteria,	92% sensitivity for the need for ICU admission

(Continued)

Table 6: (*Continued*)

Scoring system	Determinants of the scoring system	Criteria for admission
	Confusion, B**U**N > 30 mg/dL, **R**espiratory rate > 30/minute, Multilobar infiltrates on chest **X**-ray, Pa**O**$_2$/FiO$_2$ ratio < 250, age **80** years or older	
A-DROP (Japanese scoring system)	**A**ge (male ≥ 70 years, female ≥ 75 years) **D**ehydration (BUN ≥ 210 mg/L) **R**espiratory failure SaO$_2$ ≤ 90% or PaO$_2$ ≤ 60 mmHg) **O**rientation disturbance (confusion) low blood **p**ressure (systolic BP ≤ 90 mmHg)	Similar to CURB-65
REA-ICU (**R**isk of **E**arly **A**dmission to **ICU**)	Male gender, age < 80 years, comorbid conditions, respiratory rate ≥ 30 cpm, heart rate ≥ 125 bpm, multilobar infiltrate or pleural effusion, WBC count < 3 or > 20,000/μL, hypoxemia (oxygen saturation < 90% or arterial partial pressure of oxygen (PaO$_2$) < 60 mmHg), blood urea nitrogen ≥ 11 mmol/L, pH < 7.35 sodium < 130 mEq/L	Developed from a cohort of 5,000 ICU patients. Better performance than PSI for predicting the need for ICU stay. Classifies patients into four classes with an increased risk of mortality in higher classes

Management

Anti-infectives remain the cornerstone in the treatment of CAP. Table 7 summarizes site-specific and pathogen-specific treatments for CAP. Anti-influenza therapy is recommended as it shortens the time to clinical recovery in patients who test positive for influenza even though spontaneous recovery is the norm in influenza pneumonia. Peramivir, zanamivir, oseltamivir phosphate, and baloxavir marboxil are currently approved drugs for anti-influenza therapy. Although studies have shown that coadministration of corticosteroids decreased in time to clinical stability and length of hospital stay, the risks of increased chances of secondary infection and

Table 7:

Outpatient empirical treatment	
Previously healthy with no risk factors for drug-resistant *S. pneumoniae* (DRSP) infection or no use of antimicrobials within the previous 3 months	**Macrolide:** • Azithromycin, clarithromycin, or erythromycin **Alternative:** doxycycline.
Comorbid conditions: Diabetes, chronic heart, lung, liver, or renal disease, alcoholism, malignancies, asplenia, immunosuppressive conditions or drugs, use of antimicrobials in the previous 3 months, or other risks for DRSP infection	**Respiratory fluoroquinolones:** Moxifloxacin, gemifloxacin, or levofloxacin (750 mg) OR **Beta-lactam PLUS macrolide:** Amoxicillin — 1 g TID or Amoxicillin/clavulanate — 2 g BID or Cefpodoxime, ceftriaxone, or cefuroxime — 500 mg BID PLUS Azithromycin, clarithromycin, or erythromycin **Alternative to macrolide:** doxycycline.
Regions with high rate (> 25%) of macrolide-resistant *S. pneumoniae*	**Consider alternative agents: e.g.,** beta-lactams or respiratory fluroquinolones

(*Continued*)

Table 7: (*Continued*)

Inpatient empirical treatment	
Non-ICU	
Recommendations:	**Respiratory fluroquinolones OR** **Beta-lactam PLUS macrolide** • Cefotaxime, ceftriaxone, or ampicillin **PLUS** • Ertapenem (selected patients) **Alternative to the macrolide: doxycycline** **Penicillin allergy — use respiratory fluoroquinolone**
ICU	
Minimal recommendations:	Beta-lactam PLUS azithromycin OR Fluoroquinolone: • Cefotaxime, ceftriaxone, ampicillin/sulbactam **Penicillin allergy — use respiratory fluoroquinolone AND aztreonam are recommended**
Additional recommendations or modifications: If *Pseudomonas* infection	**Antipneumococcal antipseudomonal beta-lactam PLUS ciprofloxacin OR levofloxacin (750 mg):** • Piperacillin–tazobactam, cefepime, imipenem, meropenem OR • Above beta-lactam PLUS aminoglycosides AND azithromycin OR • Above beta-lactam PLUS aminoglycoside AND anti-pneumococcal fluoroquinolone **Penicillin allergy-substitute aztreonam for the above beta-lactam**

Table 7: (*Continued*)

If community-acquired MRSA	Add vancomycin or linezolid
Pathogen-specific treatment	
S. pneumoniae PCN susceptible (MIC < 2 μg/mL)	**Preferred:** penicillin G, amoxicillin **Alternative:** macrolide, cephalosporins (cefpodoxime, cefprozil, cefuroxime, cefdinir, ceftriaxone, cefotaxime), clindamycin, doxycycline, respiratory fluoroquinolone
S. pneumoniae PCN resistant (MIC > 2 μg/mL)	**Preferred:** based on susceptibility, including cefotaxime, ceftriaxone, fluoroquinolone **Alternative:** vancomycin, linezolid, high-dose amoxicillin (3 g/day with PCN MIC < 4 μg/mL)
H. influenzae non-beta-lactamase producing	**Preferred:** amoxicillin **Alternative:** fluoroquinolone, doxycycline, azithromycin, clarithromycin
H. influenzae beta-lactamase producing	**Preferred:** second- or third-generation cephalosporin, amoxicillin/clavulanate **Alternative:** fluoroquinolone, doxycycline, azithromycin, clarithromycin
Legionella species	**Preferred:** fluoroquinolone, azithromycin **Alternative:** doxycycline
Mycoplasma pneumoniae, *Chlamydophila pneumoniae*	**Preferred:** macrolide, tetracycline **Alternative: fluroquinolone**
Influenza A	**Preferred:** Initiate oseltamivir or zanamivir within 48 hours if influenza A identified. Not recommended if uncomplicated influenza and symptoms ongoing for > 48 hours
H5NI influenza	**Preferred:** oseltamivir 75 mg twice daily for 5 days

hyperglycemia outweigh the benefits, and the use of steroids is not recommended in CAP.

Time to clinical stability is one of the most important factors that determine recovery in CAP. It is dependent on several factors like the host-pathogen interaction, early appropriate antibiotic therapy, presence of prior comorbid disease, and development of local or systemic complications. Empirical antibiotic therapy once initiated should lead to clinical stability in a non-immunocompromised host within 3–4 days. Achievement of clinical stability is the most important guide to switching to oral therapy. Several other parameters are recommended as per various societal guidelines to assess the achievement of clinical stability which is summarized in Table 8. The appropriate duration of antibiotic therapy should be based on clinical stability criteria and the development of complications. Short-course therapy of fewer than 7 days has benefits of similar cure rates with lesser side effects of the emergence of antibiotic resistance and lesser adverse drug events. A longer duration of therapy (≥ 14 days) is recommended in cases of complications like empyema, lung abscess, and other extrapulmonary complications or infection with MDR organisms.

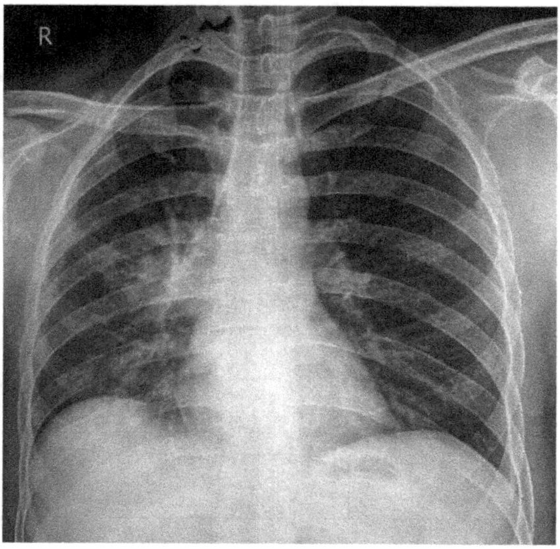

Figure 6: CAP before antibiotics.

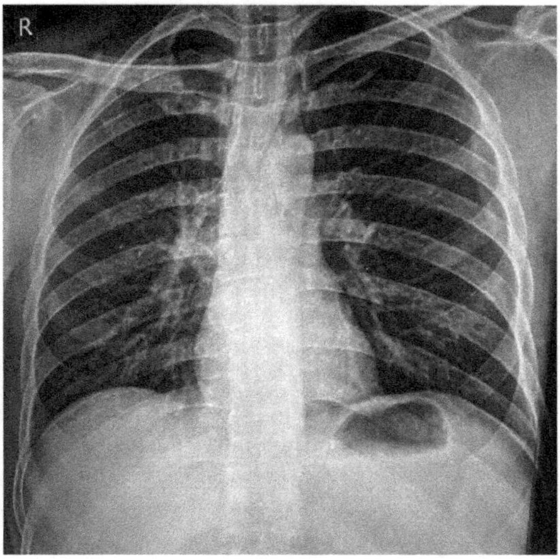

Figure 7: CAP after antibiotics resolved.

Table 8:

Guidelines	Parameters for clinical stability
ATS/IDS 2007	Temperature ≤ 37·8°C Heart rate ≤ 100 beats/minute Respiratory rate ≤ 24 beats/minute Systolic blood pressure ≥ 90 mmHg Arterial oxygen saturation ≥ 90% or PaO_2 ≥ 60 mmHg on room air Normal mental status
BTS 2009	Resolution of fever for > 24 hours Pulse rate < 100 beats/minute Resolution of tachypnea Clinically hydrated and taking oral fluids Resolution of hypotension Absence of hypoxia Improving white cell count Non-bacteremic infection No microbiological evidence of *Legionella*, *Staphylococcal*, or Gram-negative enteric bacilli infection

Complications

The following are the complications that can develop in a patient with CAP.

1. Acute respiratory failure
2. Sepsis with septic shock
3. Massive pleural effusion
4. Lung abscess
5. Empyema
6. Lung cavitation
7. Cholestasis
8. Mild anemia
9. Arthritis
10. Encephalopathy

Management of complications like acute respiratory failure requires invasive mechanical ventilation. Noninvasive ventilation and high-flow nasal oxygenation have shown some promise in treating respiratory failure, but they should not be tried for prolonged periods as it is shown to worsen mortality. The treatment of septic shock with vasopressors, fluids, and steroids along with supportive care like **f**eeding, **a**nalgesia, **s**edation whenever necessary, **t**hromboprophylaxis, **h**ead-end elevation, **u**lcer prophylaxis, and **g**lycemic control (mnemonic — FAST HUG) is important to bring down ICU mortality. Despite these measures, mortality is high (up to 50%), especially in those who develop multiorgan dysfunction syndrome.

Summary

The etiology of CAP is varied and dependent on several factors like geography, host immune status, and prior antibiotic use. Early appropriate antibiotic therapy based on history, risk factors, and severity of pneumonia lead to improved outcomes. Studies have shown that short-course antibiotic therapy has similar cure rates when compared to a longer duration of antibiotic therapy with lesser side effects. The use of steroids is not recommended in the treatment of CAP. Studies have not shown substantial evidence for the use of procalcitonin to support the diagnosis and escalate antibiotics in the treatment of bacterial pneumonia.

References and suggested readings

1. Nair GB, Niederman MS. Updates on community acquired pneumonia management in the ICU. Pharmacol Ther. 2021 Jan;217:107663. doi: 10.1016/j.pharmthera.2020.107663. Epub 2020 Aug 15. PMID: 32805298; PMCID: PMC7428725.
2. Pernica JM, Harman S, Kam AJ, Carciumaru R, Vanniyasingam T, Crawford T, Dalgleish D, Khan S, Slinger RS, Fulford M, Main C, Smieja M, Thabane L, Loeb M. Short-course antimicrobial therapy for pediatric community-acquired pneumonia: the SAFER randomized clinical trial. JAMA Pediatr. 2021 May 1;175(5):475–482. doi: 10.1001/jamapediatrics.2020.6735. PMID: 33683325; PMCID: PMC7941245.
3. Marin-Corral J, Pascual-Guardia S, Amati F, Aliberti S, Masclans JR, Soni N, Rodriguez A, Sibila O, Sanz F, Sotgiu G, Anzueto A, Dimakou K, Petrino R, van de Garde E, Restrepo MI; GLIMP investigators. Aspiration risk factors, microbiology, and empiric antibiotics for patients hospitalized with community-acquired pneumonia. Chest. 2021 Jan;159(1):58–72. doi: 10.1016/j.chest.2020.06.079. Epub 2020 Jul 17. PMID: 32687909.
4. Torres A, Garrity-Ryan L, Kirsch C, Steenbergen JN, Eckburg PB, Das AF, Curran M, Manley A, Tzanis E, McGovern PC. Omadacycline vs moxifloxacin in adults with community-acquired bacterial pneumonia. Int J Infect Dis. 2021 Mar;104:501–509. doi: 10.1016/j.ijid.2021.01.032. Epub 2021 Jan 20. PMID: 33484864.
5. Eraikhuemen N, Julien D, Kelly A, Lindsay T, Lazaridis D. Treatment of community-acquired pneumonia: a focus on Lefamulin. Infect Dis Ther. 2021 Mar;10(1):149–163. doi: 10.1007/s40121-020-00378-3. Epub 2021 Feb 2. PMID: 33528794; PMCID: PMC7851634.
6. Qu J, Zhang J, Chen Y, Huang Y. Aetiology of severe community acquired pneumonia in adults identified by combined detection methods: a multi-centre prospective study in China. Emerg Microbes Infect. 2022

Dec;11(1):556–566. doi: 10.1080/22221751.2022.2035194. PMID: 35081880; PMCID: PMC8843176.

7. Falcone M, Tiseo G, Menichetti F. Community-acquired pneumonia owing to multidrug-resistant pathogens: a step toward an early identification. Ann Am Thorac Soc. 2021 Feb;18(2):211–213. doi: 10.1513/AnnalsATS.202009-1207ED. PMID: 33522876; PMCID: PMC7869783.
8. Ensinck G, Lazarte G, Ernst A, Romagnoli A, López Papucci S, Aletti A, Chiossone A, Pigozzi F, Sguassero Y. Community-acquired methicillin-resistant Staphylococcus aureus pneumonia in a children's hospital. Our ten-year experience. Arch Argent Pediatr. 2021 Feb;119(1):11–17. English, Spanish. doi: 10.5546/aap.2021.eng.11. PMID: 33458975.
9. Gillet Y, Tristan A, Rasigade JP, Saadatian-Elahi M; PVL Pneumonia Study Group. Prognostic factors of severe community-acquired staphylococcal pneumonia in France. Eur Respir J. 2021 Nov 11;58(5):2004445. doi: 10.1183/13993003.04445-2020. PMID: 33833037; PMCID: PMC8859977.
10. Shoar S, Centeno FH, Musher DM. Clinical features and outcomes of community-acquired pneumonia caused by *Haemophilus* Influenza. Open Forum Infect Dis. 2021 Apr 8;8(4):ofaa622. doi: 10.1093/ofid/ofaa622. Erratum in: Open Forum Infect Dis. 2021 Jun 26;8(6):ofab226. PMID: 33855100; PMCID: PMC8028099.
11. Toro MS, Martínez JLV, Falcão RV, Prata-Barbosa A, Cunha AJLAD. Point-of-care ultrasound by the pediatrician in the diagnosis and follow-up of community-acquired pneumonia. J Pediatr (Rio J). 2021 Jan–Feb;97(1):13–21. doi: 10.1016/j.jped.2020.07.003. Epub 2020 Aug 9. PMID: 32781037; PMCID: PMC9432299.
12. El Gharib K, Masri K, Daoud Z, Sfeir T. Community-acquired *Acinetobacter calcoaceticus* pneumonia in a patient with agammaglobulinaemia. New Microbes New Infect. 2021 Mar 19;41:100870. doi: 10.1016/j.nmni.2021.100870. PMID: 33898044; PMCID: PMC8056432.
13. Ao XX. The epidemiology of hospital death following pediatric severe community acquired pneumonia. Ital J Pediatr. 2021 Feb 8;47(1):25. doi: 10.1186/s13052-021-00966-0. PMID: 33557900; PMCID: PMC7869472.
14. Kuluöztürk M, İne E, Telo S, Karabulut E, Geçkil AA. Efficacy of copeptin in distinguishing COVID-19 pneumonia from community-acquired pneumonia.

J Med Virol. 2021 May;93(5):3113–3121. doi: 10.1002/jmv.26870. Epub 2021 Feb 17. PMID: 33570194; PMCID: PMC8013559.

15. Pagliano P, Sellitto C, Conti V, Ascione T, Esposito S. Characteristics of viral pneumonia in the COVID-19 era: an update. Infection. 2021 Aug;49(4):607–616. doi: 10.1007/s15010-021-01603-y. Epub 2021 Mar 29. PMID: 33782861; PMCID: PMC8006879.
16. Oppen K, Ueland T, Siljan WW, Skadberg Ø, Brede C, Lauritzen T, Aukrust P, Steinsvik T, Husebye E, Michelsen AE, Holter JC, Heggelund L. Hepcidin and Ferritin predict microbial etiology in community-acquired pneumonia. Open Forum Infect Dis. 2021 Feb 18;8(4):ofab082. doi: 10.1093/ofid/ofab082. PMID: 33880390; PMCID: PMC8043258.
17. Sando E, Suzuki M, Ishida M, Yaegashi M, Aoshima M, Ariyoshi K, Morimoto K. Definitive and indeterminate *Pseudomonas aeruginosa* infection in adults with community-acquired pneumonia: a prospective observational study. Ann Am Thorac Soc. 2021 Sep;18(9):1475–1481. doi: 10.1513/AnnalsATS.201906-459OC. PMID: 33565942; PMCID: PMC8489873.

https://doi.org/10.1142/9789811271410_0031

31 Nosocomial pneumonia

Abstract

Poor economic resources and overpopulation is indirectly related to overcrowding in hospitals in Low and middle income countries. Underfunding and poor hygiene conditions are responsible for casualties in hospitalized patients, significantly due to infections. Proper interaction among physicians, microbiologists, and hospital staff of operative, dialysis, and oncology units and direct access to hospital administrative units for implementing the recommendations have been found to be fruitful in bringing down hospital-infection-related morbidity and mortality. The organism's prevalence, their sensitivity pattern, the check on ensured asepsis through a watch and surveillance on handwashing, rational antibiotics, use of disinfectant, biomedical disposals, and barrier nursing can help ultimately reduce the financial burden of the patients.

Nosocomial pneumonia is an acquired infection, localized to the gas exchanging units of the lungs, occurring during hospitalization, just after 48–72 hours of admission. Gram-negative bacteria accounts for two-third of nosocomial pneumonia cases. Since the infections are predominantly acquired in hospitalized patients having a pre-existing cardiorespiratory illness, and the organisms have varied resistance to various antimicrobials being in use in that hospital, the management of infections poses a great challenge. An increasing number of immunocompromised patients developing pneumonia as hospital-acquired infection makes the situation more difficult.

Introduction

Conflict between man and microbes is known since centuries, each one trying to gain ascendence over the other but victory eluding each one at the end of the day. However, man gathered experience of these years to carry out his struggle against these microbes, and this builds the basis of present-day control of hospital infections. Nosocomial pneumonia is a hospital-acquired respiratory infection that does not present any signs and symptoms during the first 48–72 hours after hospitalization.[1] These are the most common infections in the United States, next to urinary tract infections and top the list in most of the cancer centers. The risk increases up to 20 folds in patients on mechanical respirator, and a varied mortality rate of 20%–50% has been reported, with as higher as 80% mortality in cases infected with pathogens like *Pseudomonas aeruginosa*.[2] The situation is still worse in those associated with AIDS.[3,4]

The risk of contracting nosocomial infection increased by the use of sophisticated invasive devices in a seriously ill patient with impaired defense mechanisms. Management becomes difficult because of difficulty in diagnosing the condition. It requires meticulous care, high degree of skill, and proper ventilator and hemodynamic support to seriously ill patients, with constant watch, besides drugs and early enteral feeding. Both clinical and radiological findings are difficult to interpret and correlate, especially in patients at risk, for most of the patients have concomitant cardiopulmonary aliments such as ARDS, COPD, CCF, and so on. Where new or progressive pulmonary infiltrates along with fresh symptoms like fever, yellow sputum, and leukocytosis often point toward nosocomial pneumonia, diagnosis is always difficult in the presence of ARDS or other diffuse pulmonary diseases, and purulent tracheobronchitis poses a great differential challenge in almost one-third of cases cannot be rules out.

Usually, LMICs are a land of conflict a land of conflict and contrasts. A crop of healthcare workers is scattered between doctors and patients. The overcrowded hospitals, ill-designed wards and intensive care units, and multi-punctured veins with fluids and antibiotics which are being pushed, replacing many a times the normal flora by a tougher and resistant microbes and still on certain occasions, intestinal immunosuppression for certain serious ailments, sometimes precipitate the situation, making the patient vulnerable to secondary nosocomial infection. For such hazardous situations to face and tackle, Hospital Infection Society of India ets guidelines for prevention of hospital infections.

Microbes

Microbial diagnosis poses a great challenge. Many aids to recognize pathological organisms, such as using expectorated sputum, endotracheal suctioning, blood culture, pleural fluid, and bronchoalveolar lavage studies and isolating bacterial components like lipid A for *P. aeruginosa* have been utilized, but no specific microorganism could be reliably implicated despite the advancement in diagnostic facilities. Different clinical settings and hospitals are to have their own antibiotic policy, according to the nature of the organism isolated in that hospital. Most often, resistant microbes are seen in nosocomial infections; the mechanisms that determine resistance, such as extended-spectrum beta lactamases in Gram-negative bacilli, resistance to beta lactams, glycopeptides, and high levels of amino glycosides among enterococci, quinolone resistance in isolates of methicillin-resistant strains of *Staphylococcus aureus*, and Tn-21-related genetic resistance in Gram-negative organisms, demand an interactive and rational approach both by physicians and microbiologists to prevent the spread of resistant pathogens in hospitals.

Infection control

Selection of proper antibiotics in a proper dosage schedule may have potential utility, when used in combination regimes that include third-generation cephalosporins, extended-spectrum penicillins, imipenem–cilastatin, and ticarcillin–clavulanate, all with or without aminoglycoside and Aztreonam and clindamycin combination. These regimens must have a potent in vitro activity against *P. aeruginosa* that forms the major cause of nosocomial infections in most of the hospitals. The infection control committee has its core committee, consisting of physician, surgeon, microbiologist, senior nurse, and representatives from operation theater, dialysis room, and ICUs. To coordinate activities, there is the infection control sister. There is direct access to the chief administrative officer to urgently implement the decision. Functions of the committee are to collect data, carry out surveillance, and to enforce good infection control practices, for example, isolation of infectious patients, barrier nursing, disinfection of clothes of health workers, and proper disposal of the patient's excreta.[5,6] Necessary precautions against HIV spread, considering every patient to be a potential source of infection, by the health workers must be ensured. Unnecessary disinfection of hospital walls and floors should be avoided. Simple soap and water cleansing is cheap and best.

Adjuvant measures

Adjuvant measures to meet the challenge of nosocomial infections that are being explored include: primary prevention against *P. aeruginosa* through vaccination, and the use of murine and human monoclonal antibodies directed against the lipopolysaccharide component of *P. aeruginosa*, both for treatment and prophylaxis against nosocomial infection. Importance of prevention of development of nosocomial infection is an equally important challenge that attains significance, especially in a clinical setting, like ours, with special precaution in high-risk patients, such as those receiving respiratory interventional therapy, those on ventilators or with tracheostomies done, and with emergency intubations.[2] The risk is increased by 5–65 folds. Other high-risk patients are those undergoing major surgery, where the increased duration of surgery, followed by hospital stay would enhance the chances of nosocomial infection and subsequent difficulty in its management. The risk may be increased by 35 folds. Still further, intravascular catheters are likely to increase the risk of nosocomial infection. Old age, overuse of microbial agents, aspiration, congenital malformation of palate, immunosuppressants, impaired consciousness, low-birth-weight neonates, obese patients, systemic disorders like diabetes, chronic respiratory diseases, and so on. are the risk factors that pose a lot of challenge in precipitation as well as in management of nosocomial infections. In an Indian setup, Gram-negative pathogens pose a great challenge as hospital-acquired pneumonia, especially in patients suffering from chronic lung disease, malignancy, septicemia, and those with ventilatory support.

Despite a significant progress in detecting these pneumonia cases and their management by using numerous potent broad-spectrum antimicrobial agents has been made, nosocomial pneumonia cases pose a great challenge even today. The key to success lies in preventing the infection by selecting and caring the high-risk patients with proper interaction of doctors and nursing and finally of physicians and microbiologists. Management of nosocomial pneumonia grills the skill even of an adept pulmonologist. Despite continuous patrolling and check by mechanical barriers, reflex actions, and components of the immune system all along the respiratory tract, a large variety of microbes make a smooth landing on the moist landscape of alveolus, and despite lungs being highly vascularized and a rapid as well complete drug delivery system is expected, antibiotics access and action" is interfered by various factors such as local pH, oxygen concentration, and tissue debris and is further influenced by the type of pneumonia (i.e., necrotizing), host defense (i.e., inadequate), the pathogens (i.e., highly resistant), and the patient affected (i.e., mostly debilitated).

Certain important points are:

1. In hospital-acquired pneumonia, common etiological agents are endogenous *Enterobacteriaceae*, environmental *Pseudomonas*, and staphylococci, where environmental *Pseudomonas* and Staphylococcus are shown in Table 1.

Table 1: Nosocomial pneumonia; common etiological agents

1. Gram-negative bacilli: *Klebsiella pneumoniae, Enterobacter, Escherichia coli, Proteus, Serratia, Pseudomonas*
2. *S. aureus*
3. Anaerobes
4. *Streptococcus pneumoniae*

Table 2: Predisposing factors in nosocomial pneumonia[8]

Old age (more than 60 years)
Coexisting fatal disease
Thoracic or upper abdominal surgery
H-blocker therapy
Intubations, nasogastric tube, or recent bronchoscopy

2. There are problems in distinguishing other causes of infiltrates like acute lung injury and edema, hemorrhage as well as colonization versus tracheobronchitis versus pneumonia.
3. Unlike single-agent standard treatment for community-acquired pneumonia, combination therapy is required in nosocomial pneumonia.
4. Treatment duration may be prolonged sometimes to 1 month.
5. Initial treatment is empiric, based on the setting in which it occurs and the clinical features.[7]

Common causes that are listed in Table 2, which predispose to nosocomial pneumonia, many a times are found to be responsible for causing difficulty in the management of infection. Prognosis, as shown in Table 3, is poor in the presence of systemic illness, old age, altered consciousness, lowered BP, or rapidly spreading infection.

Management

Management modalities should be based on empiric therapy[9] based on the knowledge of likely pathogens, especially the ones known to cause

Table 3: Prognosis in nosocomial pneumonia

Prognosis is poor in the presence of:
A. *Co-existing*
a. Old age, co-existing cardiorespiratory illness or systemic disease, immunosuppression, extrapulmonary infections
B. *Clinically*
a. Altered consciousness, temperature more than 38.3°, respiration rate more than 30 per minute, blood pressure lower than 90/60 mmHg
C. *Investigation-wise*
a. Multiple-lobe involvement or rapidly spreading infection or effusion
b. Total count of white cells more than 30,000 or less than 4,000/cumm, raised creatinine, hematocrit lower than 30%, or PaO_2 less than 60 mmHg

infection in hospitalized patients in that particular setup. Supportive therapy in the form of oxygenation, antipyretics, intravenous hydration, and vasopressin agents may be required. Look for other causes of fever like catheter infections as well. Diagnosis and antibiotics can be revised as per culture and sensitivity. But one should never be taken away by fallacies in antimicrobial therapy such as broader antibiotic is always good, when in doubt, change the drug' failure to response is a failure to cure, more disease, more drugs; bigger disease, bigger drug or bigger diagnosis, newer drugs (antibiotic), and so on.[10]

Suggested regimens include b-lactam b-lactamase inhibitor in combination with third-generation cephalosporin, cefotaxime with an aminoglycoside (amikacin) or aztreonam + clindamycin or imipenem statin + aminoglycoside ticarcillin clavulanate + aminoglycoside. Ciprofloxacin in combination with amikacin is also effective. Culture and sensitivity reports should guide the treatment further. To start with, drugs against specific organisms, as has been shown in Table 4, can be started. Constant observation and treatment review by an attending physician in continuous interaction with a microbiologist may be rewarding.

Table 4: Drugs in nosocomial pneumonia[11]

Specific organisms	
Pseudomonas	1. Carbenicillin 2. Gentamicin or Tobramycin
Klebsiella	1. Gentamicin or Tobramycin 2. Cephalothin
S. aureus	1. Cloxacillin 2. Cephalothin or Vancomycin 3. Ampicillin 4. Aminoglycoside

Comments

It is difficult to totally eliminate hospital infections; but an aggressive approach can help to put a control-check. The enhanced invasive procedures[12] and ventilator-associated pneumonia,[13–15] however, have increased the chances of increasing nosocomial infections, the incidence of which is 5%–10% with nearly 1% mortality. This number has to be reduced further unreciprocated to the number of lives being saved by intensive care.[16,17] The invaluable fact of yesteryears in true *even* today sick to universal precautions, barrier nursing, near total asepsis and judicious use of antibiotics[18] Hand washing, and strict respiratory precautions for any contact health workers[19,8] and spot surveillance that how many doctors hand wash and alcohol rub and then examine the patient in ICU shall give quicker and cheaper check-results.[20]

References and suggested readings

1. Bennett JV, Brachman PS. Hospital infection. 4th ed. Philadelphia: Lippincott-Raven. 1998.
2. Fink MP, Snydman DR, Niederman MS, *et al.* Treatment of serve pneumonia in hospitalized patients. Anti-micro Agents Chemother. 1994;38:547–557.
3. Lee SC, *et al.* Nosocomial infection with Ceflzidime-resistant peudomonas aeroginosa: risk factors and outcome. Int Cont Hosp Epidemiol. 1999;20:205.

4. Smith RL, Meiler SM. Simbrx off MS: Excess mortality in critically ill patients with nosocomial blood stream infections. Chest. 1991;100:164.
5. Vincent J. Unfection in adult intensive care units. Lancet. 2003;361:2068–2076.
6. Cunha BA. Antibiotic resistance-control strategies. Crit Care Clin. 1998;8:309.
7. Soman R. Rational use of antibiotics in lower respiratory tract infection. IN: VP Munjal, ed. Med Update; API. Mumbai. 1997;7:769–771.
8. Sets WH, *et al.* Effectiveness of precautions against droplets and contact in prevention of nosocomial transmission of SARS. Lancet. 2003;361:1519–1520.
9. Sharma BK, Manju Nath S, Verma S, *et al.* Profile of pneumonias in hospitalized Indica patients. Ind J Chest Dis All Sci. 1998;30:199.
10. Joshi JM. Pneumonia. Med Update. 1997;5(8):542–546.
11. Hakim A, Deo A, Mehta P1. Treatment of resp. tract infections. Med Update. 1993;1(6):90–93.
12. Vigg A, *et al.* Fiberoptic bronchocopy. IN: LA Pathak, ed. PG Med; API. 2004;18:66–70.
13. 8andovin SV. Ventilator associated pneumonia. Thorax. 2001;56:5–50.
14. Fajon 1Y, *et al.* Ventilator associated pneumonia. Ann Intern Med. 2000;132–621.
15. Hayon J, *et al.* Role of serial routine microbiologic culture results in the management of VAP. AJRCCM. 2002;165:115.
16. Cherian Rohini, *et al.* Risk factors of nosocomial infections in medical intensive care units. Ind J Crit Care Med. 2001;5:4.
17. Mishra MP. Infections in intensive care. IN: NP Mishra, ed. Med Update; API. 2000;0:469–472.
18. Dastur FD. Hospital infection-how far can good practices reduce them? IN: SB Gupta, ed. Med Update.
19. Gawande A. On wasging hands. N Engl Med. 2004;350:1283–1286.
20. Farr BM. Reasons for non-compliance with infection control guidelines. IdCont. Hospital. 2000;21:141–16.
21. Bhatia RS. Challenges in the management of nosocomial pneumonia. IN: MM Singh, ed. Med Update; API. 1999;9:377–382.
22. Burke P. Infection control-a problem for patient safety. N Eng J Med. 2003;348:651–655.
23. Egglman R, Pitter D. Infection control in ICU. Chest. 2001;120:2059–2093.

24. Cunha BA. The antibiotic therapy of community acquired atypical and nosocomial pneumonia. IN: BA Cunha, ed. Antimicrobial therapy. Med Clin N Amer. 1995;79:581–597.
25. Betes JH, Campbell GD, Barron AL, *et al.* Microbial aetiology of acute pneumonia in hospitalised patients. Chest. 1992;101:1005–1012.
26. Joshi N, Lucalio AR, Hamory BH. A predictive risk for nosocomial pneumonia in the intensive care unit. AM J Med. 1992;93:135–142.
27. Ami Raj 5, *et al.* Infections in ICU and management. IN: S Das, ed. Med Update; API. 2003;13:18996.
28. Xu E, Pérez-Torres D, Fragkou PC, Zahar JR, Koulenti D. Nosocomial pneumonia in the era of multidrug-resistance: updates in diagnosis and management. Microorganisms. 2021 Mar 5;9(3):534. PMID: 33807623; PMCID: PMC8001201.
29. Bardi T, Pintado V, Gomez-Rojo M, Escudero-Sanchez R, Azzam Lopez A, Diez-Remesal Y, Martinez Castro N, Ruiz-Garbajosa P, Pestaña D. Nosocomial infections associated to COVID-19 in the intensive care unit: clinical characteristics and outcome. Eur J Clin Microbiol Infect Dis. 2021 Mar;40(3):495–502. Epub 2021 Jan 3. PMID: 33389263; PMCID: PMC7778834.
30. El-Mokhtar MA, Daef E, Mohamed Hussein AAR, Hashem MK, Hassan HM. Emergence of nosocomial pneumonia caused by colistin-resistant escherichia coli in patients admitted to chest intensive care unit. Antibiotics (Basel). 2021 Feb 24;10(3):226. PMID: 33668302; PMCID: PMC7996192.
31. Johnson MG, Bruno C, Castanheira M, Yu B, Huntington JA, Carmelitano P, Rhee EG, De Anda C, Motyl M. Evaluating the emergence of nonsusceptibility among pseudomonas aeruginosa respiratory isolates from a phase-3 clinical trial for treatment of nosocomial pneumonia (ASPECT-NP). Int J Antimicrob Agents. 2021 Mar;57(3):106278. Epub 2021 Jan 9. PMID: 33434676.

https://doi.org/10.1142/9789811271410_0032

32 Atypical pneumonia

Introduction

Pneumonitis is an inflammation and consolidation of the lung tissue, which can be lobar as in streptococcal pneumonia or a patchy consolidation on an X-ray that is produced by most other bacterial organisms. Atypical pneumonia is caused by non-bacterial organisms such as *Legionella*, *Mycoplasma*, *Chlamydia*, and *Coxiella*. Worsening of the clinical status despite adequate therapy requires a reinvestigative approach to reach a conclusive diagnosis for an appropriate therapy.

Clinical presentation

Unlike bacterial typical pneumonia which has high fever of sudden onset with shiver, chest pain, and viscous yellowish excitation with a segmental or lobar consolidation on chest X-ray, atypical pneumonia manifests with clinically recognizable symptoms of chest infection. Sputum is rarely present, pleural effusion is uncommon, and peripheral leukocyte count is within normal limits. It is important not to overstress the term atypical pneumonia; it is better to reconfine as mycoplasma, chlamydial pneumonia, legionnaires disease, Q fever (rickettsiosis), or *Coxiella burnetii* infection. Common differentiating features of typical and atypical pneumonia are shown in Table 1.

Legionnaires disease

It is suspected when there is recent plumbing work being done at the workplace or at home or there is a history of poorly maintained bathroom tubs.

Table 1: Characteristics of typical and atypical pneumonia

Feature	Typical pneumonia	Atypical pneumonia
Fever	Fever with chills	Fever without chills
Cheshlan/ cough	Pleuritic pain with productive cough	Upper airway symptoms and myalgias with unproductive cough
TLC, ESR, chest X-ray	Normal or consolidation in 780%	A little altered consolidation in less than 50% and ground glass appearance more common
Causative organism	*Streptococcus pneumoniae*	*Viruses Mycoplasma pneumoniae*
	Staphylococcus aureus	*Legionella pneumophila*
	Klebsiella pneumoniae	*Chlamydia psittaci*
	Haemophilus influenzae	*Coxiella burnetii*

Diabetes mellitus, old age, tobacco smoking, renal dialysis, immunosuppressive therapy including corticosteroids, chemotherapy with cytotoxic drugs, lung cancer, retroviral disease, and chronic heart or lung disease are often taken as precipitating or risk factors. Buffered charcoal–yeast extract agar medium with iron-1-cysteine and alpha ketoglutarate is used to grow *Legionella.* Often, polymyxin B, cefamandole, and vancomycin are used in the culture medium to prevent the growth of their competing microflora. Hypophosphatemia favors the diagnosis of *Legionella.* An incubation period of 2–10 days is followed by cough, dyspnea, fever, and prostration. Relative bradycardia may be encountered. Chest examination shows the presence of nodules and later signs of consolidation. Severity of the disease ranges from a trivial cough to a rapidly progressive and fatal pneumonia. Death may occur from respiratory failure, shock, hypotension, and acute renal failure. Supportive therapy with oxygen, mechanical ventilation, volume replacement, vasoactive agents, and diagnosis may be required.

Mycoplasmal pneumonia

Most of these organisms are commensals within the human host. As they become invaders, patient manifests with headache, malaise, cough, and chest tightness. A chest X-ray initially shows reticular interstitial infiltrates, and chest auscultatory findings are near normal. Pneumonia develops later. Pneumonitis with varicella zoster, herpes simplex, Epstein–Barr virus, enterovirus, adenovirus, and measles are often accompanied with maculopapular rash. Erythema multiforme, erythema nodosum, and urticaria may also accompany. Complications such as respiratory failure may require mechanical ventilation. Hemolytic anemia may also complicate. Other atypical pneumonia are kept as differentials.

Chlamydial pneumonia

Infection may initiate with sinusitis, pharyngitis, and bronchitis and may end up as pneumonitis. Conjunctival involvement may be accompanied by chronic follicular conjunctivitis where subconjunctival lymphoid follicles are grossly visible. Genital manifestations in the form of urethritis, epididymitis, parotitis, Reiter's syndrome, cervicitis, endometritis, salpingitis, lymphogranuloma venereum, and pelvic inflammatory disease are present.

Psittacosis

Chlamydia psittaci may involve the interstitium and alveoli of the lungs, producing non-productive cough, with bilateral basal crackles on auscultation. There can be signs of consolidation on auscultation of a pleural rub. A chest X-ray reveals single or multiple patches of bronchopneumonia. Systemic reticuloendothelial system is involved by this systemic infection. After an incubation period of 1–2 weeks, patients may present with fever, myalgia, headache, photophobia, and non-productive cough. Hemoptysis or skin rash may occur. /Patient's examination may reveal hepatosplenomegaly and erythema nodosum. A fourfold rise in complement fixation antibody titer in the era drawn during acute and convalescent phases is diagnostic.

Queensland fever (Q fever)

It is a rickettsial infection which, unlike other rickettsial infections that are transmitted by vectors, is disseminated by aerosol or blood transfusion. Rash is absent despite the presence of endothelial vasculitis. Contact history with goats, sheep, cats, rabbits, dogs, and cattle is a diagnostic contributor. After an incubation period for 1–2 weeks, lung affection presents with bronchiolitis and pneumonitis showing rounded opacities on the chest X-ray and may take longer time to resolve with antibiotics. Systemic infection may present with hepatitis, and subacute or chronic endocarditis. In that case, liver enzymes may be elevated. Complement fixation test shows a rising antibody titer.

Treatment

Legionella can be treated with macrolides, tetracycline, doxy or minocycline, quinolones, and rifampicin. *Mycoplasma* may require erythromycin, azithromycin, clarithromycin, and tetracycline. *Chlamydia* gives a slow treatment response to erythromycin and tetracycline. *C. burnetii* infection should be treated with a combination of two antibiotics using tetracycline, doxycycline, and quinolone.

Classification to determine diagnosis can be achieved by clinical and laboratory examination. However, classifying community-acquired pneumonia (CAP) into typical or atypical may not be a determining path for the management plan of CAP. Clinicoradiological picture may not offer conclusive evidence. Typical pneumonias often respond well as to beta-lactam antibiotics as compared to atypical pathogens which are effectively treated with macrolides, tetracyclines, and some quinolones and do not respond to beta-lactam because of being intracellular. Apart from infections like pyogenic CAP, followed by tuberculosis, malignancy and vasculitis are important etiologies. FOB and CT-guided FNAC, when combined, improved the diagnostic yield.

References and suggested reading

1. Mac Farlane IT, et al. Comparative radio graphic features of community acquired Leginnaires' disease, pneumococcal pneumonia, mycoplasma pneumonia and psittacosis. Thorax. 1984;39:28–33.
2. Bedi RS. CAP-typical or atypical. Lung India. 2006;23:130–131.

3. Chandrasekhran S. Atypical pneumonia. IN: SB Gupta, ed. Med Update; API. 2005;15:558–559.
4. Sarosi GA. Atypical preumonia-why this term may be better left unsaid. PG Med. 1999;105:131–138.
5. Bhatia RS. Community aquiredpnemonia. IN: VP Munjal, ed. PG Med; API. 1999;13:375–382.
6. Sorabjeei, MV. Non-resolving pneumonia. IN: SB Gupta, ed. PG Med; API. 2014;28:556–569.
7. Chaudhuri AD, et al. A study on non-resolving pneumonia with special reference to role of FOB. Lung India. 2013;30:27–32.
8. Ceylan N, Çinkooğlu A, Bayraktaroğlu S, Savaş R. Atypical chest CT findings of COVID-19 pneumonia: a pictorial review. Diagn Interv Radiol. 2021 May;27(3):344–349. doi: 10.5152/dir.2020.20355. PMID: 33032981; PMCID: PMC8136535.
9. Ville S, Le Bot S, Chapelet-Debout A, Blancho G, Fremeaux-Bacchi V, Deltombe C, Fakhouri F. Atypical HUS relapse triggered by COVID-19. Kidney Int. 2021 Jan;99(1):267–268. doi: 10.1016/j.kint.2020.10.030. Epub 2020 Nov 11. PMID: 33188793; PMCID: PMC7657017.
10. Westblade LF, Simon MS, Satlin MJ. Bacterial coinfections in coronavirus disease 2019. Trends Microbiol. 2021 Oct;29(10):930–941. doi: 10.1016/j.tim.2021.03.018. Epub 2021 Apr 8. PMID: 33934980; PMCID: PMC8026275.
11. Frohnhofen H, Stieglitz S. PneumonieimhohenLebensalter [Pneumonia in old age]. Pneumologe (Berl). 2021;18(3):174–181. German. doi: 10.1007/s10405-021-00388-z. Epub 2021 Mar 16. PMID: 33746676; PMCID: PMC7963464.
12. Toraih EA, Hussein MH, Elshazli RM, Kline A, Munshi R, Sultana N, Taghavi S, Killackey M, Duchesne J, Fawzy MS, Kandil E. Multisystem inflammatory syndrome in pediatric COVID-19 patients: a meta-analysis. World J Pediatr. 2021 Apr;17(2):141–151. doi: 10.1007/s12519-021-00419-y. Epub 2021 Feb 20. PMID: 33608839; PMCID: PMC7895741.
13. Watson A, Wilkinson TMA. Respiratory viral infections in the elderly. Ther Adv Respir Dis. 2021 Jan–Dec;15:1753466621995050. doi: 10.1177/1753466621995050. PMID: 33749408; PMCID: PMC7989115.
14. Ng SL, Ong YS, Khaw KY, Teh SP, Tan CS, Ming LC, Chan KG, Lee LH, Goh BH. Focused review: potential rare and atypical symptoms as indicator for

targeted COVID-19 screening. Medicina (Kaunas). 2021 Feb 23;57(2):189. doi: 10.3390/medicina57020189. PMID: 33672384; PMCID: PMC7927030.

15. Thakur V, Ratho RK, Kumar P, Bhatia SK, Bora I, Mohi GK, Saxena SK, Devi M, Yadav D, Mehariya S. Multi-organ involvement in COVID-19: beyond pulmonary manifestations. J Clin Med. 2021 Jan 24;10(3):446. doi: 10.3390/jcm10030446. PMID: 33498861; PMCID: PMC7866189.

https://doi.org/10.1142/9789811271410_0033

33 Acute respiratory failure

Introduction

Physiology of the respiratory system includes supply of oxygen to and elimination of carbon dioxide from the cells and maintenance of the normal acid–base balance of the body. This is achieved by coordinated functioning of multisystems of the body like the central nervous system, chest wall and muscles, airways and lungs, and the cardiovascular and endocrine systems. Respiratory failure occurs if any of these systems is diseased and is unable to provide an effective exchange of oxygen and carbon dioxide between the external environment and body tissues in quantities sufficient to sustain life. Diminution of arterial oxygen tension below 60 mmHg with or without an elevation of carbon dioxide tension above 45 mmHg in a person at rest points toward respiratory failure. Acute respiratory failure (ARF) has sudden onset but may develop over days, especially in patients with pre-existing lung disease.

It is a common clinical emergency encountered in the medicine department. It has a higher rate of mortality where 55.6% survival is reported despite best service in hospitalized patients. Alveolar hypoventilation leads to type 2 hypercapnic respiratory failure as acute exacerbation of chronic obstructive pulmonary disease (COPD) brings protective ventilation improves outcome in acute respiratory distress syndrome (ARDS) patients. NIPPU helps in cutting down the complications of intubation, nosocomial pneumonia, and mortality.

Hypoxemia

Hypoxemia due to acute or acute chronic respiratory failure can occur and often it is sudden in onset, presenting with restlessness, palpitation, headache, sweating, confusion and even cyanosis. The initial rise in blood pressure falls with worsening of severity of hypoxemia which is often accompanied with hypercapnia, whenever there is hypoventilation.

Hypoxemia results from hypoxia — a natural consequence of most of the diffuse lung diseases, and the degree of hypoxemia and chronicity of the disease determine the need for supplemental oxygen therapy, which is considered for its tissue utilization and not simply correcting the blood $PaCl_i$.

Classification of respiratory failure

Respiratory failure can be classified into the following two types:

a. Type 1: It is defined by $PaO_2 < 60$ mmHg with a normal or low $PaCO_2$.
b. Type 2: It is defined by $PaO_2 < 60$ mmHg and a $PaCO_2 > 45$ mmHg. It is further classified as acute, subacute, and chronic. The etiology is diverse. Type 1 hypoxemic respiratory failure occurs in pneumonia, pulmonary edema, pulmonary embolism, pulmonary fibrosis, asthma, chronic bronchitis and emphysema, pneumothorax, ARDS, pulmonary AV fistula, pneumoconiosis, thromboembolic pulmonary hypertension, fat embolism, granulomatous lung disease, and cyanotic congenital heart disease.

Type 2 respiratory failure is commonly seen in chronic bronchitis and emphysema, asthma, drug overdose, poisoning, poliomyelitis, polyneuropathy, porphyria, primary muscle disorder, primary alveolar hypoventilation, ARDS, pulmonary edema, laryngeal edema, sleep apnea syndrome, and foreign body causing obstruction.

Table 1: Common causes of ARF

1. Ventilation defect
   a. Depression of the respiratory center
      1. Cerebral trauma/infarction
      2. Drugs such as sedatives, narcotics, anesthetics, etc.
   b. Neuromuscular disorder
      1. Brain/spinal injury
      2. Guillain–Barre syndrome
      3. Myasthenia gravis
      4. Botulism, polio, porphyria
   c. Obstruction of airways
      1. Acute severe asthma
      2. COPD
   d. Restrictive defect
      1. Obesity
      2. ILDS
      3. Bilateral palsy of the diaphragm
      4. Kyphoscoliosis, ankylosing spondylitis
2. Impaired diffusion and gas exchange
   a. ARDS
   b. Pulmonary edema
   c. Pulmonary thromboembolism
   d. Pulmonary fibrosis
3. Abnormal ventilation–perfusion (V/Q)
   a. COPD
   b. ARDS
   c. Thromboembolism
   d. Pulmonary fibrosis

**Source*: Andel SK. Oxygen therapy for pulmonary disorders. IN: SK Jindal, R Agarwal, eds. Oxygen therapy; 2nd ed; Jay Pee Public. 2008;10:157–182.

ARF and COPD

Hypercarbia effects are variable from patient to patient, but coma is uncommon in patients with respiratory failure with COPD. Hypoxia results primarily from ventilation–perfusion (V/Q) mismatch. Type 2 hypercapnic failure in an exacerbation of COPD is by far more common. Hypercapnia results from airways obstruction, alveolar hypoventilation, central hypoventilation, and chronic respiratory muscle fatigue. Hypoxemia leads to reflex pulmonary vasoconstriction that worsens pulmonary hypertension. Oxygen therapy effectively treats hypoxemia of COPD and is the only strategy to improve survival in a COPD patient, of course apart from the total cessation of tobacco smoking. NIPPU obviates intubation in >50% of appropriately selected patients.

Acute respiratory distress syndrome

Genetic susceptibility plays a key role in ARDS pathogenesis, especially genes encoding angiotensin-converting enzyme (ACE), interleukin (IL)-10, tumor necrosis factor (TNF) alpha, and vascular endothelial growth factor.

Increased levels of biomarkers like IL-6 and angiopoietin 2 are associated with adverse outcomes in ARDS and are under genetic control.

Human mesenchymal seen in lung injury caused by bacteria in areas of future research.

Thompson BT, et al. ARDS. NEJM. 2017;377:562–572.

Mechanical ventilation has to be supplemented with bronchodilator therapy, corticosteroids, and antibiotics, where it becomes mandatory in severe COPD, since NIPPV has not shown convincing benefits.

Pulmonary edema and ARF

Immediate treatment of hypoxemia associated with pulmonary edema is to increase the FiO_2, and using an appropriate pattern of ventilation, however, success depends on the etiology of pulmonary edema. In the absence of pulmonary capillary damage, diuretics and fluid restriction do help in improvement, but with the presence of pulmonary capillary lesions with loss of capillary integrity and loss of proteins, Starling's law no longer pertains, and even rigorous dehydration prove ineffective. Unfortunately, pulmonary water is poorly mobilizable even with overdiuresis and dehydration. CPAP and nasal BIPP have been shown to improve $PaCO_2$ pH levels, respiratory rate, and dyspnea.

ARF in bronchial asthma

Patients in acute exacerbation have low levels of $PaCO_2$, and hypoxemia occurs even on mild exertion. Gas exchange in asthma is affected when the disease is relatively severe, due to airways diffuse obstruction. Mismatch of ventilation to perfusion is present, but CO_2 retention is not a usual feature. Humidified oxygen should be administered to reduce hypoxic pulmonary vasoconstriction, thereby improving pulmonary hypertension which is usually present during an attack of bronchial asthma. In addition, oxygen exerts a bronchodilatory effect also on the severely constricted bronchi. Arterial blood gas (ABG) analysis may be essential if the patient deteriorates on oxygen therapy, possibly because of CO_2 being retained: Failing all measures of high humidity O_2 bronchodilation, corticosteroids, hydration and treatment of infection, intubation, and mechanical ventilation are instituted. Bronchial lavage under general anesthesia is rarely required. NIPPV has been found to be successfully effective treatment modality to correct gas exchange in asthma. Complications of ARF become part and parcel of complications resulting from care of the critically ill and those of the underlying disease itself. These include complications of high-tech services of ICU like ventricular tachycardia during the passage of a flow-directed catheter through the right ventricle or barotrauma from the use of PEER. Other complications that do not occur because of the disease or care being delivered include gastrointestinal bleeding from stress ulceration and nosocomial infections. Yet another group of complications like psychological stress occur because of new environments of hospital and risk of exposure to various infections like hepatitis, tuberculosis, and HIV disease. The ethical question regarding acute care in ICU or ICU and about the socioeconomic cost benefit salsoft part of the complications of ARF, especially in a setup like ours.

Hypoxia

There is acute worsening of pre-existing hypoxia or redevelopment of hypoxia may occur, possibly because of retention of secretions in the tracheobronchial tree or endotracheal tube, premature extubation, ventilator failure or disconnection, gastric distention, and atelectasis. Hypoxia is clinically signaled by changes in the heart rate, respiratory rate, or blood pressure or by the presence of cyanosis. Severe hypoxia may lead to cardiac arrest.

Complications of endotracheal tube

Difficult intubation may account for gastric distension or convulsions. Malpositioning of the tube detected physically or on chest roentgenography may confine to one side, mostly right hemithorax. Cuff rupture can lead to severe leaks, and overinflation may cause cuff herniation to obstruct the flow or compress the tube. Even a kinked tube can cause obstruction.

Nasal injury at the site of contact is common. This happens because of excessive pressure on external nares from the tape or equipment attached to the tube. Rarely erosion of the esophagus (tracheoesophageal fistula) or of the neighboring artery (innominate artery) may occur. Laryngeal ulceration may develop as early as 6 hours after endotracheal intubation. The severity of damage is directly related to the duration of intubation and presents as hoarseness, stridor, and dysphagia. Vocal cords when affected can result in hoarseness and dysphagia; airways obstruction may occur when the subglottic area is affected, and healing with fibrosis results in adhesions and serious sequelae. Injuries are due to mechanical, chemical, and reactionary ethylene oxide used for sterilization trauma.

Barotrauma

Sudden catastrophic worsening of the clinical course of a patient on a mechanical ventilator, especially PEEP, should arouse suspicion of pneumothorax. Look for physical findings, and in case of emergency, insert a needle into each of the hemithoraces to search for air in the pleural cavity. Roentgenography is always helpful, and if confirmed, tube thoracostomy is indicated. Pulmonary barotrauma (pneumothorax, pneumomediastinum, subcutaneous emphysema) is related directly to maximum distending volume than to the peak inspiratory pressure.

Oxygen toxicity

Oxygen toxicity is a complication of artificial ventilation in ARF. Pulmonary lesions are quite characteristic. Lungs are heavy, "beefy," and edematous. Histologic examination reveals during exudative phase, congestion, alveolar edema, intraalveolar hemorrhage, and fibrinous exudate with the formation of prominent hyaline membranes without any associated inflammatory component, and during late proliferative phase, pronounced alveolar and intraalveolar septal edema, fibroblastic proliferation with early fibrosis, and prominent hyperplasia of alveolar lining cells. Morphological changes are unrelated to the duration of artificial ventilation but to correlate with the prolonged use and high-inspired oxygen concentration.

Oxygen toxicity can develop within 48 hours of exposure to pure oxygen. Physiological complications such as suppression of hypoxic ventilatory drive, absorption atelectasis, effect on circulation, and a marginal decrease in diffusion capacity are generally clinically insignificant.

Oxygen toxicity includes the formation of several types of free radicals, tissue damage due to toxic oxygen metabolites, emergence of clinical syndromes of oxidant injury and pulmonary oxygen toxicity presenting *either* as tracheobronchitis or acute lung injury (ALI) or bronchopulmonary dysplasia (chronic lung injury), depending on the duration and concentration of oxygen used (normobaric/hyperbaric hyperoxia). Unequivocal decrease in PaO, with pure O_2, in patients without any preexisting cardiopulmonary disease, increased intrapulmonary shunt and increased VD/VT ratio, as well as increased lung weight on autopsy have been demonstrated. This is influenced by many factors; however, tolerance is known to develop in lungs. Newborn and premature babies are more prone to some effects like retinal damage. With prolonged positive pressure ventilation, a clinical syndrome characterized by positive water balance and radiologically consistent with pulmonary edema in the absence of cardiac failure or elevated central venous pressure is observed. The reason for this is not known, but there is evidence of decreased compliance and altered gas exchange associated. Diuretics and a check on the total fluid intake can print this transudative fluid collection that causes hemodilum and relative hyponatremia. The potential dangers of oxygen toxicity underscores the need for controlled oxygen therapy, especially when it is required for more than 24 hours.

Acid–base imbalance leads to multiorgan involvement and may become life threatening; simple steps to interpret ABG analysis are highly useful.

Exogenous antioxidant enzymes, chelation therapy, enzyme induction, and modulation of inflammatory response as cofactors have been tried, but most of the approaches to treat oxygen toxicity are still in infancy. Better not to exceed the lowest possible concentration required to correct tissue hypoxia.

Infection

Nosocomial infections are common and form serious complications. Many reports have been documented where aerobic Gram-negative infections resulted from the use of contaminated ventilators or other respiratory equipment. Therefore, sterilization rather than disinfection, use of disposable items, and rigorous periodical infection surveillance can help, if not completely, to eliminate the problem. Infection can occur from indwelling arterial, venous, or urinary catheters also. Rarely, nosocomial infection may transform normal oropharyngeal floras to floras containing aerobic Gram-negative bacilli and staphylococci in severely ill patients even after hospitalization and remain vulnerable to pneumonia if they happen to aspirate these secretions. Such infections often worsen or precipitate respiratory failure in an otherwise stable patient of COPD. The role of supplemental oxygen as supportive therapy cannot be ruled out. The role of oxygen is determined by the severity of pneumonia, the extent of lung involvement, and the presence of hypoxemia and not by the etiology of the infection causing pneumonitis.

Hyper/hypoventilation

Inappropriate adjustment or changed distribution of ventilation can affect CO_2 elimination resulting in hyper- or hypocarbia. Accompanying acid–base or electrolyte shire may cause hypo- or hypertension, cardiac arrhythmias, convulsions, or other neurologic abnormalities.

Fluid, electrolyte, and acid disturbances

Respiratory acidosis is frequent with hypokalemic metabolic alkalosis. Potassium deficit is common, especially when corticosteroids and diuretics have been used. Intravenous correction with KCL 20–60 mEg in 500 mL of glucose will tackle this iatrogenic complication until the blood reports of electrolyte are available.

Cardiac arrhythmias

Almost all varieties of cardiac arrhythmias such as atrial extrasystoles, multifocal atrial tachycardia, atrial tachycardia with block, atrial fibrillation, AV dissociation, ventricular extrasystole, and so on have been documented in ARF. Mortality rate increases in these patients if not adequately treated.

Pulmonary thromboembolism

It is an important and yet common complication in ARF. Heparin 5,000 units 6 hourly, guided by periodic clotting time, is given. Secondary polycythemia occurs, adding to the gravity of thromboembolism. Phlebotomies may rarely be required. Thrombosis, ischemia, and cerebral embolization are known to occur in radial artery cannulation, the former two increase with the duration of cannulation; therefore, arterial catheters used for pressure monitoring, if being left for days, just for ABG analysis specimens, is not justified. Hypoxia occurs due to V/Q abnormality or due to the presence of pulmonary edema. Hypoventilation results in hypoc-risy. Pulmonary infarction occurs in about 10% of cases. Oxygen therapy corrects arterial hypoxemia and prevents further extension of pulmonary infarction. In addition, oxygen therapy helps in absorbing embolism (in case of air embolism) as a primary method of treatment.

Miscellaneous

Acute lobar or whole lung atelectasis form important complications in ARF, especially when the patient is comatose or paralyzed. Hypoxemia, if persists, can lead to pneumonia. Therefore, keystone relief measures are relief of hypoxemia, bronchospasm, and retained secretions. In ALI, oxygen therapy provides adequate tissue oxygen. In ARF due to an infection episode in bronchiectasis, oxygen.

Use of water within plasma to generate oxygen and hydrogen using light energy is the emerging concept in case of gas exchange failure at the alveolar capillary membrane. Efficacy of O_2 depends on photocatalyst, using nano-thin films of titanium dioxide with indium tin oxide.

Therapy is useful for hypoxemic correction. Hypoxemia in pneumothorax, especially if the lung functions are already compromised, has to be essentially treated with oxygen therapy. It also helps in absorption of any abnormal presence of air.

Patients with kyphoscoliosis may face acute worsening of chronic respiratory failure following a lower respiratory tract infection or during pregnancy, and oxygen therapy often helps in minimizing dyspnea. Patients with obstructive sleep apnea developing respiratory failure due to associated problems or complications do improve arterial oxygenation by oxygen therapy during sleep.

Alveolar hypoxia in pulmonary hypertension is relieved by selective primary vasodilator effect of 100% oxygen, regardless of the primary diagnosis, especially with documented resting hypoxemia.

Hypoxemia in interstitial lung disease occurs due to V/Q mismatch and impaired diffusion which may further be increased following exercise due to diffusion limitation. And in advanced cases, CO_2 tension may occur, Hence, oxygen therapy is required in higher concentrations at high flow rates in most of the cases. Inadequate clearance of secretions may occur because of many factors such as (a) increased viscosity due to local and systemic dehydration, (b) central depression of cough reflex, (c) loss of glottic function and airway drying due to endotracheal I tube, and (d) gravitational secretional pooling due to the supine position of the patient.

Clearing of secretions is, thus, as important as is the kind and efficient nursing care to prevent many complications and help in making patients early ambulatory. Chest physiotherapy or bronchoscopically, secretions can be cleared, but an unskilled use of bronchoscopic trauma may be hazardous as it may contribute to further edema and increased airways obstruction.

Comments

Despite increased understanding regarding the pathophysiology of ARF, the golden molecule is yet to come to stop or reverse the same. Management targets at maintaining gas exchange and minimizing the complications arising out of the process of correcting ARF until lungs are opportunities to recover. Judicious use of oxygen therapy is supportive and supplemental in various situations. Many patients may remain refractory to the therapy, and in an exercise to achieve the target, newer modalities are being tried, but these do add to consequent therapeutic complications such as oxygen toxicity and alveolar injury. Still more and more modes such as pressure-controlled ventilation, airway pressure release ventilation, and

Table 2: Criteria for ABG analysis for ARF (with few exceptions)

Oxygenation: An acute decrease in arterial PO to 50 mmHg or below
Ventilation: An acute increase in arterial PCO such that the pH drops below 7.30

Table 3: Black and white criteria of OD of hypoxemic ARF $PCO_2 < 40$ mmHg

<table>
<tr><td>Black</td><td>White</td></tr>
<tr><td>1. Acute pulmonary embolism</td><td>a. If diffuse, ARDS, cardiopulmonary edema</td></tr>
<tr><td>2. Other vascular obstruction</td><td>b. If localized, pulmonary fibrosis with acute insult</td></tr>
<tr><td colspan="2">Simple fine steps to acid–base analysis

Step I: Acidemia or alkalemia pH < 7.38, pH > 7.42
Step II: Primary respiratory or metabolic disturbance KCO_2 on ABG HCO-3
Step III: Metabolic acidosis PCO_2 = (1.5 serum HCO-3 + 8(±2)
Metabolic acidosis ↑PCO_2 = 0.8 × ↑ HCO-3 + 8 + 20
Respiratory acidosis: ↑ PaO_2 = 10, ↑ HCO-3 by 1 acute chronic
Respiratory acidosis: ↓ PaO_2 = 10, ↓ HCO-3 by 2 acute chronic
Step IV: Anion (AGMA) anion gap metabolic acidosis or 5 (chronic)
AG=Na-(HCO3 + Cl, if > 12, AGMA)
Step V: If metabolic acidosis, find out delta ratio to mixed in order
Delta ratio = AG/HCO3</td></tr>
<tr><td>3.Circulatory failure</td><td>a. If diffuse, ARDS, cardiopulmonary edema with respiratory depression, pulmonary fibrosis with end-stage airways disease</td></tr>
<tr><td>4. Anatomic right to left shunt (PCO_2 >40 mmHg) Black
Status asthmaticus
Alveolar hypoventilation drug overdose
Neuromuscular weakness or paralysis</td><td>b. If localized, pneumonia with COPD, respiratory depression, drugs</td></tr>
</table>

Table 4: Treatment order

Treatment order
Arterial blood gas (ABG) repeatedly obtained in ICU.
Chest X-ray, followed by 24 hours O_2 Venturi mask and respiratory therapy called IPPB. Ventilation.
Suction 2 hourly; if needed, nebulized acetylcysteine.
Semi-Fowler's position, rotating 2 hourly.
Sputum sent for culture and sensitivity: Antibiotics started for infection suspected.
Input/output chart.
Blood gas studies 2 hourly with pH, PaCO, and PAO.
NaHCO is given, pH is 7.10–7.20.
Deflate the endotracheal cuffed balloon 2 hourly.
ECG.
Tranquilizer/muscle relaxant if the patient is fighting ventilation.
Ventilation without low-pressure cuff, if needed, for more than 5 days, tracheostomy may be performed.

Table 5: Major complications of acute respiratory failure respiratory: hypoxia

- Poorly positioned and malfunctioning endotracheal tube
- Airway injury, barotrauma
- Oxygen toxicity
- Nosocomial pneumonia and other infections
- Lobar atelectasis
- Mechanical failure of the ventilator/alarm
- Hypo/hyperventilation
- Circulatory:
- Decreased cardiac output
- Cardiac arrhythmias
- Vascular damage
- DIC
- Malpositioned aortic catheter pulsation balloon

(*Continued*)

Table 5: (*Continued*)

Adverse effects of vasopressors and vasodilators
Gastrointestinal:
Gastrointestinal bleeding renal aspiration of gastric contents
• Renal failure
Electrolyte imbalance
Complication of dialysis Nutritional: Malnutrition
Metabolic disturbances Complications of ICU/ICPU:
Fluid overload
Electrolyte imbalance Physical deconditioning Depression: ICU psychosis
(pneumothorax, pneumomediastinum, subcutaneous emphysema, bronchopleural fistula)

Table 6: Management of complications of ARF

1. Retained secretions: (suppressed coughing) bronchoscope aspiration/ aspiration via endotracheal tube
2. Hypoxias: Graduated 0, therapy
3. Alveolar hypoventilation: assisted ventilation, respiratory stimulants
4. Respiratory: antibiotics
5. Bronchospasm: bronchodilator aerosol IA/aminophylline line and corticosteroids
6. Cardiac failure: diuretics, digoxin.
Clumsy attempt on endotracheal intubation should be avoided to avoid laryngeal edema.

volume-controlled ventilation with a modified decelerating flow waveform are being utilized in an attempt to bring down mortality due to ARF and its complications during management.

Acute respiratory distress syndrome

Treatment

Management of ARDS focuses on treating the underlying cause of lung injury as well as providing supportive care. It has been shown that pharmacologic interventions may provide additional benefit by maintaining adequate oxygenation and ventilation while reducing the duration of ventilator use and decreasing morbidity and mortality. To date, corticosteroids, neuromuscular blocking agents (NMBAs), nitric oxide (NO), surfactants, and beta$_2$-adrenergic agonists (beta$_2$-agonists) have been theorized to improve outcomes.

Oxygen therapy

Indications for oxygen therapy

Oxygen can be given in high or low concentration in all the conditions associated with hypoxemia. In conditions like COPD in which there is a risk for hypercarbia, low concentration should be used. In acute lung conditions (without underlying chronic lung disease) like pulmonary embolism, pneumonia, tension pneumothorax, acute severe asthma, pulmonary edema, or myocardial infarction, a higher concentration of oxygen can be given. Similarly, in fibrosing alveolitis, there is no retention of CO_2, so high concentration can be given as in these conditions, there is no danger of induction of hypoventilation. Maintaining PaO_2 above 60 mmHg gives O_2 saturation of 90%. During acute exacerbation of COPD, chemoreceptor drive for ventilation is eliminated which leads to reduced alveolar ventilation. Hypoxemia should be reduced immediately by giving oxygen generally in a concentration of 24% to improve oxygenation without losing the respiratory stimulant effect.

Goals of oxygen therapy

The goal is to relieve hypoxemia by increasing alveolar tension, to reduce the work of breathing, and to decrease the work of myocardium. Oxygen should be used like a drug in various conditions, and its dose should be individualized. ABGs should be measured repeatedly in patients with ARF on oxygen therapy. The goal is to maintain PaO_2 above 60 mmHg. Oxygen should be given in low doses continuously since a small increase in FiO_2 causes an increase in PaO_2 as most patients of COPD lie on the steep part of the oxyhemoglobin curve.

Monitoring oxygen therapy

Oxygen therapy should be given continuously and should not be stopped abruptly until the patient has recovered, since sudden discontinuation can wash out small body stores of oxygen, resulting in the fall of alveolar oxygen tension. The dose of oxygen should be calculated carefully. Partial pressure of oxygen can be measured in the arterial blood. Complete saturation of hemoglobin in arterial blood should not be attempted. Arterial PO_2 of 60 mmHg can provide 90% saturation of arterial blood, but if acidosis is present, PaO_2 more than 80 mmHg is required. In a patient with respiratory failure, anemia should be corrected for proper oxygen transport to the tissue. A small increment in arterial oxygen tension results in a significant rise in the saturation of hemoglobin. Under normal situations, no additional benefit is secured by raising PaO_2 level to greater than 60–80 mmHg. An increase of 1% oxygen concentration elevates oxygen tension by 7 mmHg. It is necessary to maintain normal hemoglobin level in the presence of respiratory disease as proper oxygen transport to the tissues is to be maintained. Measurement of ABGs repeatedly is difficult, so a simple and noninvasive technique like pulse oximeter may be used to assess oxygen therapy.

When to stop oxygen therapy

Weaning should be considered when the patient becomes comfortable, his underlying disease is stabilized, and his BP, pulse rate, respiratory rate, skin color, and oximetry are within normal range. Weaning can be gradually attempted by discontinuing oxygen or lowering its concentration for a fixed period, for example, 30 minutes, and reevaluating the clinical parameters and SpO_2 periodically. Patients with chronic respiratory disease may require oxygen at lower concentrations for prolonged periods. Prospects of long-term domiciliary oxygen need to be discussed with the patient after the acute need is over.

Dangers of oxygen therapy

There are three types of risks associated with oxygen use.

1. **Physical risks**: Oxygen being combustible, fire hazard and tank explosion is always there. This is more with high concentration of oxygen, use of pressure chambers, and in smokers. Catheters and masks can cause injury to the nose and mouth. Dry and nonhumidified gas can cause dryness and crusting.
2. **Functional risks**: Patients who have lost sensitivity to CO_2 and are upon the hypoxic drive are in danger of ventilatory depression as seen in patients of COPD. Hypoventilation can lead to hypercapnia and CO_2 narcosis, although the risk is small with low-flow oxygen therapy. Arterial pH may be a better guide than $PaCO_2$ for monitoring oxygen therapy. As long as pH does not suggest acidosis, long-term oxygen therapy can benefit the patients with CO_2 retention.
3. **Cytotoxic damage**: COPD patients on long-term oxygen therapy, on autopsy, show proliferative and fibrotic changes in their lungs. In acute conditions, most of the structural damage occurs from high FiO_2 as the oxygen can lead to the release of various reactive species which attack the DNA, lipids, and SH-containing proteins.

Neuromuscular blockade

NMBAs are commonly used in ARDS, but their use remains controversial. Muscle relaxants have been shown to be beneficial as adjunct therapy to ventilation in the management of ARDS. NMBAs work by antagonizing the actions of acetylcholine by binding to cholinergic receptors leading to decreased muscle responsiveness to presynaptic excitation. These agents improve patient–ventilator synchrony, aid with lung-protective ventilation, and improve the overall survival rate when used early (within 48 hours) and in severe ARDS (i.e., PaO_2/FiO_2 <150 mmHg). However, limited evidence is available to dictate which specific agent within the class proves more beneficial.

Guidelines from the Society of Critical Care Medicine outline the use of NMBAs, favoring the use of cisatracurium or atracurium in patients with hepatic or renal dysfunction. In contrast, the guidelines discouraged the use of pancuronium in patients who exhibited signs of vagolytic effects.

Fluid-conservative therapy

In ARDS patients, due to increased alveolar vascular permeability, there is the presence of alveolar edema, which may get worsened as a consequence of fluid overload. The conservative approach of fluid management in ARDS has been proven to be beneficial in reducing ventilator days but does not improve survival.

β-2 agonist in ARDS

These agents are theorized to aid in ARDS by reducing pulmonary edema via fluid reabsorption. Beta$_2$-agonists upregulate the Na^+/K^+ ATPase pump, which transports electrolytes, accompanied by water, across the epithelial membrane. Additionally, beta$_2$-agonists minimize the permeability of pulmonary vasculature. In randomized controlled trials, salbutamol (known as albuterol in the United States) was poorly tolerated and did not improve mortality.

Corticosteroids in ARDS

The anti-inflammatory properties of corticosteroids make these medications reasonable pharmacologic options. Corticosteroids exert their anti-inflammatory effect through both genomic and nongenomic mechanisms. The two genomic anti-inflammatory mechanisms are described as transrepression and transactivation. Transrepression, occurring within a few hours after corticosteroid administration, directly inhibits NF-KB from migrating to the cell nucleus and transcribing genes for proinflammatory cytokines. In contrast, transactivation occurs within days after glucocorticoid administration and involves the activation of glucocorticoid receptor-α. Once activated, the glucocorticoid receptor complex migrates to the cell nucleus and transcribes genes for anti-inflammatory proteins. In addition to both of the genomic mechanisms, corticosteroids also prevent neutrophil degranulation and stabilize the cell membrane.

Nitric oxide

The mechanism by which NO exerts its pharmacologic action makes it a preferred option for management of ARDS. Inhaled NO enhances perfusion in the lungs by targeting the lungs directly and reduces systemic effects due to its short half-life. NO works by selectively dilating the pulmonary vasculature in ventilated alveoli, resulting in improvement of blood flow by enhancing V/Q matching (i.e., V/Q ratio). By improving this ratio, hypoxemia is reversed, and the pulmonary arterial pressure is lowered.

Surfactant

Depletion and inactivation of the lung surfactant occurs during the progression of ARDS. The role of a surfactant is to reduce surface tension, prevent alveolar damage, and decrease inflammation. In the pediatric population, administration of bovine lung surfactant significantly reduced 28-day mortality rates. In contrast, clinical studies in adults have shown that administration of exogenous surfactant improves oxygenation but has no effect on mortality or ventilator-free days. This may be due to several variables, including dose and type of the surfactant administered. Therefore, surfactants may be useful for a transient improvement in oxygenation for adults with ARDS.

Current therapies

Lung-protective ventilation

Mechanical ventilation with lower tidal volumes (LTVs) and airway pressures (tidal volume of 4–6 mL/kg predicted body weight and maintenance of plateau pressure between 25 and 30 cm H_2O) reduces mortality in ALI and ARDS. This lung-protective ventilation preserves barrier properties of the alveolar endothelium and alveolar epithelium by preventing alveolar over distension, which is one of the major causes of ventilator-induced lung injury. The concept of open lung ventilation uses LTV with high PEEP with the rationale that LTV will minimize the damage due to overdistension while the high PEEP will minimize the cyclic atelectasis, which has been shown to have a beneficial effect on the outcome of the patients. Lung-protective ventilation also regulates mechanosensitive proinflammatory pathways, resulting in reduced neutrophil accumulation in the alveoli and lower plasma levels of IL-6, IL-8, and TNF.

Prone ventilation

Prone ventilation showed improvement in the level of oxygenation and thus improved the outcome in patients with ARDS having severe hypoxia. This effect is due to the reduction in the transpulmonary pressure gradient on making the patient prone, which helps in recruiting the collapsed areas of the lung without causing significant increase in the airway pressures. Prone ventilation was found to be a significantly effective in obese patients with ARDS than in nonobese patients. In ARDS, dependent lung regions become consolidated as the lung collapses on its own weight. This phenomenon is exacerbated by the weight of the heart compressing adjacent lung regions. Prone positioning ameliorates these phenomena, as the weight of the lung is suspended from a larger horizontal dorsal chest wall. This homogenizes ventilation to lung areas reduces stress and strain and alleviates stress raisers. Further, perfusion is more evenly distributed, leading to better V/Q matching and consequently better gas exchange.

Extracorporeal membrane oxygenation

Extracorporeal membrane oxygenation (ECMO) is an advanced circulatory and ventilatory support system, which is used to salvage the patients with refractory hypoxemia when the conventional treatment fails. The technique has been used successfully as a rescue therapy for the severe ARDS cases. The evidence to support the use of ECMO as a primary treatment in ARDS is lacking and needs further research. Used mainly as a rescue therapy, the use of ECMO for patients with ARDS remains controversial. Many centers advocate early use and prefer it to prone positioning. The rationale is the ease of delivery of lung-protective ventilation because associated gas exchange abnormalities are corrected via the extracorporeal gas exchanger. Several reports during the H1N1 pandemic in 2009 alluded to benefit, but none of these were randomized investigations. The recently concluded ECMO to Rescue Lung Injury in Severe ARDS (EOLIA) trial randomly assigned patients with very severe ARDS (P/F of 50 mmHg or less for more than 3 hours, a P/F of less than 80 mmHg for more than 6 hours, or an arterial blood pH of less than 7.25 with a $PaCO_2$ of 60 mmHg or more for more than 6 hours) to receive immediate veno-venous ECMO (ECMO group) or continued conventional treatment (control group). Crossover to ECMO was possible for patients in the control group who had refractory hypoxemia. The trial was halted prematurely because it was determined that the futility threshold had been crossed. Although there were no differences in mortality, the results were complicated by a large number of patients (28%) in the control group who crossed over to the ECMO group because of the refractory respiratory failure. The results, however, did not show that routine use of ECMO in severe ARDS is superior to reserving ECMO as a rescue maneuver. Therefore, it may be prudent to utilize other evidence-based recommendations such as neuromuscular blockade and prone positioning prior to the initiation of ECMO.

High-frequency oscillatory ventilation

High-frequency oscillatory ventilation (HFOV) seemed ideal for lung protection in ARDS, but the OSCAR study concluded with no 30-day survival benefit or cost benefit in patients in whom HFOV was used. The meta-analysis of randomized control trials (RCTs) by Gu et al. (2014) also concluded that with the use of HFOV, there was no improvement in survival in ARDS patients, although it had no increase in the risk of barotrauma or hypotension and also reduced the risk of oxygenation failure.

Noninvasive ventilation

A single-center RCT of helmet noninvasive ventilation and face mask noninvasive ventilation in patients with ARDS who were already receiving face mask noninvasive ventilation for at least 8 hours was stopped early for efficacy after 83 of a planned 206 patients were enrolled. Patients receiving helmet noninvasive ventilation had significantly lower rates of endotracheal intubation, more ventilator-free days, and a remarkably better mortality than patients with face mask ventilation. The results of this trial should be interpreted with caution; the face mask arm had a mortality of 56% at 90 days as compared to 35% in the helmet arm, which is much higher than recent NHLBI ARDS cohorts and other epidemiological ARDS studies. This suggests that large differences in mortality may have been secondary to failure of timely intubation, especially in the face mask arm. The LUNG-SAFE study found that in patients with severe ARDS the application of noninvasive ventilation was associated with worse mortality.

Pharmacological therapies

The clinical landscape in ARDS therapy has been fraught with failure of therapeutic trials. Most recent amongst such failures are the use of statins, beta-2 adrenergic agents, and keratinocyte growth factor (KGF). A multicenter trial of aspirin to prevent ARDS in high-risk patients (lung injury prevention score over four) also failed to reduce the incidence of ARDS. A promising new paradigm in ARDS is the use of cell-based therapies to accelerate injured lung epithelium and endothelium and enhance the clearance of edema fluid. Two phase I trials of mesenchymal stem/stromal cells (MSCs) in ARDS did not report any safety events, and a phase 2a trial is currently ongoing.

The NIH NHLBI PETAL (prevention and early treatment of ALI) network is presently conducting two RCTs: Vitamin D to improve outcomes by leveraging early treatment (VIOLET) and re-evaluation of systemic early neuromuscular blockade (ROSE). Other noteworthy ongoing trials include vitamin C infusion for the treatment in sepsis-induced ALI (CITRUS-ALI), two studies looking at vitamin C in combination with corticosteroids and thiamine, liberal oxygenation versus conservative oxygenation in ARDS (LOCO2), protective ventilation with veno-venous lung assist in respiratory failure (REST), and the Strategy of Ultra Protective Lung Ventilation with Extracorporeal CO_2 Removal for New-Onset Moderate to Severe ARDS (SUPERNOVA).

References and suggested readings

1. Bhatia RS. Complications of acute respiratory failure. IN: YP Munjal, ed. Med Update; API. 1997;7:783–786.
2. Prasad R, et al. An open randomized controlled trial of NIPPV in patients of acute or chronic hypercapnic respiratory failure in a general respiratory ward setting. Lung India. 2007;24:132–138. 93,72-31-4-1r.
3. Bhatia RS. Respiratory disorders and air travel. IN: Selected topics in chest medicine. Lucknow: Arora Publ. 2005;3:19–21.
4. Soo Hoo GW, et al. Hypercapnic respiratory failure in COPD patients-response to therapy. Chest. 2000;117:169–177.
5. Brower RG, et al. Treatment of ARDS. Chest. 2001;120:1347–1367.
6. Gupta A, Jyoti B. ABG analysis. PG Med; API. 2015;29:366–372.
7. Hers DR. Evidence of NIPPU in case of patient in ARF-a systematic review of literature. Respir Care. 2004;49:810–829.
8. Greg L, et al. Managing ARF during exacerbation of COPD. Respir Care. 2004;49:766–782.
9. Bajan K. Non invasive ventilation. IN: SB Gupta, ed. Med Update; API. 2005;15:553–557.
10. Ramesh TP, et al. Nanotechnology at work, photocatalytic oxygenation blood. Med Update; API. 2013;23:505–506.
11. Sahni T, et al. Hyperbaric oxygen therapy-current trends and applications. JAPI. 2003;51:280–284.
12. Dupont M, et al. Survival of patients with bronchiectasis after the first ICU stay for respiratory failure. Chest. 2004;125:1815–1820.
13. Buyse B, et al. Treatment of chronic respiratory failure in kyphoscoliosis: oxygen or ventilation. Eurp Respir J. 2003;22:525–528.
14. Enarson PM, et al. Management of pneumonia in the child 2 to 59 months of age. Int J Tubere Lung Dis. 2005;9:959–963.
15. Sangstad OD. Oxygen for newborns-how much is too much? J Perinatal. 2005;25:S 45–549.

16. New A. Oxygen-kill or use? Pre hospital hyperoxia in COPD patients. Emerg Med J. 2006;23:144–146.
17. Todi SK. Current classification and early diagnosis of ARDS. Pa Med; API. 2013;27:226–237.
18. Synowiec A, Szczepański A, Barreto-Duran E, Lie LK, Pyrc K. Severe acute respiratory syndrome coronavirus 2 (SARS-CoV-2): a systemic infection. Clin Microbiol Rev. 2021 Jan 13;34(2):e00133–20. doi: 10.1128/CMR.00133-20. PMID: 33441314; PMCID: PMC7849242.
19. Vega ML, Pisani L. Nasal high flow oxygen in acute respiratory failure. Pulmonology. 2021 May–Jun;27(3):240–247. doi: 10.1016/j.pulmoe.2021.01.005. Epub 2021 Feb 13. PMID: 33589403.
20. Giraud R, Banfi C, Assouline B, De Charrière A, Cecconi M, Bendjelid K. The use of extracorporeal CO_2 removal in acute respiratory failure. Ann Intensive Care. 2021 Mar 11;11(1):43. doi: 10.1186/s13613-021-00824-6. PMID: 33709318; PMCID: PMC7951130.
21. Blumenthal JA, Duvall MG. Invasive and noninvasive ventilation strategies for acute respiratory failure in children with coronavirus disease 2019. Curr Opin Pediatr. 2021 Jun 1;33(3):311–318. doi: 10.1097/MOP.0000000000001021. PMID: 33851935; PMCID: PMC8117173.
22. Worsham CM, Banzett RB, Schwartzstein RM. Dyspnea, acute respiratory failure, psychological trauma, and post-ICU mental health: a caution and a call for research. Chest. 2021 Feb;159(2):749–756. doi: 10.1016/j.chest.2020.09.251. Epub 2020 Oct 1. PMID: 33011205; PMCID: PMC7528739.

https://doi.org/10.1142/9789811271410_0034

34 Commonly encountered respiratory emergencies

Introduction

Respiratory symptoms may be present for nonpulmonary disorders and vice versa. At the same time, pulmonary emergencies are often frightening and, if not attended urgently, can be life threatening and even fatal. Therefore, recognition, diagnosing, and differentiating from nonrespiratory causes is as important as management of respiratory emergencies because management modalities and line of action would tremendously be affected and directed by differential diagnosis and pinpointing toward a conclusive diagnosis and an ultimate outcome.

Hemoptysis

Hemoptysis (blood in sputum) is always an emergency (at least for the patient). Nevertheless, massive hemoptysis (200 mL of blood/24 hours) is always a life-threatening situation. Blood in streaks is suggesting infection; expectorated frank blood in an adult suggests a bronchogenic carcinoma. Recurrent bleed over a period of time suggests adenocarcinoma, and persistent bleeding despite treatment for 24 hours suggests an endobronchial tuberculosis or malignancy. Associated dyspnea should point toward cardiovascular etiology; chest pain with a history of PVD or anticoagulant therapy would point toward acute pulmonary embolism. The presence of finger clubbing favors suppurative lung disorders and lung cancer. Local chest examination would look for consolidation or pleurisy. Cutaneous rash with hematuria would point toward systemic vascular disease; signs of mitral valve disease and left ventricular failure should also be looked for. Positive laboratory tests rule out infection as well as hematological malignancy. Urinalysis differentiate vasculitis, polyarteritis nodosa, and Goodpasture's syndrome. A plain X-ray of the chest rules out consolidation, congestion, tuberculosis, bronchiectasis, lung cancer, lung abscess pleural/effusion, and so on. Bronchoscopy adds more diagnosis and reveals more locations of bleeding. The diagnostic yield is higher during the bleeding. However, there is no extra advantage of bronchoscopy if the chest X-ray is normal. Sputum analysis may give additional information for infection and malignant cells. CT pulmonary angiography is useful in diagnosing pulmonary embolism, in addition to ventilation/perfusion lung scan. CT scan can be utilized for source of bleeding from the peripheral lesion where percutaneous needle biopsy is required to be done. Management requires diagnosis to be made for the cause of bleeding in case it is mild and has not affected the gas exchange. But if it is massive and has affected gas exchange, the urgency requires prompt management in the form of advising bed rest, suppressing cough reflex, and positioning toward the dependent side, in case the cause in known, to avoid aspiration of blood to the unaffected lung. Supplement oxygen and maintenance of adequate gas exchange in case of massive hemoptysis may need incubation and mechanical ventilation. Blood transfusion may be required in such cases, along with coagulation factors and platelets if coagulopathies form an underlying etiology. Drugs and fluids may be required to resuscitate shock.

Bronchoscopic balloon tamponade is attempted to compress the bleeding site to stop bleeding. This may be assisted with laser.

Common causes of hemoptysis

A. Bronchopulmonary

- Acute bronchitis
- Bronchial adenoma/carcinoma
- Bronchiectasis
- Foreign body
- Trauma/bronchoscopy — TB

- – Suppurative/lung infections (pneumonia, abscess)
- – Parasitic/fungal lung diseases

B. Pulmonary vascular disorders

- – Polyarteritis nodosa
- – Goodpasture'ssyndrome
- – Wegener's disease
- – Pulmonary embolism

C. Hematological disorders

- – Leukemia
- – Hemophilia
- – Thrombocytopenia
- – Anticoagulant therapy

D. Cardiovascular disorders

- – Mitral stenosis
- – Acute left ventricular failure
- – Aortic aneurysm

Photocoagulation, embolotherapy, and surgical resection of the affected lung areas may be considered, if needed.

Antimicrobial prophylaxis always started. Chest physiotherapy, spirometry, and postural drainage in this situation should be avoided.

Community-acquired pneumonia (CAP) — an acute inflammation of lung parenchyma of infective or noninfective etiology — is another important pulmonary emergency attended in hospitals. Mostly, droplets inhalation is the route of infection, often precipitated due to poor host defense and impaired mucociliary clearance due to corticoid therapy and use of tobacco and alcohol.

Sudden onset of fever, chest pain, productive cough with or without blood in sputum, along with radiological evidence of consolidation point toward diagnosis. Chest X-ray provides diagnosis, extent of the lesion, and the associated involvement of the pleura and lymph nodes. Focal consolidation lesions are the usual findings, multiple areas are affected in hematogenous spread, and diffuse involvement is seen in immunocompromised hosts.

Sputum is not very contributory; sputum culture may be useful. Blood culture is positive in case there is bacteremia. Routine blood tests may show evidence of infection. Invasive procedures may be required in case hospitalization is ordered, especially when the patient is elderly, has comorbidities, accompanying leukopenia, anaerobic infection is suspected as the underlying cause, or multilobar severe pneumonia is presented with hypotension, hypoxia, tachypnea and tachycardia, or altered/confusional state, accompanying complications such as empyema, endocarditis or meningitis, and/or not responding to OPD treatment. Outdoor empirical antibiotic management includes high-dose amoxicillin/doxycycline or macrolide and quinolone. Hospitalized patients are treated with intravenous beta-lactam plus macrolide or in fluoroquinolone. Intravenous fluids, supplemental oxygen, and relief of pleuritic pain are other comanagement measures. Acute severe bronchial asthma is another emergency faced in respiratory medicine where severe airway obstruction with pulsus paradoxus and the use of accessory respiratory muscles and failure to maintenance therapy demands urgent aggressive therapy to cut down both morbidity and mortality. Such an attack is often precipitated by sudden exposure to smoke/changed environment, sudden stress, tobacco smoke, drugs like aspirin, NSAIDS, beta blockers, and so forth, or respiratory tract infections. The early symptom of cough and wheeze becomes feeble or missing, and patients often gasp for air. The patient is unable to speak, consciousness is altered, chest is silent, central cyanosis appears, and there is bradycardia with PEP < 100 </minute. Chest X-ray may be normal or have accompanying complications such a collapse, pneumonia, or pneumothorax. PEFR < 50% of the predicted value suggests severe obstruction. Arterial gas analysis shows hypoxemia (PaO_2 < 60 mmHg [sessions]), acidosis (pH < 7.38), and hypercapnia ($PaCO_2$ > 40 mmHg). Acute severe asthma has to be differentiated from cardiac asthma due to acute left ventricular failure, pulmonary embolism, vocal cord dysfunction, laryngeal edema, eosinophilic (hypersensitivity) pneumonia, or endobronchial obstruction due to foreign body, bronchial stenosis, or neoplasm. Management includes urgent institution of therapy to overcome airway obstruction, correcting hypoxemia, and preventing precipitating factors to reduce relapse or recurrence. Prednisolone orally or IV along with nebulized bronchodilator solution of salbutamol/terbutaline, with supplemental oxygen are given. In the hospital emergency, IV fluids, antimicrobials (if infection is present), and addition of ipratropium bromide in nebulized form are given. PGFR recording, arterial blood gas (ABG) analysis, and pulse oximetry are valuable in assessing therapeutic response. Sedation and triggering agents have to be avoided. Pneumothorax — the entry of air into the pleural space — is another respiratory emergency which may be spontaneous, without an overt lung disease cause primary or secondary, with an underlying etiology commonly chronic obstructive pulmonary disease (COPD) or TB, as well as asthma, abscess, carcinoma, pulmonary infarction and fibrotic and cystic lung lesions and secondary it may, occur posttraumatic following chest trauma or iatrogenic following biopsy or thoracic surgery. Risk factors in primary form include heavy tobacco inhalation, high altitude, congenital bronchial anomalies, thin and tall body-built, mitral valve prolapse, and Marfan's syndrome. Secondary form may occur in addition to abovementioned causes, in necrotizing pneumonia, LDS, silicosis, coal worker's pneumoconiosis, eosinophilic granuloma, postirradiation, catamenial, and tuberous sclerosis. It can be of closed, open, and tension (valvular) variety. Unilateral, localized sharp chest pain with dyspnea proportional to the size of pneumothorax are the usual symptoms, which are more prominent in secondary types due to the preexisting lung disease.

Reduced chest movement, full intercostal space, hyperresonant percussion, and lung sounds and vocal fremitus (reduced) in the closed type and increased in open pneumothorax. Recurrence is common in patients with emphysema. Bilateral spontaneous pneumothorax is rare. Chest X-ray offers the diagnosis in a clinically suspected patient, and a lateral decubitus film offers to delineate free air in the pleural cavity.

Less than 20% (a small pneumothorax) is left as such to absorb and resolve spontaneously. More than 20% (pneumothorax) is usually symptomatic and is treated with (16/18 G) needle or an IV cannula catheter using a 50-mL syringe having three-way valve; when no air comes, leave the catheter for 4–6 hours (tightly used) and repeat chest X-ray. If air is less than 20%, remove the catheter, and if recurrence occur, intercostal tube drainage is considered. Third or fourth intercostal space in the mid-axillary line is selected for tube inspection, dissecting through to the parietal pleura; advanced with apical direction and connected to underwater seal. Lung expansion and no recurrence is checked by repeat chest X-ray. Clamping of the tube is dangerous and should not be attempted. Lung reinflation and stoppage of bubbling for 24 hours requires the tube to be blocked or displaced.

Supplemental oxygen is useful to accelerate air resorption by pleura. Prevention of recurrence demands total abstinence from smoking: Diving and flying should be avoided for 3–6 months.

Due to seriousness of the condition and higher rate of recurrence, especially in primary pneumothorax, pleurodesis is usually recommended in all the cases. Chemical pleurodesis is done with tetracycline/doxycycline institution and talc insufflation. Thoracoscopic surgical pleurodesis can be attempted causing pleural abrasion or parietal pleurectomy.

Re-expansion pulmonary edema should be suspected if there is a sudden onset of cough and dyspnea following sudden withdrawal of air in pneumothorax. Treatment is supportive; slow withdrawal of air is the best preventive measure.

Asphyxia is yet another emergency in pulmonary medicine where lungs are less/not receiving atmospheric O_2, leading to retention of CO_2. It can be mechanical obstruction by closing of face, mouth, or nostrils, or obstruction by food or a foreign body in the airways, gagging, hanging, strangulation, throttling (manual neck compression), drowning, or traumatic asphyxia.

Nonmechanical suffocation may be caused by infections (diphtheria, infectious mononucleosis, *Haemophilus influenzae*) in children, rupture of aortic aneurysm, massive hemoptysis in TB/carcinoma, pharyngeal abscess, laryngeal tumor or laryngeal edema, and blunt frontal neck injury.

Partial obstruction may lead to the person to struggle, while complete airway obstruction may press the patient to use sign language as he is unable to speak or breathe; pallor followed by cyanosis or loss of consciousness or collapse may occur. In case urgent relief of obstruction is not offered, cardiac arrest and even death can occur.

History is therefore very important. Vital signs, such as pulse, heart, and respiratory rates, and of course, cyanosis are very important. It may be useful to help the person to expel the obstructing foreign body by artificial coughing. This can be attempted by using the fingers to dislodge the foreign body by giving abdominal thrust by placing the hand beneath the xiphisternum. Alternatively, back slaps can be given. Cardiac arrest if suspected, precordial thump should also be delivered.

Pulmonary embolism due to acute hemodynamic disturbance causing pulmonary vascular occlusion by embolus is another important emergency in pulmonary medicine. It originates from deep vein thrombosis in 95% of cases, from leg veins in more than 80% of cases, and 10%–15% of cases have emboli from pelvic veins. Predisposing factors are obesity, immobility, diabetes, varicose veins, drugs, pregnancy, hypercoagulable state, and congestive heart failure.

Increased pulmonary vascular resistance, impaired gas exchange, increased airways resistance, decreased pulmonary compliance, and right ventricular dysfunction eventually lead to circulatory collapse and death. So, two principle criteria include cardiogenic shock (hypotension) and right ventricular dysfunction (or failure). Acute cor pulmonale is encountered in case of massive pulmonary embolism. Triad of hemoptysis, pleuritic chest pain, and wheeze are seen in pulmonary infarction; dyspnea, syncope/shock, or hypotension are features seen in massive embolization compared to small embolization which produces symptoms like cough, hemoptysis, wheeze, and pleuritic pain.

Routine blood examination shows raised ESR and leukocytosis; chest X-ray may be normal or offers varied radiological appearances such as cardiomegaly, raised hemidiaphragm, atelectasis, enlarged pulmonary conus/descending pulmonary artery, consolidation, or pleural effusion. These changes are nonspecific. Similarly, nonspecific ECG changes such as ischemia, RBBB, and right axis deviation with or without right ventricular strain may be seen, appearing and disappearing on subsequent ECG. At the same time, normal ECG does not rule one pulmonary embolism. ABG analysis shows hypoxemia with respiratory alkalosis. A normal nuclear lung scan (perfusion scan) virtually excludes pulmonary embolism, but CT pulmonary angiography is a better choice than ventilation/perfusion scan in pulmonary embolism. D-dimer test and echocardiography also have diagnostic value.

Being mortal in first 2 hours in almost 80% of cases, massive pulmonary thromboembolism is urgently attended with oxygen administration through mask and IV fluids with drugs such as norepinephrine and dobutamine to raise of shocked/hypotensive (generally in acute massive pulmonary embolism). Caution is not to use diuretics and vasodilators. Anticoagulant therapy using heparin or LMWH S/C and thrombolysis can be attempted if diagnosis is confirmed, using streptokinase, urokinase, or tPA. In that case, heparin should be given subsequently.

Refractory hypotension despite thrombolytic therapy or contraindication to thrombolytic therapy opens options for life-saving catheter/surgical embolectomy.

Follow-up prophylaxis therapy in all cases of deep vein thrombosis must be mandatorily advised. And those having contraindications to anticoagulation therapy or having recurrence despite continued anticoagulation therapy can be benefitted from insertion of filter, placed in inferior vena cava below the origin of renal vessels.

Acute empyema thoracis, mostly due to bacterial pneumonia, forms another emergency in chest medicine where pus get collected in the pleural cavity; infection may travel from lungs, blood-borne, abdominal viscera, or following some procedures. Malnutrition, diabetes, alcoholism, drug abuse, malignancy, and immunosuppression due to cytotoxic drugs, corticoids, and HIV disease often predispose to acute empyema.

Fever with chills, cough with often purulent expectoration, unilateral chest discomfort, and dyspnea are the presenting symptoms; on examination, fever tachypnea and tachycardia with tenderness on percussion are encountered. Digital clubbing appears.

Raised ESR and leukocytosis are present in acute empyema. Chest X-ray gives a picture of fluid in the pleural space. Ultrasound is useful in guiding the site of aspiration, especially in loculated empyema. CT scan differentiates from peripheral parenchymal lesions.

Management aims at relieving the symptoms, and to sterilize the pleural space, allow full lung expansion and avoid complications such as fistula formation, pleural thickening, fibrosis, chronic sinus, and preventing dissemination of infection in the form of meningitis, pericarditis, brain abscess, and so on.

Antimicrobials should be broad spectrum based on the culture and sensitivity with thorough and adequate pus drainage under aseptic precaution and with observing guidelines and keeping a watch on the development of respiratory distress, which, in case if develops, needs immediate suspension of aspiration procedure. Successful drainage shows clinicoradiological improvement within 24 hours.

Thrombolytic therapy can be attempted for better results; in case there is no contraindication such as the presence of recent injury, bronchial suturing of bronchopleural fistula is done.

Thoracoscopy is useful to inspect the pleural surface, in case there is need for decortication. Lung resection is attempted if the lung does not expand after decortication.

Acute hypoxic lung injury producing acute respiratory distress syndrome is an important respiratory emergency, having fatality in more than 50% of cases. There is refractory hypoxemia, respiratory distress with reduced lung compliance, and bilateral extensive pulmonary infiltrates on chest X-ray. It results from shock, sepsis, embolism, trauma, inhaled toxic smoke, and so on, resulting in a nonspecific reaction called ARDS, which has pneumonia as its common complication. It has exudative, proliferative, fibrotic, and repairing (recovery) phases. It clinically manifests as unexplained dyspnea and dry cough with bilateral fine crackles in both the lungs. Agitated/disoriented behavior (usually after 24 hours), tachycardia, tachypnea, and cyanosis appear later. Chest X-ray reveals bilateral patchy ill-defined opacities initially, which become massive consolidations as they rapidly coalesce. ABG analysis shows refractory hypoxia, hypocapnia, and alkalosis; CT scan chest initially reveals nonuniform diffuse ground glass opacification, which becomes reticular as the disease progresses. Polymorphs are increased in BAL fluid analysis. Differential diagnosis include acute left ventricular failure (cardiogenic pulmonary edema) which has elevated (more than 18 mmHg) pulmonary capillary wedge pressure and secondary diffuse alveolar hemorrhage, where BAL fluid analysis has the presence of blood and hemosiderin-laden macrophages.

Management included monitoring of pulmonary and systemic fluids and gas with adequate nutrition and empirical antimicrobial cover until culture and sensitivity reports are available. Pulmonary capillary wedge pressure guides fluids/vasopressors drugs and face mask or supplementation is used to improve PaO_2, without increasing Fi 0, and if needed, endotracheal intubation can be considered. Patients can be kept in a prone position; nitric oxide and antioxidants have been used; steroids have no role in ARDS, except when hypereosinophilia exists in blood and lungs.

Respiratory failure

Failure to keep gas exchange within normal range leads to the failure of the respiratory system. This emergency is clinically suspected and is confirmed by ABG analysis and is often indicated by PaO_2 less than 60 mmHg or $PaCO_2$ more than 50 mmHg. It can either be hypoxic or hypercapnic; however, hypoxemic respiratory failure can progress to hypercapnic with the fatigue of respiratory muscles.

Acute respiratory failure can develop in severe bronchial asthma, laryngeal edema, foreign body in airways, pulmonary embolism, and multiple rib fractures, and also due to myxedema, myasthenia gravis, metabolic alkalosis, Guillain–Barre syndrome, brain stem infarct, respiratory muscle paralysis, and overdose of narcotics.

Clinically, tachycardia, tachypnea, confusion, agitated/restless behavior, and cyanosis are observed in hypoxia and flapping tremors, headache, disorientation, somnolence, bounding pulse, and papilledema are present in hypercapnia.

Etiology can be differentiated with a history of wheeze and cough, followed by silent chest in acute severe asthma, fever and chest pain without stained sputum in case of pneumonia, dry cough with exertional dyspnea in ILD, breathlessness and chest discomfort in pneumothorax, and neuro-details to differentiate myopathy, neuropathy, and other CNS disorders.

Management includes urgent O_2 administration to correct lung hypoxemia along with correction of the underlying cause, such as bronchodilation and systemic steroids in asthma, bronchodilator and antimicrobials in COPD, bronchiectasis, and pneumonia, LMWH in pulmonary embolism, intercostal tube drainage in pneumothorax, and diuretics along with digitalis and antihypertensives (if hypertension accompanies) in left ventricular failure.

Sedatives and depressants should be avoided. Management of hypercapnic respiratory failure needs noninvasive positive pressure oxygen, along with stopping narcotic drug, removing the foreign body from larynx/airways, treating acute severe asthma, fixing the failing chest, and treating infections in case of acute exacerbation in COPD.

Continuous monitoring of pulse, BP, respiratory rate, temperature, and a watch on urinary output along with routine TLC and DLC testing, and ECG and ABG analysis serve as good guides. Blood urea/creatinine and electrolytes are other parameters.

Acute chest pain

Respiratory conditions causing acute chest pain is often presented as an emergency. Common causes of chest pain of respiratory conditions presenting as an emergency are pleurisy where the pain increases with breathing and often a pleural rub is present, and secondly, pneumothorax, where the patient presents with sudden onset of pain with breathlessness. Percussion note is hyperresonant, and chest X-ray is diagnostic.

Chest pain can also occur in pneumonia as has been discussed. It can also occur in malignancy of lung/mediastinum, in tracheitis, and in massive pulmonary embolism, which has been described earlier.

Acute pulmonary edema is another important cardiorespiratory emergency where elevated left atrial pressure leading to elevated pulmonary capillary venous pressure (more than 25 mmHg) consequently result in transudation of fluid into alveoli, its wall, and alveolar sacs. Apart from cardiac causes, pulmonary edema may get precipitated by infections, severe anemia, pregnancy, rapid IV infusion, and even undue physical exertion.

Chest X-ray may show cardiomegaly in addition to pulmonary edema (haziness). ECG may reveal arrhythmia, infarction, or LBBB. Pulmonary capillary wedge pressure is more than 25 mmHg. Noninvasive echography is very useful to reveal valvular defect, cardiac aneurysm, hypertrophy or dilated cardiomyopathy, and left ventricular dysfunctions.

Management includes prop up position of the patient, 100%0, through mask and injection IV morphine S10 mg (with antiemetic) and sodium nitroprusside (20% g) and furosemide (40 mg).

In addition, nitrates, digitalis, and bronchodilators such as aminophylline should be added.

High-altitude pulmonary edema

It is an emergency when a young person rapidly ascends at high altitude, with a little heavy exertion. Mechanism is not clear. The patient becomes breathless; mucoid expectoration with blood stains may follow. Chest discomfort may accompany. The patient is ill looking, in a panic situation, with tachycardia and tachypnea.

Bilateral coarse crepitations due to noncardiogenic edema are present. Leukocytosis in blood film and generally bilateral diffuse haziness on chest X-ray are present. Cardiorespiratory failure, collapse, and even death can occur if not urgently managed. Immediate descent to a lower altitude is very important. High-flow-rate oxygen supplementation with a face mask should be done. Morphine, bronchodilators, and corticoids are not indicated. Diuretics play a limited role. Sublingual nifedipine reduces pulmonary arterial pressure and subsequently pulmonary edema. Nitroxide can be combined with O_2 therapy. Mortality can be reduced from 50% (if not treated) to less than 10% if treated urgently.

References and suggested readings

1. Jean-Baptistic E. Clinical assessment and management of massive haemoptysis. Crit Care Med. 2000;28:1642–1647.
2. Hicks K, et al. Treatment of diffuse alveolar hemorrhage after allogeneic bone marrow transplant with recombinant factor VII a. Bone Marrow Transplant. 2002;30:975–978.
3. Haponik EF, et al. Managing life threatening haemoptysis — has anything really changed? Chest. 2000;18:1431–1435.
4. Nair G, et al. Haemoptysis — a rare presentation of aortic aneurysm. Lung India. 2008;25:20–21.
5. Bhatia RS. Community aquired pneumonia-emerging etology with institution of therapy. IN: YP Munjal, ed. Med Update; API. 1999;977–982.
6. Casey KR, Winterbauer RH. Acute severe asthma: how to recognize and respond to a life threatening attack. PG Med. 1995;97:71–78.
7. Bhatia RS, Singal M. Acute bronchial asthma-current trends. Med Update. 1999;6:783–784.
8. Beth RS. Managing acute severe asthma-nebulizer or MDI? Lung India. 2005;22:4.
9. Shankar PS. Tooling trends in the management of COPD. IN: YP Munjal, ed. PG Med; API. 2007;21445–21454.
10. Sharma, A. Pneumothorax. IN: RK Singal, DG Jain, ed. Med Update; API. 2007;17:813–817.
11. Bhatia RS, Sibia SS. Management of spontaneous pneumothorax. IN: S Vankataraman, ed. Med Update; API. 2004;14:221–226.
12. Murat A, et al. Re expansion pulmonary edema. Acta Radial. 2004;45:431–433.
13. Digonnet A, et al. Acute pulmonary embolism-current surgical approach. Interact Cardio-Vast Surg. 2007;6:27–29.
14. Piazza G, Goldhaber SZ. Acute pulmonary embolism. Circulation. 2006;114:E 42–E 47.

15. Lohan DG, et al. Massive pulmonary embolism with haemodynamic compromise-therapeutic options. Emerg Radiology. 2007;13:161–169.
16. Khoja AM. Bronchial artery embolization-life saving therapy for haemoptysis. Jonsn Bronchol. 2003;10:22–29.
17. Sarkar SK. Current aspects in the surgical management of TB. IN: RS Bhatia, ed. Tuberulosis. New Delhi: Pee PeePubl. 2007;17:96–101.
18. Bhatia RS. TB and AIDS. JAPI. 2000;48:613–616.
19. Bhatia RS, Nigam P. Pulmonary tuberculosis. Curr Med Trends. 1997;3:19–24.
20. Desai SR, et al. ARDS caused by pulmonary and extra pulmonary injury — a comparative CT study. Radiology. 2001;218:689–693.
21. Sinha S, Sharma SK. Severe acute respiratory syndrome. IN: S Vankataraman, ed. Med Update; API. 2004;14:214–220.
22. Mishra NP. Diagnostic approach to bronchial asthma. IN: S Vankataraman, ed. Med Update; API. 2004;14:227–230.
23. Reng M, et al. Pumpless extracorporeal lung assist and ARDS. Lancet. 2000;356:219–220.
24. Saili A. Approach to respiratory distress in newborns. Ind J Pract Pediat. 2005;7:187–191.
25. Bhatia RS, Sibia SS. Therapeutic use of FOB. Lung India. 1994;12:138–139.
26. Khan GQ, Bhatia RS. FOB. IN: RS Bhatia, GO Khan, ed. Pulmonary Med. Pee Pee Publ. 2007;1:1–5.
27. Bhatia RS. Complications of ARF. IN: YP Munjal, ed. Med Update; API. 1997;783–786.
28. Sahni T, et al. Recent advantes in hyperbaric oxygen therapy. IN: S Venkataraman, ed. Med Update; API. 2004;14:632–639.
29. Koyuncu N, et al. An unusual cause of chest pain-foreign body in oesphagus. Emerg Med J. 2007;24:65.

https://doi.org/10.1142/9789811271410_0035

35 Sleep apnea syndrome

Introduction

Sleep apnea is a sleep-induced pulmonary disorder characterized by snoring and respiratory pauses,[1] often accompanied with respiratory obstruction. Two-thirds of patients are obese, and male population is 20 times more frequently affected as compared to females. Idiopathic sleep apnea syndrome (SAS) afflicts 1% of the adult population in the United States, affecting more commonly in the age-group between 40 and 60 years. Nevertheless, the gravity of morbidity and mortality caused by the disease has not been realized by physicians in this part of the country, where 5% of adults are suffering from this condition.

SAS is defined as the presence of more than five apneas or hypopneas per hour of sleep in young or middle-aged patients in conjunction with at least two major symptoms. There is cessation of airflow for at least 10 seconds and hypopnea as a 50% reduction in thoracoabdominal movements for at least 10 seconds. Respiratory disturbance index (RDI) is the number of apneas or hypopneas per hour of sleep. In other words, SAS is diagnosed if respiratory events occur during both non-rapid eye movement (NREM) and rapid eye movement (REM) sleep with an RDI of greater than 5. The severity of SAS is denoted by RDI and the degree of oxygen desaturation accompanying apneic episodes. Mild cases have RDI below 20/hour with oxygen saturation remaining above 85%, while severe cases of SAS have RDI above 50/hour with oxygen saturation falling below 65% or cardiac arrhythmia accompanying apneic episode.

There are two types of sleep apneas: obstructive variety characterized by frustrated respiratory efforts to breathe against blocked upper airways; and central apnea (Figure 2), where there is a simple cessation of breathing without ventilatory efforts, that is, cessation of all airflow simultaneous with cessation of respiratory muscle activity. Those with obstructive apnea (Figure 3) having no initial respiratory efforts, when they start

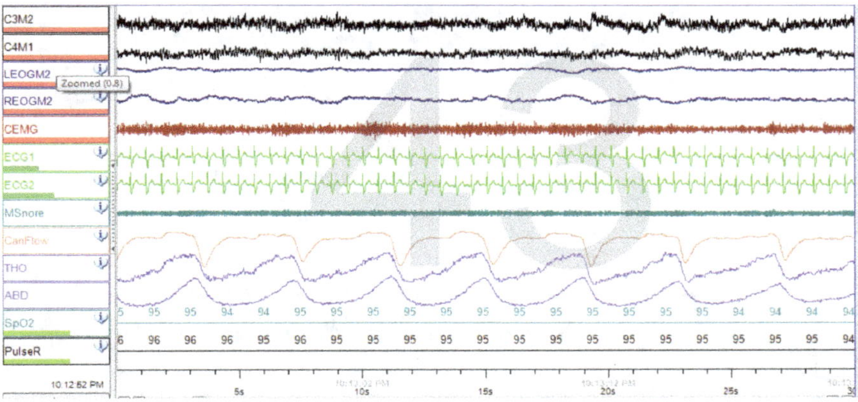

Figure 1: Normal.

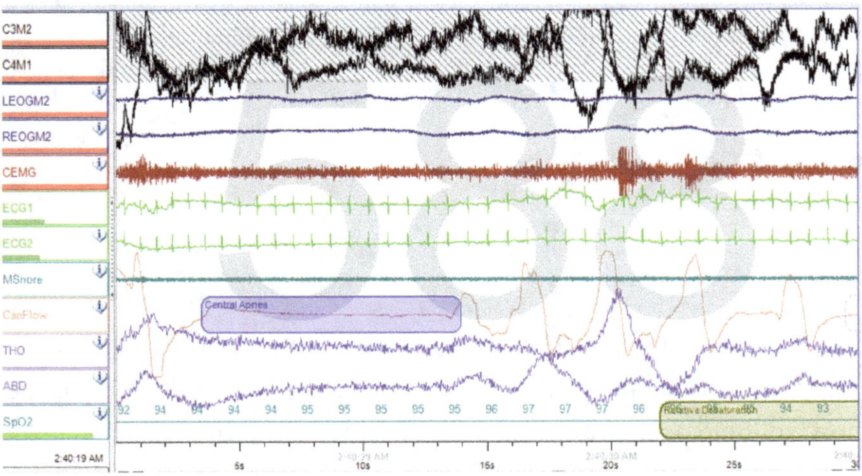

Figure 2: Central apneas.

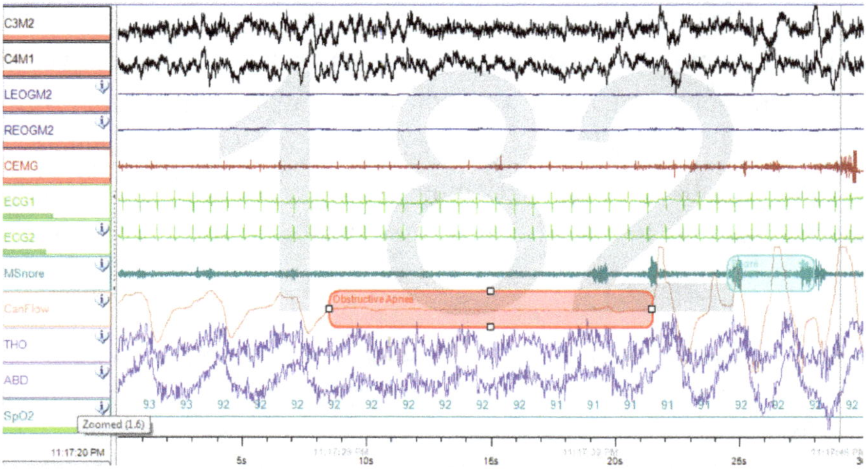

Figure 3: Obstructive apneas.

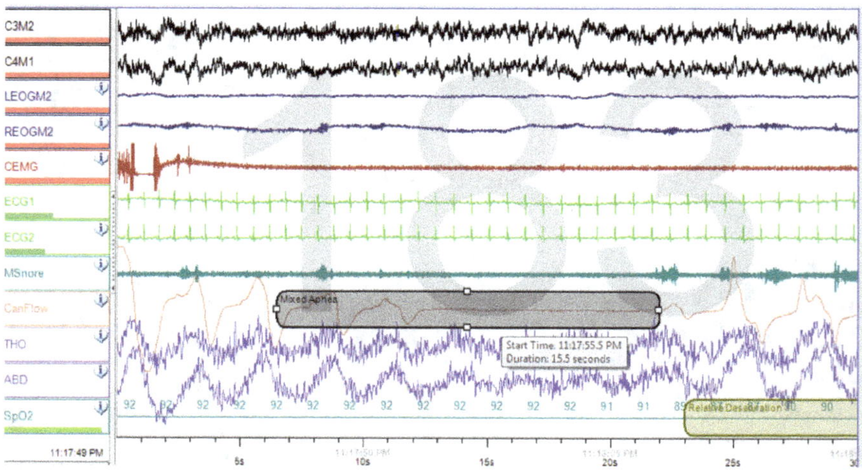

Figure 4: Mixed apneas.

having thoracic effects with the progress of apnea, are called mixed apnea (Figure 4). All the apneas can occur in SAS; the obstructive variety is the most common one. Familial tendency in SAS has also been documented.[2] Obstructive variety has only been recognized in the past decade, although it is as common as asthma.[3] The exact prevalence of obstructive variety is not known; it is roughly estimated around 1%–5%. In India, prevalence of sleep-related disordered breathing is 19.5% while that of obstructive sleep apnea/hypopnea syndrome (OSAHS) is 7.5%.[4]

Pathophysiology

Almost all the apneas originate from airway occlusion around the level of soft palate. There is an active contraction of muscles such as genioglossus, geniohyoid, and omohyoid with each inspiration. During sleep, the muscle tone drops, creating a greater tendency of the upper airway to narrow on inspiration. Turbulent flow occurs, resulting in the vibration sound of snoring. If the airway narrows subcritically, hypopnea results, and if the airway occludes almost totally, apnea results with total occlusion.

Predisposing factors include obesity, enlarged tonsils, hypothyroidism macroglossia, retrognathia, and so forth for pharyngeal encroachment, recurrent rhinitis and deviated nasal septum for nasal obstruction, and alcohol, benzodiazepines, and so forth for decreased activity of the upper airway dilator muscle. Possibly, the upper airway behaving like a starling resistor may tend to collapse within a limited upper airway segment in sleep apnea/hypopnea patients. Anatomical and functional mechanisms

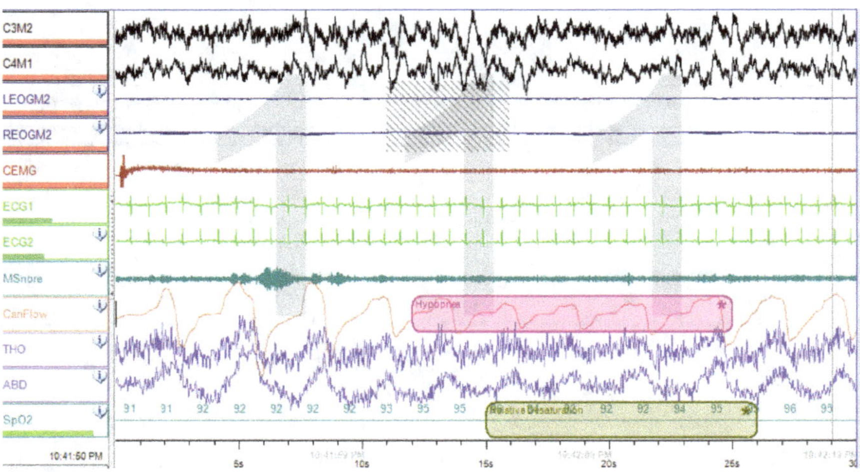

Figure 5: Hypopnea.

lead to the development of critical collapsing pressure, the most important being a small lumen in the upper airways and the reduction and instability of drive to the dilator and abductors of the upper airways. The latter is the characteristic of REM sleep and light NREM sleep.

Excessive daytime sleepiness (EDS) and snoring are the clinical hallmarks of SAS. Most of the patients find falling asleep while being idle or doing monotonous work such as driving a vehicle on lonely road. Vehicular accidents are likely to be more is such cases. Often there is a history of snoring in these patients is quite old and may be intermittent; absence of snoring, however, does not exclude SAS. In children, snoring in usually due to enlarged tonsils and adenoids. OSAHS in children can cause learning disabilities.[5] In adults, there is often a history of unsatisfying sleep, unrefreshed awakening, disorientation, and generalized headache. Gradual onset of EDS keeps it underdiagnosed for years. Occasional episodes of nocturnal choking are quite disturbing. Even homicidal behavior has been described during sleep apnea.[6] Possibly because of atrial natriuretic peptide secretion being stimulated by apnea, nocturia may appear due to excess of salt and water excretion.[7] Enuresis has been documented in younger patients. Recently, association of cherubin with obstructive sleep apnea (OSA) (Figure 6) and mental retardation has been documented.[8,9]

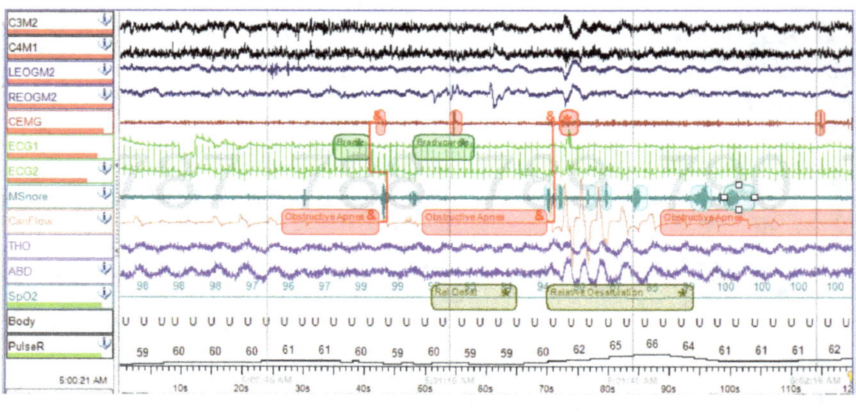

Figure 6: OSA with bradycardia.

Decrease in libido is yet another problem; impotence in males is often associated with long-lasting and severe SAS. Majority of the patients with SAS are males; the role of testosterone may be important both in hypogonadal patients of both sexes.[1]

Although SAS is commonly seen in overweight patients, obesity is not a prerequisite to establish the diagnosis. When sleep apnea is associated with a significant fall of 74% in arterial oxygen saturation, this leads to repeated apnea. Long-standing severe cases, however, precipitate hypoxemic complications of cor pulmonale, secondary polycythemia, and daytime carbon dioxide retention, especially in the presence of coexisting pulmonary disease.[10] Coexisting systemic as well as pulmonary hypertension and cardiac arrhythmias have been documented with SAS. Higher incidence of SAS in chronic obstructive pulmonary disease (COPD) as overlap syndrome has been recorded, and these patients hence are at a higher risk of developing respiratory insufficiency and cor pulmonale.[11] Personality changes, impaired memory, and motor performance are often encountered in SAS. An evidence of a link between OSA and insulin resistances, independent of the degree of obesity,[12,13] has been observed. Significant higher levels of fasting glucose and insulin levels have been demonstrated when compared with weight-matched controls. Further studies have identified impaired metabolism as one of the consequences of sleep loss, suggesting that decrements in sleep duration and/or quality may increase the severity of metabolic disorders, particularly diabetes mellitus. Sleep disturbances *are* common in type 2 diabetes mellitus. In fact, there has been a significant association of sleep disturbances with the presence of dyspnea, nocturnal cramps, paresthesia, and burning of the sole.[14] But findings of sleep-disturbed breathing in these patients are mostly observed in obese patients with a mean body mass index (BMI) of 35.6 (SD:9.9) kg/m' in an Indian study. Therefore, a large community-based epidemiological study is required to identify the true prevalence of sleep apnea in Indian population.

During clinical examination, obesity should be noticed, nose and oropharynx should be examined, especially by an ENT surgeon, and assessment for hypothyroidism and acromegaly and for complications such as cyanosis and congestive cardiac failure should be made. There will be sleep fragmentation also. Observations should be recorded, leaving the patient alone on the examination table, especially for induction of sleep while sitting idle (waiting for the doctor).

When airflow stops at the mouth and nose for a period of 10 seconds or more (apnea) and is accompanied by continuing respiratory movement, it is called obstructive apnea. An occurrence of five apneas/hour or more than 35/night, during sleep, with frequent arousals. Unrestful sleep, followed by daytime hypersomnolence, constitutes OSAHS. The classic patient with OSAHS is an overweight, middle-aged person (although it can occur at any age and obesity is not necessarily present). Majority of these patients have some degree of upper airway obstruction. Alcohol is often a cofactor. Apnea is associated with oxygen denaturation and a marked fall in tissue oxygen concretion during sleep. Snoring to OSAHS is a spectrum; it is a preapneic marker of OSAHS. But it is rare to find snoring progressing to OSAHS after the age of 65 years. Typical snoring of OSAHS is loud and spouse-disturbing. With the progress of the disease, periods of silence may alternate with vigorous breathing efforts of irregular intervals, with a terminal explosive snoring, accompanied with restlessness and flailing of limbs. Recurrent arousals and insomnia cause unrefreshing effects of sleep, leading to mental fogginess, disorientation, and tiredness during the day. Even a headache is noted in one-fifth of these patients. Intermittent snoring and arousals occur due to a combination of hypoxia and hypercapnia.[15] Daytime excessive sleepiness may result in social consequences due to deterioration in intelligence, impaired memory, and decreased sense of appropriate judgment. These patients may become unstable, irritable, and lose temper on little provocation.

Systemic hypertension may be associated in 50% of these patients. Progressive asphyxia is associated with pulmonary hypertension. Though pulmonary artery pressure returns to a normal level during wakefulness in majority of cases, the nocturnal event may be accentuated in patients with obstructive airway disease, associated with sustained daytime hypoxemia, hypercapnia, and polycythemia in 10%–15% of patients. Such an event leads to right heart failure, cardiac arrhythmia such as ventricular premature beats and ventricular tachycardia, and may cause death during sleep (but further corroborate data are lacking). Nevertheless, daytime sleepiness has to be differentiated in case of narcolepsy, hypometabolic states such as hypothermia and hypothyroidism, uremia, cerebrovascular disease, and depression and are shown in the following table of sedatives (Table 1).

Table 1: Consequences of ASA/HS[16]

a. Cardiovascular
— Nocturnal angina, CAO
— Hypertension
— Heart failure
— Cardiac arrhythmias
— Myocardial infarction/death
— Pulmonary hypertension
— Cor pulmonale
— Thromboembolism (in veins)
b. Neurological
— Anxiety, depression
— Cephalalgia, delirium
— TIA/ischemic stroke
— Epilepsy
c. Endocrinal
— Hypogonadism
— Hyperthyroidism
— Insulin resistance
— Acromegaly
d. Miscellaneous
— Impotence/erectile dysfunction
— Esophageal reflux
— Nocturia
— Polycythemia
— Nocturnal dyspnea/respiratory failure

Management

Major advances in understanding the morbidity caused by OSAHS have been observed in the last decade. Since the clinical history or clinical observation are not sufficient to diagnose SAS, oximetry has been applied to observe the characteristic pattern of recurrent arterial oxyhemoglobin desaturation. Again, simple pulse oximetry is not disease-pictorial, although it may be useful for population screening. At the same time, false negative results are obtained when oximetry is employed even for screening. Ideal diagnostic choice for SAS includes overnight polysomnography, recording oxygen saturation by an oximeter, thoracoabdominal movement by surface techniques, airflow by temperature or carbon dioxide sensors, electroencephalogram, electromyogram, and electro-oculogram. This helps in differentiating other causes of excessive daytime sleep, that is, narcolepsy. It is observed that the severity of apnea increases as the night progresses, possibly due to the lengthening of mean apnea duration. Forced oscillation technique has recently been used as a diagnostic tool to accurately and non-invisibly quantify respiratory obstruction during sleep.[17] Elevated serum amyloid has been suggested to be a risk factor for cardiovascular and neuronal dysfunction in patients with OSA.[18]

Avoid alcohol intake and sedative use. Weight reduction is important. This is sufficient for mild form of disorder; sleep apnea may get cured if obesity as an important associated etiology is brought down by bariatric surgery.[19] Appropriate treatment should be provided for myxedema, acromegaly, retrognathia, and nasopharyngeal problems. Drug therapy as such has found no place in the treatment of SAS.[1] However, tricyclic antidepressant protriptyline has been used. It is thought to increase the tone of the upper airway muscles and also help in reducing REP sleep. Tracheostomy that used to be the original 100% effective treatment has now *been* obsolete. Increasing the pharynx size through surgical operation may be considered. Uvulopalatopharyngoplasty prevents snoring, but it is not effective in treating SAS.

Improvement in symptoms, cognitive function, mood, and quality of life has been observed in patients with two major features of OSAHS who have more than 15 respiratory events/hour during sleep.[20] When treated with continuous positive airway pressure (CPAP), use positive pressure *between* 7.5 and 20 cm H_2O. It works by physically blowing the back of the throat open. It acts by splinting the upper airways and preventing its collapse during inspiration. OSAHS can be managed using a combination of surgical technique and oxygen therapies.[21,22] Nocturnal intermittent positive pressure ventilation, using a nasal or face mask, has good patient compliance, when used at home in patients suffering from COPD and sleep apnea.[23] CPAP therapy improved subjective and objective measures of sleepiness more than placebo in OSA.[24] Short-term beneficial effect on blood pressure and cardiac functions has been observed in these patients; long-term vascular consequences of OSAHS are influenced by CPAP is yet to be confirmed.[25,26] Improvement in arterial blood pressure is small but significant on CPAP or with mandibular advancement device and is greatest in those who are most hypoxemic during sleep.[27–29] Regression in left ventricular hypertrophy in patients with severe OSAHS has also been observed after 6 months of nasal CPAP therapy.[30] However, CPAP therapy is ineffective in those who have not been benefited by uvulopalatopharyngoplasty. Cost factor is another major hurdle in our country.

Treatment of central sleep apnea is more difficult. Often seen in the elderly, it is associated with a little snoring. There is a lack of drive to the upper airway muscles and diaphragm, which may be primary or due to reflex elicited by stimulation of mucosal sensory receptors by passive airway closure. Earlier treatment included diaphragm pacing with tracheostomy. Recently, CPAP has been effectively used along with acetazolamide in low dose to reduce the number of apneas.[31] In clinical practice, only sleeted patients get benefit from therapies other than CPAP,[32] although alternatives to CPAP in the treatment of OSAS have been studied.[33] Bariatric surgery is suggested in obese patients. Modafinil helps daytime sleepers in OSA.

Suspecting and diagnosing SAS early and referring to a sleep clinic and seeking advice to benefit from modern, *effective*, and straightforward treatments to lead a better social life is the need of the present time. The advancement in sleep medicine in diagnosing and treatment in recent years should reach to primary care and specialty physicians so as to enable them to educate patients on the health effects of sleep disorders. Despite the increasing evidence of the need of treatment, it is, however, being delivered at an unacceptably slow time scale.[34] Let us ensure to accord OSAHS a priority in healthcare and further research its prevalence and consequence.[35,36] Indian guidelines initiative has been rolled.[37]

References and suggested readings

1. Singh RK. OSA in India — prevalence, profile & management. Med Update; API. 2016;26:1038–1042.
2. Guilleminault C, Partinen M, Hollman K, et al. Familial aggregates in obstructive sleep apnoea syndrome. Chest. 1995;107:1045–1051.
3. Douglas MI, Polo 0. Pathogenesis of obstructive sleep apnoea/hypopnoea syndrome. Lancer. 1994;344:653055.
4. Udwadia ZF, et al. Prevalence of sleep disordered breathing and sleep apnoea in middle aged urban India men. Am J Respir Crit Care Med. 2004;169:168–173.
5. Lyer SR, Iyer RR. Snoring-harmful effects. IN: SB Gupta, ed. Med Update; API. 2005;15:541–544.
6. Nefxinger EA, et al. Homicidal behaviour and sleep apnoea. Sleep. 1995;18:776–782.
7. Warley ARH, et al. Abnormal diurnal variation in salt and water excretion in patients with OSAS. Clin Sci. 1988;74:183–185.
8. Ladhani S, et al. Sleep disordered breathing in an adult with cherubism. Thorax. 2003;58:552.
9. Battaglia A, et al. Cherubism and upper airway obstruction. Otolaryngol Head Neck Surg. 2000;122:673–674.
10. Bardly TO, et al. Role of daytime hypoxemia in the pathogenesis of right heart failure of OSAS. Am Rev Respir Dis. 1985;131:835–839.

11. Chaonat A, et al. Association of COPD and OSAS. Am J Respir Crit Care Med. 1995;151:82–86.
12. Punjabi NM, et al. Sleep disordered breathing and insulin resistance in middle aged and overweight men. Am J Respir Crit Care Med. 2002;165:677–682.
13. Bhatia RS. Sleep apnoea syndrome. IN: LA Pathak, ed. PG Med; API. 2004;18:79–83.
14. Vigg A, et al. Sleep in type 2 diabetes. JAPI. 2003;51:479–481.
15. Sharma SK, et al. Prediction of OSA in patients presenting to a tertiary case centre. Sleep Breath. 2006;10:14754.
16. Gupta D, Handa A. Consequences of OSA/HS. IN: RK Singal, DG Jain, ed. Med Update; API. 2007;17:768–771.
17. Forced oscillation technique in the sleep apnoea/hypoapnoea syndrome. Physiol Meas. 2003;24:11–25.
18. Satikova A, et al. Serum amyloid in OSA. Circulation. 2003;108(2):1451–1454.
19. Chowbey PK. Bariatric surgery importance in obesity management. IN: YP Munjal, ed. PG Med; AFT. 2007;21:413–.
20. Douglas N. Recent advances in SAHS. IN: SI3 Gupta, ed. Med Update; API. 2005;15:446.
21. Gupta YK, et al. Pattern of sleep disordered breathing in obese Indians. Ind J Sleep Med. 2009;4:19–31.
22. Garg, et al. A comparative study on the clinical & polysomnographic pattern of OSA among obese & non obese subjects. Ann Thorac Med. 2012;7:26–30.
23. Goel AK, et al. Evaluation of short term use of nocturnal nasal continuous positive pressure for OSA HS. Lung India. 2015;32:225–232.
24. Patel SR, et al. CPAP therapy improves subjective and objective sleepiness in OSA. Evidence-Based Med. 2003;8:112.
25. Kaneko V, et al. Cardiovascular effects of CPAP in patients with heart failure and OSA. N Engl J Med. 2003;348:1233–1241.
26. Cloward TV, et al. LVH is a common echocardiographic abnormality in severe OSA and reversed with nasal CPAP. Chest. 2003;124(2):594–601.
27. Pepperail JC, et al. Ambulatory blood pressure after therapeutic and sub-therapeutic nasal continuous positive airway pressure for obstructive sleep apnoea: a randomised parallel trial. Lancet. 2002;359:204–210.

28. Becker HF, et al. Effect of nasal CPAP treatment on blood pressure in patients with obstructive sleep apnoea. Circulation. 2003;107:68–73.
29. Gotsopolos H, et al. Oral appliance therapy reduces blood pressure in obstructive sleep apnoea — a randomized controlled trial. Sleep. 2004;24:934–941.
30. Lanfranchi P, Somers K. OSA and vascular disease. Respir Res. 2001;2:315.
31. Debacker WA, et al. Central apnoea index decreases after prolonged treatment with acetazolamide. Am J Respir Crit Care Med. 1995;151:87–91.
32. Chhajed PN, et al. Obstructive sleep apnoea-therapies other than CPAP. JAPI. 2004;52:143–151.
33. Block KE. Alternatives to CPAP in the treatment of OSAS. Swiss Med Weekly. 2006;136:261–267.
34. Mehta N, Vanani V. Prevalence, implications & management. Med Update; API. 2016;26:610.
35. Bhatia RS, Khan GO. Sleep apnoea syndrome. IN: Pulmonary Med. New Delhi: Pee Pee Publ. 2007;11:98–109.
36. Bhatia RS. Sleep apnoea syndrome — pathophysiology and management. Curr Med Trends. 2005;9:1769–1774.
37. Sharma SK, et al. Consensus & evidence-based Indian initiative on OSA guidelines 2014. Lung India. 2015;32:422–434.
38. Ip SM, et al. Obstructive sleep apnoea is independently associated with insulin resistance. Am Respir Crit Care Med. 2002;165:670–676.
39. Salzano G, Maglitto F, Bisogno A. Obstructive sleep apnoea/hypopnoea syndrome: relationship with obesity and management in obese patients. Acta Otorhinolaryngol Ital. 2021 Apr;41(2):120–130.
40. Leung TN, Cheng JW, Chan AK. Paediatrics: how to manage obstructive sleep apnoea syndrome. Drugs Context. 2021 Mar 26;10:2020-12-5.
41. Chasens ER, Imes CC, Kariuki JK, Luyster FS, Morris JL, DiNardo MM, Godzik CM, Jeon B, Yang K. Sleep and metabolic syndrome. Nurs Clin North Am. 2021 Jun;56(2):203–217.
42. Malhotra A, Ayappa I, Ayas N, Collop N, Kirsch D, Mcardle N, Mehra R, Pack AI, Punjabi N, White DP, Gottlieb DJ. Metrics of sleep apnea severity: beyond the apnea-hypopnea index. Sleep. 2021 Jul 9;44(7).

https://doi.org/10.1142/9789811271410_0036

36 Noninvasive mechanical ventilation

Introduction

Noninvasive ventilation (NIV) refers to the delivery of mechanical ventilation without the use of an invasive artificial airway. The greatest advantage of NIV is avoiding the complications of invasive mechanical ventilation. Other advantages are summarized in Table 1. Different approaches to negative pressure ventilation include the use of pneumo belts, rocking beds, negative pressure ventilators, and noninvasive positive pressure ventilation (NIPPV) delivered using an interface. NIPPV using face masks has become the predominant form of NIV in the past few decades. Continuous positive airway pressure (CPAP) is a form of NIPPV where the positive pressure is constant irrespective of the phase of respiration (expiration or inspiration). Bi-level positive airway pressure (BiPAP) is a proprietary name for NIV delivered via a portable ventilator (Respironics/Philips). The term is inappropriately used interchangeably with NIV.

The evidence for NIV use is robust in patients with restrictive lung diseases, neuromuscular disorders, acute exacerbation of chronic obstructive pulmonary disease (AE-COPD), and acute cardiogenic pulmonary edema. It can also be used in acute hypoxemic respiratory failure under certain conditions with closed monitoring in ICU. The use of NIV in ICU for acute respiratory failure increased by 10%–200% between 1990 and 2000 according to a worldwide survey. NIV can also be used for transient respiratory support during short procedures like bronchoscopy and intubation and prehospital transport. It is also being used increasingly for respiratory support during palliative care.

Table 1: Advantages of NIV

Advantages of noninvasive ventilation over invasive mechanical ventilation
Better patient comfort
Preserved ability to communicate, eat, and drink
Lesser cost
No intrusion in upper airway defense mechanisms
Reduce infectious complications like nosocomial pneumonia or sinusitis
Ability to deliver respiratory support in non-ICU settings also
No sedation requirements

Mechanism of action and changes in respiratory physiology during NIV

In acute respiratory failure

NIV has similar physiological effects as invasive mechanical ventilation. The increase in transpulmonary pressure due to positive pressure ventilation increases tidal volume and minute ventilation. The positive pressure during inspiration (IPAP) unloads the respiratory muscles and decreases the Work of Breathing (WOB). This is helpful in patients who develop respiratory failure due to neuromuscular disorders. CPAP increases the Functional Residual Capacity (FRC). This causes a redistribution of ventilation by the opening of collapsed alveoli and a decrease in ventilation–perfusion mismatch which in turn improves oxygenation. CPAP also has beneficial cardiac effects including a decrease in venous return and a decrease in afterload which aids the ailing left ventricle. In cases of acute pulmonary edema, this is the main mechanism for left ventricular offloading. In cases of COPD, CPAP offsets the effects of auto-positive end-expiratory pressure (PEEP). A combination of inspiratory support and CPAP reduces dyspnea, respiratory rate, and WOB in COPD patients.

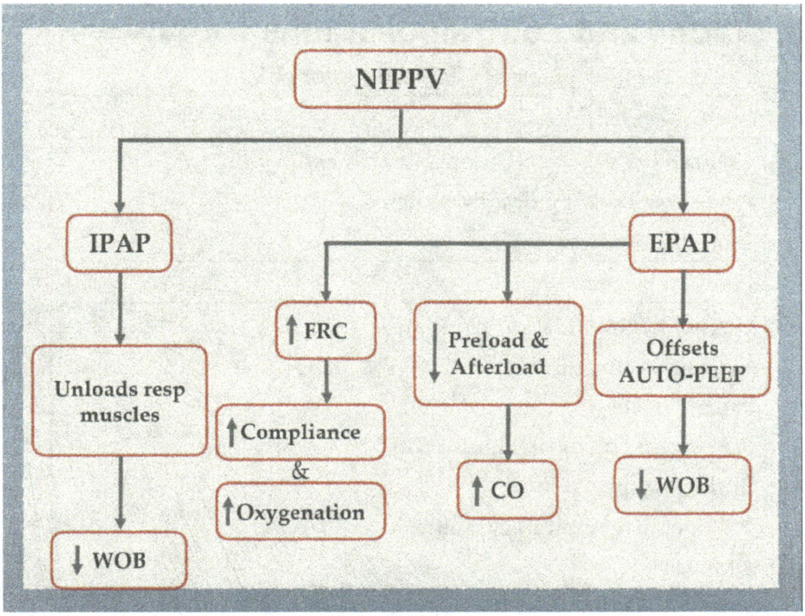

Figure 1: Mechanism of action of NIV in acute respiratory failure.

Image courtesy — Dr. Jagadish Chandran

In chronic respiratory failure

Few theories explain the improvement in respiratory functions with the use of nighttime NIV in patients with chronic respiratory failure. First, it is postulated that nighttime NIV rests the chronically fatigued respiratory muscles. This helps in improved function in daytime, thereby alleviating the symptoms of respiratory failure. Other theories include decreased microatelectasis due to improvement in FRC, improved gas exchange, and better daytime lung function. Third, NIV is presumed to lower the medullary respiratory center's set point sensitivity to carbon dioxide. Fourth, NIV prevents nocturnal hypoventilation-related sleep disturbances like sleep fragmentation, leading to decreased daytime somnolence in obesity hypoventilation syndrome (OHS). However, all the above theories lack high-quality clinical evidence.

Indications and contraindications for NIV

Table 2: Indications for NIV

Level-A evidence
COPD — acute exacerbation and early extubation Acute cardiogenic pulmonary edema Immunocompromised state
Level-B evidence
Obesity hypoventilation syndrome Neuromuscular disorders Palliative care Preoxygenation during intubation Bronchoscopy Postoperative respiratory failure Asthma
Level-C evidence (may be harmful)
Postextubation failure Moderate and severe acute respiratory distress syndrome (ARDS)

Table 3: Contraindications for NIV

Contraindications
Shock Cardiopulmonary resuscitation Nonrespiratory organ failure Copious secretions Unstable cardiac rhythm Upper airway obstruction Obtunded mentation Raised intra-abdominal pressure High risk for aspiration and vomiting Noncooperative or agitated patient Bulbar dysfunction Upper gastrointestinal hemorrhage

NIV in acute hypoxemic respiratory failure

a. Acute cardiogenic pulmonary edema

CPAP has consistently been shown to decrease the respiratory rate, alleviate dyspnea, improve oxygenation, and reduce the need for invasive mechanical ventilation when compared to conventional oxygen therapy in acute cardiogenic pulmonary edema. Multiple meta-analyses have shown that NIV alleviates the symptoms of respiratory distress earlier or better compared to CPAP due to additional support during inspiration as explained earlier. Improvement in biochemical parameters like pH and $PaCO_2$ is faster when compared to CPAP alone. Randomized controlled trials comparing NIV and CPAP did not show any difference in the reduction of respiratory distress, intubation rates, or mortality when used in these patients. Furthermore, the prehospital use of CPAP or NIV has also shown similar effects as in ICU like a decrease in intubation rates and a reduction in mortality in these patients. NIV may also reduce the length of ICU stay and decrease mortality. However, these benefits were not consistently seen in all studies. There appears to be some controversy in an increase in myocardial infarction rates in patients on NIV with acute pulmonary edema when compared to CPAP alone, but this finding has not been consistently replicated in further trials. Thus, NIV has become a standard and first-line modality of respiratory support in acute cardiogenic pulmonary edema.

b. Acute respiratory distress syndrome

The use of NIV in acute respiratory distress syndrome (ARDS) is controversial. While the use of NIV in mild and moderate ARDS has some benefits, its use in severe ARDS has been shown to increase mortality and delay invasive mechanical ventilation. Especially those patients having ARDS who present with shock, multiorgan involvement, and respiratory acidosis are poor candidates for a trial of NIV. In these patients, NIV has been shown to increase mortality. But in patients with mild and moderate ARDS, NIV has been found to decrease the respiratory rate and the need for invasive mechanical ventilation. The same finding has been replicated in the COVID pandemic. However, NIV has been found to be inferior to High-Flow Nasal Oxygenation (HFNO) in mild and moderate ARDS due to COVID-19 pneumonia. Thus, HFNO is preferred over NIV in ARDS, and it should be used with caution in mild and moderate ARDS only. The trial of NIV should not last for more than 6 hours, and if there is no symptomatic improvement within this window, the patient should receive invasive mechanical ventilation.

c. Immunocompromised patients

The use of NIV in immunocompromised patients has various benefits. It prevents the risk of nosocomial pneumonia and severe sepsis which can be deadly due to pathogens being commonly multidrug resistant. Evidence has shown that the trial of NIV can be safely extended to 48 hours in these patients. NIV has been shown to reduce the need for invasive mechanical ventilation and mortality in immunocompromised patients. This finding has been consistently seen in multiple small trials. Thus, NIV is the preferred modality of treatment in immunocompromised patients with acute hypoxemic respiratory failure. However, these benefits are seen in patients with respiratory failure alone. The failure rate of NIV is higher in patients with multiorgan involvement and hence should be used with caution in this subset of patients.

d. Pneumonia

NIV may not be helpful in patients with pneumonia and acute respiratory failure. It decreases respiratory rates and improves oxygenation but does not prevent the eventual need for invasive mechanical ventilation. It may increase the aerosol transmission of pathogens and can cause barotrauma. But it can be used in patients with pneumonia and COPD. In COPD patients who developed pneumonia, NIV has been shown to decrease the need for invasive mechanical ventilation and the length of ICU stay.

e. Trauma

NIV can be safely used in patients with thoracic trauma and the flail chest. Patients with trauma-associated mild ARDS also respond favorably to either NIV or HFNO.

f. Prevention of extubation failure

NIV can be prophylactically used to prevent extubation failure in at-risk patients. Preemptive application of NIV before respiratory failure sets in after extubation is shown to prevent reintubation rates and reduce mortality.

g. Treatment of extubation failure

Patients who suffer from extubation failure have higher mortality compared to those with successful weaning and extubation. NIV has been tried in these patients but has been shown to worsen mortality. The delay in intubation was found to be the reason for higher mortality in clinical trials by Esteban. Thus, it is better to avoid NIV in these patients and treat them with reintubation and invasive mechanical ventilation unless they have coexisting COPD or pulmonary edema.

NIV in acute hypercapnic respiratory failure

a. Acute exacerbation of COPD

These patients show good response to NIV due to the following reasons: acute exacerbations are short-lived and reversible within a few days of therapy. Hypoxemia in AE-COPD is usually mild. NIV offsets the effects of auto-PEEP and helps alleviate dynamic hyperinflation. Clinical trials have consistently shown reduced respiratory rates, reduction in $PaCO_2$, and the need for intubation. The success rate of NIV has been reported from 50% to 90% in these patients in clinical trials. Hence, NIV should be attempted as a first choice in all conscious AE-COPD patients before instituting invasive mechanical ventilation. Meta-analysis has shown a reduction in the cost of hospitalization, heart rate, and dyspnea scores with the use of NIV in AE-COPD patients.

However, NIV cannot function as a substitute for invasive mechanical ventilation in advanced severe acute hypercapnic respiratory failure (pH < 7.25, $PaCO_2$ > 70 mmHg, and respiratory rate > 35 cycles/minute).

b. Asthma

The use of NIV in acute severe asthma has been controversial. NIV has been shown to decrease gas exchange abnormalities, provide bronchodilatory effects, alleviate respiratory distress, and decrease the need for invasive ventilation in a few clinical trials when compared to the conventional oxygen therapy. Many of these trials are of low quality and have small sample sizes. These findings were not corroborated by the Cochrane meta-analysis. Hence, more data are needed to ascertain the benefits of NIV in acute severe asthma. Also, trials comparing NIV and invasive mechanical ventilation in acute severe asthma have shown reduced hospital stay and improved pH and $PaCO_2$ in invasively ventilated patients over NIV.

c. Postoperative respiratory failure

Although high-quality studies specific to the type of surgeries performed are lacking, smaller trials have found NIV to be beneficial in acute respiratory failure, especially the hypercapnic type in postoperative patients.

d. Do-not-intubate patients

Although the use of NIV may prolong the dying process, it helps to reduce respiratory distress and preserves communication in a dying patient. Thus, goals of care for a do-not-intubate (DNI) patient on NIV should be clearly established after consultation with the patient and caregivers before the start of therapy. NIV should be discontinued if the interface hinders communications or increases discomfort and adds to suffering instead of alleviating it.

Table 4: Predictors of success/failure of NIV in an acute care setting

Predictors of success during NIV
Lower APACHE II or SOFA scores
Cooperative patient with absence of anxiety or delirium
Good fitting interface
Respiratory failure alone (single organ involvement)
pH between 7.25 and 7.34
$PaCO_2$ less than 70 mmHg
Respiratory rate between 25 and 35
Good response to NIV within 1 hour of initiation (alleviation of tachypnea, tachycardia, and respiratory distress)
Good ability to clear airway secretions and protect the airway
Predictors of failure of NIV
pH < 7.25
Respiratory rate > 35
APACHE score > 25
Multiorgan involvement
Frailty
High rapid shallow breathing index on NIV

NIV in chronic respiratory failure

a. Restrictive lung disease, secondary chest wall abnormalities, and neuromuscular disorders

The use of NIV improves the symptoms of fatigue, daytime hypersomnolence, and morning headache in patients with OHS and obstructive sleep apnea (OSA). It also improves the quality of sleep by decreasing night desaturations and improving gas exchange.

In patients with neuromuscular disorders, improvement in the quality of life was noted despite a continued decline in the functional status due to disease progression. Long-term cohort series show improvement in survival with the use of NIV in these patients compared to those receiving medical therapy alone. Available data, although limited, show that the use of NIV along with cough augmentation devices improves survival in patients with respiratory failure due to neuromuscular disorders.

b. Obstructive lung disease

There is a clear lack of high-quality trials evaluating the use of long-term NIV in chronic stable COPD patients. Most of the studies have small sample sizes and high drop-out rates. Available evidence shows a decrease in the rate of worsening of respiratory rates, dyspnea scores, and $PaCO_2$ levels in patients treated with NIV over those receiving oxygen alone. This benefit is greater in patients with higher $PaCO_2$ and the presence of uncompensated respiratory acidosis. Initiation of NIV in patients with compensated respiratory acidosis may not be beneficial. Some trials have shown improved mortality and quality of life, but the results have not been replicated in similar studies. Evidence for the use of NIV in cystic fibrosis and diffuse bronchiectasis comes from case series and meta-analysis based on these case series. These have reported improved gas exchange and clearance of secretions. NIV seems to have a role in those patients with cystic fibrosis who develop CO_2 retention, especially awaiting lung transplantation.

c. Congestive cardiac failure

NIV or CPAP has shown similar effects on cardiac function in patients with congestive cardiac failure (CCF) as seen in acute pulmonary edema. Nocturnal NIV or CPAP improves left ventricular systolic function.

NIV for patients undergoing procedures

NIV delivered via face mask and T-tube has been successfully used for respiratory support during bronchoscopy, endoscopy, and transesophageal echocardiography, especially in patients with neuromuscular disorders, pneumonia, and cystic fibrosis. It also has been used for preoxygenation before intubation in similar patient populations.

Table 5: Practice points for successful use of NIV

Diagnosis	Acute conditions — acute exacerbation of COPD, cardiogenic pulmonary edema respond better to NIV
Patient selection	A conscious and cooperative patient with the ability to clear airway secretions ensures better success rates
Site of care	Acute conditions — emergency or intensive care unit Chronic conditions — NIV can be initiated in the ward for chronic stable COPD patients Initiation of NIV in patients with acute respiratory failure in the ward is shown to increase mortality
Initiation criteria	Acute — refer to Table 4 Initiation of long-term NIV for chronic respiratory failure depends on specific diagnosis and goals of care Obstructive lung diseases • Presence of symptoms like daytime somnolence, fatigue, and dyspnea • Presence of symptoms despite maximal medical therapy and supplemental oxygen • Persistent hypercapnia ($PaCO_2$ > 55 mmHg) and hypoxemia despite supplemental oxygen Restrictive lung disease (OSA/OHS) • Confirmed OSA as per polysomnography • Failure to improve with CPAP alone • Significant improvement in oxygenation during NIV trials
Interfaces	Acute — full face mask/helmet Chronic — nasal interfaces/full face mask
Mode selection	No studies have shown that one ventilator mode is superior to another in the acute setting for preventing intubation or mortality
Settings	High–low approach • begins with higher inspiratory pressure (between 20 and 25 cm H_2O) and then decreases it if the patient is tolerant • alleviates respiratory distress early Low–high approach • begins with low inspiratory pressure (8–10 cm H_2O) and gradually increases it to a level the patient can tolerate • ensures better patient acceptance

Table 6: Complications with the use of NIV

Complications
Major complications
Pneumothorax Hypotension Aspiration pneumonia
Minor complications
Discomfort Erythema on the face Claustrophobia Bridge of the nose ulceration Nasal clogging Ear and sinus pain Nasal and oral drying Eye irritation Gastric distention

Adverse effects and complications

NIPPV is safe and well tolerated in carefully selected patients. Major complications are seen more in patients with acute respiratory failure, especially in those who continue to receive NIV despite no signs of improvement. Hence, it is imperative to recognize the failure of NIV and institute invasive mechanical ventilation in such patients. Minor complications are usually related to the interface, and appropriate selection of the interface and modification in size decreases these types of complications.

Summary

The benefits of NIV lie in avoiding the complications of invasive mechanical ventilation. These are greatest in acute cardiogenic pulmonary edema, immunocompromised patients, and patients with acute exacerbations of COPD. Judicious use of NIV and appropriate patient selection has shown to decrease the cost of hospitalization without compromising patient outcomes. Long-term NIV in select patient populations prolongs survival, improves dyspnea scores, and improves the quality of life while decreasing hospitalization rates.

Suggested reading

Principles and Practice of Mechanical Ventilation by Martin J. Tobin
NIV in Acute Respiratory Failure by Dean R Hess
Ventilator Modes and Settings During Non-invasive Ventilation by Claudio Rabec
Guidelines for NIV by ISCCM

References and suggested readings

1. Guia M, Ciobanu LD, Sreedharan JK, Abdelrahim ME. International Association of Non Invasive Ventilation. The role of non-invasive ventilation in weaning and decannulation critically ill patients with tracheostomy: a narrative review of the literature. Pulmonology. 2021 Jan–Feb;27(1):43–51. doi: 10.1016/j.pulmoe.2020.07.002. Epub 2020 Jul 25. PMID: 32723618.
2. Radovanovic D, Coppola S, Franceschi E, Gervasoni F, Duscio E, Chiumello DA, Santus P. Mortality and clinical outcomes in patients with COVID-19 pneumonia treated with non-invasive respiratory support: a rapid review. J Crit Care. 2021 Oct;65:1–8. doi: 10.1016/j.jcrc.2021.05.007. Epub 2021 May 21. PMID: 34052780; PMCID: PMC8137355.
3. Amirfarzan H, Cereda M, Gaulton TG, Leissner KB, Cortegiani A, Schumann R, Gregoretti C. Use of helmet CPAP in COVID-19 — a practical review. Pulmonology. 2021 Sep–Oct;27(5):413–422. doi: 10.1016/j.pulmoe.2021.01.008. Epub 2021 Feb 1. PMID: 33583765; PMCID: PMC7849604.
4. Saeed H, Harb HS, Madney YM, Abdelrahim MEA. Aerosol delivery via noninvasive ventilation: role of models and bioanalysis. Ann Transl Med. 2021 Apr;9(7):589. doi: 10.21037/atm-20-1261. PMID: 33987287; PMCID: PMC8105861.
5. O'Toole C, Joyce M, McGrath JA, O'Sullivan A, Byrne MA, MacLoughlin R. Fugitive aerosols in the intensive care unit: a narrative review. Ann Transl

Med. 2021 Apr;9(7):592. doi: 10.21037/atm-20-2280. PMID: 33987290; PMCID: PMC8105852.

6. Martins IPM, Nakato AM, Heimbecker PK, Ioshii SO, Nohama P. Correlation of end-tidal carbon dioxide with arterial carbon dioxide in mechanically ventilated neonates: a scoping review. Glob Pediatr Health. 2021 May 17;8: 2333794X211016790. doi: 10.1177/2333794X211016790. PMID: 34036124; PMCID: PMC8132087.
7. Singh A, Khanna P, Sarkar S. High-flow nasal cannula: a boon or a bane for COVID-19 patients? An evidence-based review. Curr Anesthesiol Rep. 2021;11(2):101–106. doi: 10.1007/s40140-021-00439-4. Epub 2021 Mar 2. PMID: 33679254; PMCID: PMC7921283.
8. Masip J, Peacock WF, Price S, Cullen L. Acute Heart Failure Study Group of the Acute Cardiovascular Care Association and the Committee on Acute Heart Failure of the Heart Failure Association of the European Society of Cardiology. Indications and practical approach to non-invasive ventilation in acute heart failure. Eur Heart J. 2018 Jan 1;39(1):17–25. doi: 10.1093/eurheartj/ehx580. PMID: 29186485; PMCID: PMC6251669.
9. Bittencourt HS, Reis HF, Lima MS, Gomes-Neto M. Non-invasive ventilation in patients with heart failure: a systematic review and meta-analysis. Arq Bras Cardiol. 2017 Feb;108(2):161–168. doi: 10.5935/abc.20170001. Epub 2017 Jan 16. PMID: 28099587; PMCID: PMC5344662.
10. Moran F, Bradley JM, Piper AJ. Non-invasive ventilation for cystic fibrosis. Cochrane Database Syst Rev. 2017 Feb 20;2(2):CD002769. doi: 10.1002/14651858.CD002769.pub5. PMID: 28218802; PMCID: PMC6464053.
11. Luo F, Annane D, Orlikowski D, He L, Yang M, Zhou M, Liu GJ. Invasive versus non-invasive ventilation for acute respiratory failure in neuromuscular disease and chest wall disorders. Cochrane Database Syst Rev. 2017 Dec 4;12(12):CD008380. doi: 10.1002/14651858.CD008380.pub2. PMID: 29199768; PMCID: PMC6486162.
12. Radunovic A, Annane D, Rafiq MK, Brassington R, Mustafa N. Mechanical ventilation for amyotrophic lateral sclerosis/motor neuron disease. Cochrane Database Syst Rev. 2017 Oct 6;10(10):CD004427. doi: 10.1002/14651858.CD004427.pub4. PMID: 28982219; PMCID: PMC6485636.

13. Slain KN, Shein SL, Rotta AT. The use of high-flow nasal cannula in the pediatric emergency department. J Pediatr (Rio J). 2017 Nov–Dec;93(Suppl 1):36–45. doi: 10.1016/j.jped.2017.06.006. Epub 2017 Aug 15. PMID: 28818509.
14. Castro-Codesal ML, Dehaan K, Featherstone R, Bedi PK, Martinez Carrasco C, Katz SL, Chan EY, Bendiak GN, Almeida FR, Olmstead DL, Young R, Woolf V, Waters KA, Sullivan C, Hartling L, MacLean JE. Long-term non-invasive ventilation therapies in children: a scoping review. Sleep Med Rev. 2018 Feb;37:148–158. doi: 10.1016/j.smrv.2017.02.005. Epub 2017 Mar 2. PMID: 28410811.
15. Ou J, Chen H, Li L, Zhao L, Nie N. The role of non-invasive ventilation used immediately after planned extubation for adults with chronic respiratory disorders. Saudi Med J. 2018 Feb;39(2):131–136. doi: 10.15537/smj.2018.2.21942. PMID: 29436560; PMCID: PMC5885088.
16. Faverio P, De Giacomi F, Sardella L, Fiorentino G, Carone M, Salerno F, Ora J, Rogliani P, Pellegrino G, Sferrazza Papa GF, Bini F, Bodoni BD, Messinesi G, Pesci A, Esquinas A. Management of acute respiratory failure in interstitial lung diseases: overview and clinical insights. BMC Pulm Med. 2018 May 15;18(1):70. doi: 10.1186/s12890-018-0643-3. PMID: 29764401; PMCID: PMC5952859.

https://doi.org/10.1142/9789811271410_0037

37 Invasive mechanical ventilation

History

The history of mechanical ventilation dates back to Galen who described ventilating an animal as follows: "If you take a dead animal and blow air through its larynx, you will fill its bronchi and watch its lung attain the greatest distension." The first use of artificial respiration in humans is documented in apparently drowned patients using mouth-to-mouth respiration by the mid-17th century. By the early 19th century, techniques of resuscitation using tracheal intubation and bellows ventilation were gaining acceptance. However, experiments by Leroy showed pneumothorax which was fatal due to overzealous ventilation. Consequently, positive pressure ventilation was banned and not used until the early 20th century. But experiments on negative pressure ventilators continued, and the iron lung was the first negative pressure ventilator used successfully in clinical practice in 1928. Despite being cumbersome and inconvenient, the iron lung saved a lot of lives during polio epidemics. Positive pressure ventilators were reintroduced in clinical medicine by the 1950s, first in the operating room for thoracic surgery and later in nonoperative patients. A significant increase in the number of patients requiring mechanical ventilation in the 1960s led to the development of modern ventilators.

Physical principles of ventilatory support

A ventilator is a machine that converts electrical energy or energy from compressed gas in a controlled predetermined manner that supplements or completely replaces a patient's respiratory muscles, thereby assisting or entirely performing the work of breathing. This can be mathematically described by the equation of motion for the respiratory system which is derived from **Newton's third law of motion**.

$$P_{vent} + P_{mus} = \text{Elastance} \times \text{Volume} + \text{Resistance} \times \text{Flow}$$

where P_{vent} represents the transrespiratory pressure generated by the ventilator, and P_{mus} represents the transrespiratory pressure generated by respiratory muscles. The product of elastance and volume represents the elastic load, whereas the product of resistance and flow represents the resistive load against which the transrespiratory pressure acts to bring about inspiration.

Since expiration is passive (even in a patient on a ventilator), the equation becomes

$$-\text{Resistance} \times \text{Flow} = \text{Elastance} \times \text{Volume}$$

The negative sign indicates the opposite direction of airflow which is now generated by the energy stored in the lungs and chest wall (elastic compartment) during inspiration.

Thus, the equation of motion represents various combinations of the ventilator and respiratory muscle work done for infinite combinations of elastic and resistive loads. In a patient where a ventilator must generate all the work, the muscle pressure will be zero, and the other extreme is a spontaneously breathing patient who does not require a ventilator. In between these two extremes lies the concept of assisted breaths or partial ventilatory support. The same is true for the load against which these forces act. For example, a patient with asthma has a high resistive load, whereas a patient with acute respiratory distress syndrome (ARDS) has a high elastic load. Other lung pathologies like pneumonia, large pleural effusions, and pulmonary edema represent various combinations of resistive and elastic loads. Understanding these concepts will help in the diagnosis of a patient's pulmonary pathology at the bedside using the ventilator graphs.

The basic design of a ventilator

A ventilator is a machine that has three basic components.

1. An input source of energy to power the device.
2. A processing unit that converts the input energy into pressure and generates flow into the patient's lungs along with means to regulate the timing and duration of the generated flow.
3. A monitoring unit to check the output from the ventilator to evaluate the performance of the device along with monitoring the patient's lung mechanics.

1. Input source

Usually, electricity powers the compressors and control circuitry in mechanical ventilators. They also have batteries as an alternative power source for emergency use or transport. Compressors provide compressed air for ventilation of the patient and provide energy to drive the flow of gas. Alternatively, compressed gas (oxygen) can also be supplied via wall-mounted gas outlets in hospitals. These separate sources of compressed air and oxygen permit the delivery of a wide range of FiO_2 (fraction of inspired oxygen) to the patient.

Some transport and emergency ventilators are powered by compressed gas alone. Since both lung inflation and control circuit used compressed gas, additional gas consumption should be factored in for the safe transport of the patient.

2. Processing unit

These are parts of the ventilator that convert electrical energy into pressure that generates airflow in a controlled and predetermined manner as set by the clinician. These include compressor or blower, flow control valves, and control systems like microprocessors, control software, and pressure and flow sensors.

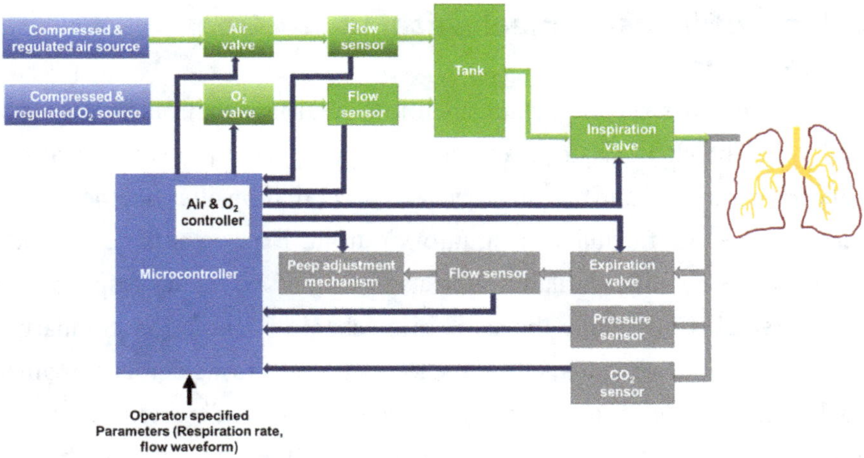

Figure 1: The basic design of a ventilator.

3. Output and monitoring unit

These include the pressure, volume, flow scalars (output variables graphed over time), loops, trends, and various numbers displayed on the user interface. Collectively, these scalars and values (inspired and expired tidal volume, resistance, compliance, work of breathing, time constant, $P_{0.1}$, peak airway, plateau pressures, etc.) help in monitoring the ventilator performance, recognizing changes in the patient's respiratory mechanics, triggering appropriate safety alarms, preventing lung damage, and alerting the clinician to possible adverse events.

Indications for mechanical ventilation

Physiological effects of mechanical ventilation

Mechanical ventilation has profound effects on various systems in the body, and knowledge of these effects is essential for a clinician to make appropriate decisions to improve patient outcomes. The effects can be classified and studied as follows:

1. Effects of mechanical ventilation on the lungs
2. Effects on heart–lung interaction
3. Effects on other organ systems

Effects of invasive mechanical ventilation on the lungs

Respiration relies on important chemical, neuromechanical, and reflex feedback. The chemical feedback includes pH, partial pressures of arterial carbon dioxide, and oxygen. Mechanical ventilation alters all the above and modifies the medullary respiratory output. Experiments performed on conscious healthy ventilated subjects show that medullary response to $PaCO_2$ remains essentially the same in mechanical ventilation. Similarly, the sensitivity of medullary centers for hypoxia and acidemia remains unaltered as in nonventilated patients. Hypoxia and acidemia increase the intensity of respiratory efforts without affecting the rate, whereas $PaCO_2$ alters the rate of respiration. The implications of these findings at the bedside are

a. A ventilated patient who has bradypnea at the bedside has possible carbon dioxide washout.
b. A ventilated patient who is using accessory muscles of respiration has possible hypoxemia or acidemia.

Also, there is no difference noted in medullary response to this chemical feedback on different modes of ventilation. However, this experimental evidence is from healthy volunteers, and there is limited evidence from diseased patients and patients on sedatives. In contrast to medullary response, the respiratory muscle output varies significantly in critically ill patients in response to changes in pH, $PaCO_2$, and PaO_2. It depends on the mode of ventilation, disease pathophysiology, and use of sedatives.

The neuromechanical feedback includes changes in respiratory muscle activation in response to lung volume and flow changes. With increasing lung volume, respiratory muscle output decreases in spontaneously breathing patients more so in mechanically ventilated patients as the pressure generated by the ventilator leads to additional lung expansion.

Animal studies have shown that vagally mediated reflexes and Hering–Breuer reflexes remain active even in mechanically ventilated patients, preventing lung overdistension and injury. Still, the magnitude of the reflex response has been unpredictable.

Effects of invasive mechanical ventilation on heart–lung interaction

The heart and lungs are intimately connected not only via blood vessels but also by the intrathoracic location. The pressure changes in one organ usually affect pressures in the other. Knowledge of heart–lung interactions during mechanical ventilation is, therefore, a vital skill.

Cyclical changes in intrathoracic pressure that occur due to positive pressure ventilation have effects on preload and afterload of the right ventricle and left ventricle. This is summarized in Figure 2.

In a patient with hypervolemia, invasive mechanical ventilation has far less effect on cardiac output as the effect on venous return is blunted. If there is associated left ventricular dysfunction, the reduction in afterload improves left ventricular performance.

Effects of mechanical ventilation on other organs

The positive end-expiratory pressure (PEEP) and raised intrathoracic pressure are known to decrease venous return. This can cause raised

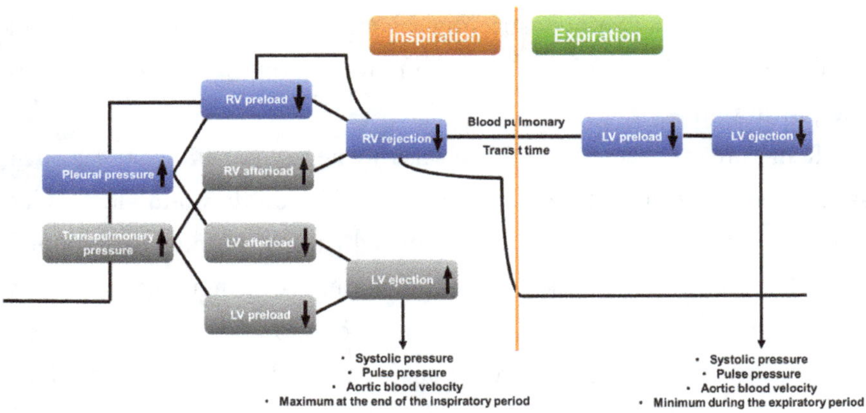

Figure 2: Effect of mechanical ventilation on other organs.

intracranial pressure and intra-abdominal pressure. It can be detrimental in patients with a head injury, acute kidney injury, or abdominal compartment syndrome. Mechanical ventilation increases central venous pressure which may reduce venous return from the head, increase intracranial pressure, and reduce cerebral perfusion pressure, thus resulting in cerebral hypoxia from reduced perfusion and increased cerebral edema from increased intracranial pressure. Patients with head injury, cerebral tumors, and post neurosurgery fall in this category.

In normal intracranial dynamics, when mechanically hyperventilated, cerebral perfusion is reduced due to lowering of arterial carbon dioxide partial pressure ($PaCO_2$) to 25–30 mmHg, which causes alkalosis that brings about cerebral vessels constriction. This in turn reduces the intracranial pressure and augments cerebral perfusion. Patients with refractory hypoxemia may require PEEP for maintenance of life-saving oxygen; need to be monitored for intracranial pressure (since PEEP can increase the intracranial pressure).

Mechanical ventilation may cause gastric mucosal ischemia due to reduced splanchnic venous flow because of increased splanchnic resistance and may precipitate gastrointestinal bleeding. Hepatic dysfunction may occur because of increased splanchnic resistance or reduced portal venous flow or downward diaphragm movement against liver. It can also occur because of arteriolar vasoconstriction during positive pressure ventilation or effect of intrathoracic increased mean pressure on sinusoidal capillaries and portal vein.

Renal effects include renal response to hemodynamic changes such as reduced urine output due to reduced renal blood flow and glomerular filtration rate (GFR) as a result of reduced cardiac output. Antidiuretic hormone release is increased, resulting in oliguria. Oliguria also results due to reduction in atrial-natriuretic factor due to positive pressure ventilation, which also stimulates renin angiotensin system to enhance aldosterone level, causing retention of sodium and water. Renal functions are also reduced due to changes in arterial blood gases. Though not clinically significant, mechanical ventilation, especially PEEP, enhances the release of plasminogen-activating factor in lungs which increases fibrinolysis which prevents intravascular coagulation.

Classification of modes of ventilation

The mode of ventilation is defined as the predetermined pattern of interaction between the ventilator and the patient. It is set by the clinician and defines how a breath is delivered. To understand the modes of ventilation familiarity with the below terminologies is essential.

Table 1: Common terminologies used to describe mechanical ventilation

Term	Description
Control variable	It is the primary variable the ventilator influences to bring about inspiration. For example, PCV is pressure control ventilation, a basic mode of ventilation. Here, the control variable is pressure. There are three primary control variables: pressure, volume, and flow (because the equation of motion has only these three variables).
Limit variable	There is an upper ceiling fixed for this variable. For example, if pressure is limited in a mode of ventilation, then during inspiration, irrespective of the set tidal volume, the airway pressure is not allowed to cross the threshold set by the clinician. The delivery of tidal volume stops once this ceiling is reached. It acts as a safety mechanism to prevent lung damage by excessive peak pressure.
Trigger variable	This variable initiates inspiration. It is time for mandatory breaths, and pressure or flow in spontaneous or assisted breaths.
Cycle variable	This variable decides the change from inspiration to expiration. In mandatory breaths, time is the cycle variable. After a set time, the ventilator stops inspiration, and expiration happens passively. In spontaneous breath, flow acts as a cycle variable.

(*Continued*)

Table 1: (*Continued*)

Term	Description
Baseline variable	Positive end-expiratory pressure is also called the baseline variable as this pressure is maintained even throughout the expiration.
Target variable	Same as limit variable except that the term limit variable is used for those that trigger alarms and target variable to those that have an upper bound without initiating an alarm.
Breath	A breath is one cycle of positive flow (inspiration) and negative flow (expiration).
Assisted breath	A breath is assisted if pressure rises above the baseline during inspiration or falls during expiration. An assisted breath is when a ventilator performs some portion of the work of breathing.
Spontaneous breath	A spontaneous breath is patient triggered and patient cycled.
Mandatory breath	Any machine involvement in triggering or cycling is a mandatory breath.
Breath sequence	It describes the pattern of breaths delivered by ventilation during a particular mode of ventilation.
Targeting scheme	It is the type of feedback control system ventilator used to deliver breaths during a particular mode of ventilation. The targeting scheme can be a set point, servo, dual, adaptive, and intelligent. A detailed discussion is presented in the suggested reading.
Scalars	These are pressure–volume or flow graphs plotted over time.
Loops	These are graphs of two variables plotted against each other. Examples are pressure–volume loops and flow–volume loops.

There are three possible sequences of breaths that can be delivered.

a. Continuous mandatory ventilation — All breaths delivered by the ventilator are mandatory.
b. Continuous spontaneous ventilation — All breaths during the mode of ventilation are patient triggered and patient cycled.
c. Intermittent mandatory ventilation — Both mandatory and spontaneous breaths are delivered.

There are more than 150 modes of ventilation described so far. Each ventilator manufacturer uses different nomenclature to describe the available options in a particular product to make them sound more attractive. However, this has led to much confusion due to the lack of a standardized system describing the modes. For beginners, all modes of ventilation can be classified in a simple manner using a control variable and breath sequence.

The above classification helps the clinician to convert the mode name (usually proprietary) into mode classification. This helps in understanding the operational logic and the patient–ventilator interaction in any mode on any ventilator. For example, pressure-regulated volume control (PRVC) has volume control along with pressure being limited. It delivers mandatory breaths alone. Hence, it is a form of dual control continuous mandatory ventilation.

Table 2: A basic classification scheme for modes of ventilation

Control variable	Breath sequence
Pressure	Continuous mandatory ventilation (PC-CMV) Intermittent mandatory ventilation (PC-IMV) Continuous spontaneous ventilation (PC-CSV)
Volume	Continuous mandatory ventilation (VC-CMV) Intermittent mandatory ventilation (VC-IMV)
Dual	Continuous mandatory ventilation (DC-CMV) Intermittent mandatory ventilation (DC-IMV) Continuous spontaneous ventilation (DC-CSV)

It is interesting to note that volume control continuous spontaneous ventilation does not exist because once the size of breath is controlled (volume control), the breath becomes mandatory.

A more detailed classification system includes a targeting scheme for primary and secondary breaths, conditional variable, operational logic, along with control variable and breath sequence.

Conventional modes of ventilatory support

Although no standardized definition of conventional modes exists, those modes that have a set-point targeting scheme (pressure, volume, or flow) are generally considered conventional. The commonly used conventional modes of ventilation include volume control ventilation, pressure control

Table 3: Modes of mechanical ventilation

1. Pressure control ventilation: Useful in minimizing barotraumas.
2. Pressure support ventilation: Specially designed for weaning purpose.
3. Inverse ratio ventilation.
4. Airway pressure release ventilation: Largely used experimentally.
5. High-frequency ventilation: It can provide
   a. High-frequency positive pressure ventilation.
   b. High-frequency jet ventilation.
   c. High-frequency oscillation.

Table 4: Comparison of volume control versus pressure control mode of ventilation

Parameter	Volume control	Pressure control
Control variable	Volume	Pressure
Preset variables	Tidal volume/minute ventilation, I:E ratio, respiratory rate (RR), PEEP	Peak inspiratory pressure, I:E ratio, RR, PEEP
Inspiratory flow	Fixed	Variable (decelerating)

Table 4: (*Continued*)

Parameter	Volume control	Pressure control
Dependent variables (based on resistance and compliance of the patient)	Peak airway pressure, plateau pressure	Tidal volume
Mean airway pressure for the same tidal volume	Lower	Higher
Advantages	Guaranteed minute ventilation	Airway pressure is always below the set point
Disadvantages	Risk of barotrauma	Risk of hypoventilation/ hyperventilation
Indications	Desired more in whom minute ventilation should be precise and volume should be assured (head injury and neuromuscular diseases) and those with unstable lung mechanics (asthma)	Desired in whom more even distribution of ventilation is required (ARDS) and those patients with volume leaks (peri-tracheostomy/small bronchopleural fistula)

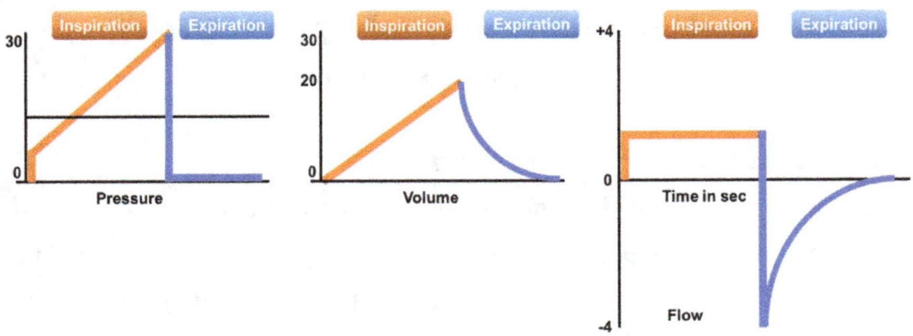

Figure 3: Scalars on volume control ventilation.

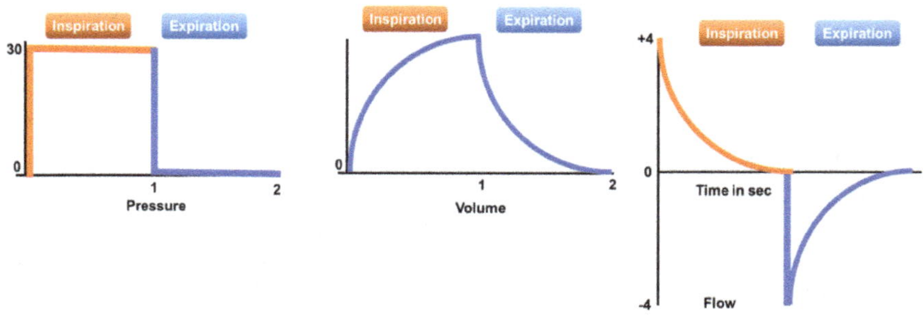

Figure 4: Scalars on pressure control ventilation.

ventilation, synchronized intermittent mandatory ventilation (SIMV), and pressure support.

Synchronized intermittent mandatory ventilation

This mode comes under VC-IMV. True to the classification system, this mode delivers both mandatory (with the preset tidal volume/pressure) and spontaneous breaths; mandatory breaths are delivered only if the patient fails to generate spontaneous efforts within a specified interval (the so-called SIMV interval). Hence, the name. SIMV mode was introduced as a mode for weaning from mechanical ventilation allowing patients to breathe spontaneously, while mandatory breaths ensured adequate minute ventilation. However, a randomized control trial by Esteban et al showed that SIMV delayed weaning when compared to pressure support mode as it increased the work of breathing and asynchrony.

Pressure support ventilation

This is a form of PC-CSV. The breaths delivered are spontaneous, and inspiratory support depends on the pressure support set by the clinician. At a low level of support, it helps the patient to compensate for increased resistive work of breathing due to the presence of an endotracheal tube. At a higher level of support, the ventilator may completely perform the work of breathing. The advantages of the pressure support mode lie in the fact that it ensures patient comfort and synchrony. Hence, it is one of the most commonly preferred modes for weaning from a ventilator.

Advanced modes of ventilatory support

Generally, the term advanced mode refers to a mode with dual control or other means of advanced closed-loop (servo, adaptive, intelligent, or optimal) targeting schemes. In dual control mode, the operator sets both pressure and tidal volume along with rate, and the ventilator adjusts the tidal volume to change lung mechanics without crossing the set pressure limit. The ventilator can deliver either volume preset mandatory breaths or pressure control breaths depending on the lung mechanics of the patient. So far there is no convincing evidence that dual control modes decrease mortality. Readers are referred to the suggested reading for a detailed description of advanced closed-loop targeting schemes. Some commonly used advanced modes of ventilatory support are described below.

Pressure regulated volume control

This is a commonly used dual-mode, especially in ARDS patients. The targeting scheme is DC-IMV, but some consider it under the adaptive targeting scheme. The operator first sets a target tidal volume and pressure. The ventilator delivers initially a volume control breath during which the patient's pulmonary resistance and compliance are calculated. In the next breath, it delivers a pressure control breath at the least pressure that can achieve the set tidal volume for that particular resistance and compliance. If the set tidal volume targets are not met, then it gradually increases the pressure to achieve the targeted tidal volume over the next few breaths. This process ensures minimal airway pressures for a guaranteed tidal volume for specific pulmonary resistance and compliance. These changes are made over a few consecutive breaths, whereas some modes make such changes within a single breath. Adaptive Pressure Ventilation, Autoflow, and Volume Control Plus (VC+) are different proprietary names for the PRVC mode.

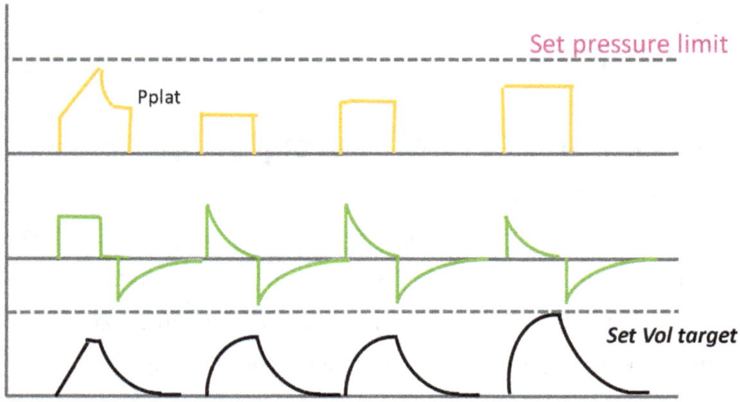

Figure 5: The operating principles in the PRVC mode. The first breath is a volume-controlled mandatory breath that assesses the patient's pulmonary mechanics. Over the next few pressure control breaths, the desired tidal volume is achieved with minimum possible airway pressure limiting lung injury. Image courtesy — Dr. Manu Verma, associate professor, Department of Critical Care Medicine, Dayananda Sagar Medical College.

Airway pressure release ventilation

This mode has a PC-IMV breath sequence with inverse ratio ventilation (wherein the duration of inspiration is larger than expiration), sometimes used in ARDS patients. The advantage of the APRV mode is that it allows spontaneous breaths during the inverse ratio ventilation. The operator sets P_{high} and P_{low}. These are the pressures at which the ventilator operates for the duration of T_{high} and T_{low}, respectively. The difference between P_{high} and P_{low} is akin to pressure control set on PC-IMV, and P_{low} is akin to PEEP. T_{high} is the inspiratory time, and T_{low} is the duration of expiration. During inspiration, the patient is allowed to breathe spontaneously. The spontaneous breaths are pressure supported. The advantages of the APRV mode are that it allows for less sedation; posterior and dependent parts of the lungs are better ventilated, and hemodynamic stability is better when compared to the inverse ratio ventilation. However, too low T_{low} can lead to significant auto-PEEP.

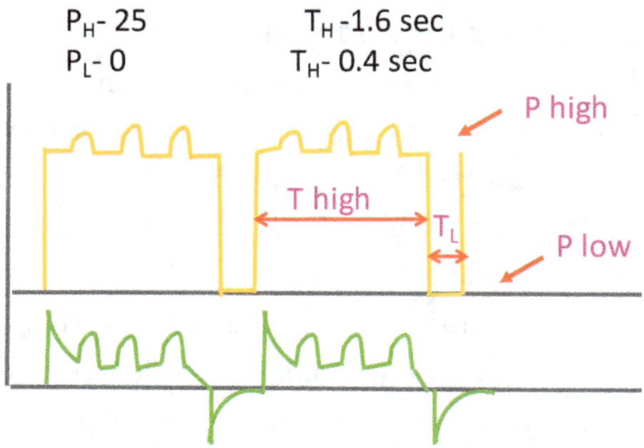

Figure 6: An example setting with pressure-time and flow-time scalars on APRV. Image courtesy — Dr. Manu Verma, associate professor, Department of Critical Care Medicine, Dayananda Sagar Medical College.

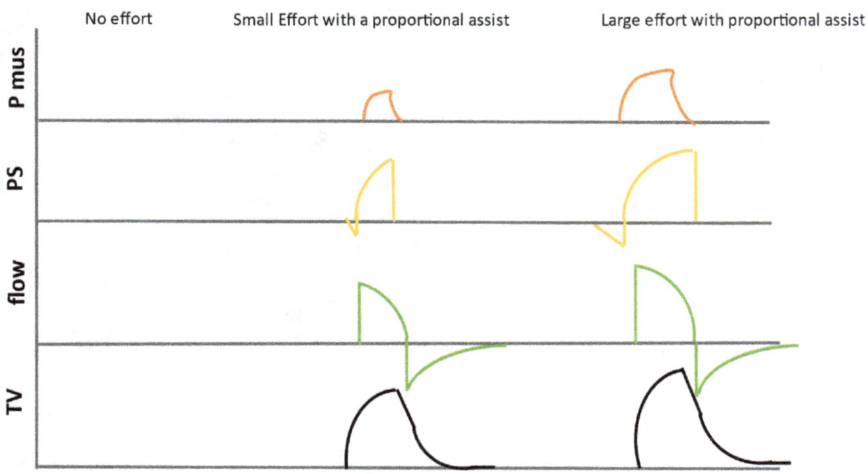

Figure 7: The operating principles of proportional assist ventilation. Image courtesy — Dr. Manu Verma, associate professor, Department of Critical Care Medicine, Dayananda Sagar Medical College.

Proportional assist ventilation

It has a CSV breath sequence, but the targeting scheme is a servo control closed-loop system. As the name suggests, the pressure support is directly proportional to the patient's efforts. The operator sets the proportion of volume and flow support to be given by the ventilator. This is termed gain. This gain amplifies the patient's tidal volume. The gain is set individually as flow proportional assist (to overcome the resistive workload) and volume proportional assist (to overcome the elastic workload). The final tidal volume is determined by the combination of the patient's effort and proportional assist ventilation (PAV) support (PS in Figure 8). There is no minimum support provided. Tidal volume can be large if the patient's efforts are more (P_{mus} in Figure 7) or less if the patient's efforts are less. This preserves the biological variability in respiration which is considered lung protective.

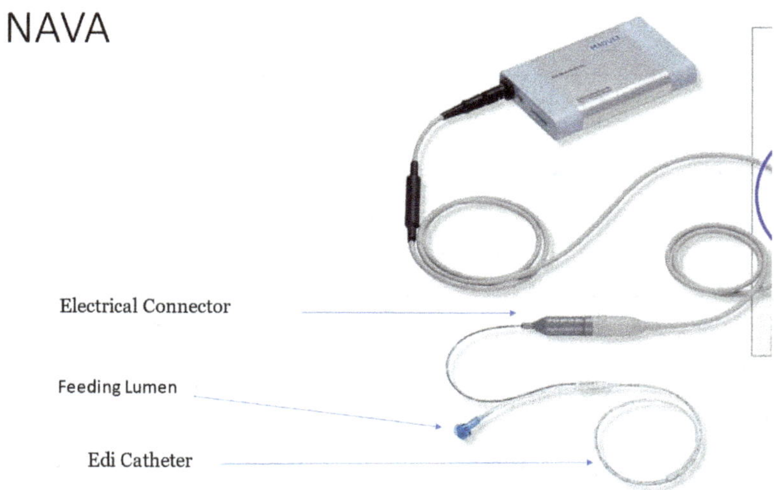

Figure 8: Parts of NAVA hardware. Image courtesy — Dr. Manu Verma, associate professor, Department of Critical Care Medicine, Dayananda Sagar Medical College.

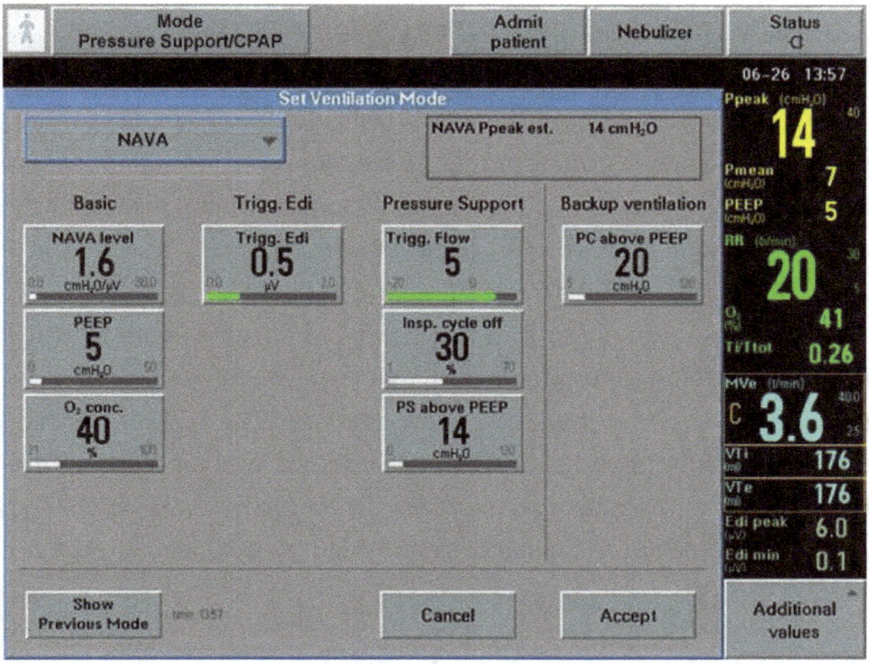

Figure 9: The user interface of a ventilator in NAVA mode. Image courtesy — Dr. Manu Verma, associate professor, Department of Critical Care Medicine, Dayananda Sagar Medical College.

Adaptive support ventilation

This mode has a PC-IMV breath sequence with an optimal targeting scheme. Here, the operator inputs the patient's weight from which the required alveolar ventilation is calculated (after deducting the anatomical dead space). Based on an equation by Otis et al, the required respiratory rate (RR) for which there is least work of breathing is calculated, and the machine sets the tidal volume also. Along with the above, the machine adjusts the required pressure to the varying lung mechanics of the patient in between breaths (similar to the PRVC mode). This mode of ventilation was designed to decrease the work of breathing, imitate natural breathing, and decrease the weaning time.

Neurally adjusted ventilatory assistance

This mode has a CSV breath sequence with an intelligent targeting scheme (uses artificial intelligence techniques). Unlike other modes, there is no targeted tidal volume or flow or minute ventilation, or pressure. It has an Edi catheter that detects electrical signals from the diaphragmatic activity of the patient and proportionally assists a patient's effort by a factor called neurally adjusted ventilatory assistance (NAVA) level.

NAVA is also available as a noninvasive ventilation mode and for neonatal ventilation. Advantages of NAVA over conventional modes are decreased periods of over-assist or under-assist, decreased patient–ventilator asynchrony, improved patient comfort, reduced need for sedation, and better quality of sleep. Recent studies have shown that NAVA can be used as a weaning mode for spontaneous breathing trials similar to pressure support modes.

Complications associated with invasive mechanical ventilation

Invasive mechanical ventilation is associated with infectious complications because it breaches the protection given by upper airway mucosal immunity, depressed ciliary action of trachea and bronchi, colonization of the endotracheal tube by pathogenic bacteria, and biofilm formation, microaspiration despite cuffed endotracheal tubes and chances of infection during suctioning.

Noninfectious complications are mainly due to positive pressure ventilation and its adverse effects. The injury due to excessive tidal volume (volutrauma), excess airway pressure (barotrauma), the release of inflammatory mediators (biotrauma), and repeated collapse (atelectrauma) together leads to ventilator-induced lung injury (VILI). Mechanical ventilation itself releases inflammatory mediators like myeloperoxidase, tumor necrosis factor-α, and interleukin-6, enhancing neutrophil infiltration and cellular response due to any infection. There is some evidence that even

Table 5: Summary of the complications due to invasive mechanical ventilation

Pulmonary complications	Extrapulmonary complications
Ventilator-induced lung injury (VILI)	Pressure sores due to sedation and paralysis
Ventilator-associated pneumonia (VAP)	Muscle atrophy
Pneumothorax	Raised intracranial pressure decreases cerebral venous drainage
Pneumomediastinum	Raised intra-abdominal pressure can cause decreased perfusion to all abdominal organs
Tracheal mucosal injury	Decreased venous return can cause decreased cardiac output
Tracheobronchial injury	Decreased coronary blood flow if cardiac output is decreased
Auto-PEEP	Increased risk of deep vein thrombosis
Aspiration pneumonia	Increased risk of pulmonary embolism
Sinusitis	Exacerbation of hypotension in the hypovolemic patient

24 hours of mechanical ventilation induces deconditioning in the diaphragm and respiratory muscles. There is also recent evidence showing ergotrauma due to the transfer of mechanical energy from the ventilator to the lung causing stress and strain-induced injury to the lung, especially in patients with ARDS. Asynchrony during mechanical ventilation can cause raised intracranial pressure, delayed weaning, and hyper- or hypoventilation. Unrecognized tube migration and a damaged cuff in a sedated patient can lead to hypoventilation.

Weaning/liberation from invasive mechanical ventilation

There are no rigid defined criteria for initiating weaning from mechanical ventilation. Generally, the patient should meet the following criteria to initiate weaning:

a. The underlying disease for which a patient was put on invasive mechanical ventilation should have been resolved.
b. There should be minimal or no requirements for vasopressors.
c. Oxygenation should be adequate (minimal requirement of PEEP and fraction of inspired oxygen).

Once these above basic criteria are met, there are well-defined indices of weaning to help the clinician to decide on successful extubation (rapid shallow breathing index, $P_{0.1}$, CROP index, integrated weaning index). However, extensive studies have not shown high specificity for any single weaning index so far, and hence, it remains a clinical decision. Nevertheless, there is evidence for the following:

1. Protocol-based weaning leads to favorable outcomes.
2. Spontaneous breathing trials on pressure support mode are superior to the SIMV mode.
3. Prolonging the duration of the spontaneous breathing trial from 30 to 120 minutes does not change outcomes.
4. Daily interruption in sedation and assessment for readiness to weaning leads to better outcomes.
5. Early tracheostomy reduces ventilator days and the length of stay in ICU.

Summary

Invasive mechanical ventilation is life-saving organ support. In-depth knowledge of ventilator functioning and interpretation of scalars helps in the understanding of a patient's lung mechanics at the bedside. Timely recognition and treatment of complications and timely weaning of the patient will lead to successful outcomes.

Clinical aspects of mechanical ventilation in acute respiratory failure

Acute respiratory failure manifests with the feature of hypoxemia and/or hypercapnia; the presence of either is determined to the well-being of the person. Clinically, hypoxia presents with tachypnea, dyspnea, pallor, and cyanosis in the patient who is restless, disoriented, and confused, and complaining of headache, lassitude, somnolence, blurred vision, patch of consolidation, show reaction time, impaired judgment and may have manic depression psychosis and coma. Hypercapnia is associated with tachypnea, dyspnea, vasodilation, tachycardia, hypertension, headache, hallucination, drowsiness, hypomania, sweating, and convulsions,

Mechanical ventilation may be required in acute respiratory failure in the following conditions:

Central nervous system disorders

Brain or brainstem lesions (hemorrhage, infarction, tumors, encephalitis)

Depression drugs (barbiturates, sedatives, anesthetics)

Pickwickian syndrome

Central sleep apnea syndrome

Inappropriate O_2 therapy

Neuromuscular disorders

Tetanus

Botulism

Myasthenia gravis

Guillain–Barre syndrome

Poliomyelitis

Muscular dystrophy

Drugs (curare, succinylcholine, insecticide poison, nerve gas)

Others

Pleural effusion, hemothorax, pneumothorax

Kyphoscoliosis, rib fracture, flat chest, chest wall deformity

Interstitial lung disease

Asthma, COPD, aspiration pneumonia

ARDS

Cardiopulmonary edema

Pulmonary thromboembolism

Postoperative complications

Asthma: Mechanical ventilation has absolute indication in asthma when the patient is unable to speak or gasping air (i.e., not cardiorespiratory arrest) or in cardiorespiratory arrest or in coma. Mechanical ventilation for severe asthma has reduced mortality to 6%–10%. If it should be utilized only for respiratory muscle fatigue, pCO_2 is rising and pO_2 is reducing. The narrow airways in asthma may result in very high peak airways pressure; thus, selection of mode of ventilation is important. Ventilator management strategies during positive pressure ventilation in acute severe asthma include selecting mode that provides initial substantial muscle unloading, minimizes dynamic hyperinflation (DHI), and attempts to keep airway pressure down to minimum. Use assisted controlled mode, both pressure- and volume-targeted modes are effective. Barotrauma has been found complicating status asthmaticus in 14%–27% of cases. Minimum effective dose of muscle relaxant will not contribute to difficulty in weaning. Bronchodilators can be delivered through ventilator circuits; in case of refractory bronchospasm, mixture of helium and O_2 can be used to reduce airways muscle tone. Median duration of 3 days of mechanical ventilation is sufficient. Gastrointestinal bleeding, venous thromboembolism, and sepsis are the potential complications. Other situations when mechanical ventilation is required are refractory hypoxemia, arterial $pH < 7.21$, and progressive hypercapnia despite bronchodilator therapy; endotracheal tube is contraindicated in patients with nasal polyp and sinusitis, but it is a good option for obese patients with short neck. A wide bore of >8 mm endotracheal tube can be introduced orally that allows suction as well as bronchoscopy. Sedation is needed for better compliance, decreases O_2 consumption, decreases CO_2 consumption, and minimizes barotraumas. A volume-cycled ventilator delivering as VT 4–6 mL/kg, or RR of 6–10 breaths/minute with maximum inspiratory pressure of <50 cm H_2O is usually recommended. Asthmatics are vulnerable to development of auto-PEEP or DHI, which can in turn produce hypotension and barotraumas exhaustion, and altered mental status. However, all patients with rising $PaCO_2$ level need not be intubated, as the majority will respond to conservative approaches.

Noninvasive mechanical ventilation involves using continuous positive airway pressure (CPAP at 5–7.5 cm H_2O, indicated in patients with hypercapnic ventilatory failure, not responding pharmacologically to treatment alone). Such patients can sedate well, irritation is decreased, and chances of infections in the hospital, such nosocomial pneumonia, sinusitis, and so forth, are decreased. Disadvantages include increased risk of aspiration of gastric contents, facial pressure necrosis, and lesser control of the patient's mechanical ventilation. Mechanical ventilation requires intubation through the nasal or oral route. Nasal route allows only a small bore (<7.5 mm). Noninvasive ventilation seems to have a role in selected cases of severe acute asthma not responding to optimal pharmacotherapy.

Case discussion

A: COPD

A 72-year-old man with h/o COPD was brought to casualty with complaints of severe shortness of breath. The patient is alert and oriented but shows signs of fatigue, speaking in halting sentences.

Vitals: PR: 134/minute, RR: 38/minute, BP: 180/100 mmHg, Height: 170 cm, Weight: 70 kg

SpO_2: 75%@RA, 80%–84%@5 L oxygen via mask

ABG: pH: 7.14, pCO_2: 97, pO_2: 42, HCO_3: 44

Patient was started on noninvasive ventilation: 10/6 cm of water, rate: 12/minute with FiO_2 titrated to maintain SpO_2 > 90%.

The patient was later shifted to ICU, and noninvasive ventilation continued for 4 hours. The patient is restless and tries to remove the mask;

finally intubated with ET tube number 8 and put on volume control mode.

Settings: tidal volume: 500 mL, rate: 24, PEEP: 8, FiO_2: 100%, PEFR: 60 L/minute, I:E — 1:2.2

Immediately post intubation, the patient developed hypotension.

1. What are the causes of hypotension in this patient?
   - Hypovolemia
   - Drug-induced (drug used while intubation)
   - Cardiac event — acute coronary syndrome
   - Dynamic hyperinflation

Dynamic hyperinflation

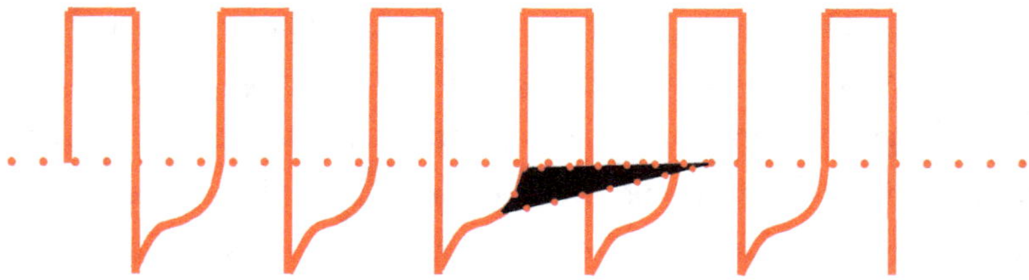

2. How do you manage the hypotension?
   - Fluid resuscitation
   - ECG, cardiac enzymes
   - Look at the mechanical ventilator graph to see auto-PEEP
3. How do you identify auto-PEEP?

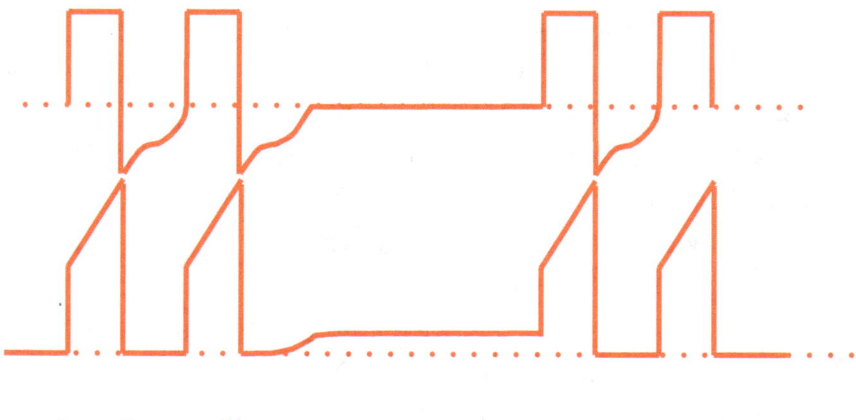

In flow-time scalar, peak inspiratory flow rate will be reduced, and expiratory flow will not touch the baseline, before it touches the baseline, another breath is triggered, so there is no complete exhalation. Some amount of air is trapped in each breath. If the patient is tachypneic, after sometime, the trapped amount of air will increase significantly which will in turn increase the intrathoracic pressure. This is called dynamic hyperinflation. This will be identified in a flow-time scalar easily.

4. What are the causes and consequences of auto-PEEP/DHI?
   - Auto-PEEP/DHI increases the intrathoracic pressure reducing venous return, RV output, and **LV cardiac output** causing hypotension.
   - In severe forms, if not recognized early, it may lead to bradycardia and cardiac arrest.
5. How do you measure auto-PEEP?
   - Auto-PEEP can be measured by applying end expiratory pause in deeply sedated and relaxed patients.
   - Look into pressure-time scalar, where the baseline pressure increases above PEEP. That is auto-PEEP.
   - In most of the ventilators, the auto-PEEP will be displayed on the monitor; some ventilators will display total PEEP, where we have to subtract extrinsic PEEP to get auto/intrinsic PEEP.
6. How do you treat auto-PEEP?
   - Auto-PEEP is mainly because of inadequate expiratory time.
   - It can be minimized or avoided by:
   - Reducing RR with adequate sedation and/or relaxation.
   - By increasing the peak inspiratory flow rate to reduce the inspiratory time.
   - By reducing the tidal volume.
7. In this patient, what ventilator setting should be changed?
   - Rate can reduced be to 12.
   - Tidal volume can be reduced to 400 mL.
   - Peak inspiratory flow rate increased from 60 to 80 L/minute.
   - I:E ratio 1:3.3
   - FiO_2 reduced to 60% to maintain SpO_2 88%–90%.

B: ARDS

A 24-year-old student found unresponsive at a party with vomitus in mouth was brought to casualty.

- Height: 168 cm, weight: 72 kgs
- Vitals: PR: 120/minute, RR: 12/minute, SpO_2: 84% at room air, 88%–90% with 5 L room air intubated in casualty with settings

mode-volume control	FiO_2:100%
tidal volume: 550 mL	I:E — 1:2.6
PEEP: 5 cm H_2O	Peak: 50 cm of H_2O
	Plateau: 48 cm of H_2O
	Investigations

- 2D-ECHO: normal
- CXR: B/L infiltrates
- ABG: pH: 7.38, pCO_2: 38, pO_2: 59, HCO_3: 23.1

1. How do you diagnose ARDS?
    - Acute onset: within 7 days of some defined event. It may be pneumonia, sepsis, or the patient's recognition of worsening of symptoms.
    - Bilateral opacities consistent with pulmonary edema must be present on CXR and CT thorax.
    - "Acute lung injury" no longer exists. Under the BERLIN ARDS definition, patients with PaO_2/FiO_2 200–300 would now have "mild ARDS."
    - There is no need to exclude heart failure; in the new ARDS criteria, patients with high pulmonary capillary wedge pressures or congestive heart failure with left atrial hypertension can still have ARDS.
2. What are the ventilator settings strategy in ventilator patient?
    - Protective lung ventilation with low tidal volume of 6 mL/kg of ideal body weight and plateau pressure less than 30 cm of H_2O has been shown to improve survival benefit.
    - Keep PEEP above the lower inflection point.

- Settings: tidal volume: 400 mL, rate: 20/minute (increased from 10 to maintain minute ventilation), PEEP: 8, FiO_2: 100%, I:E — 1:2.6

3. What is the role of PEEP in ARDS?

   It acts by

   - Recruitment of collapsed alveoli
   - Preventing atelectasis
   - Improving V/Q mismatch
   - Improving hypoxia
   - Improving V/Q mismatch
   - ARDS network trial alveoli study 2004, high PEEP versus low PEEP has not shown clinical outcome which emphasis on the identification of recruitable alveoli in ARDS patients. PEEP works better in a recruitable than a non-recruitable lung.
   - If the patient is having an identifiable lower inflection point in the PV loop which is usually seen in 20%–30% of patients, keeping PEEP 2 cm above the lower inflection point may help in atelectatic trauma and improves oxygenation. In rest of the patients where it is difficult to identify optimal PEEP, ARDS network trial tables can be used for the same.

4. How do you treat refractory hypoxia?

   - In spite of increasing FiO_2 and PEEP to the maximal level, if oxygenation is not improving, it is considered as refractory hypoxia; these patients should be considered for early proning with longer duration which has shown to increase survival benefits in such patients.

5. What are the precautions to be taken during proning?

   - Proning should be considered if health care workers are familiar with the procedure.
   - Patient should be hemodynamically stable.
   - Adequate sedation of the patient.
   - Check the endotracheal tube and all other lines.
   - Suctioning prior to proning.
   - Coordination between team members.

- Hyperoxygenation with 100% oxygen.
- Moving the patient to one side of the bed and tilting to the other side.
- Monitor vital signs.
- Pillow should be placed on each side of the chest and forehead for the endotracheal tube to not be compressed.

6. In spite of proning abg showing hypoxia what next?
   - ECMO

C: Head injury

A 34-year-old man is admitted to casualty after an RTA, unconscious on admission, no fractures to his head, neck, thorax, and limbs.

Admission: Vitals: BP: 180/90 mmHg, HR: 124/minute, RR: 14/minute, afebrile, height: 160 cm, weight: 60 kg

RS: B/L AE+, clear

Patient withdraws limbs to painful stimuli.

Pupils respond unequally to light.

E1M3V1

Patient intubated to keep his airway patent in the emergency department.

Ventilator settings

Volume control mode FiO_2: 100%, PEEP: 5 cm of water, rate: 15/minute

Tidal volume: 480 mL

ABG after 30 minutes of initial setting

pH: 7.28, pCO_2: 50, pO_2: 145, HCO_3: 18

1. What are the initial ventilator strategy in this head injury patient and why?
   - In this patient, it appears is having traumatic brain injury with increased intracranial pressure and coming. Our goal is to minimize increase and reduce the intracranial pressure.
   - So avoiding hypercapnia is priority as it may cause cerebral vasodilation and increased intracranial pressure.

- As in this patient pCO_2 is 50 rate is increased to maintain pCO_2 between 35 and 45.

2. What is the role of prophylactic hyperventilation?
   - In earlier days, prophylactic hyperventilation was done to reduce pCO_2 in turn causing cerebral vasoconstriction and decrease in the intracranial pressure, but later, it was found that a significant drop in pCO_2 causes intense vasoconstriction aggravating cerebral ischemia causing more damage, so prophylactic hyperventilation is not done.
   - It is done only in rare cases as the patient is coning and about to shift to OT for craniotomy for a brief period.
   - So it is always better to maintain normocapnia to avoid cerebral vasoconstriction.
3. What are other causes that may increase the intracranial pressure in such patients?
   - Restlessness and irritability — the patient to be kept calm by sedation and/or relaxation
   - Inadequate analgesia
   - Positioning of the patient — the patient to be kept in neutral posture avoiding extreme lateral position which hampers the drainage of venous return from the brain
   - Full bladder which causes pain
4. What is the effect of the PEEP on intracranial pressure?
   - Modest PEEP less than 10 cm of H_2O will rarely affect the intracranial pressure.
   - Animal studies have not proven high PEEP causing increased intracranial pressure, but still if higher PEEP levels are required, monitoring intracranial pressure is a better option.
   - Elevating the head end of the bed and maintaining euvolemic will reduce PEEP effect on the intracranial pressure.

References and suggested readings

1. Sindhwani G, Rawat J. Ventilator dependence-role of nutrition and airway clearance therapy. Lung India. 2006;23:39–41.
2. Troche G, Moine P. Is the duration of mechanical ventilation predictable? Chest. 1997;112:745–751.
3. Hira HS, Mittal A. Evaluation of the predictors or duration of mechanical ventilation in respiratory intensive care unit. Lung India. 2006;23:70–74.
4. Bhasin A. ABG analysis for physicians. Med Update; API. 2016;26:1600–1604.
5. Rippe JM. Mechanical ventilation. IN: Manual of intensive care medicine. 1989:P60–P80.
6. Arulraj S. Mechanical ventilation-mechanical 300. IN: YP Munjal, ed. Med Update; API. 1997;7:787–793.
7. Antonelli M, et al. A comparison of NIPPU and COMENTIONAL mechanical ventilation in patient with ARF. New Engl J Med. 1998;339:429.
8. Bandovin SV. Ventilator associated pneumonia. Thrax. 2001;56:500.
9. Fajon JY, et al. Ventilator associated pneumonia. Ann Intern Med. 2000;132:621.
10. Bhatia RS. Challenges in the management of nosocomial pneumonia. IN: MM Singh, ed. Med Update; API. 1999;9:377–382.
11. Hayon J, et al. Role of serial routine microbiologic culture results in the management of ventilator associated pneumonia. AJRCCM. 2002;165:115.
12. Scneihora DJ, et al. Weaning from prolonged mechanical ventilation. Chest. 1994;105:534–539.
13. Prayag S. Ventilator support. IN: LA Pathak, ed. PG Med; API. 2004;18: 94–100.
14. Jain CK. Ventilator associated pneumonia. IN: SR Joshi, ed. Med Update; API. 2014;24:606–613.
15. Kollef MH. What is ventilator associated pneumonia and why is it important? Respir Care. 2005;50:714–721.
16. Ambrosino N, Gabbrielli L. The difficulty to wean patient. Expert Rev Respir Med. 2010;4:685–692.
17. Lim ZJ, Subramaniam A, Ponnapa Reddy M, Blecher G, Kadam U, Afroz A, Billah B, Ashwin S, Kubicki M, Bilotta F, Curtis JR, Rubulotta F. Case fatality rates for patients with COVID-19 requiring invasive mechanical ventilation. A meta-analysis. Am J Respir Crit Care Med. 2021 Jan 1;203(1):54–66.

18. Lai CC, Yu WL. COVID-19 associated with pulmonary aspergillosis: a literature review. J Microbiol Immunol Infect. 2021 Feb;54(1):46–53.
19. MacLeod M, Papi A, Contoli M. Chronic obstructive pulmonary disease exacerbation fundamentals: diagnosis, treatment, prevention and disease impact. Respirology. 2021 Jun;26(6):532–551.
20. Fainardi V, Abelli L, Muscarà M, Pisi G, Principi N, Esposito S. Update on the role of high-flow nasal cannula in infants with bronchiolitis. Children (Basel). 2021 Jan 20;8(2):66.
21. Lin HL, Fink JB, Ge H. Aerosol delivery via invasive ventilation: a narrative review. Ann Transl Med. 2021 Apr;9(7):588.

https://doi.org/10.1142/9789811271410_0038

38 Interstitial lung diseases

Abstract

Interstitial lung disease, also called diffuse parenchymal lung disease, is actually a group of disorders that involves the distal lung parenchyma and was earlier classified into four main groups. There are more than 250 lung disorders with interstitial involvement and with similar clinicoradiological manifestations.[1] Hamman and Rich described diffuse parenchymal lung fibrosis as early as in 1944.[2] The term idiopathic interstitial pneumonia in Japan was also called idiopathic pulmonary fibrosis (IPF) in the United States and cryptogenic fibrosing alveolitis (CFA) in the United Kingdom, and the earlier classification by Leibow and Carsington, Katzenstein and Muller, and Colby[3–5] has been revised as the new classification proposed by the American Thoracic Society and the European Respiratory Society, describing seven histological patterns: But for histological pattern of usual interstitial pneumonia which is reserved for idiopathic intestinal pneumonia or CFA. IPF is considered as a distinctive type of chronic fibrosing interstitial pneumonia of unknown cause, limited to the lungs, and rest of the varieties are considered as separate entities.[6]

Introduction[7]

Interstitial lung disease (ILD) is a diffuse parenchymal lung disease involving the distal lung parenchyma and is a heterogeneous group of noninfectious and nonmalignant disorders of the lower respiratory tract. There is a resultant restrictive ventilatory impairment, diffuse interstitial opacities, granulomatous or interstitial inflammation, and fibrosis which is often

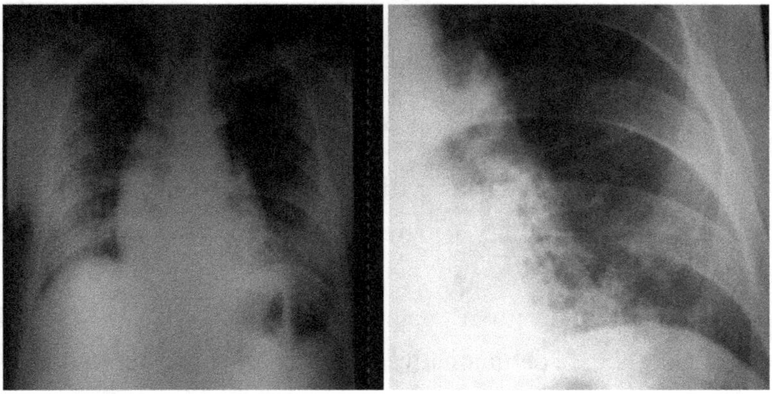

Figure 1: Early ILD with bilateral reticulonodular opacities and close-up view.

progressive and fatal. Idiopathic interstitial pneumonia is the most common variety, involving varying combinations of fibrosis and inflammation in lung parenchyma in contrast to the airspace disease typically seen in bacterial pneumonia where the etiology is known, such as drug induced, occupational, environmental, and systemic disorders like sarcoid or pulmonary hemorrhage or vasculitis or connective tissue disease. All these cause injuries that lead to lung fibrosis which can lead to progressive end-stage fibrosis called the honeycomb lung.

Etiopathogenesis[8–11]: Disorders such as idiopathic interstitial pneumonia, sarcoidosis, hypersensitivity pneumonitis, eosinophilic granuloma, silicosis, asbestosis, drug-induced pneumopathy, pulmonary edema, miliary TB, lymphangitis carcinomatosis, and tropical eosinophilia form almost 85.90 of diagnosis of ILDs. Prevalence of IPF is 13–20/100,000 in the United States, and the disease onset is usually between 50 and 70 years. Seven potential causes and categories of ILDs have been described:

1. Organic inhalation: animal/bird antigen, farm antigen; inorganic inhalation: silica, asbestos, beryllium.
2. Drug: anti-inflammatory, antibiotics, antiarrhythmics, antidepressants, anticancer (chemotherapy), radiation, and oxygen.

3. Infection: TB, PCP, atypical pneumonia, HIV infection.
4. Malignancy: lymphangitic carcinomatosis, bronchoalveolar cell carcinoma.
5. Connective tissue disorder: systemic lupus erythematosus (SLE), RA, mixed connective tissue disease, scleroderma, polymyositis/dermatomyositis, primary Sjogren's syndrome, Behcet's syndrome, ankylosing spondylitis.
6. Idiopathic: usual interstitial pneumonia (UIP), nonspecific interstitial pneumonia (NSIP), desquamative interstitial pneumonia (DIP), respiratory bronchiolitis-ILD (RB-ILD), lymphoid interstitial pneumonia (LIP), 1300P, acute interstitial pneumonia, eosinophilic granuloma, sarcoidosis lymphangioleiomyomatosis.

Histological patterns as proposed by the American Thoracic Society (ATS)/EF5 are UIP, NSIP, organizing pneumonia (OP), diffuse alveolar damage (DAD), RB, DIP, and LIP. The term UIP is reserved for those cases in which the lesion is idiopathic and is currently called as idiopathic pulmonary fibrosis (IPF) or cryptogenic fibrosing alveolitis (CFA). IPF or CFA, thus, is a distinctive variety of chronic fibrosing interstitial pneumonia of unknown cause, limited to the lungs, with a histological pattern of UIP. The rest six varieties are separate entities and need not be included in the group of patients with IPF.

Lung involvement in SLE and value of high-resolution computed tomography

Introduction

Indian studies reveal the prevalence of SLE as 3.2/100,000, with a predominance of the infection in females. Thus, complex, multifactorial, multisystem disorder has variable incidence of distinct pulmonary manifestation in 30%–60% of SLE patients having direct or consequential involvement from the disease affecting other organ systems. Awareness of lung infection and the pattern of the disease would help early detection of the disease and influence the therapeutic strategies as well. Serum ferritin levels offer an excellent marker of SLE with hematological manifestations.

Pulmonary manifestations

Cough, chest pain, and exertional dyspnea are the common presenting features of the respiratory system infection clinically affecting in less than one-fourth number of cases. Clinical examination may detect suspected abnormalities in one-sixth number of cases. Only 20% of cases show radiological abnormality on a plain chest X-ray in the form of reticular opacity, atelectasis, or pleural effusion. Pulmonary function tests (PFTs) may reveal restrictive patterns in one-fourth number of cases.

High-resolution computed tomography (HRCT) provides diagnostic yield in more than 50% of cases which is likely to increase with the increasing duration of the disease. Pleural infection may be accompanying in almost 20% of cases, although pathological pleural involvement has been documented in more than three-fourth number of cases at autopsy. HRCT reveals the diagnosis of ILD in more than one-third of cases, and ground-glass pacification can be observed in more than one-fourth of cases.

HRCT findings are thickened interlobular septa, parenchymal bonds, and ground-glass opacification, most of which suggest ILD.

Comments

HRCT is a useful diagnostic test for assessing lung involvement in SLE, which can help in clinching early diagnosis to evolve management strategies, even in asymptomatic cases, having normal chest X-ray and PFTs. Definite HRCT abnormalities may be observed in nearly half the number of cases, where more than one-fourth of cases have features of ILD. Pleural infection may be accompanying in less than 20% of cases.

Histopathology[6,2,12–14]

UIP: This has insidious onset, slow progress, marked fibrosis, and poor progression. There is a patchy involvement with areas of marked fibrosis and areas of less fibrosis and more inflammation, often progressive to the end-stage disease — honeycombing of the lung. Subpleural I and paraseptal areas are more affected, showing alternating areas of normal tissue interstitial inflammation, fibrosis, and honeycombing. The interstitial inflammation occurs in the form of alveolar septal infiltrate of lymphocytes, plasma cells, and histiocytes, associated with hyperplasia of type 2 pneumocytes. Areas of honeycomb and fibrosis show smooth muscle hyperplasia.

NSIP (in HIV disease): Suggested by Katzenstein and Fiorelli[13] in 1944, it occurs in HIV disease when the CD4 cell count is still preserved. Its incidence in AIDS patients is 4.6%–38%, more so in Africa where the incidence of PCP is low.

Patients present with cough, fatigue, breathlessness, and in some of cases with weight loss. Clinically, lymph nodes of axilla and groins may be palpable. Chest auscultation may reveal bilateral basal crepitations and widespread inspiratory rhonchi. Routine investigations may show low Hb and raised ESR. Serum hypoalbuminemia maybe observed. Blood test for HIV is positive, and CD4 cell count is decreased but not less than 200 cells/cu mm. Chest X-ray may be normal. HRCT may reveal diffuse ground-glass alternation with few reticulonodular infiltration.

PFTs show a restrictive ventilatory defect. Arterial blood gas analysis may reveal mild hypoxemia. Bronchoscopy may be normal, bronchoalveolar lavage (BAL) may reveal predominant lymphocytes, and transbronchial biopsy shows reduced alveolar spaces, with thickened septae and presence of lymphocytes and plasma cells in interstitial tissue with areas of fibrosis and alveolar pneumocytic hyperplasia. Absence of granuloma, *Pneumocystis carinii*, inclusion body, or tumor favors the diagnosis of NSIP in HIV disease. Spontaneous resolution or responding to corticosteroids along with HAART shows its better prognosis as compared to other ILDs such as DIP and UIP.

OP: This is characterized by intraluminal OP in the distal airspaces such as bronchioles, alveolar duct, and alveoli. Mild patchy interstitial inflammation with preserved lung architecture is observed. The same was earlier referred to as BOOR.

NSIP: This is characterized by uniform lymphocytic interstitial inflammation with rare plasma cells. Cellular pattern has mild to moderate chronic inflammation with type 2 pneumocyte hyperplasia, while fibrosing pattern has loose or dense fibrosis that lacks the temporal patchy feature of UIP. Hematoxylin and eosin staining shows loss of lung architecture, but elastic strains are kept preserved. Differential diagnosis includes NSIP in HIV disease which simulates *P. carinii* pneumonia in presentation, but diagnosis is by exclusion and by histological pattern which is different from classical ILD. What is most important is the better prognosis as compared to other.

RB-ILD: This is commonly seen in smokers. Focal bronchiolar–alveolar and pigmented macrophages accumulation is observed, mostly in first- and second-order bronchioles. Chronic inflammation and mild bronchiolar fibrosis are also present. Minor small airway dying functioning is present. Patients are rarely symptomatic. DIP has been suggested to be an extensive form of RB-ILD.

DIP: Uniform distribution of nonpigmented macrophages in the alveoli along with mild interstitial fibrosis is observed. Because of similar pathology and association with smoking, both active and passive, it is considered to be an extensive form of RB-ILD.

LIP: There is prominent alveolar septa distribution of interstitial infiltration of T-lymphocytes, grouped into germinal centers.

Acute interstitial pneumonia (AIP): This is a rarely fulminant form of lung injury, originally described as Hamman–Rich syndrome, which has acute presentation in a previously healthy person. The DAD is indistinguishable from acute respiratory distress syndrome (ARDS) caused by sepsis and shock. The term AIP is reserved for cases of unknown etiology.

Histological pattern reveals exudation and proliferation, and for fibrotic phases of DAD, along with the presence of focal or diffuse hyaline membrane, an airspace organization, diffuse or patchy, may be seen.

Comparison of histopathologic features of chronic idiopathic interstitial pneumonia

	UIP	NSIP	OP	RB-ILD	DIP	LIP
Temporal appearance	Variegated	Uniform	Uniform	Uniform	Uniform	Uniform
Spatial appearance Patchy		Uniform	Patchy	Patchy	Uniform	Patchy
Interstitial inflammation	Scanty	Prominent	Mild	Mild	Moderate	Alveolar septal cells
Collagen deposition		Variable	Occasional	Variable	Rare	Rare
Fibrosis	Present	Patchy	Diffuse		Peribronchial	
Fibroblast proliferation	Prominent	Rare	No diffuse	No	No	No
Organizing pneumonia	No	Variable	Yes	No	No	No
Microscopic honeycombing	Yes	Rare	Rare	No	No	No
Macrophage accumulation	Variable	Variable	No	Peribronchial	Alveolar Nonpigmented	No

Comparative pathological features of chronic idiopathic interstitial pneumonia are shown in the table. A small subgroup of patients with interstitial pneumonia still remains unclassified even after this exhaustive clinicoradiological cum pathological evaluation.[6]

Two major histological patterns of diffuse lung parenchymal disease are granulomatous process and interstitial inflammation and fibrosis. Granulomatous process can be seen in sarcoidosis, hypersensitive pneumonitis (organic dusts), berylliosis and silicosis (inorganic dust), and vascular vasculitides such as Wegener's granulomatosis and Churg–Strauss syndrome. Interstitial inflammation and fibrosis is commonly seen in drug-induced (chemotherapy) pulmonary radiation.

CD4 and CD25 lymphocytopenia can be used as reliable, sensitive, and valid markers for activity of disease and in its follow-up in SLE during disease flares.

Limited physical activity in RA as well as drug therapy impairs bone mineral density, causing osteopenia and osteoporosis, especially in early active, erosive disease. So, bone mineral density test can be a useful marker.

Chest CT is useful for diagnosing lung lesions; MRCT scan can differentiate ILDs from alveolar lesions.

Head cheese sign is the commonest appearance in hypersensitivity pneumonitis, due to prolonged exposure to an allergen such as jute, fiber, or wool. Fluffy opacities on both lung fields on chest X-ray would show on thorax HRCT, a heterogenous appearance of low, normal, and high attenuated regions called head cheese sign. Tuiz can also be present in atypical lung infections with bronchiolitis or sarcoidosis.

Pirfenidone is effective only in early stage and not of use in advanced disease.

lung effects, inorganic drugs such as asbestos, fumes, gases, collagen vascular disease, pulmonary hemorrhage syndrome, lymphocytes infiltration disorders, eosinophilic pneumonia, inherited disease such a tumors sclerosis and idiopathic interstitial pneumonia like UIP, DIP, NSIP, BOOP.[14]

Clinical presentation[13]

This is always nonspecific and consists of progressive exertion dyspnea, nonproductive paroxysmal coughing, and fine, dry, and inspiratory crackles in the lower chest. If the symptoms are of few weeks to months, consider the probability of sarcoidosis, drug-induced lung disease, alveolar hemorrhage syndrome, or connective tissue disease. If the symptoms are chronic, that is, few months to years, consider the probability of sarcoidosis, IPF, or pulmonary histiocytosis. If the chest examination reveals basal fine crackles, it is more in favor of inflammatory disease and rarely in favor of granulomatous lung disease. Often signs of systemic disorders may give a diagnostic clue such as arthritis in rheumatoid arthritis (RA) and skin changes in scleroderma. With the progression of the disease, signs such clubbing and cor pulmonale may be seen.

Investigations (1S-20)

Antineutrophilic cytoplasmic antibody is useful in Wegener's disease or vasculitis. Similarly, ANA, RA factor, ACE may be value in collagen disease and sarcoidosis (may be nonspecific). PFTs predominately show a restrictive pattern. The flow of all lung volumes is markedly increased. Diffusing capacity is reduced due to loss of functioning alveolar capillary units. Lung compliance is reduced due to lung stiffness; very low levels of TLCO (<40%) point toward pulmonary hypertension. Arterial gas analysis shows that partial pressure of arterial oxygen is decreased, and alveo-arenagraient is increased. Chest X-ray shows bilateral lower zone nodular or reticular opacities or honeycombing. Thus, on a plain chest X-ray, ILDs can be recognized as well as characterized[15,16] The characterization is done on the basis of pattern of the interstitial disease, where nodular lesions are mainly seen in miliary TB, silicosis, miliary metastases, and sarcoidosis. The rest of the diseases have reticulonodular or reticular appearance. Second, distribution of the disease gives a diagnostic clue, such as central distribution is observed in sarcoidosis, pulmonary edema, and lymphangitis carcinomatosis, while the rest of the diseases have peripheral distribution.

Similarly, if the upper zones are involved, differential diagnosis tilts toward TB, silicosis, eosinophilic granuloma, end-stage hypersensitivity pneumonitis, and ankylosing spondylitis, while other ILDs have mid or lower zone involvement. If the lung volume is increased or near normal, sarcoidosis, eosinophilic granuloma, or lymphangioleiomyomatosis can be considered, while lung volumes are reduced in the rest of ILDs. Accompanying lymphadenopathy brings diagnostic differential in favor of TB, sarcoidosis, silicosis, berylliosis, lymphoma, and metastasis. Similarly, accompanying other features also give diagnostic clue, for example, pleural effusion in RA and lymphoma, pericardial effusion in scleroderma, pneumothorax in eosinophilic granuloma, and lymphangioleiomyomatosis and arthritis in RA and scleroderma.

CT scan shows bilateral, subpleural reticular opacities or honeycombing, mainly in the lower zones. Ground-glass opacities are suggestive of alveolitis and mostly favor NSIP. RCT confirms the presence or absence of ILDs. Also, it differentiates emphysema which presents with restrictive lung disease pattern on PFTs.[17–19] Diagnostic accuracy of the tune of 70% is achieved by HRCT, especially in cystic lung disease and in idiopathic interstitial pneumonias, where various varieties of the latter can also be differentiated. HRCT also helps in evaluation of therapy. It can reliably guide localization of the segment for lung biopsy. HRCT signs that offer diagnostic clues include septal thickening of the interlobular septa, resulting in septal lines that occur usually in interstitial pneumonia, asbestosis, lymphangitis, alveolar proteinosis, and pulmonary edema.

Nodular pattern is seen in metastases, sarcoidosis, TB, lymphangitis, silicosis, eosinophilic granuloma, and hypersensitivity pneumonitis. Random distribution of nodules favors the diagnosis of miliary TB, while distribution along the bronchovascular bundles favors the diagnosis of sarcoidosis. Cystic lesions may rarely be seen outpost of end-stage disease due to intra-alveolar cystic degeneration may be in lymphangioleiomyomatosis and eosinophilic granuloma. Ground-glass attenuation signifies the presence of acute stage or alveolitis. Central distribution is better appreciated by HRCT as compared to the plain X-ray. Transbronchial or thoracoscopic lung biopsy may be useful diagnostically, especially when CT shows ground-glass opacity or airspace consolidation. Diagnostic value of transbronchial lung biopsy is very appreciable in diseases such as sarcoidosis, alveolar proteomics, lymphatic carcinomatosis, bronchoalveolar carcinoma, berylliosis, and eosinophilic pneumonia. It can be of some diagnostic utility in few disorders such as eosinophilic granuloma, hypersensitivity pneumonitis, amyloidosis, pulmonary lymphoma, lymphocytic interstitial pneumonia, Wegener's granulomatosis, and BOOP. Nevertheless, this is not useful in IPF.

HRCT and ILD

Introduction

HRCT is one of the most sensitive tool for noninvasive imaging of the lung, pleura, and of abnormalities on the chest radiographs that may ultimately prove to be nonspecific but similar number of cases having normal chest radiographs that have been detected by HRCT to been having diffuse parenchymal lung disease, ultimately histological proved.

HRCT utilized thin collimation and image reconstruction with spatial frequency algorithm. The technique consists of narrow 1–2 mm collimation scans and narrow field of vision of 20–25 mm. HRCT gives a detailed image of the lung with characteristics pattern, and thus, an optimal site for lung biopsy can be determined. Apart from its use in studying the lungs for bronchial abnormalities, interstitial fibrosis, miliary disease, or emphysema, its diagnostic role in diffuse lung disease has made the need of conventional CT almost obsolete.

Common indications

a. To evaluate unexplained pulmonary function abnormalities, in the presence of normal chest radiographs, especially in the situations like chronic dyspnea and hemoptysis.
b. To determine the presence and extent of parenchymal disease.
c. To assess the disease activity and response to therapy.
d. To assess the requirement and optimal site of biopsy. Four different types of findings observed in different lung disorders are classified as follows:

   1. Reticular opacities
   2. Nodular opacities
   3. Increased lung opacities
   4. Decreased lung opacities

There can be homogenous or ground-glass opacity without obscuring the underlying vessels. Ground-glass opacity is a nonspecific finding seen in an acute and active process such as pulmonary edema, alveolitis, hypersensitive pneumonitis, lymphocytic interstitial pneumonitis, active IPF, alveolar proteinosis, pneumonia, and sarcoidosis.

HRCT: Activity of the disease and pulmonary disorders

In IPF, HRCT can demonstrate the foci of active alveolitis, which are therapeutically responding to corticosteroid therapy. Similarly, activity of the disease can be correlated in sarcoidosis on HRCT.

In a short study in SLE patients, HRCT demonstrated abnormalities (in the form of ILD and bronchiectasis) in 70% of cases, compared to only 24% abnormalities observed on plain chest radiography and 41% abnormalities detected on pulmonary function testing. Diagnostic clues offered by HRCT include septal thickening as in interstitial pneumonia, asbestosis, lymphangitis, alveolar proteinosis, and pulmonary edema.

Cystic appearance may be seen in as a part of end stage due to intra-alveolar degeneration in lymphangioleiomyomatosis and eosinophilic granuloma.

Chest findings suggestive of active TB by HRCT are given below:

1. Centrilobular nodule with branching linear structures.
2. Tree-in-bud appearance — a form of bronchiolar impaction with branching linear structures having more than one contiguous branching site.
3. Cavitary nodules/consolidation.
4. 5–8 mm diameter poorly defined nodules.
5. Bronchial wall thickness with or without bronchiectasis.
6. Lobar consolidation with thickening of inter lobular septae.

HRCT offers >70% of diagnosis of primary or secondary spontaneous pneumothorax, and COPD is found as a major frequent abnormality in secondary spontaneous pneumothorax. It detects the emphysema as well as gives valuable information regarding the extent and nature of the underlying disease.

In fibrosing alveolitis or interstitial pulmonary fibrosis (IPF), the crescentic subpleural distribution, mostly concentrated in the posterobasal segment, is virtually pathognomonic on HRCT. In the later stage of IPF, a course reticular pattern followed by honeycombing results in giving a nonspecific appearance.

Active alveolitis — a feature of hypersensitivity pneumonitis — gives nodular and ground-glass opacification predominantly affecting the midzone with relative sparing of bases and apices.

In lymphocytic interstitial pneumonitis, often associated with HIV infection, Sjogren's syndrome, and hypogammaglobulinemia, bilateral patchy ground-glass opacification may be demonstrated on HRCT.

Peribronchial nodules and airspace consolidation on HRCT may yield the diagnosis of bronchogenic tuberculosis. Similar picture may be obtained in BOOP and chronic eosinophilic pneumonia. HRCT has greater sensitivity in yielding the diagnosis of bronchiectasis and reduces the risk of radiation. It reveals bronchial dilation with translucencies like signet ring shape. There is loss of tapering bronchus. In sarcoidosis, HRCT reveals nodules, ground-glass opacification, consolidation with hilar adenopathy, especially in the upper and mid lung zone. And in the advanced stage, irreversible changes like fibrocystic lesions, bullae, bronchiectasis, and cavities may be seen.

HRCT can demonstrate pulmonary complications in ulcerative colitis, both due to colitis or due to sulfasalazine therapy, as well as bronchial abnormalities and extensive steroid response alveolitis.

HRCT can be of diagnostic value in diffuse infiltrative lung disease "mimics" such as cystic bronchiectasis, constrictive bronchiolitis, respiratory bronchiolitis, histiocytosis, tuberous sclerosis, and lymphangioleiomyomatosis. The common HRCT appearance in various ILDs are presented in the following table.

Types	CT appearance
Usual interstitial pneumonia (UIP)	Honeycomb appearance Subpleural Basal predominance
Nonspecific interstitial pneumonia (NSIP)	Ground-glass appearance
Acute interstitial pneumonia (AIP)	Ground-glass opacities which appear rapid, diffuse damage seen
Desquamative interstitial pneumonia (respiratory bronchiolitis-ILD)	Ground-glass opacities with slight upper zone predominance
Lymphoid interstitial pneumonia	Diffuse infiltration of the interstitium and alveolar spaces (associated with HIV and Sjogren's)

HRCT and lung biopsy

It is useful in selecting the site for transbronchial biopsy. In certain situations like IPF, hypersensitivity pneumonitis, pneumoconiosis, lymphangitic carcinomatosis, and sarcoidosis, HRCT has obviated the need for biopsy, although biopsy remains the only definitive diagnostic means in chronic ILD. At the same time, the presence of emphysematous or bronchiectatic changes in HRCT does not require further histologic confirmation gives rise to an increase in reticular lung opacities in HRCT. The thickened interlocular septa are abnormal findings. These thickened septa are smooth in pulmonary edema, nodular in sarcoidosis, smooth, nodular, and beaded in lymphangitis and carcinomatosis, and irregular in interstitial fibrosis.

There can be peribronchovascular interstitial thickening due to fibrosis, infiltration, or due to bronchiolar abnormalities such as dilatation or wall thickening. Such a centrilobular abnormality in the form of "airspace

Table 1: HRCT findings in various pulmonary disorders

A. Reticular opacities Pulmonary edema Sarcoidosis Coal workers' pneumoconiosis Lymphangitis carcinomatosis Interstitial fibrosis Asbestosis Silicosis Allergic alveolitis Histiocytosis X
B. Nodular opacities Sarcoidosis, silicosis, coal workers' pneumoconiosis, tuberculosis, metastatic tumors, histiocytosis X, lobar pneumonia, pulmonary edema, transbronchial tuberculosis, organizing pneumonia, bronchiolitis obliterans
C. Increased normal lung architecture Acute pulmonary edema Alveolitis Desquamative interstitial fibrosis Active idiopathic pulmonary fibrosis Alveolar allergic alveolitis pneumonia Sarcoidosis
D. Decreased lung opacities Honeycomb lung lesions — a predictor of poor prognosis Emphysema Lung cysts

nodule" or ground-glass opacity may be visible in sarcoidosis, pulmonary edema, and allergic alveolitis. Lobule architecture is maintained in edema and infiltrated and distorted in fibrosis. Extensive fibrosis with destruction of lung tissue results in honeycombing and gives a cystic reticular appearance on HRCT.

Open lung biopsy is the gold standard test for diagnosing ILDs in more than 90% of cases. It is indicated only histological pattern influence the treatment regimen or HRCT is suggestive of an active disease. However, it is contraindicated in patients with serious pulmonary or cardiovascular comorbidity, or honeycombing with diffuse end-stage disease. Open biopsy is undertaken when all other diagnostic procedures have been exhausted. But definitely, it can clinch the diagnosis of a treatable pulmonary disease much as BOOP, sarcoidosis, and hypersensitivity pneumonitis, and it can rule out neoplastic/infectious disorders mimicking ILDs and even early definitive diagnosis of ILDs so as to plan lung transplantation.[20]

Management[21–24]

Treatment of ILDs involves treating the systemic cause or removing the offending agent if any. Supportive treatment and anti-inflammatory drugs are used. Oral prednisolone can be given as 0.5 mg/kg/day for 4–6 weeks, followed by gradually tapering down to half the dose on alternate day. Oral azathioprine or cyclophosphamide can be started as 2 mg/kg/day, starting with 25–50 mg/day, increasing 25 mg every week or 10 days until maximum of 100–150 mg/day is reached or results are obtained. Adverse effects of these drugs must be kept in mind. Newer drugs such as acetylcysteine, pirfenidone, relaxin, and interferon beta and gamma are being tried.[20,21] Doxycycline as an MMPS inhibitor can be used for at least up to 2 years in treating IPF.[22] Both single and double lung transplantation[23,24] has been indicated on ILDs in cases where PaO_2 is <55 mmHg. To provide management of pulmonary hypertension and right-sided heart failure. Futurology: FDA has approved nintedanib and pirfenidone for patients of IPF. Nintedanib is not given for patients with severe liver problems and in pregnancy. Pirfenidone has immunosuppressant action on fibroblast proliferation, reducing the production of fibrosis. Current guidelines address many issues which were not addressed in 2011 IPF guidelines, especially regarding strong recommendations not to use agents like warfarin and prednisolone in combination with azathioprine, acetylcysteine, ambrisentan, and nintedanib and also regarding single v/s double lung transplantation.[7]

Conclusion

The histological pattern of UIP is reserved for idiopathic interstitial pneumonia or CFA. IPF or CFA is a distinctive type of chronic fibrosing interstitial pneumonia of unknown etiology, limited to the lungs, in which lung biopsy shows a histological pattern of UIP. The rest of the patterns proposed by ATS and European Respiratory Society (ERS) are considered separate entities.[6,25] IPF is a chronic fibrosing ILD, affecting older adults. The recent international guidelines give a weak recommendation for the use of corticosteroids in patients during periods of acute exacerbations of IPF.

References and suggested readings

1. Park IN, Jegal Y, Kim DS, et al. Clinical course and lung function change of idiopathic nonspecific interstitial pneumonia. Eur Respir J. 2009;33(1):68–76.
2. Im JG, et al. Pulmonary TB: CT findings-early active disease and sequential change with anti TB therapy. Radiology. 1993;186–653.
3. Koyama M, et al. Chronic cystic lung disease-diagnostic accuracy of HRCT in 92 patients. AJR. 2003;180:827–835.
4. Wittram C, et al. CT histologic correlation of ATS-ERS 2002 classification of idiopathic interstitial pneumonias. Radiographics. 2003;23:1057–1071.
5. Kant S, Bhatia RS. ILDS. Lucknow: JB Foundation. 2015.
6. Kakati S, et al. Pulmonary manifestations in SLE with special reference to HRCT. JAPI. 2007;55:839–841.
7. Malaviya AN, et al. SLE in India. Lupus. 1997;6:690–700.
8. Fenlon HM, et al. HRCT chest in SLE. AIR. 1996;166:301–307.
9. Sant SM, et al. Pleuropulmonary abnormalities in patients with SLE-assessment with HRCT, chest radiography and pulmonary function tests. Clin Exp Rheumato. 1997;14:507–513.
10. Pradhan V, et al. Association of ferritin levels with hematological manifestations in SLE. JAPI. 2016;64:14–18.

11. Singh H, et al. SLE. Med Update; API. 2014;24:409–417.
12. Raja Adhyaksha AG, et al. Biologica in CLE. JAPI. 2013;61:262–267.
13. Brigilite ARA, van der Brugen-Bogavts BA, Hein MJG, et al. Assessment of bronchiectasis: comparison of HRCT and spiral volumetric CT. J Comp Asst Tomogr. 1996;20:15–19.
14. Park JJ, Lee KS, Kin JS, et al. Nonspecific interstitial pneumonia with fibrosis: radiographic and CT findings in seven patients. Radiology. 1995;195:645–648.
15. Shankar PS. HRCT of lungs. IN: BC Bansal, ed. PG Med. Mumbai: API. 1997;11:353–359.
16. Joshi JM, Sundaram P, Mania R Dr. DILD and HRCT: an initial experience. JAPI. 1997;45:436–439.
17. Collins J, et al. CT patterns of bronchiolar disease: what is tree-in-bud? AiR. 1998;171:365–370.
18. Flaherty KR, Martinez FJ. Diagnosing interstitial lung disease–a practical approach to a difficult problem. Cleve Clin Med. 2001;68:33–49.
19. Hamman L, Rich AR. Acute diffuse interstitial fibrosis of lungs. Bull Johns Hopkins Hasp. 1944;74:177.
20. Leibow AA, Carrington CB. The interstitial pneumonia. IN: M Simon, et al., ed. Frontiers of pulmonary radiology, 1st ed. New York: Gurney and Stratton. 1969;102–141.
21. Katzenstein AI. Katzenstein and Askin's surgical pathology of non-neoplastic lung diseases. Philadelphia: WB Saunders. 1997.
22. Lynch DA, et al. HRCT in IPF — diagnosis and prognosis. Am J Respir Care Med. 2005;172:488–493.
23. AT SIERS. International multidisciplinary consensus classification of idiopathic interstitial pneumonia. Am J Respir Crit Care Med. 2002;165:277–304.
24. Kant S, Bhatia RS. ILD. NATCON. 2005.
25. Bhatia RS. Pulmonary involvement in connective tissue disorders. IN: Selected topics in chest medicine. Arora Publishers. 2005;13:77–74.
26. Arjun P, et al. Undifferentiated connective diseases with pulmonary involvement. JAPI. 2011;59:175–178.
27. Badyal D, Bhatia RS. ADR. New Delhi: PP Publishers. 2006;8:101–114.
28. Shanker PS. IPF-what is new. IN: MS Rao, ed. Med Update; API. 2010; 20:795–801.

29. Katzenstein AL, Meyers JL. IPF: clinical relevance of pathologic classification. Am J Respir Crit Care Med. 1998;157:1301–1315.
30. Vijayan VK. Classification of interstitial lung disease. IN: S8 Gupta, ed. Med Update; API. 2005;15:522–525.
31. Wittrem C, et al. CT-histologic correlation of the idiopathic interstitial pneumonia. Radiographics. 2003;23:1057.
32. Mahashur AA. ILD — management. IN: S8 Gupta, ed. Med Update; API. 2005;15:530–531.
33. Bhattacharya P, et al. Role of long term doxycycline in patients of IPF. Lung India. 2009;26:81185.
34. Felson DT, et al. ACR/ELAR provisional definition. Arch Rheum. 2011;63:573.
35. Gauri LA, et al. Study of bone mineral density in patients with RA and its correlation with severity of disease. JAPI. 2017;65:26–30.
36. Sonawala A, et al. Evaluation of CD4, CD8 and CD25 cell counts and SLE in active disease and in remission. JAPI. 2017;65:37–42.
37. Ghosh VC, et al. Chest radiography. Med Update; API. 2016;26:472–478.
38. Sarkar R, et al. Head cheese sign. JAPI. 2017;65:76.
39. Shankar PS. ILD recent trends in its management. Med Update; API. 2016; 26:1028–1032.
40. Suraj KP, et al. Role of pirfenidone in IPF. JAPI. 2016;64:36–41.
41. Yoo H, et al. Connective tissue disease-related interstitial lung disease (CTD-ILD) and interstitial lung abnormality (ILA): evolving concept of CT findings, pathology and management. Eur J Radiol Open. 2020;16(8):100311.
42. Fujisawa T. Management of myositis-associated interstitial lung disease. Medicina (Kaunas). 2021 Apr 3;57(4):347.
43. Guler SA, Corte TJ. Interstitial lung disease in 2020: a history of progress. Clin Chest Med. 2021 Jun;42(2):229–239.

https://doi.org/10.1142/9789811271410_0039

39 Sarcoidosis

Introduction

Sarcoidosis is a granulomatous disease of unknown etiology, characterized by the formation of immune, noncaseating granulomas in various organs, predominantly in the lungs and intrathoracic lymph nodes, occurring worldwide, having a variable clinical course with diverse clinical manifestations, thereby posing challenges in therapeutic management.

Jonathan Hutchinson was the first to describe a case of sarcoidosis in 1887. He coined the term "Mortimer's Malady" after the name of his patient Mrs. Mortimer who presented with multiple, raised, dusky-red, nonulcerative, and persistent patches, which Hutchinson considered different from tuberculous affliction.

Epidemiology

The data on the prevalence of sarcoidosis vary across the world and are influenced by the high diagnostic dilemma and lack of a uniform reporting system. Sarcoidosis has heterogeneous presentations across the world, varying with race, ethnicity, gender, age, and so forth; thus, it has multifactorial causation that includes genetic, environmental, and microbiological factors. It can affect people of all ages but mostly develops in young and middle-aged adults. The incidence has been reported to peak at 30–50 years of age in men and at 50–60 years of age in women. Lung transplantation remains the only hope in cases of irreversible advanced sarcoidosis. Post-transplant survival and graft outcomes remain unclear, as the disease is known to recur,[1] and also because of extrapulmonary involvement and chronic lung infections.[2]

Etiopathogenesis

Genetic predisposition for sarcoidosis has been supported by

1. Familial clustering (5%–16% of cases).
2. Increased concordance in monozygotic twins.
3. Large ethnicity-driven variations in disease frequency, clinical expression, and outcomes.
4. Genetic studies that have identified human leukocyte antigens (HLAs) and non-HLA alleles as associated with sarcoidosis susceptibility, phenotype, and prognosis. The *HLA-DRB1*03* allele has strong association with acute and self-limiting sarcoidosis (i.e., Löfgren's syndrome), particularly in Scandinavians, whereas *HLA-DRB1*14* and *-DRB1*15* predispose to a chronic disease course. Additional genes associated with sarcoidosis risk include butyrophilin-like 2 gene and annexin A11. In combination, the above findings suggest a heterogenous genetic profile composed of multiple gene variants, each potentially contributing to disease susceptibility.

Environmental triggers

As pulmonary involvement is seen in most of the patients with sarcoidosis, it indicates that exposure to airborne agents in susceptible individuals might play a role in the etiopathogenesis of the disease. Among the organic environmental agents, *Mycobacterium* and *Propionibacterium* have both been implicated in sarcoidosis. Of the inorganic triggers, metal exposures to beryllium, zirconium, and aluminum have traditionally been associated to the development of a sarcoidosis-like granulomatous disease. Granulomatous pulmonary disease with features of sarcoidosis also developed in the firefighters exposed to World Trade Center "dust."

Pathology

The pathological hallmark of sarcoidosis is the presence of discrete, non-caseating, epithelioid cell granulomas. Cytoplasmic inclusions include "asteroid bodies" seen in 2%–9% of sarcoid granulomas and "Schaumann bodies"/"conchoidal bodies" seen in 44%–88% of cases of sarcoidosis and are lamellated calcifications. "Birefringent calcium oxalate crystals" poorly stained lucent material with irregular configuration seen in over two-thirds of lung biopsies in sarcoidosis. "Hamazaki–Wesenberg (H–W) bodies are lysosomal inclusions containing hemolipofuscin, usually found extracellularly in the sinusoids of granuloma containing lymph nodes.

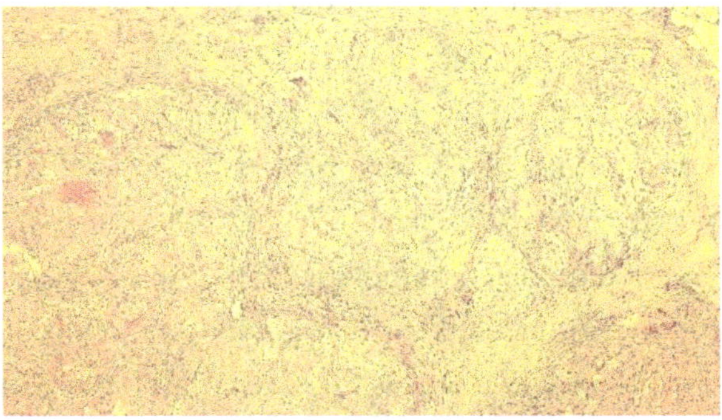

Figure 1: Multiple discrete noncaseating granulomas with giant cells.

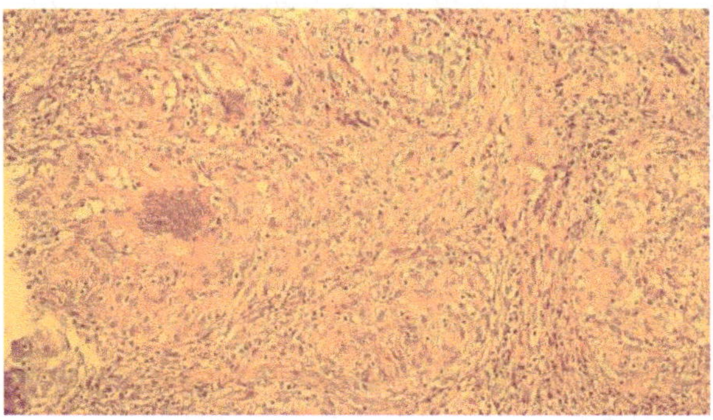

Figure 2: Higher power of granuloma with multinucleated giant cells.

As there are little evidence-based treatment guidelines, for most clinical manifestations of sarcoidosis, patients are best evaluated by a multidisciplinary approach to their care. Comprehensive care should not be just limited to pharmacological interventions, but also supportive measures aimed at relieving symptoms and improving quality of life (QoL). In general, sarcoidosis leads to a substantial economic burden, mainly because of hospitalizations, medication costs, and sickness absenteeism.

The diagnosis of sarcoidosis is based on three major criteria: compatible clinical characteristics, identification of non-necrotizing granulomas in one or more tissue samples, and the ruling out of other causes of granulomatous disease. In about 60% of patients, remission occurs spontaneously or after treatment within 10 years after diagnosis.

All patients with suspected sarcoidosis should undergo a comprehensive evaluation, including a detailed history, physical examination, a chest radiograph, pulmonary function tests, peripheral blood counts, serum angiotensin-converting enzyme (ACE) levels, urinalysis, electrocardiogram, ophthalmologic examination, and a tuberculin skin test. Comprehensive evaluation helps to provide additional data supporting the diagnosis of sarcoidosis and to assess the severity and extent of the disease while eliminating alternative diagnoses.

The diagnosis of sarcoidosis requires histopathological evidence of noncaseating granulomatous inflammation in one or more organs coupled with compatible clinical and radiological features and the exclusion of other causes of granulomatous inflammation; however, in the presence of typical disease manifestations such as Löfgren's syndrome, Heerfordt's syndrome, lupus pernio, and asymptomatic bilateral and symmetrical hilar lymphadenopathy, the diagnosis can be established with high level of certainty on clinical grounds alone. Future research should be aimed at identification of environmental triggers, genetic associations, biomarkers for treatment response, and newer treatment options.

Pulmonary sarcoidosis

Although sarcoidosis is a multisystem disease, pulmonary involvement is the most common cause of morbidity and mortality. The clinical presentations of pulmonary sarcoidosis can vary from an asymptomatic state detected on a chest radiograph to a progressive, debilitating pulmonary disorder causing respiratory failure.

Symptoms of pulmonary sarcoidosis are nonspecific; dyspnea and cough are the most common, with the latter being reported in over 90% of patients with an acute pulmonary exacerbation of the disease or nonspecific chest discomfort. Spontaneous resolution of the disease is common, but progressive lung disease occurs in approximately 25% and disabling organ failure in up to 10%.

Systemic constitutional symptoms such as fever, fatigue, malaise, and weight loss are seen in over 50% of patients and may be disabling. Other symptoms including muscle weakness and exercise intolerance, visual changes, dry eyes or mouth, parotid swelling, palpitations, syncope, joint pain, or swelling are also observed.

Sarcoidosis may manifest with the acute onset of erythema nodosum associated with bilateral hilar adenopathy, fevers, polyarthritis, and often uveitis, known as Löfgren's syndrome. Diffuse interstitial lung disease (ILD) is the classic type of lung involvement; other less common pulmonary manifestations include pneumothorax, pleural thickening, chylothorax, and pulmonary hypertension (PH). Even in the presence of lung parenchymal sarcoidosis, crackles are not commonly heard on chest examination. Wheezing may be present when there is endobronchial involvement or traction bronchiectasis due to scarring. Digital clubbing is rare and typically associated with advanced pulmonary fibrosis.

The natural course of pulmonary sarcoidosis tends to follow three general paths.

1. Benign course that presents in asymptomatic individuals undergoing a screening test: these patients tend to remain asymptomatic and usually require no therapeutic interventions.
2. A nonfibrotic symptomatic course, where the patient presents with pulmonary symptoms, intraparenchymal granulomatous inflammation in the lungs, and mild decrements in pulmonary function. These patients rarely experience progressive pulmonary deterioration. The disease can however last for months, years, or lifelong and might require immunosuppressive therapy.
3. Progressive fibrotic disease, and it accounts for ~10%–20% of sarcoidosis patients. The overwhelming majority of respiratory deaths occur in this subgroup of patients.

Pulmonary imaging in sarcoidosis includes

1. Chest radiographs are typically abnormal in >90% of pulmonary sarcoidosis patients. In 1961, Scadding reported on a radiographic staging system for sarcoidosis using chest X-ray and classified into five stages.

   Stage 0 (seen in 5%–15% of patients with sarcoidosis) refers to sarcoidosis that is occult on the chest.

   In stage 1 sarcoidosis, chest radiographs show only thoracic adenopathy (in 25%–65% of patients with radiographic sarcoidosis).

   In stage 2, chest radiographs show thoracic adenopathy and pulmonary infiltrates (in 25%–65% of patients).

   Stage 3 shows parenchymal infiltrates without hilar adenopathy.

   Stage 4 shows upper lobe predominant fibrotic changes with volume loss (least common).
2. High-resolution chest computed tomography (HRCT) scans better identify parenchymal details so that sarcoidosis may often be distinguished from other diffuse lung diseases. The characteristic features of pulmonary sarcoidosis on HRCT include (a) mediastinal (usually bilateral hilar) lymphadenopathy, (b) nodular and micronodular opacities along the bronchovascular bundle, pleural, and subpleural locations as

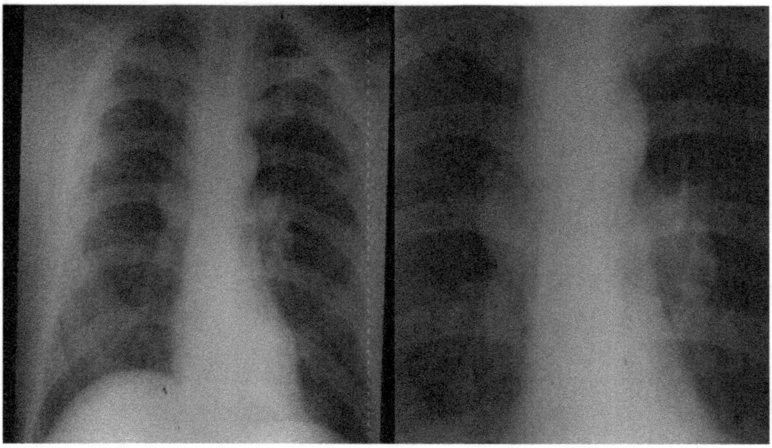

Figure 3: Stage 1 chest X-ray of a patient with arthralgia with bilateral enlarged hilar lymph node with associated arthralgia — sarcoidosis.

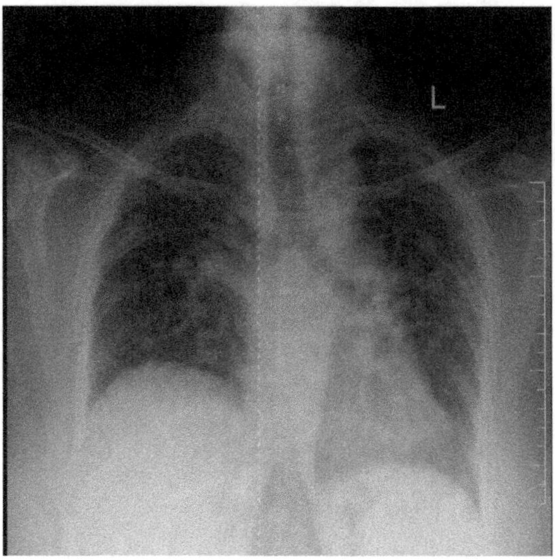

Figure 4: Stage 3 bilateral interstitial infiltrates in sarcoidosis.

well as the fissure lines, (c) a confluence of micronodules into conglomerate larger masses, and (d) pulmonary fibrosis more easily detected on HRCT than the chest radiograph. Showing fibrocystic disease, architectural distortion, hilar retraction, and traction bronchiectasis. These fibrotic changes are most common in the upper lobes.

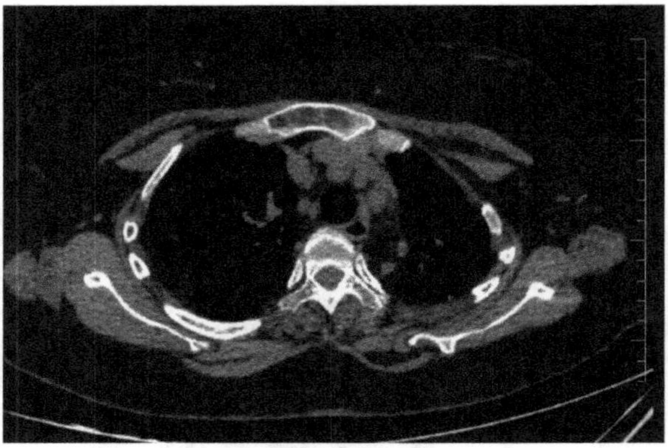

Figure 5: Calcified lymph nodes in sarcoidosis.

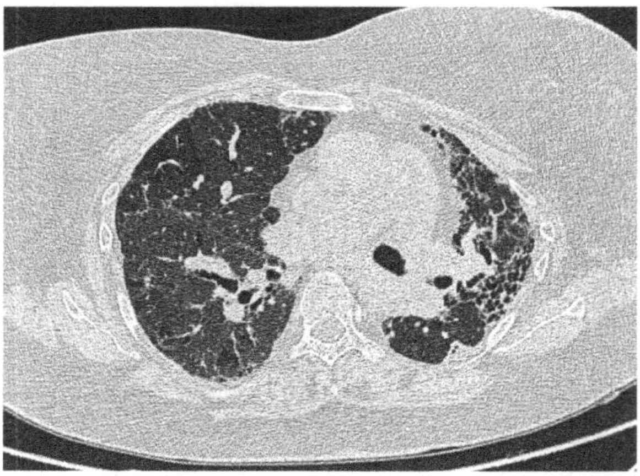

Figure 6: Ground-glass opacity, reticulation, suggesting interstitial thickening and honeycombing in the left lung in sarcoidosis.

3. Pulmonary function tests

   Spirometry of pulmonary sarcoidosis patients generally reveals modest abnormalities showing either restrictive, obstructive, or mixed patterns. Reduced DLCO in the presence of ILD. The diagnosis, assessment, and management of pulmonary sarcoidosis have evolved as new technologies and therapies have been adopted.
4. EBUS-TBNA

   Transbronchial needle aspiration guided by endobronchial ultrasound has replaced mediastinoscopy in many centers.

Complications of pulmonary sarcoidosis

1. Bronchiectasis leading to severe lung infection.
2. Mycetoma colonization triggering life-threatening infection hemoptysis.
3. PH[3]: Sarcoidosis-associated pulmonary hypertension (SAPH) is a complication associated with significant morbidity and increased mortality. SAPH is categorized as group 5 PH and is associated with poor prognosis, conferring up to a 10-fold increase in mortality in patients with sarcoidosis.
4. Chronic type 2 respiratory failure.
5. Cor pulmonale.

All newly diagnosed case of pulmonary sarcoidosis must undergo at baseline extrapulmonary organ screening test even if asymptomatic. Patients, with sarcoidosis even without any ocular symptoms, should undergo a baseline eye examination to screen for ocular sarcoidosis. As there is no universal standardization in the diagnosis of sarcoidosis, it is based on the following three major criteria: a compatible clinical presentation, the finding of non-necrotizing granulomatous inflammation in one or more tissue samples, and the exclusion of alternative causes of granulomatous disease two new guidelines were published by the American and European Thoracic societies in 2020.

The decision of who and when to treat an individual sarcoidosis patient depends on two major factors: risk for death or organ failure and impairment of QoL. All patients with sarcoidosis may not require the treatment. The decision to treat and the strategy for how to treat usually require input and shared decision-making by the patient. Many patients with sarcoidosis have favorable outcomes, with a significant proportion showing spontaneous remission without systemic therapy. However, a small number of cases progress to advanced sarcoidosis, which is the end-stage of sarcoidosis associated with significant mortality.[4–7] Pharmacological treatment of sarcoidosis is directed at decreasing granulomatous inflammation.[8] Adverse events are common with steroids, and many of the side effects are dose dependent. Careful titration of dose and strategies to minimize toxicity are essential when glucocorticoids are used.

According to the American Thoracic Society Clinical Practice Guideline released in 2020, the following recommendations were made for the diagnosis of sarcoidosis:

1. In patients for whom there is a high clinical suspicion for sarcoidosis (e.g., Löfgren's syndrome, lupus pernio, or Heerfordt's syndrome), there is no indication for lymph node sampling. However, these patients require close clinical follow-up.
2. In asymptomatic bilateral hilar lymphadenopathy, there are no recommendations for or against obtaining a lymph node sample. These patients do require close clinical follow-up.
3. In suspected sarcoidosis with mediastinal and/or hilar lymphadenopathy who need tissue sampling, EBUS-guided lymph node sampling is recommended.
4. In sarcoidosis patients without ocular symptoms, baseline eye examination is suggested to screen for ocular sarcoidosis.
5. In sarcoidosis without any renal symptoms or established renal sarcoidosis, baseline serum creatinine testing is suggested.
6. In sarcoidosis without hepatic symptoms or established hepatic sarcoidosis, baseline serum alkaline phosphatase testing is suggested.
7. In all patients with sarcoidosis, baseline serum calcium testing to screen for abnormal calcium metabolism is recommended even in the absence of symptoms or signs of hypercalcemia.
8. When assessment of vitamin D metabolism is deemed necessary in sarcoidosis, measuring both 25- and 1, 25-OH vitamin D levels is suggested, before vitamin D replacement.

Other suggestions include

1. Baseline complete blood cell count testing to screen for hematological abnormalities.

2. For patients with extracardiac sarcoidosis, the following tests are suggested.
3. Baseline ECG to screen for possible cardiac involvement. For patients with suspected cardiac involvement, cardiac MRI is recommended to obtain diagnostic and prognostic information.
4. If cardiac MRI is not available, dedicated cPET is recommended to obtain diagnostic and prognostic information.
5. For patients with sarcoidosis in whom PH is suspected, initial testing with transthoracic echocardiogram is suggested, and if it identifies PH, right heart catheterization to definitively confirm or exclude SAPH is suggested. In patients in whom PH is clinically suspected and a transthoracic echocardiogram is NOT suggestive of PH, the need for right heart catheterization should be determined on an individual basis.
6. PH is suspected refers to clinical manifestations, including exertional chest pain and/or syncope, exam findings of a prominent P2 or S4, reduced 6-minute walk distance, desaturation with exercise, reduced DL_{CO}, increased pulmonary artery diameter relative to ascending aorta diameter (e.g., by CT scan), elevated brain natriuretic factor, and fibrotic lung disease. Routine screening for SAPH is not necessary in patients who are asymptomatic.

ERS clinical practice guidelines on treatment of sarcoidosis

The management of sarcoidosis can be challenging. The clinician must remember not to focus on a single manifestation, but to look at the various manifestations both initially and over time. The outcome of the disease is variable. Some patients have a very good outcome and never require treatment. Less than 10% of patients die, mostly from advanced lung disease. For many patients, the response to anti-inflammatory treatment can readily be seen. However, recurrence of disease is common if treatment is withdrawn too soon, and at least a quarter of patients require treatment for more than 2 years.

Role of biomarkers in the diagnosis and assessment of pulmonary sarcoidosis

Biomarkers should be viewed as evidence of active inflammation, not as pathognomonic tests.[9] Serum biomarkers for pulmonary sarcoidosis usually reflect total body granuloma burden and are not specific for lung involvement. Pulmonary specific biomarkers include bronchoalveolar lavage (BAL) specimens, pulmonary function tests, and chest imaging studies. Although approximately 90% of pulmonary sarcoidosis patients demonstrate a BAL lymphocytes at the time of diagnosis, this finding is observed in several other lung diseases and, therefore, is not a useful diagnostic biomarker. The role of the BAL T-lymphocyte CD4/CD8 ratio remains also controversial, with some studies suggesting ratios greater than 3–4 have a >95% specificity for sarcoidosis and others disputing it. Regardless, it would be impractical to perform these tests serially to monitor pulmonary sarcoidosis activity. Pulmonary function tests and, specifically, spirometry are often used to monitor pulmonary sarcoidosis clinically and in research trials. The serum ACE level is elevated in 50%–60% of patients with sarcoidosis. However, this biomarker lacks diagnostic specificity, so its use is limited to evaluating the therapeutic response. Other biomarkers such as soluble interleukin-2 receptor, C-reactive protein, serum amyloid A, and chitotriosidase are generally useful for assessing disease activity, but FDG PET-CT is most effective for detecting tissue-specific inflammatory activity and identifying sites for diagnostic biopsies. ^{18}F-FDG PET scanning frequently demonstrates ^{18}F-FDG uptake in active lung lesions. Parenchymal lung FDG-PET uptake has been found to correlate with improvement in pulmonary function in symptomatic pulmonary sarcoidosis patients who require therapy, including corticosteroid-refractory patients treated with infliximab. Gallium-67 scintigraphy was historically used to identify active pulmonary sarcoidosis but has fallen out of favor because of its lower sensitivity/specificity compared to ^{18}F-FDG-PET higher radiation exposure and lengthy acquisition protocols.

Lastly, somatostatin receptor scintigraphy is a relatively new imaging technique to detect active sarcoid inflammatory lesions that has shown promise[3,9] in single-center retrospective studies.

Treatment of pulmonary sarcoidosis

Factors to be considered before initiation of treatment

a. indications for treatment,
b. initial anti-granulomatous therapy,
c. therapy for chronic and fibrotic disease,
d. glucocorticoid therapy,
e. alternative therapy to glucocorticoids,
f. nongranulomatous therapies, and
g. managing the complications of the disease.

Indications for treatment in patients with pulmonary sarcoidosis are the balance of

1. The minimization of risk of disability, loss of life due to pulmonary involvement, or loss of QoL, and
2. The risk of comorbidities and loss of QoL due to glucocorticoid and other therapies.

   General treatment goals are to achieve either disease regression or short-term disease stabilization (when irreversible) with higher dose glucocorticoid treatment and to identify the minimum long-term glucocorticoid dose required for stabilization of sarcoidosis.

   In sarcoidosis, lifelong exercise intolerance can result from ILD or PH which are the main causes of sarcoidosis-related mortality.

European Respiratory Society (ERS) clinical practice guidelines on treatment of sarcoidosis

The current task force committee has put more emphasis on patient-tailored choice than the 1999 guidelines. They used the GRADE (Grading of Recommendations Assessment, Development and Evaluation) methodology to develop 12 specific treatment recommendations for the management of sarcoidosis. All recommendations were based on very low to low quality of evidence.

ERS Task Force recommendations — 2021

New guidelines for treating sarcoidosis using a standardized methodology were developed by ERS Task Force in 2021. Specific recommendations for each PICO (Patients, Intervention, Comparison, Outcomes) question using GRADE (Grading of Recommendations, Assessment, Development and Evaluations) criteria have been developed, which is summarized below.

ERS Task Force gives the following recommendations:

1. For untreated patients with major involvement from pulmonary sarcoidosis who may be at higher risk of future mortality or permanent disability from sarcoidosis, steroids should be introduced to improve and/or preserve forced vital capacity (FVC) and QoL.
2. For symptomatic pulmonary sarcoidosis patients at higher risk of future mortality or permanent disability from sarcoidosis treated with glucocorticoids and suffer from continued disease or unacceptable side effects from steroids, methotrexate should be added to improve and/or preserve FVC and QoL.
3. For symptomatic pulmonary sarcoidosis patients at higher risk of future mortality or permanent disability from sarcoidosis treated with glucocorticoids or immunosuppressive agents and suffer from continued disease, addition of infliximab to improve and/or preserve FVC and QoL can be considered.
4. For patients with cutaneous sarcoidosis and cosmetically important active skin lesions which cannot be controlled by local treatment, Task Force suggested addition of oral glucocorticoids be considered to reduce skin lesions.
5. For patients with cutaneous sarcoidosis who have been treated with glucocorticoids and/or other immunosuppressive agents and have

continued cosmetically important active skin disease, addition of infliximab should be considered against no additional treatment to reduce skin lesions.

6. For patients with evidence of functional cardiac abnormalities, including heart block, dysrhythmias or cardiomyopathy, steroids are recommended (if necessary, other immunosuppressives can be added).
7. For clinically significant neurosarcoidosis, treat with steroids. Methotrexate can be added if the patient still has continued/progressive disease. If disease is still not under control, infliximab should be added along with a second-line immunosuppressive agent such as methotrexate, azathioprine, and mycophenolate mofetil.
8. In sarcoidosis with severe fatigue, pulmonary rehabilitation program for limb and inspiratory muscle strength training for 6–12 weeks can improve fatigue. If patients are not benefited by this, d-methylphenidate or armodafinil should be tried for 8 weeks.

Flow chart depicting the diagnostic approach to sarcoidosis

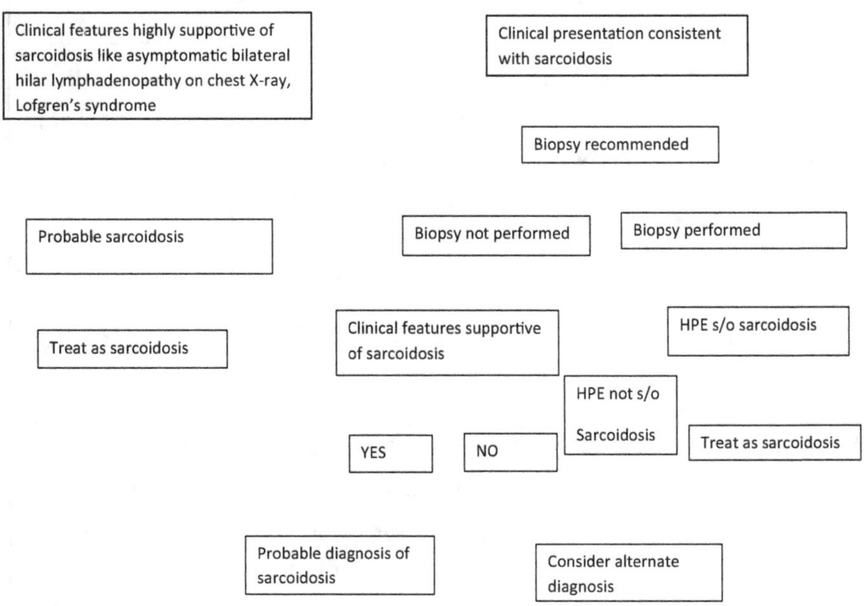

Anti-inflammatory drugs used in the treatment of sarcoidosis

Drugs	Dosage	Carefully monitor	Contraindications
Prednisone/ prednisolone	Initial 20 mg/ day; follow-up 5–10 mg	Bone density, blood pressure, and blood glucose	As steroids are known to cause cumulative toxicity, chronic steroid therapy requires close monitoring
Methotrexate	10–15 mg once a week	CBC, SGOT, SGPT, serum creatinine	Renal failure
Leflunomide	10–20 mg once a day	CBC, SGOT, SGPT, serum creatinine	Renal failure
Azathioprine	50–250 mg once a day	CBC	Allergic reactions which may be sometimes life threatening
Mycophenolate mofetil	500–1,500 mg twice a day	CBC	Less experience in sarcoidosis than other conditions
Infliximab or other similar biologicals	3–5 mg/kg initially and after 2 weeks once every 4–6 weeks	Rule out active TB before starting the treatment; other contraindications include congestive heart failure (CHF), prior malignancy, demyelinating neurologic disease, deep fungal infections	Possibility of life-threatening allergic reactions
Adalimumab	40 mg every 1–2 weeks	Active TB should be ruled out before starting the therapy; other contraindications include CHF, prior	Less toxic than infliximab

(*Continued*)

Drugs	Dosage	Carefully monitor	Contraindications
		malignancy, demyelinating neurologic disease, deep fungal infections	
Rituximab	500–1,000 mg every 1–6 months	Screening should be done for active viral hepatitis Monitor IgG levels	Reactivation of viral infections can cause IgG deficiency
Repository corticotropin injection (RCI)	50–80 units twice a week	Monitor BP and blood glucose levels	Toxic effects are more on the day of injection
HCQ	200–400 mg/day	Periodic eye examination	Impact on cardiac and neurological disease is less

Biologicals and RCI are reserved for patients who did not respond to prior treatment with steroids and antimetabolites.

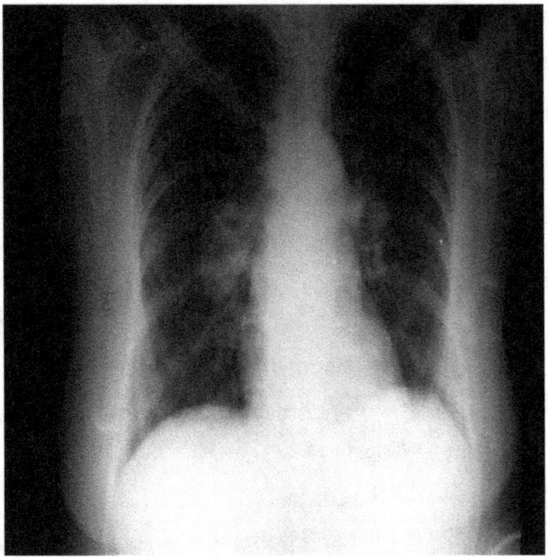

Figure 7: Enlarged bilateral hilar lymph node.

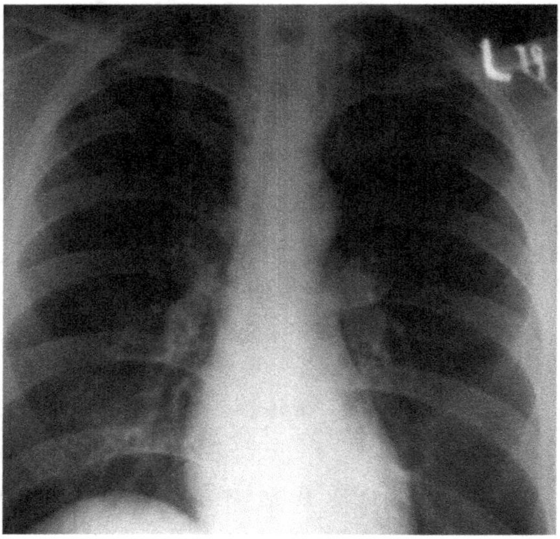

Figure 8: Chest X-ray of sarcoid arthralgia which shows hilar lymph. nodes have reduced in size after 6 months of steroids.

Challenges in sarcoidosis

Diagnostic uncertainty and treatment delays, because of its varied presentation and resemblance to more common diseases, and possibility of recurrence of sarcoidosis though rare should be kept in mind.

Reference and suggested readings

1. Crouser ED, Maier LA, Wilson KC, Bonham CA, Morgenthau AS, Patterson KC, Abston E, Bernstein RC, Blankstein R, Chen ES, Culver DA, Drake W, Drent M, Gerke AK, Ghobrial M, Govender P, Hamzeh N, James WE, Judson MA, Kellermeyer L, Knight S, Koth LL, Poletti V, Raman SV, Tukey MH, Westney GE, Baughman RP. Diagnosis and detection of sarcoidosis. An official American Thoracic Society clinical practice guideline. Am J Respir Crit Care Med. 2020 Apr 15;201(8):e26–e51.
2. Scadding JG, Mitchell DN. Sarcoidosis. Springer. 2013 Nov 11.
3. Denning DW, Pleuvry A, Cole DC. Global burden of chronic pulmonary aspergillosis complicating sarcoidosis. Eur Respir J. 2013 Mar 1;41(3):621–626.

4. Rybicki BA, Iannuzzi MC, Frederick MM, Thompson BW, Rossman MD, Bresnitz EA, Terrin ML, Moller DR, Barnard J, Baughman RP, DePalo L, Hunninghake G, Johns C, Judson MA, Knatterud GL, McLennan G, Newman LS, Rabin DL, Rose C, Teirstein AS, Weinberger SE, Yeager H, Cherniack R. ACCESS Research Group. Familial aggregation of sarcoidosis: a case–control etiologic study of sarcoidosis (ACCESS). Am J Respir Crit Care Med. 2001 Dec 1;164(11):2085–2091.
5. Spagnolo P, Grunewald J. Recent advances in the genetics of sarcoidosis. J Med Genet. 2013 May 1;50(5):290–297.
6. Valeyre D, Prasse A, Nunes H, et al. Sarcoidosis. Lancet. 2014;383(9923):1155–1167.
7. Judson MA, Baughman RP, Thompson BW, et al. Two year prognosis of sarcoidosis: the ACCESS experience. Sarcoidosis Vasc Diffuse Lung Dis. 2003;20(3):204–211. PubMed: 18996998.
8. Drent M, Crouser ED, Grunewald J. Challenges of sarcoidosis and its management. N Engl J Med. 2021 Sep 9;385(11):1018–1032.
9. Parikh KS, Dahhan T, Nicholl L, Ruopp N, Pomann GM, Fortin T, Tapson VF, Rajagopal S. Clinical features and outcomes of patients with sarcoidosis-associated pulmonary hypertension. Sci Rep. 2019 Mar 11;9(1):1–7.
10. Danbolt N. The historical aspects of sarcoidosis. Postgrad Med J. 1958 May;34(391):245.
11. Berlin M, Fogdell-Hahn A, Olerup O, Eklund A, Grunewald J. HLA-DR predicts the prognosis in Scandinavian patients with pulmonary sarcoidosis. Am J Respir Crit Care Med. 1997 Nov 1;156(5):1601–1605.
12. Valentonyte R, Hampe J, Huse K, Rosenstiel P, Albrecht M, Stenzel A, Nagy M, Gaede KI, Franke A, Haesler R, Koch A. Sarcoidosis is associated with a truncating splice site mutation in BTNL2. Nat Genet. 2005 Apr;37(4):357–364.
13. Hofmann S, Franke A, Fischer A, Jacobs G, Nothnagel M, Gaede KI, Schürmann M, Müller-Quernheim J, Krawczak M, Rosenstiel P, Schreiber S. Genome-wide association study identifies ANXA11 as a new susceptibility locus for sarcoidosis. Nat Genet. 2008 Sep;40(9):1103–1106.
14. Drake WP, Pei Z, Pride DT, Collins RD, Cover TL, Blaser MJ. Molecular analysis of sarcoidosis tissues for mycobacterium species DNA. Emerg Infect Dis. 2002 Nov;8(11):1334.

15. Song Z, Marzilli L, Greenlee BM, Chen ES, Silver RF, Askin FB, Teirstein AS, Zhang Y, Cotter RJ, Moller DR. Mycobacterial catalase–peroxidase is a tissue antigen and target of the adaptive immune response in systemic sarcoidosis. J Exper Med. 2005 Mar 7;201(5):755–767.
16. Rosen Y. Pathology of sarcoidosis. Semin Respir Crit Care Med. 2007 Feb;28(1):36–52. Copyright© 2007 by Thieme Medical Publishers, Inc., 333 Seventh Avenue, New York, NY 10001, USA.
17. Izbicki G, Chavko R, Banauch GI, Weiden MD, Berger KI, Aldrich TK, Hall C, Kelly KJ, Prezant DJ. World Trade Center "sarcoid-like" granulomatous pulmonary disease in New York city fire department rescue workers. Chest. 2007 May 1;131(5):1414–1423.
18. McKinzie BP, Bullington WM, Mazur JE, Judson MA. Efficacy of short-course, low-dose corticosteroid therapy for acute pulmonary sarcoidosis exacerbations. Am J Med Sci. 2010 Jan 1;339(1):1–4.
19. Lynch JP, Ma YL, Koss MN, White ES. Pulmonary sarcoidosis. Semin Respir Crit Care Med. 2007 Feb;28(1):53–74. Copyright© 2007 by Thieme Medical Publishers, Inc., 333 Seventh Avenue, New York, NY 10001, USA.
20. Baughman RP, Grutters JC. New treatment strategies for pulmonary sarcoidosis: antimetabolites, biological drugs, and other treatment approaches. Lancet Respir Med. 2015 Oct 1;3(10):813–822.
21. Judson MA, Boan AD, Lackland DT. The clinical course of sarcoidosis: presentation, diagnosis, and treatment in a large white and black cohort in the United States. Sarcoidosis Vasc Diffuse Lung Dis. 2012 Oct 1;29(2):119–127.
22. Moller DR. Pulmonary fibrosis of sarcoidosis: new approaches, old ideas. Am J Respir Cell Mol Biol. 2003 Sep 1;29(3):S37.
23. Lewis MM, Mortelliti MP, Yeager Jr H, Tsou E. Clinical bronchiectasis complicating pulmonary sarcoidosis: case series of seven patients. Sarcoidosis Vasc Diffuse Lung Dis. 2002 Jun 1;19(2):154–159.
24. Scadding J. Prognosis of intrathoracic sarcoidosis in England. Br Med J. 1961 Nov 11;2(5261):1165.
25. Abehsera M, Valeyre D, Grenier P, Jaillet H, Battesti JP, Brauner MW. Sarcoidosis with pulmonary fibrosis: CT patterns and correlation with pulmonary function. Am J Roentgenol. 2000 Jun;174(6):1751–1757.

26. Handa T, Nagai S, Miki S, Fushimi Y, Ohta K, Mishima M, Izumi T. Incidence of pulmonary hypertension and its clinical relevance in patients with sarcoidosis. Chest. 2006 May 1;129(5):1246–1252.
27. Nardi A, Brillet PY, Letoumelin P, Girard F, Brauner M, Uzunhan Y, Naccache JM, Valeyre D, Nunes H. Stage IV sarcoidosis: comparison of survival with the general population and causes of death. Eur Respir J. 2011 Dec 1; 38(6):1368–1373.
28. Baughman RP, Engel PJ, Taylor L, Lower EE. Survival in sarcoidosis-associated pulmonary hypertension: the importance of hemodynamic evaluation. Chest. 2010 Nov 1;138(5):1078–1085.
29. Simonneau G, Robbins IM, Beghetti M, Channick RN, Delcroix M, Denton CP, Elliott CG, Gaine SP, Gladwin MT, Jing ZC, Krowka MJ. Updated clinical classification of pulmonary hypertension. J Am Coll Cardiol. 2009 Jun 30;54(1_Supplement_S):S43–S54.
30. Baughman RP, Teirstein AS, Judson MA, et al. Clinical characteristics of patients in a case control study of sarcoidosis. Am J Respir Crit Care Med. 2001;164:1885–1889.
31. Grunewald J, Eklund A. Lofgren's syndrome: human leukocyte antigen strongly influences the disease course. Am J Respir Crit Care Med. 2009;179(4):307–312.
32. Walsh SL, Wells AU, Sverzellati N, et al. An integrated clinicoradiological staging system for pulmonary sarcoidosis: a case-cohort study. Lancet Respir Med. 2014;2(2):123–130.
33. Uzunhan Y, Nunes H, Jeny F, et al. Chronic pulmonary aspergillosis complicating sarcoidosis. Eur Respir J. 2017;49(6):49-6-2016.
34. Kirkil G, Lower EE, Baughman RP. Predictors of mortality in pulmonary sarcoidosis. Chest. 2018;153(1):105–113.
35. Rizzato G, Montemurro L, Colombo P. The late follow-up of chronic sarcoid patients previously treated with corticosteroids. Sarcoidosis. 1998;15:52–58.
36. Gottlieb JE, Israel HL, Steiner RM, et al. Outcome in sarcoidosis. The relationship of relapse to corticosteroid therapy. Chest. 1997;111(3):623–631.
37. Judson MA, Boan AD, Lackland DT. The clinical course of sarcoidosis: presentation, diagnosis, and treatment in a large white and black cohort in the United States. Sarcoidosis Vasc Diffuse Lung Dis. 2012 Oct 1;29(2):119–127.

38. Bergin CJ, Bell DY, Coblentz CL, Chiles C, Gamsu G, MacIntyre NR, Coleman RE, Putman CE. Sarcoidosis: correlation of pulmonary parenchymal pattern at CT with results of pulmonary function tests. Radiology. 1989 Jun;171(3):619–624.
39. Baughman RP, Wells A. Advanced sarcoidosis. Curr Opin Pulm Med. 2019 Sep 1;25(5):497–504.
40. Shlobin OA, Nathan SD. Management of end-stage sarcoidosis: pulmonary hypertension and lung transplantation. Eur Respir J. 2012 Jun 1;39(6):1520–1533.
41. Thillai M, Atkins CP, Crawshaw A, Hart SP, Ho LP, Kouranos V, Patterson KC, Screaton NJ, Whight J, Wells AU. BTS clinical statement on pulmonary sarcoidosis. Thorax. 2021 Jan 1;76(1):4–20.
42. Drent M, Crouser ED, Grunewald J. Challenges of sarcoidosis and its management. N Engl J Med. 2021 Sep 9;385(11):1018–1032.
43. Baughman RP, Valeyre D, Korsten P, Mathioudakis AG, Wuyts WA, Wells A, Rottoli P, Nunes H, Lower EE, Judson MA, Israel-Biet D. ERS clinical practice guidelines on treatment of sarcoidosis. Eur Respir J. 2021 Dec 1;58(6). doi: 10.1183/13993003.04079-2020.
44. Kirkil G, Lower EE, Baughman RP. Chest CT scan: the best predictor of mortality in advanced pulmonary sarcoidosis? Respir Med. 2020 Aug–Sep; 170:106059. doi: 10.1016/j.rmed.2020.106059.
45. Baughman RP, Judson MA, Teirstein A, Yeager H, Rossman M, Knatterud GL, Thompson B. Presenting characteristics as predictors of duration of treatment in sarcoidosis. J Assoc Physicians. 2006 May 1;99(5):307–315. doi: 10.1093/qjmed/hcl038.
46. Nagai S, Izumi T. Bronchoalveolar lavage: still useful in diagnosing sarcoidosis? Clin Chest Med. 1997 Dec 1;18(4):787–797.
47. Costabel U, Bonella F, Ohshimo S, Guzman J. Diagnostic modalities in sarcoidosis: BAL, EBUS, and PET. Semin Respir Crit Care Med. 2010 Aug; 31(4):404–408. © Thieme Medical Publishers.
48. Malinowska E, Doboszyńska A, Śliwińska A, Buscombe JR, Kulesza G, Moczulska B, Ćwikła JB. The use of 67Ga scintigraphy in patients with sarcoidosis. Nucl Med Rev. 2018;21(1):59–65.

49. Kamphuis LS, Kwekkeboom DJ, Missotten TO, Baarsma GS, Dalm VA, Dik WA, Timmermans WM, Van Daele PL, van Hagen PM, van Laar JA. Somatostatin receptor scintigraphy patterns in patients with sarcoidosis. Clin Nucl Med. 2015 Dec 1;40(12):925–929.
50. Martinez FJ, Orens JB, Deeb M, Brunsting LA, Flint A, Lynch III JP. Recurrence of sarcoidosis following bilateral allogeneic lung transplantation. Chest. 1994 Nov 1;106(5):1597–1599.
51. Amin EN, Closser DR, Crouser ED. Current best practice in the management of pulmonary and systemic sarcoidosis. Ther Adv Respir Dis. 2014 Aug;8(4):111–132.
52. Treglia G, Annunziata S, Sobic-Saranovic D, Bertagna F, Caldarella C, Giovanella L. The role of 18F-FDG-PET and PET/CT in patients with sarcoidosis: an updated evidence-based review. Acad Radiol. 2014;21(5):675–684.

https://doi.org/10.1142/9789811271410_0040

40 Pharmacological options in the management of nonspecific interstitial pneumonia

Glucocorticoids

The optimal dose and duration of glucocorticoid therapy remains unknown, and a variety of regimens have been tried in patients with idiopathic nonspecific interstitial pneumonia (NSIP).

Dose: Prednisone 0.5–1 mg/kg ideal body weight/day up to a maximum of 60 mg/day for 1 month followed by 30–40 mg/day for an additional 2 months can be given.

For patients who respond or stabilize with treatment, the dose is gradually tapered and could be reached to 5–10 mg daily or on alternate days, by the end of 6–9 months, with attempted cessation after at least 1 year of therapy.

For patients who relapse when prednisone is tapered or discontinued, low-dose prednisone can be maintained for a longer period. For patients with severe NSIP requiring hospitalization, pulse intravenous methylprednisolone may be preferred for initial therapy. A typical regimen is 1,000 mg/day for 3 days followed by oral prednisone described above. The key issue with long-term steroids is HPA suppression, osteoporosis, muscle weakness, and induction or worsening of diabetes and hypertension.

Azathioprine

Azathioprine is a prodrug which is metabolized to 6-mercaptopurine, its active form. It blocks enzymes such as amidophosphoribosyltransferase, thereby inhibiting the synthesis of purines adenine and guanine. This results in the formation of nonfunctional nucleic acid strands. The proliferation of fast-growing cells like lymphocytes is inhibited by the disruption of de novo purine synthesis. Since lymphocytes relatively lack the purine "salvage" pathway, they are particularly susceptible to the effects of de novo pathway inhibition. 6-MP inhibits the activity of T cells and, to a lesser extent, B cells, by interfering in the early phase of lymphoid cell proliferation; however, further evidence on more detailed mechanism of action is needed. Other possible mechanisms of azathioprine include blockage of T cell activation and stimulation of T cell apoptosis.

Azathioprine is metabolized and inactivated by thiopurine methyltransferase (TPMT). Hence, toxicities due to azathioprine, like bone marrow suppression, are experienced by patients who lack this enzyme (1 in 300). It is also found that 6-MP interacts with Rac1, blocking up the regulation of Bcl-xL messenger RNA and protein, which leads to the suppression of delayed hypersensitivity reactions and cell-mediated cytotoxicity. Low levels of this enzyme have been associated with severe gastrointestinal (GI) distress and bone marrow suppression.

Dose: A common regimen is to start with 25–50 mg/day and increase by 50 mg increments every 7–14 days up to 1.5–2.0 mg/kg/day, but not exceeding a maximum total dose of 200 mg/day. A lower dose is indicated in renal insufficiency.

ADR: Leukopenia, pancreatitis, hepatitis, bone marrow suppression.

Mycophenolate mofetil

Mycophenolate mofetil (MMF) is a prodrug of mycophenolic acid (MPA), an inhibitor of inosine monophosphate dehydrogenase (IMPDH), a rate limiting enzyme in the de novo synthesis of guanosine nucleotides. MPA depletes guanosine nucleotides preferentially in T and B lymphocytes causing the suppression of glycosylation as they are more dependent on this enzyme than other cell types. Another reason is that the type I isoform of IMPDH present in other cells is weakly inhibited compared to the type II isoform of IMPDH present in the lymphocytes. This is the main mechanism by which MPA inhibits the proliferation of T and B lymphocytes, thereby suppressing cell-mediated immune responses and antibody formation.

Apart from this, there are other mechanisms that contribute to the efficacy of MMF. In activated T-lymphocytes, MPA induces apoptosis, eliminating clones of cells responding to stimulation from particular antigens. MMF inhibits the expression of adhesion molecules, thus reducing the recruitment of lymphocytes and monocytes into areas of inflammation. MPA depletes tetrahydrobiopterin, a cofactor for inducible form of nitric oxide synthase (iNOS), decreasing the production of nitric oxide by iNOS. This generally does not affect the activity of constitutive NO synthases. This, therefore, has an effect also on the activated macrophages that produce NO and superoxide, which interact to produce peroxynitrite, with a significant tissue damaging potential.

Dose: The target dose of MMF is generally between 1.5 and 3 g daily, usually in two divided doses (e.g., 0.75–1.5 twice daily). Starting with lower doses, such as 500 mg twice daily, and increasing to the target dose over 3–4 months may improve a patient's gastrointestinal tolerance of MMF.

ADR: Hyperglycemia, hypercholesterolemia, hypomagnesemia, dyspnea, increased BUN, leukopenia, hyperkalemia, anemia, hypocalcemia, progressive multifocal leukoencephalopathy, increased susceptibility to infections, increased risk of lymphoma and skin malignancy, pure red-cell aplasia in patients treated with MMF in combination with other immunosuppressants, neutropenia, and serious infections.

Cyclophosphamide

Cyclophosphamide (CYC) is an alkylating agent related to the nitrogen mustards.

The most significant metabolite of CYC is considered to be 4-hydroxycyclophosphamide as it has a property to distribute throughout the body including the tumor where it immediately degrades to form phosphoramide mustard or nor-nitrogen mustard. These two forms have a chloroethyl moiety which is transformed to a highly reactive alkylating aziridinium ion. Since both, the phosphoramide and nor-nitrogen mustard have chloroethyl groups, a bifunctional reaction takes place, forming an interstrand cross-link between the two strands of DNA. This cross-link formation prevents the two strands from separating during replication which inhibits DNA synthesis.

Dose: When using CYC for NSIP, a monthly intravenous dosing over daily oral dosing is preferred, due to the lower risk of bladder toxicity.

The initial dose is based on body surface area (BSA) and adjusted for age, obesity, and renal impairment. Subsequent dosing is based on response to therapy and monitoring of hematologic toxicity.

Adequate hydration should be given prior to and for 24 hours after infusion of CYC to reduce the risk of hemorrhagic cystitis.

A trial of at least 3–6 months of CYC is needed to ensure an adequate opportunity for clinical response. The drug can be discontinued after 6–12 months due to toxicities.

ADR: Infections, myelosuppression, leukopenia, neutropenia, immunosuppression, hepatic function abnormalities, alopecia, cystitis, microhematuria, hemorrhagic cystitis, macrohematuria, impairment of spermatogenesis, fever, chills, asthenia, malaise.

Cyclosporine

Cyclosporine is an important immunosuppressive agent and blocks the transcription of inflammatory genes in activated T cells. This happens due to the cyclosporine–cyclophilin complex that inhibits the phosphatase activity of calcineurin (a regulator of nuclear translocation and activation of NFAT transcription factors), as well as blocking the activation of JNK and p38 signaling pathways triggered by recognition of specific antigens.

Dose: In acute interstitial pneumonia, the dose of cyclosporine was 50–200 mg/day, trough level 100–150 ng/mL. In a study of interstitial lung disease associated with polymyositis/dermatomyositis (PM/DM), cyclosporine was titrated to a trough level of 150 ng/mL and 2-hour peak level of 1,000 ng/mL.

ADR: Nephrotoxicity; hypertension; tremor; hyperkalemia; hypomagnesemia; hepatotoxicity; CNS (headache, tremor, seizure, coma, encephalopathy, leukoencephalopathy); hirsutism; gingival hyperplasia; burning sensation in the eye.

Tacrolimus

Tacrolimus is a macrolide antibiotic with immunosuppressive properties. It exerts its effects principally through impairment of gene expression in target cells. Tacrolimus forms a complex with an immunophilin, FK506-binding protein (FKBP). This complex inhibits calcineurin phosphatase. The drug not only inhibits calcium-dependent events like interleukin-2 gene transcription, NOS activation, cell degranulation, and apoptosis but also potentiates the actions of glucocorticoids and progesterone by binding to FKBPs contained within the hormone receptor complex, preventing degradation. The drug is also known to enhance the expression of the transforming growth factor beta-1 gene. It also plays a role in suppression of type 1 T helper cells and B cell growth and antibody production.

Dose: A starting dose of 1–3 mg/day may be given.

ADR: Cardiac (prolonged QT interval, hypertension, cardiomegaly); diabetes mellitus; nephrotoxicity; hypomagnesemia; hyperkalemia; neurologic (headache, tremor, insomnia, paresthesia, coma); leukoencephalopathy; skin (alopecia, pruritus, rash); GI upset; anemia; thrombocytopenia.

Pharmacological options in the management of Idiopathic pulmonary fibrosis

Pirfenidone

Mechanism of action

Pirfenidone is an orally active molecule that shows a wide range of biologic activity. In vitro evidence has shown that pirfenidone inhibits collagen synthesis, downregulates profibrotic cytokines, and decreases fibroblast proliferation. Pirfenidone leads to a reduction of TGF-beta2 mRNA levels and of the mature TGF-beta2 protein due to decreased expression and direct inhibition of the TGF-beta pro-protein convertase furin. In addition, pirfenidone reduces the protein levels of the matrix metalloproteinase (MMP)-11, a TGF-beta target gene and furin substrate involved in carcinogenesis.

Brand name	Dosage form	Strength
Esbriet	Capsule	267 mg
Esbriet	Tablet	267 mg
Esbriet	Tablet, coated	801 mg

Common side effects of pirfenidone include the following:

Nausea, vomiting, diarrhea headache, rashes, indigestion, stomach pain, and dizziness.

Pirfenidone can cause liver injury and as well as sensitivity to light.

The mechanism of pirfenidone-induced photosensitivity is likely to be phototoxic and is related to the drug's ability to absorb ultraviolet A and ultraviolet B. Absorption of ultraviolet light in the skin tissue could result in skin lesions due to generation of reactive oxygen species and lipid peroxidation.

The mechanism by which pirfenidone might cause liver injury is not known. It is metabolized in the liver largely via the cytochrome P450 system, predominantly CYP 1A2, and liver injury may be due to the production of a toxic or immunogenic metabolite.

Nintedanib

Mechanism of action

Nintedanib targets multiple receptor tyrosine kinases (RTKs) and non-receptor tyrosine kinases (nRTKs). Nintedanib inhibits the following RTKs: platelet-derived growth factor receptor (PDGFR) α and β, fibroblast growth factor receptor (FGFR) 1–3, vascular endothelial growth factor receptor (VEGFR) 1–3, and Fms-like tyrosine kinase-3 (FLT3). Among them, FGFR, PDGFR, and VEGFR have been implicated in idiopathic pulmonary fibrosis (IPF) pathogenesis. Nintedanib binds competitively to the adenosine triphosphate (ATP)-binding pocket of these receptors and blocks the intracellular signaling which is crucial for the proliferation, migration, and transformation of fibroblasts representing essential mechanisms of the IPF pathology. In addition, nintedanib inhibits the following nRTKs: Lck, Lyn, and Src kinases. The contribution of FLT3 and nRTK inhibition to IPF efficacy is unknown.

Brand name	Dosage form	Strength
Ofev	Capsule	150 mg
Ofev	Capsule	100 mg

Common side effects of nintedanib

Diarrhea, nausea, vomiting, abdominal pain, liver enzyme elevation, headache, decreased weight, decreased appetite, and hypertension.

Nintedanib can also cause fetal harm when administered to a pregnant woman.

Important clinical trials

Name of the trial	Patient centers	Outcome
Pirfenidone: an update on the clinical trial data and insights from everyday practice	**CAPACITY, RECAP**—multicenter, randomized, placebo-controlled trials consisting of 779 patients	Support the clinical profile of pirfenidone in adult patients with mild-to-moderate IPF. Sub-analyses of the CAPACITY studies and data from the RECAP extension study might suggest that the benefits of pirfenidone can be maximized, particularly in patients at a greater risk of FVC decline. Data from patients completing the CAPACITY studies who continued on treatment in RECAP also highlight the positive longer-term continuation rates on treatment.
Clinical use of nintedanib in patients with idiopathic pulmonary fibrosis	**TOMORROW**—multicenter, randomized control trials consisting of 1,061 patients treated with nintedanib 150 mg twice daily or placebo. Dose interruption or reduction to 100 mg twice daily was allowed for the management of adverse events	The clinical trial program for nintedanib included an international phase II trial known as the TOMORROW trial. Placebo-controlled trials have shown that nintedanib reduces the rate of disease progression in patients with IPF, with adverse events that are manageable in

(*Continued*)

(*Continued*)

Name of the trial	Patient centers	Outcome
		most patients through dose reduction, treatment interruption, and symptomatic management of diarrhea. Nintedanib has been shown to be effective across a wide range of subgroups of patients with IPF.
Clinical use of nintedanib in patients with idiopathic pulmonary fibrosis	**INPULSIS TRIALS—** multicenter, randomized control trials consisting of 1,066 patients. Across the two INPULSIS trials, a total of 1,066 patients were randomized and treated with nintedanib 150 mg twice daily or placebo. Dose interruption or reduction to 100 mg twice daily was allowed for the management of adverse events	Placebo-controlled trials have shown that nintedanib reduces the rate of disease progression in patients with IPF, with adverse events that are manageable in most patients through dose reduction, treatment interruption, and symptomatic management of diarrhea. Nintedanib has been shown to be effective across a wide range of subgroups of patients with IPF.

References and suggested readings

1. Taniguchi H, Kondoh Y. Acute and subacute idiopathic interstitial pneumonias. Respirology. 2016 Jul;21(5):810–820. doi: 10.1111/resp.12786. Epub 2016 Apr 28. PMID: 27123874.
2. Cavagna L, Monti S, Grosso V, Boffini N, Scorletti E, Crepaldi G, Caporali R. The multifaceted aspects of interstitial lung disease in rheumatoid arthritis.

Biomed Res Int. 2013;2013:759760. doi: 10.1155/2013/759760. Epub 2013 Sep 25. PMID: 24205507; PMCID: PMC3800606.

3. Nishino M, Ramaiya NH, Awad MM, Sholl LM, Maattala JA, Taibi M, Hatabu H, Ott PA, Armand PF, Hodi FS. PD-1 inhibitor-related pneumonitis in advanced cancer patients: radiographic patterns and clinical course. Clin Cancer Res. 2016 Dec 15;22(24):6051–6060. doi: 10.1158/1078-0432.CCR-16-1320. Epub 2016 Aug 17. PMID: 27535979; PMCID: PMC5161686.
4. Grecuccio S, Sverzellati N, Uslenghi E, Caminati A, Pedrazzi G, Zompatori M. Prognostic value of mediastinal lymph node enlargement in chronic interstitial lung disease. Diagn Interv Radiol. 2021 May;27(3):329–335. doi: 10.5152/dir.2021.19585. PMID: 34003121; PMCID: PMC8136534.
5. Schupp JC, Köhler T, Müller-Quernheim J. Usefulness of cyclophosphamide pulse therapy in interstitial lung diseases. Respiration. 2016;91(4):296–301. doi: 10.1159/000445031. Epub 2016 Apr 16. PMID: 27082957.

https://doi.org/10.1142/9789811271410_0041

41 Lungs and rheumatological diseases

Introduction

Rheumatological diseases have protean manifestations and can affect any organ system in the body either at the onset of the disease or as part of progression of the disease. The lung is one of the major organ involved in many rheumatological conditions in which there can be parenchymal involvement, pleural involvement, or a vascular component occurring in various degrees in isolation or as a combination. Drug-induced lung diseases have also been reported, especially with the widespread use of biological agents more commonly with the use of anti-TNFs. Lung infections (bacterial or viral) are commonly seen in many rheumatic diseases, especially amongst those of immunosuppressive agents.

Rheumatological problems are broadly divided into two categories, namely, connective tissue diseases and vasculitis (Table 1).

Diseases like relapsing polychondritis (RP), rheumatoid arthritis (RA), and granulomatous polyangiitis without eosinophilia may have upper airway involvement as well. It is pertinent to note that a combination of pulmonary manifestations may be present in a single disease phenotype, and hence, it is necessary to investigate for all the pulmonary manifestations despite clinical evaluation suggestive of a clinical phenotype.

Progressive lung disease is one of the leading causes of morbidity in these diseases; however, better control of infection with timely vaccination, immunosuppression, rehabilitation, and cardiopulmonary transplant in selected scenarios has vastly improved the overall outcome of connective tissue-associated lung diseases.

Table 1: Broad classification of rheumatological disorders

Connective tissue disorders	Vasculitis
Rheumatoid arthritis*	Primary
Sjogren's syndrome*	A: Large vessel
Systemic lupus erythematosus*	— Takayasu's aortoarteritis
Polymyositis/dermatomyositis*	— Giant cell arteritis
Systemic sclerosis*	— Relapsing polychondritis
Spondyloarthropathies	— Cogan's syndrome
	— Behcet's syndrome
	B: Medium vessel
	— Polyarteritis nodosa
	— Kawasaki disease
	C: Small vessel
	ANCA associated*
	— Granulomatous polyangiitis without eosinophilia (Wegener's granulomatosis)
	— Granulomatous polyangiitis with eosinophilia (Churg–Strauss vasculitis)
	— Microscopic polyangiitis
	Non-ANCA associated
	— Essential mixed cryoglobulinemia
	— Hepatitis B and C associated
	— IgA vasculitis (Henoch–Schonlein purpura)
	— Leukocytoclastic vasculitis
	Secondary
	SLE/rheumatoid arthritis/dermatomyositis

*Conditions in which lungs can be commonly affected.

Table 2: Pulmonary involvement in rheumatological diseases

Upper airway	Pleural	Parenchymal	Nodular	Vascular	Miscellaneous
— Sinus involvement granulomatosis with polyangiitis (GPA) — Nasal septal and cartilage (RP/GPA/ Cogans) — Nasal polyposis (GPA with eosinophilia) — Cricoarytenoid joint (RA) — Laryngeal involvement (GPA/RP)	— Pleural effusion (RA/SLE/ Infections) — Fistulous diseases (GPA)	— Interstitial lung diseases A: Usual interstitial pneumonias (RA/SSc) B: Nonspecific interstitial pneumonias (RA/SSc/DM/ MCTD) C: Bronchiolitis obliterans with organizing pneumonia (RA/SLE) — Cavitary lung diseases (RA/ GPA) — Diffuse alveolar hemorrhage (SLE/GPA/MPA/ Goodpasture's syndrome) — Shrinking lung syndrome (SLE) — Hyperreactive airway disease (GPA with eosinophilia)	— Rheumatoid nodules — Sarcoidosis — GPA	— Thromboembolic disease (SLE/ APS) — Pulmonary arterial hypertension (SSc/MCTD/RA/ SLE) — Pulmonary aneurysms (Behcet's syndrome, Takayasu's aortoarteritis)	— Infections — Drugs — Malignancy — Thoracic cage restriction (SpA, SSc) — Respiratory muscle weakness (PM/DM/ SSc/SLE)

RA: Rheumatoid arthritis, RP: relapsing polychondritis, GPA: granulomatosis with polyangiitis (Wegener's granulomatosis), GPA with eosinophilia: granulomatous polyangiitis with eosinophilia (Churg–Strauss), SSc: systemic sclerosis, PM: polymyositis, DM: dermatomyositis, SLE: systemic lupus erythematosus, APS: antiphospholipid antibody syndrome, MPA: microscopic polyangiitis, MCTD: mixed connective tissue disorder, SpA: spondyloarthropathies.

The spectrum of interstitial lung diseases

The spectrum of interstitial lung diseases (ILDs) or diffuse lung diseases encompasses (Figure 1) idiopathic variety (idiopathic pulmonary fibrosis, desquamative interstitial pneumonia (DIP), bronchiolitis obliterans with organizing pneumonia, and acute interstitial pneumonias), hypersensitivity pneumonitis, drug-induced ILD, Langerhans cell histiocytosis, and ILD related to occupational hazards. Connective tissue disease-associated interstitial lung disease (CTD–ILD) accounts for nearly 15%–20%,[1] and some ILDs may be a formes frustes of future CTD depending on the histology, distribution pattern, and the presence of autoantibodies.[2]

In clinical practice, autoantibodies are routinely ordered in a patient with ILD even without any clear features suggestive of CTD or vasculitis. The most common autoantibodies ordered are ANA and rheumatoid factor, the positivity of which may vary between 20% and 40%.[3] Whether these antibodies in a patient with ILD is a harbinger of future definitive connective tissue disease remains an enigma and is dependent on follow-up time.

Investigations/tissue diagnosis and bronchoscopy with respect to lung manifestations may be mandated where the pattern of ILD or the presence of a connective tissue disease is not ominous. However, exclusion of infection either at presentation or during the course of treatment is a definitive indication for targeted investigation with respect to the type of presentation.

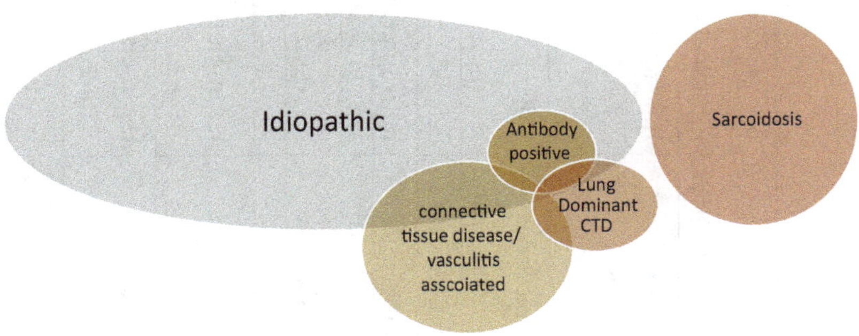

Figure 1: Spectrum of interstitial lung diseases.

Table 3: Diseases associations and pattern distribution

Clinical phenotype	Clinical features	Autoantibodies	Time to development of ILD	Lung manifestations
Rheumatoid arthritis	Inflammatory arthritis	Rheumatoid factor Anticyclic citrullinated peptide antibody	Later stages of the disease	Variable
Systemic lupus erythematosus	Malar rash, oral ulcers, associated nephritis	ANA, dsDNA, anti-SSA/SSB/u1RNP/nucleosomes	Variable	Variable
Systemic sclerosis	Sclerodactyly, Raynaud's	ANA/SCL70, CENP B	Variable	ILD
MCTD	Puffy fingers, arthritis	ANA/U1RNP	Variable	ILD
Inflammatory myositis	Muscle weakness	Myositis-specific antibody	Variable	ILD
Vasculitis	Fever/constitutional symptoms/varied organ involvement	Antibodies may be absent ANCA/ANA may be sometimes positive	Variable	Variable
Sarcoidosis	Uveitis/erythema nodosum/fever	Angiotensin-converting enzyme levels	Variable	Mediastinal adenopathy/ILD/nodules

Symptomatology and pattern overlap

A disease phenotype in connective tissue disorders may have protean manifestations and a plethora of antibodies. More often, there is going to be an overlap of symptomatology as shown in the figure vis-à-vis the presence of ILDs except in the distinct symptomatology and presentation of sarcoidosis (Figure 2). Fever, arthralgia/arthritis, nonspecific rash, and weight loss may be some of the clinical pointers toward the presence of a connective tissue disease. A proper history, clinical examination, and the pattern distribution along with serologies most often clinch the diagnosis in most connective tissue disorders.

Case scenario A

A 57-year-old gentleman, diagnosed to be having RA since the past 6 years, has been having cough with scanty expectoration since 3 months. The cough is nonepisodic with no diurnal or postural variation. He is having associated progressive breathlessness such that he is unable to climb a flight of stairs which he was able to do 2 months back. He does not report any fever but has been having loss of appetite and is has lost 5 kg in the past 6 months. He is a smoker and does not consume alcohol. He has been on regular follow-up with his physician and is currently taking methotrexate 20 mg/week along with leflunomide 10 mg/day. In addition, he has been on folic acid along with calcium and vitamin D supplementations.

On examination, he was afebrile, and pulse rate was 94/min and BP was 118/70 mmHg. Respiratory rate was 20 cycles/minute, and saturation

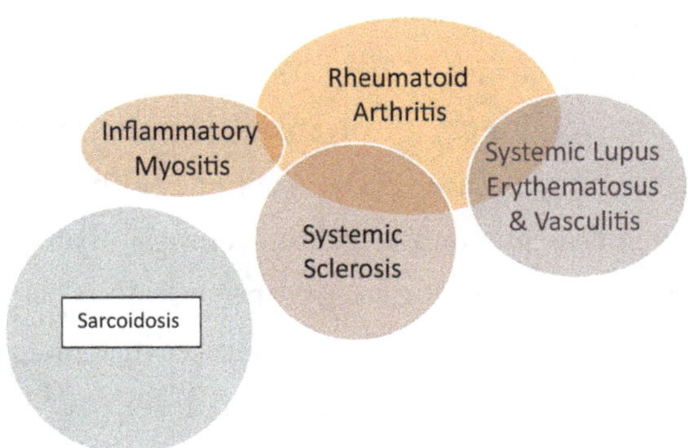

Figure 2: Disease phenotype and overlap pattern based on symptomatology of connective tissue disease and antibodies.

on room air was 96%. General physical examination was unremarkable for pallor, icterus, cyanosis, clubbing, lymphadenopathy, or pedal edema. He had deforming arthritis of the hands and feet along with nodules over the elbows. Cardiovascular examination was normal, and S1S2 was heard normally without any murmurs. Respiratory system: the upper respiratory tract was normal, and the lower respiratory tract examination was remarkable for decreased chest expansion of 2 cm and fine end inspiratory crackles in bilateral lung fields.

Rest of the examination was normal.

Questions:

How do we proceed?

What would be your clinical impression?

How do we investigate?

Clinical assessment — Middle-aged male with RA with probably active disease, with extraarticular manifestations in the form of rheumatoid nodules and probably a parenchymal lung disease.

RA and lung diseases

Most of the extraarticular manifestations are seen in the late stages of RA rather than early phases. Extra-articular manifestations are more common in patients who are antibody positive (rheumatoid factor [RF] and anticyclic citrullinated peptide antibody[ACPA]).

Upper airway involvement: Patients with longstanding RA can have involvement of the cricoarytenoid joints and can present with hoarseness of voice and very rarely stridor.

More common respiratory involvement is pulmonary parenchymal disease (interstitial lung disease [ILD]), rheumatoid nodules in the lungs and inflammation of the pleura (pleural thickening and effusions), airways, and pulmonary vasculature (vasculitis and pulmonary hypertension). Although rheumatoid arthritis is more common in females, rheumatoid arthritis associated-ILD (RA-ILD) occurs more frequently in males, with a male-to-female ratio as high as 2:1 in some studies.[4,5] Pleural involvement is a common pulmonary manifestation of rheumatoid arthritis, with small pleural effusions noted in up to 70% on autopsy studies.[6,7] However, only about 3%–5% of patients are symptomatic.[6,7] Most effusions are unilateral, which may or may not be associated with fever and pleuritic chest pain. Coexistent pericardial effusion may also be present. The typical "rheumatoid effusion" is a sterile exudative fluid with low pH (<7.3), low glucose (<60 mg/dL), and elevated lactate dehydrogenase (may be >700 IU/L) along with neutrophilic leucocytosis and the presence of ragocytes. The effusions may be pseudochylous and sometimes empyematous. It is essential to diligently look for any infections in a case of suspected rheumatoid pleural involvement.

Rheumatoid nodules can occur in the lungs, particularly in patients with longstanding disease and subcutaneous nodules. They are typically located along the interlobular septa or in subpleural regions. Nodules may be single or multiple, ranging in size from a few millimetres to several centimetres.[8]

It is important to note that methotrexate, which is the anchor drug for the treatment of RA does not seem to be truly related to the development of ILD observed in some patients as part of the natural history of RA (RA-ILD).[9]

Discussion: case scenario A

Undoubtedly, this patient is having RA with risk factors, namely, male sex, smoking, middle to elderly age-group, and longstanding disease for the development of pulmonary manifestations of RA and in this case, ILD.

When considering a diagnosis of RA-ILD, knowledge of the histopathological pattern of ILD by surgical lung biopsy may provide information that assists in the diagnosis and prognostication and has been considered the "gold standard" for diagnosis by some. While knowledge of the specific histopathological patterns of interstitial pneumonias may clarify histopathological diagnosis and be of prognostic value, this knowledge is usually not essential to determining a treatment regimen, which is invariably made up of immune modulating agents. Thus, in patients with known RA, and in the absence of clinical suspicion for infection and/or other respiratory complications, high-resolution computed tomography (HRCT) may be used to make a diagnosis of interstitial pneumonia. A variety of patterns are seen on HRCT scans in RA, with the most common being usual interstitial pneumonia (UIP), which occurs in 40%–62% of cases.[10,11] This is a notable difference from other connective tissue disorders, in which a nonspecific interstitial pneumonia (NSIP) pattern is most frequently seen.[10,12] NSIP is the second most common pattern, occurring in ~11%–32% of patients.[12] Additional patterns less commonly seen in RA include other patterns of interstitial pneumonia, including organizing pneumonia, diffuse alveolar damage (DAD), lymphocytic interstitial pneumonia (LIP), and DIP-like patterns. Combined pulmonary fibrosis and emphysema (CPFE) has also been demonstrated on HRCT scans in patients with RA.

Treatment with anti-inflammatory and/or immunosuppressive agents is recommended regardless of the pattern of fibrosis. This is in contrast to IPF, in which the use of immunosuppressive therapy has not demonstrated any clinical benefit. Steroids form the mainstay of treatment and steroid-sparing agents in the form of azathioprine, cyclophosphamide, mycophenolate, and rituximab have been used. The choice of agents in connective tissue disease related ILD depends on the pattern of ILD and overall disease activity. Agent switch may be often deemed necessary depending on the progression of ILD on serial functional assessments.

Case scenario B

A 23-year-old female patient comes to the emergency with a history of cough with hemoptysis since 3 months. There is a history of low-grade fever and generalized fatigue. There is history of swelling of both the feet since the past 15 days. There is no history of any decreased urine output. There is no history of any other bleeding tendencies. She was evaluated at a local hospital, and sputum smears were negative for AFB and was started on empirical ATT. She reports worsening of symptoms after commencement of ATT, and breathlessness has been progressively increasing.

On examination, she was pale with a respiratory rate of 26 cycles/second. Pulse rate was 120/minute, and she was unable to lie down supine. Accessory muscle of respiration were in use. There were nasal crusts and thick purulent secretions from the nasal cavity. Respiratory system involvement showed bilateral coarse crackles. Cardiac and other systems were normal except for bilateral pitting pedal edema.

Investigations showed a hemoglobin 7 g%, total WBH of 13,700/cu mm, and platelet of 256,000 cu mm with normal PT and APTT. Creatinine was 2.3 mg% with a BUN of 60 mg%. Potassium was 5.6 mEq/L. Urine routine microscopy was evident for albuminuria ++, no sugars with RBS of 50–60/HPF with 100 pus cells/HPF.

How do we approach this case?

Discussion: case scenario B

Case B has historical and clinical upper and lower respiratory disease along with pedal edema which is unresponsive ATT. Pan-airway involvement in Tb is, however, uncommon. This patient in addition to a respiratory disease has an ongoing renal disease as evident by pedal edema and decreased GFR along with albuminuria and sedimenturia. The possibility of pulmonary renal syndrome will need to be considered in such a scenario. A drop in hemoglobin and saturation along with fleeting pulmonary infiltrates is commonly seen in patients with an ongoing pulmonary hemorrhage.

Pulmonary–renal syndromes or lung–kidney syndromes[13] are clinical syndromes defined by a combination of diffuse alveolar hemorrhage (DAH) and glomerulonephritis. Pulmonary–renal syndromes are not a single entity but are caused by a wide variety of diseases, including various forms of primary systemic vasculitis (especially granulomatosis with polyangiitis [GPA] without eosinophilia and MPA), Goodpasture's syndrome (associated with autoantibodies to the alveolar and glomerular basement membrane), and SLE. The diagnosis rests on the identification of particular patterns of clinical, radiologic, pathologic, and laboratory features. Serologic testing is important in the diagnostic workup of patients presenting with a pulmonary–renal syndrome. The majority of cases of pulmonary–renal syndrome are associated with ANCAs, either c-ANCA or p-ANCA, due to autoantibodies against the target antigens proteinase-3 and myeloperoxidase respectively, ANA which is seen in patients with SLE or anti-GBM antibodies in Goodpasture's syndrome.

Apart from Goodpasture's syndrome, in SLE and ANCA-associated vasculitis, it is always recommended to have a tissue diagnosis which may help prognosticate the disease. However, this may not be possible in an acute situations as in the case in discussion. The treatment of choice in such a situation may be plasmapheresis, high-dose corticosteroids along with rituximab or cyclophosphamide. This is along with supportive measures such as mechanical ventilation and hemodialysis.

GPA without eosinophilia is a relapsing disease, and serial follow-up for disease assessment indices and a multidisciplinary approach is absolutely essential in improving the patient survival.

Case C

A 30-year-old patient has been having recurrent episodes of breathlessness since the past 1 month. There is no history of fever, cough with expectoration. There is no history of any chest pains or palpitations. There is no history of any bowel or bladder complaints. She has had three spontaneous abortions, and she had a history of left lower limb swelling 3 years back about which the details are unavailable.

On examination, she was afebrile with a respiratory rate of 22 cycles/minute with intermittent episodes of regular tachycardia of 130/minute. BP was 130/80 mmHg. JVP was raised with a prominent a wave. Cardiovascular and respiratory system were unremarkable. Breathing was abdominothoracic. There was no proximal muscle weakness.

Chest X-ray was normal; ECHO showed evidence of increased RV systolic pressure to 35 mm.

Discussion: case C

This patient gives a history of intermittent episodes of breathlessness. With a normal chest X-ray and features suggestive of right ventricular strain in the form of raised a wave on JVP and ECHO showing increased right ventricular systolic pressures. The general examination being normal with no evident skin changes takes the thoughts away from diseases like SSc, wherein skin tightening is evident. Breathing was abdominothoracic with no evidence of muscle weakness in diseases like inflammatory muscle disorders (PM/DM) which can lead to diaphragmatic muscle weakness causing respiratory difficulty.

The investigation of choice in this case scenario is D-dimer followed by CT pulmonary angiogram and Doppler to look for lower limb deep vein thrombosis as historically, intermittent leg swelling and spontaneous abortions in a female are pointers toward a pulmonary thromboembolic disease.

Pulmonary thromboembolic diseases

De novo pulmonary thromboembolic disease is more common in patients with and underlying pre-existing prothrombotic states. In the rheumatological setting, APS which may be primary or secondary, or diseases like inflammatory myopathies in which prolonged immobilization due to muscle weakness can give rise to spontaneous de no thrombosis.

Rheumatologic conditions are often inflammatory by nature. However, despite this mechanistic link between rheumatologic diseases and VTEs, these highly inflammatory conditions may be under-recognized as risk factors for hypercoagulability. The only exception is the well-known association between antiphospholipid antibodies in SLE and both venous and arterial thromboses. There are several case reports, retrospective cohort studies, and prospective observational analyses highlighting the increased risk of VTE in patients with rheumatologic diseases.[14–18] Most of the data in the literature reveal this concern in patients with RA and SLE, and the

SLE studies are focused mostly on increased risks associated with positive antiphospholipid status rather than on the innate hypercoagulability nature of this inflammatory disease.[18,19] VTEs seem to be linked to disease activity and/or inflammation in many of the inflammatory rheumatologic diseases.

Patients who develop VTEs have high rates of morbidity and mortality.[5] The incidence of first-time VTE in the United States is about 1 in 1,000 person-years.[4] Therefore, it is important to understand the excess magnitude of this issue in patients with inflammatory rheumatologic diseases. Ideally, the modifiable risk factors would be known and altered and poor outcomes mitigated.

Treatment of lung in rheumatic diseases

Most of the lung manifestations in rheumatologic diseases will require an intensifications of immunosuppression after ruling out an underlying infection or sometimes neoplastic conditions.

Azathioprine, cyclophosphamide, mycophenolate, and rituximab have been tried individually or sequentially depending on the response. The treatment outcomes especially in ILD is dependent on the initial mount of disease activity, serial functional assessments, and pre-existing underlying cardiac diseases.

Second-line agents are given in disorders which require long-term immunosuppression to prevent the progression of parenchymal pulmonary diseases, for example, SSc with ILD, DM with ILD, SLE with bronchiolitis obliterans, and so forth. The choice of agents will be dependent of the accompaniments of lung diseases, for example, azathioprine may be the drug of choice in patients with RA with ILD, cyclophosphamide (pulse therapy: 15 mg/kg body/dose or oral cyclophosphamide: 1–2 mg/kg)/azathioprine (2–3 mg/kg) or mycophenolate (2–3 g/day) in DM, rituximab (1 g × 2 doses given 2 weeks apart or 375 mg/m^2 × 4 doses) in pulmonary hemorrhage. However, it is important to note that the choice of second-line

Table 4: Therapeutics in CTD-associated lung diseases

Drug	Dose	Duration	Indications for lung involvement
IV pulse methylprednisolone	15–20 mg/kg/day	3 days	— Pulmonary alveolar hemorrhage — Collapsing lung syndrome
Prednisolone	0.5 mg to 1 mg/kg/day	4 weeks and then taper to 5 mg/day or less over a period of 3 months	— Ground-glass opacities — Bronchiolitis obliterans with organizing pneumonia — Induction remission in pulmonary vasculitis — Polyserositis of connective tissue disorder
Anticoagulation	Coumarins	INR 2.5–3.5	— Pulmonary thromboembolic disorders — Antiphospholipid antibody syndrome
Heart lung transplantation			— Pulmonary fibrosis with pulmonary hypertension
Plasma exchange		3–7 cycles	— Pulmonary alveolar hemorrhage

agent is never a rule and switches between different agents if often considered depending on the response and the adverse effects. Additive treatment such as antifibrotics, bronchodilators, and rehabilitative measures need to constituted in all treatment protocols wherever required.

Approach to connective tissue disease with lung involvement

Flow chart: approach to CTD and lung involvement.

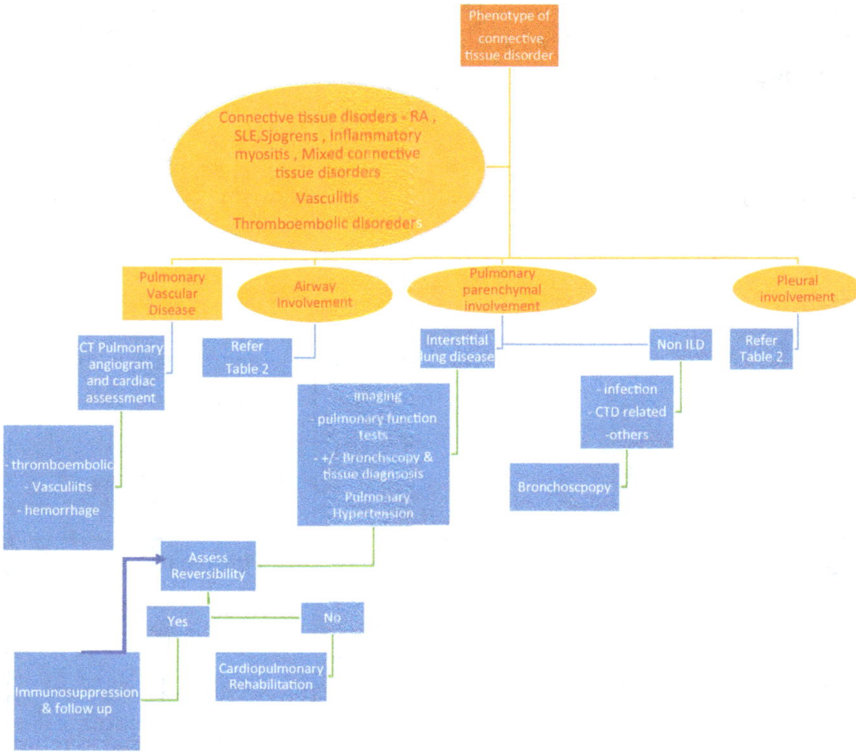

In CTD-associated ILDs, it is foremost important to identify the disease phenotype which depends on the symptomatology at presentation. Presence and pattern of joint involvement, distribution of skin rashes, muscle involvement, symptoms of Raynaud's, and ophthalmic symptoms may give some clues toward the disease phenotype. This clubbed together with the presence or absence of antibodies will help in identifying the disease phenotype and further evaluation of the organ involvement in connective tissue diseases.

Once the disease subset is identified, the pattern of respiratory involvement depending on the airway involvement, pulmonary parenchymal involvement, and pleural involvement aid in further workup of the patient.

Involvement may be unison or combined involvement of different components of the respiratory systems.

Investigations are either targeted toward exclusion of infective etiologies (pleural fluid analysis and bronchoscopy) or in aiding the diagnosis (CT/HRCT/CTPA/tissue diagnosis). It is pertinent to assess cardiac involvement at baseline and at follow-up in addition to lung functions in ILD which aid therapeutic decisions with respect to the intensity of immunosuppression (Table 4) and switch in immunosuppressive agents on need basis. During periods of flare of lung symptoms, an infective exacerbation needs to be excluded.

Pulmonary rehabilitation, vaccination for pneumococcus and influenza virus along with the use of prophylactic antibiotics of pneumocystis are essential in management of any chronic lung conditions, especially in CTD related lung diseases where immunosuppressive agents are commonly administered.

Conclusion

CTD-associated lung diseases need to encompass a significant proportion of population with chronic respiratory diseases whose incidence and prevalence varies amongst different ethnic groups and disease subsets. The manifestations are often protean, and early identification and treatment often results in favorable outcomes in these patients.

References and suggested readings

1. Antoniou KM, Margaritopoulos G, Economidou F, Siafakas NM. Pivotal clinical dilemmas in collagen vascular diseases associated with interstitial lung involvement. Eur Respir J. 2009;33:882–896.
2. Fischer A, West SG, Swigris JJ, Brown KK, du Bois RM. Connective tissue disease-associated interstitial lung disease: a call for clarification. Chest. 2010;138(2):251–256. doi: 10.1378/chest.10-0194.
3. Travis WD, Hunninghake G, King TE Jr, Lynch DA, Colby TV, Galvin JR, Brown KK, Chung MP, Cordier JF, du Bois RM, Flaherty KR, Franks TJ, Hansell DM, Hartman TE, Kazerooni EA, Kim DS, Kitaichi M, Koyama T,

Martinez FJ, Nagai S, Midthun DE, Müller NL, Nicholson AG, Raghu G, Selman M, Wells A. Idiopathic nonspecific interstitial pneumonia: report of an American Thoracic Society project. Am J Respir Crit Care Med. 2008 Jun 15;177(12):1338–1347.

4. Marigliano B, Soriano A, Margiotta D, et al. Lung involvement in connective tissue diseases: a comprehensive review and a focus on rheumatoid arthritis. Autoimmun Rev. 2013;12:1076–1084.
5. O'Dwyer DN, Armstrong ME, Cooke G, et al. Rheumatoid arthritis (RA) associated interstitial lung disease (ILD). Eur J Intern Med. 2013;24:597–603.
6. Balbir-Gurman A, Yigla M, Nahir AM, et al. Rheumatoid pleural effusion. Semin Arthritis Rheum. 2006;35:368–378.
7. Corcoran JP, Ahmad M, Mukherjee R, et al. Pleuro-pulmonary complications of rheumatoid arthritis. Respir Care. 2014;59:e55–e59.
8. Shaw M, Collins BF, Ho LA, Raghu G. Rheumatoid arthritis-associated lung disease. Eur Respir Rev. 2015;24:1–16. doi: 10.1183/09059180.00008014.
9. Fragoulis GE, Conway R, Nikiphorou E. Methotrexate and interstitial lung disease: controversies and questions. A narrative review of the literature. Rheumatology. 2019 Nov;58(11):1900–1906. doi: 10.1093/rheumatology/kez337.
10. de Lauretis A, Veeraraghavan S, Renzoni E. Review series: aspects of interstitial lung disease: connective tissue disease-associated interstitial lung disease: how does it differ from IPF? How should the clinical approach differ? Chron Respir Dis. 2011;8:53–82.
11. Hallowell RW, Horton MR. Interstitial lung disease in patients with rheumatoid arthritis: spontaneous and drug induced. Drugs. 2014;74:443–450.
12. Kim EJ, Elicker BM, Maldonado F, et al. Usual interstitial pneumonia in rheumatoid arthritis-associated interstitial lung disease. Eur Respir J. 2010;35:1322–1328.
13. Brusselle GG. Pulmonary-renal syndromes. Acta Clinica Belgica. 2007;62(2):88–96. doi: 10.1179/acb.2007.016.
14. Aviña-Zubieta JA, Lacaille D, Sayre EC, Kopec J, Choi HK, Esdaile JM. Risk of pulmonary embolism and deep vein thrombosis in systemic lupus erythematosus: a population-based cohort study. Arthritis Res Ther. 2012;14:A43. doi: 10.1186/ar3987.
15. Choi HK, Rho Y, Zhu Y, Cea-Soriano L, Aviña-Zubieta JA, Zhang Y. The risk of pulmonary embolism and deep vein thrombosis in rheumatoid

arthritis: a UK population-based outpatient cohort study. Ann Rheum Dis. 2013;72:1182–1187. doi: 10.1136/annrheumdis-2012-201669. [PubMed] [CrossRef] [Google Scholar]

16. Bacani AK, Gabriel SE, Crowson CS, Heit JA, Matteson EL. Noncardiac vascular disease in rheumatoid arthritis: increase in venous thromboembolic events? Arthritis Rheum. 2012;64:53–61. doi: 10.1002/art.33322. [PMC free article] [PubMed] [CrossRef] [Google Scholar]
17. Holmqvist ME, Neovius M, Eriksson J, Mantel Ä, Wållberg-Jonsson S, Jacobsson LTH, Askling J. Risk of venous thromboembolism in patients with rheumatoid arthritis and association with disease duration and hospitalization. JAMA. 2012;308:1350–1356. doi: 10.1001/2012.jama.11741. [PubMed] [CrossRef] [Google Scholar]
18. Calvo-Alén J, Toloza SMA, Fernández M, Bastian HM, Fessler BJ, Roseman JM, McGwin G, Jr, Vilá LM, Reveille JD, Alarcón GS; The LUMINA Study Group. Systemic lupus erythematosus in a multiethnic US cohort (LUMINA): XXV. Smoking, older age, disease activity, lupus anticoagulant, and glucocorticoid dose as risk factors for the occurrence of venous thrombosis in lupus patients. Arthritis Rheum. 2005 Jul;52(7):2060–2068.
19. Burgos PI, McGwin G Jr, Reveille JD, Vilá LM, Alarcón GS. Factors predictive of thrombotic events in LUMINA, a multi-ethnic cohort of SLE patients (LXXII). Rheumatology (Oxford). 2010 Sep;49(9):1720–1725.
20. Bax CE, Maddukuri S, Ravishankar A, Pappas-Taffer L, Werth VP. Environmental triggers of dermatomyositis: a narrative review. Ann Transl Med. 2021 Mar;9(5):434. doi: 10.21037/atm-20-3719. PMID: 33842655; PMCID: PMC8033368.

https://doi.org/10.1142/9789811271410_0042

42 Congenital lung lesions

Introduction

These are a group of rare and clinically significant congenital anomalies affecting the lungs and mediastinum. Recent advances in antenatal imaging and widespread availability have made most of these lesions being detected antenatally. A few decades ago, many of these lesions were considered fatal, and termination of pregnancy was recommended. However, now most lesions are successfully followed up perinatally and have good outcomes.

Incidence

The incidence varies from region to region. No definite data are available from India. The reported data suggest an incidence of 1:10,000 to 1:350,000. Nearly all lesions can be detected antenatally between 18 and 24 weeks of gestation. The lesions are typically classified as

1. Congenital pulmonary airway malformation (CPAM)
2. Congenital lobar emphysema
3. Pulmonary sequestration
4. Hybrid lesions

Embryology

Development of the lung begins at third week of gestation proceeding postnatally until 5–8 years of life for complete maturation. The stages of lung development are described as follows:

Stage	Gestation (weeks)	Parenchyma developed	Vasculature
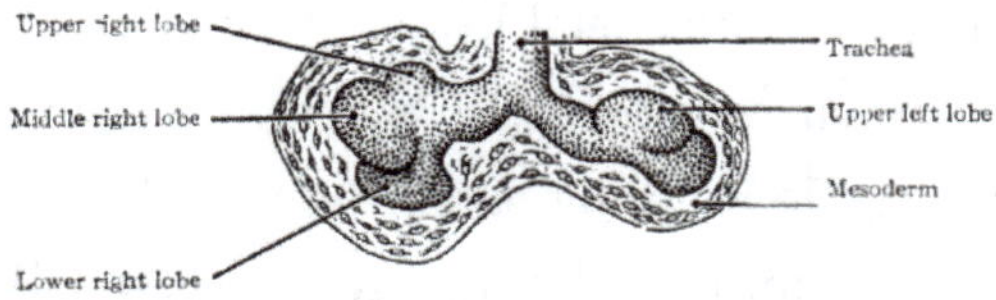 https://embryology.med.unsw.edu.au/embryology/index.php/File:Bailey287.jpg			
Embryonic	3–7 weeks	Organogenesis Lung bud as diverticula from foregut epithelium	Pulmonary artery Lobular artery
Pseudoglandular	5–16 weeks	Bronchi up to terminal bronchioles, preaching	Preacinar vessels
Canalicular	16–24 weeks	Epithelial differentiation into type 1 and 2 pneumocytes, alveolar sac starts forming	Intra-acinar arteries
Saccular	24–38 weeks	Maturation of alveoli production of surfactant	Alveolar ductal vessels
Alveolar	38 months to 8 years	Secondary septation, increase in number of alveoli	Alveolar capillary network

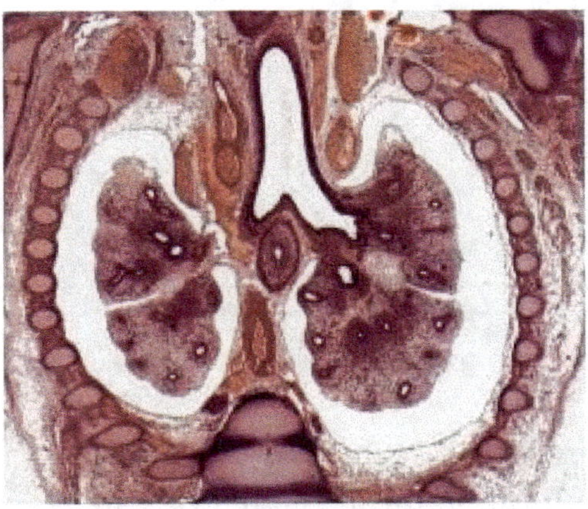

https://embryology.med.unsw.edu.au/embryology/index.php/File:ME54_001.jpg

Congenital pulmonary airway malformation

They are relatively common among the congenital lung lesions, can cause significant morbidity, hydrops, fetal loss, and hypoplasia of the adjacent lung. A CPAM is a hamartomatous mass of abnormal fetal lung tissue with a disorganized distribution of lung parenchyma and conducting airways. This results in the development of lung cysts with loss of lung tissue. The cysts may be single or multiple. The lesions are malformations since many of them were cystic and had adenomatoid tissue. However, it is not always present; hence, the newer nomenclature has been accepted.

Classification

Based on the level of origin and histological picture, they are classified into five types. With type 0 starting from trachea–bronchi to type 4 which is the alveoli. Types 1 to 3 were initially described, and types 0 and 4 were added later.

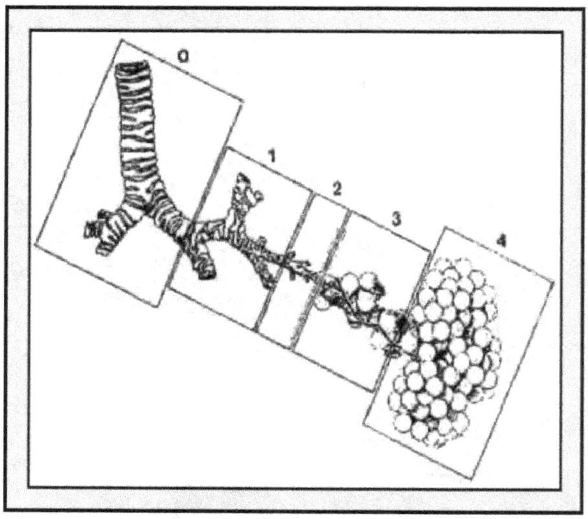

https://www.ncbi.nlm.nih.gov/pmc/articles/PMC3410507/figure/F1/

Type 0 (Tracheobronchial) — these lesions appear like a solid mass of tissue consisting of cartilage of smooth muscle reminiscent of a bronchi. Usually lethal.

Type 1 (Bronchial/bronchiolar) — large cysts 2–10 cm, most common of all types, accounting for nearly 50% of all cases.
Lined by pseudostratified columnar epithelium and covered by smooth muscles and connective tissue. Rarely, cartilaginous tissue may be found. Echolucent cysts single or multiple on USG, fills up with air after birth once the fluid within the cyst is absorbed.

Type 2 (Bronchiolar) — second most common lesions. Approximately 35% of all CPAMs. The cysts are now smaller between 0.5 and 2 cm, and the lining epithelium is cuboid or columnar. Few smooth muscles and connective tissue are found but sparse compared to type 1 lesions. The lung consistency assumes a spongy feel. Associated with other congenital anomalies.

Type 3 (Bronchiolar/alveolar) — cysts are now much smaller, less than 0.5 cm. Most of them become microscopic cysts and appear like bronchioles. They account for around 10% of cases.

Type 4 (Distal acinar) — these are alveolar in origin. It is a single large cyst with a flat epithelial lining and have been associated with pleuropulmonary blastomas.

They have also been classified into two major subgroups — bronchiolar and acinar–alveolar type depending on the epithelial differentiation. Types 1 to 3 are bronchiolar, and type 4 is acinar–alveolar.

Morphologically, they are represented as microcystic (<5 mm) and macrocystic types (>5 mm), described by Azdick et al., and are used for antenatal detection and prognostication. Macrocystic lesions are echolucent, and microcystic types appear as echogenic solid lesions interspersed between normal lung tissue.

Microcystic CPAMs are generally larger, associated with poorer outcome due to mass effect, lung hypoplasia, pulmonary vasculature anomalies, and hydrops.

Macrocystic CPAMs are slow growing, rarely cause lung compromise early in life and can be followed up for delayed surgical treatment.

Clinical features

Antenatal

CPAMs cause compression of normal lung parenchyma, leading to lung hypoplasia. Compression of vena cava leads to hydrops fetalis. Types 0 and 3 usually tend to be fatal. With fetal hydrops, the mother may develop features of mirror syndrome or Ballantyne syndrome or triple edema characterized by maternal preeclampsia and edema. Antenatal detection is usually during anomaly scans during 19–21 weeks of gestation where lung cysts — single or multiple, thin or thick walled surrounded by lung parenchyma — are reported. In solid lesions, the appearance is of echogenic tissue within the hemithoraces. In pregnancies with abnormal fetal karyotype and early-onset hydrops, termination can be discussed early.

Monitoring of nonhydrops fetuses with lung cysts

Rapid development of cysts may occur up to 20–25 weeks of gestation. Later on, nearly 20% of these lesions show regression in size and may disappear completely. Serial monitoring with 4 weekly ultrasound is done to monitor growth unless signs of hydrops or maternal PIH appear. Cases showing regression tend to have a lower CVR (CPAM volume ratio) of less than 1.6. The cause for regression of CPAM has not been determined. It is hypothesized to be due to disproportionate increase in the size of a normal lung tissue with gestation (during saccular stage) compared to a cyst. A fraction of antenatally regressing lesions may persist or progress postnatally and require follow-up imaging after birth.

Fetal intervention

Cases with evolving hydrops with polyhydramnios and large cysts are suitable for intervention in utero.

Medical management involves administration of corticosteroids — betamethasone to the mother at or after 24 weeks of gestation. The mechanism of action in these cases is not exactly known. Many lesions do show regression.

Fetal surgical interventions include:

1. Aspiration of the cyst for decompression.
2. Sclerotherapy after aspiration with ethanolamine oleate.
3. Thoracoamniotic shunts.
4. Fetal surgical excision of the CPAM.
   Surgical excision carries a high risk of fetal demise and may be suitable for selected cases with solid lesions (microcystic CPAMs).

Postnatal monitoring

Asymptomatic babies can be opted for expectant management, and further imaging is done electively. All postnatally persisting lesions require resection. Complications like pneumonia, bleeding into the cysts, and rupture of the cyst with pneumothorax. They have a predisposition to develop lung malignancy — pleuropulmonary blastoma which is similar to rhabdomyosarcoma with primitive lung tissue.

Surgical treatment

Anatomical resection — Lobectomy
Segmentectomy

Bronchopulmonary sequestration

Bronchopulmonary sequestration (BPS) is a mass of nonfunctioning lung tissue that has no connection with the tracheobronchial tree and receives its anomalous blood supply from the systemic circulation. Because of this anomalous blood supply, some argue that it should be classified as vascular anomaly. Sequestrations are usually solid in nature. Pathologically, these lesions show parenchymal maldevelopment similar to microcystic CCAMs.

There are two types of sequestrations, namely, extralobar and intralobar. Extralobar sequestrations are outside the normal lung and is surrounded by its own pleura. Intralobar sequestrations are situated within the investing pleura of the normal lung. Both varieties can occur simultaneously, or an entire lung can be sequestered. Intralobar sequestrations usually involve the basilar segments of the lower lobes more commonly on the left side. Rarely, they may occur in the upper thorax, below the diaphragm, within the mediastinum or pericardium. As they are derivatives of the foregut, BPS may communicate with the esophagus or stomach. Blood supply can come from arteries above or below the diaphragm, but the venous drainage can be either to the pulmonary or systemic venous circulation. There can be significant arteriovenous shunting leading to high-output cardiac failure or bleeding with massive hemoptysis or hemothorax.

A BPS appears as a well-defined hypodense echodense mass on prenatal ultrasonography. The pathognomonic feature of BPS is detection by color Doppler of a systemic artery supplying the fetal lung lesion. Fetal MRI is useful in differentiating CCAM from BPS where fetal Doppler fails.

Extralobar BPS is more common in males (3:1), is more common on the left side, and can be associated with other anomalies. Isolated small noncystic extralobar BPS rarely requires treatment. In contrast, intralobar BPS usually presents as recurrent pneumonia or lung abscess, thus requiring resection (lobectomy or segmentectomy). It is important to ligate the systemic feeding artery usually found in the inferior pulmonary ligament; otherwise, accidental division of feeding artery can cause uncontrolled hemorrhage.

Job's syndrome

Introduction

It is a rare idiopathic primary immunodeficiency disorder characterized by recurrent semisoft tissue infections and recurrent sinopulmonary infections, with raised IgE levels in serum. First reported in 1966, this congenital immunodeficiency disorder has peripheral and tissue eosinophilia and extrapulmonary features involving the face, teeth, and skeletal affections.[1]

Pathophysiology

Some cases may show autosomal dominant transmission with linkage to chromosome; otherwise, pathophysiology of Job's syndrome (hyper IgE syndrome) is poorly understood; cytokine and chemokine dysregulation in hyper IgE syndrome has been studied.[2] There is a delayed hypersensitivity reaction to antigens, perhaps due to defective chemotaxis of neutrophils because of defective production of gamma interferon. The disease starts in infancy, but diagnosis may be delayed up to childhood. Sex predilection is absent.

Clinical features

Clinically, mucocutaneous manifestations include chronic candidiasis/onychomycosis, eczema, and cold abscess of skin/soft tissue. Sinopulmonary involvements include recurrent *Staphylococcus aureus* pneumonia with pneumatoceles, with recurrent otitis media. Patient presents with fever, cough, and mucopurulent sputum. Patient may look pale, and clubbing is present. Chest examination may reveal coarse crepitation scattered over the affected areas. Extrapulmonary manifestations include retained primary tooth/double row of teeth or unerupted permanent teeth. Scoliosis may occur in adolescents, and they may remain short stature also.[3] Coarse face, with prominent brow and supraorbital ridge is another feature. Fracture may occur due to osteoporosis.[4]

Diagnosis

Investigations reveal eosinophilia in blood and tissues. Pyogenic organism usually *Staphylococcus* is isolated and cultured from sputum. Total leukocytosis with raised eosinophils and raised ESR and the presence of toxic granules in neutrophils are observed. Plain X-ray chest may reveal varying pictures of consolidation, pneumatoceles, bronchiectasis, and lung abscess. Lymph node biopsy shows histopathological findings such as dermatopathic lymphadenitis, and granulation tissue having an increased number of eosinophils and with put any granuloma formation.

Anti-*S. aureus* IgE and IgM are raised, and IgA is lowered. Serum IgE levels are raised. IgE directed against *S. aureus* offers a relatively specific diagnostic value. Osteoporotic changes in plain X-rays of long bone may offer additional diagnostic clue.

Management

It includes treatment of the infection and the use of prophylactic antimicrobial with extra care for personal hygiene and excellent sanitation to reduce mortality and morbidity. Bone marrow transplantation offers no relief to hyper IgE syndrome.[8] Acute pneumonia in Job's syndrome can be offered intravenous adjunct therapy.[9]

References

1. Abhilash N, et al. Congenital immunodeficiency disorder. JAPI. 2007;56: 808–809.
2. Chehimi J, et al. Cytokine and chemokine dysregulation in hyper-IgE syndrome. Philadelphia, PA: The Children's Hospital of Philadelphia. 2001;100:49–56.

Lymphangioleiomyomatosis

Introduction

Lymphangioleiomyomatosis (LAM) is a rare pulmonary idiopathic, diffuse, progressive interstitial lung disorder, primarily affecting the women of reproductive age-group, and is characterized by an abnormal nonneoplastic proliferation of smooth-muscle-like cells called LAM cells," involving the small airways, pulmonary microvasculature, and lymphatic structures, leading to airways obstruction, pulmonary hemorrhages, chylous pleural effusion, and pneumothorax. Hormonal factors are suspected to play a role since the disorder primarily occurs in pre-menopausal young childbearing women. Its prevalence in the United Kingdom, France, and the United States is one per million, its prevalence in Asia is lower, and its prevalence in Singapore and Korea is 0.24 and 0.03 per 100,000, respectively.

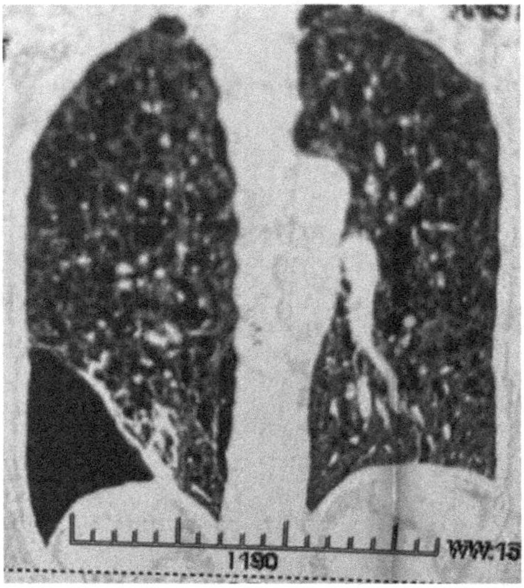

Figure 1: Lymphangioleiomyomatosis.

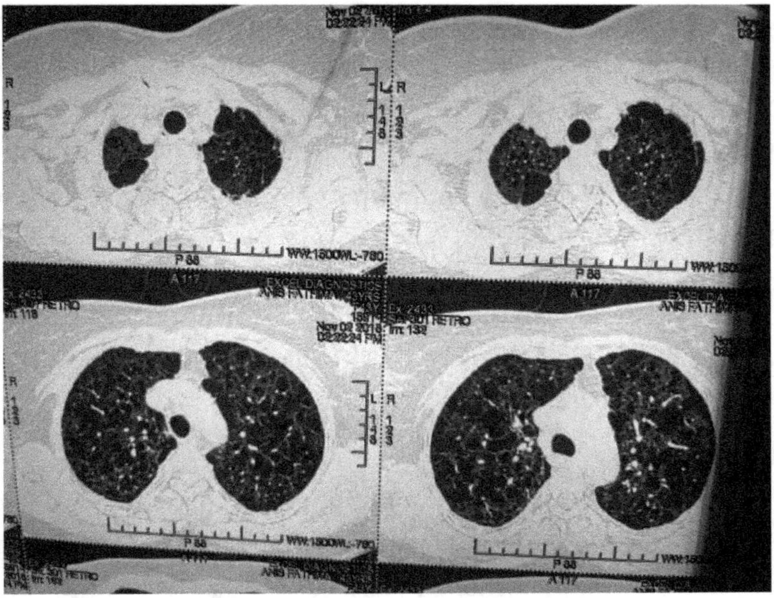

Figure 2: CT scans of LAM.

Clinical presentation

Clinically, a patient presents with progressive dyspnea.[1] Recurrent, bilateral spontaneous pneumothorax can be seen in 50% of cases.[2] Those with lymphatic disruption may present with chylothorax. Often, there is an associated wasting. Hemoptysis may occur in a few. Clinical signs are not pathognomonic. There can be features of hyperinflation, pleural effusion, or pneumothorax. Chest X-ray may reveal prominent cystic changes in addition to reticulonodular markings. Clubbing is absent. Hamartomatous tumors composed of smooth muscle, blood vessels, and adipose tissue as well as intra-abdominal or pelvic masses.[3] So, extrapulmonary features include lymph node masses, chylous ascites uterine fibroids, and renal angiomyolipomas.

Pathogenesis

It is a hormone-dependent disease, featuring smooth muscle-like cell proliferation, occurring exclusively in women, worsened by pregnancy perhaps. Lung functions slowly worsen after menopause. A marker for LAM cells is positioned on chromosome 12q 13–15.[4] Estrogens are found to accelerate the growth of the lesion. High mitotic and low apoptotic activities are seen in LAM cells with features of specific estrogen receptors.[5] Gp 100 m RNA in the lungs of LAM patients has been demonstrated by cellular and molecular studies. Gp 100 immunoreactivity in small electron-dense granules having fine lamellar structure has been seen under an electron microscope.

Pathology

Pathologically, entire pulmonary interstitium is involved by LAM and is characterized by abnormal proliferation of atypical smooth muscle cells in the peribronchial, perilymphatic, and perivascular areas which over a period of time can grow to obstruct the airways with aggregates of lymphoid cells, terminal airspaces may show diffuse cystic dilatation, the cystic walls showing lining of smooth muscle.[6] Cystic changes form the hallmark of the disease. These smooth muscle cells — LAM cells — are heterogeneous in nature. Collagen deposits are present between the muscle cells; fibrosis is, however, not seen. LAM cells may penetrate the essel wall, secondary to which microscopic hemorrhage is common. Peribronchiolar proliferating tissue may circumstantially narrow the bronchioles. Occlusion of venules may result in pulmonary venous hypertension and hemoptysis. Chylous pleural effusion may result from obstruction of lymphatic channels.

Diagnosis

Features of emphysema, recurrent pneumothorax, and a chylous effusion in a young woman should arouse the suspicion of LAM. Cystic nature of the disease can be demonstrated by HRCT,[7] in the form of diffuse, small thin-walled cysts and ground-glass appearance. Chest X-ray may be variable,[1] depending on the presence of pneumothorax or pleural effusion, exhibiting hyperinflation with cystic dilation of airspaces. Unlike other interstitial lung diseases (ILDs), lungs are hyperinflated in LAM rather than small. It is the course reticulonodular shadows that appear because of compression smooth muscle-rich interstitial tissue by dilated cystic airspaces. Lymphatic obstruction may produce Keriey B septa! lines on chest X-ray. Pulmonary function tests reveal increased total lung capacity with increased residual volume, expressing an increased gas trapping. FEV and FVC *are* deceased. So, obstructive and combined obstructive–restrictive ventilatory defects with impaired gas transfer are commonly seen in patients with LAM. Pleural fluid analysis reveals the presence of chyle (giving milky appearance), having raised triglyceride levels more than 100 mg/dL and presence of chylomicrons. Open lung or transbronchial biopsy provide sufficient characteristic histologic picture HBM 45 staining (monoclonal antibody which in the lung stains only LAM cells) further helps in diagnosing LAM. HRCT of the thorax reveals thin-walled cysts of 2 mm to an almost imperceptible thickness size distributed through and the lung fields with normal lung parenchyma in between. The cysts are differentiated from honeycombing due to ILD by their diffuse distribution (subpleural distribution in ILDs) and presence of normal lung parenchyma in between.

Differential diagnosis

These cysts can be differentiated from honeycombing due to ILDs by their diffuse distribution (subpleural location in ILDS) and the presence of relatively normal intervening parenchyma. LAM is one of the chronic ILDs that needs to be differentiated from eosinophilic granuloma. Eosinophilic granuloma exhibits the features of multiple, thin-walled cysts upper and middle lobes of the lung. Stellate pattern of fibrosis with presence of Langerhans histiocytosis can be demonstrated on histologic studies. Pulmonary involvement in tuberous sclerosis poses another difficult differential diagnosis. It is a congenital hamartoma of autosomal dominant inheritance,[8] commonly found in middle-aged females. Chylothorax is very rare. Idiopathic pulmonary fibrosis can be differentiated from LAM by its predilection for peripheral lung fields, with nonuniformly distributed cysts. Both leiomyoma and LAM affect females in their reproductive age and exhibit muscle-like cellular proliferation, perhaps both do share a genetic origin.[9] Cystic changes with preserved lung volume *can* in Langerhans cell histiocytosis, sarcoidosis, and extrinsic allergic alveolitis. In sarcoidots is, HRCT findings e linear or finely nodular interstitial shadow, ground-glass opacification, and segmental air space disease.

Treatment

No satisfactory treatment of LAM is available. Hormonal manipulation and ovarian ablation have been tried. Oophorectomy and progesterone therapy may yield stabilization. Response is better to progesterone therapy in those having impaired lung functions. Beneficial response has been obtained with tamoxifen 20 mg/day[10] and analogues of luteinizing hormone-releasing hormone (LHRH). Pleurodesis has been noted for recurrent pneumothorax or pleural effusion[11] Chylous pleural effusion should not be drained as it; to loss of proteins.

Progression of the disease, as indicated by TLC > 130%, FEV,/FVC < 50%, FEW < 30% and severe cystic disease on and can consider the candidate fit for lung transplantation." However, recurrence of the disease in transplanted lung requires to continue hormonal therapy.

Prognosis

Prognosis is variable, since the rate of progression of LAM is variable. Pregnancy and the use of estrogen preparations precipitate and accelerate the disease process. Remission of the disease may follow menopause. Severe cystic disease on biopsy, indicated by increased TLC and decreased FEV_1/FVC ratio, predicts poor prognosis. Respiratory failure and death express the ultimate of this slowly progressive disorder, that appeared in 1937 in literature; the etiology is still eluding us.

References and suggested readings

1. Singh A, Singh J. Sudden onset of dyspnea in a woman with skin lesions and lung cysts. Lung India. 2013;20:164–165.
2. Shankar PS. Lymphangioleiomyomatosis. Med Update. 2000;8(2):25–26.
3. Torres EU, et al. Extrapulmonary LAM and lymphangiomatous cysts in tuberous sclerosis complex. Mayo Clin Pract. 1995;70:641–648.
4. NHLBI workshop summary. Report of workshop on lymphangioleiomyomatosis. National Heart, Lung, and Blood Institute. Am J Respir Crit Care Med. 1999;159:679–683.
5. Usuki J, et al. Inverse correlation between markers of cell proliferation and expression of melanosomal antigens in smooth muscle melanoma cell lines (Abstract). Am J Respir Crit Care Med. 1998;157:A806.
6. Kitaichi M, et al. Pulmonary lymphangioleiomyomatosis: a report of 46 patients including a clinicopathologic study of prognostic factors. Am J Respir Crit Care Med. 1995;151:527–533.
7. Johnson SR, Tattersfields AE. Clinical experience of LAM in the UK. Thorax. 2000;55:1052–1057.

8. Castro M, et al. Pulmonary tuberous sclerosis. Chest. 1995;107:189–195.
9. Mitra S, Ghosal AG, Bhattacharya P. Pregnancy unmasking LAM. JAPI. 2004;52:828–830.
10. Verma SK, Verma SK. Pulmonary lymphangioleiomyomatosis. Lung India. 2007;24:150–152.
11. Mc Cormack FX, et al. LAM and leiomyoma: possibility of shared genetic origins? IN: J Moss, ed. LAM and other diseases characterized by smooth muscle proliferation. New York: Marcel Dekkar. 1998;373–386.
12. Trulock EP. Lung transplantation: special consideration and outcome in LAM. IN: Moss, ed. LAM and other diseases characterized by smooth muscle proliferation. New York: Marcel Dekkar. 1998;65–78.
13. Al Jadaan SA, Alaqeel SM, Alsadoun N. Clinicopathological features of resected pediatric congenital lung and mediastinal lesions: a single institution experience. Saudi Med J. 2021 Feb;42(2):209–212.
14. Ceylan KC, Batihan G, Üçvet A, Gürsoy S. Surgery in congenital lung malformations: the evolution from thoracotomy to VATS, 10-year experience in a single center. J Cardiothorac Surg. 2021 May 17;16(1):131.
15. Nathan M, Levine JC, Van Rompay MI; Pediatric Heart Network Investigators. Impact of major residual lesions on outcomes after surgery for congenital heart disease. J Am Coll Cardiol. 2021 May 18;77(19):2382–2394.

https://doi.org/10.1142/9789811271410_0043

43 Pleural effusion

Introduction

A simple definition would be "Pleural effusion is the pathological accumulation of fluid within the pleural space due a wide variety of causes. The normal pleural fluid production is around 30 mL/day, and a homeostasis is maintained. The pleural fluid is necessary to reduce the friction during the respiratory movements and has a lubricating effect. Initially, it was thought that the pleural space was a potential space, but by now, it is clear that the pleural space is approximately 18–20 μm, and the visceral and the parietal pleural actually do not touch each other during normal respiration. The normal pleural fluid at any given moment is around 1 mL or less; it just coats the visceral and parietal pleural surfaces. The normal rate of pleural fluid production per hour is around 0.01 mL/kg body weight. The removal of the fluid from the pleural space is through the pores in the parietal pleural that drain into the lymphatics. The normal pleural pressures are negative relative to the atmospheric pressure and helps to keep the lung expanded. The surface of the parietal pleura is quite large and is approximately 1,000 cm^2.

For the accumulation of the pleural fluid, usually the generation of the pleural fluid has to increase and its absorption has to decrease. Any increase in the pleural fluid generation is easily cleared. If only the increased fluid generation is the cause of pleural effusion, it has to increase more than 30 times the normal pleural fluid production rate. The following are the three common reasons for accumulation of the pleural fluid:

a. An increase in permeability, most commonly due to inflammation that leads to an exudative pleural effusion is the most common cause of pleural effusion.

b. An increase in hydrostatic pressure that leads to a transudative effusion.
c. A decrease in oncotic pressure that leads to a transudative effusion.

There are other less common causes of pleural effusion, and it is important to remember them as well.

a. Movement of the fluid from across the pores in the diaphragm. Depending on the nature of the ascetic fluid, the pleural effusion is similarly an exudate or a transudate. In some cases, both ascites and pleural effusion are detected, and it is easy to suspect an abdominal pathology. Sometimes, only pleural fluid is detected, and there is no ascites, though the primary pathology is in the abdomen and not in the lungs. There is a natural tendency for the fluid to migrate to the pleural space due to its negative pressure.
b. Increased production of pleural fluid due to malignant infiltration of the pleural surfaces, which leads to an exudative effusion.
c. Increased pleural space due to active collapse of the lung causing an increased negative pressure in the pleural space that leads to a transudative effusion.
d. Decreased clearance or drainage of the pleural fluid due to obstruction of the pores due to pleural fibrosis that leads to exudative effusion.
e. Decreased clearance of the fluid due to obstruction of the lymph channels that leads to an exudative effusion.
f. Rarely, transudative effusions can occur due to poor clearance of the fluid from the pleural surfaces. These pleural effusions are usually small in size.

Causes of pleural effusion

It is extremely important for the clinician to identify the cause of the pleural effusion. Is it due to a local cause or a systemic cause? If it is a transudate, it is very likely due to a systemic cause, and if it is an exudate, it is very likely to be due to local cause. There are exceptions of course. A collapse is an example of a local cause that can cause a transudative effusion, and collagen vascular disease is an example of a systemic disease that has caused an exudative effusion. The following table enumerates the most common causes of transudative and exudative effusions seen in the clinical practice.

Transudative effusion	Exudative effusion
Due to an increased hydrostatic pressure Cardiac failure (left sided or CCF) Glomerulonephritis Constrictive pericarditis SVC obstruction	Local inflammation increasing permeability Pneumonia and lung abscess — Bacterial — Tubercular — Fungal — Parasitic — Viral Bronchiectasis with infections
Due to a decreased osmotic pressure Cirrhosis Nephrotic syndrome Hypoalbuminemia due to any cause (malnutrition, malabsorption)	Local lesions increasing fluid production or obstructing the pleural fluid clearance Malignancy Primary lung cancer Mesothelioma Lymphoma Secondary of metastatic lung cancers
Other causes Myxedema Pulmonary embolism	Systemic inflammatory diseases Collagen vascular diseases Systemic lupus erythematosus Rheumatoid disease Wegener's granulomatosis Churg–Strauss syndrome Sjogren's syndrome
Abdominal causes Transudative ascites — cirrhosis of the liver Meigs syndrome Urinothorax	Occupational lung diseases Asbestosis

(*Continued*)

(*Continued*)

Transudative effusion	Exudative effusion
	Abdominal and pelvic causes Pancreatitis Subphrenic abscess Meigs syndrome
	Other causes Sarcoidosis Uremia Pulmonary embolism Chylothorax
	Drug-induced pleural effusion Amiodarone Drug-induced lupus (INH, hydralazine)

Mechanism of pleural effusion

1. **Increased pleural fluid formation, in turn, is attributed to the following factors:**
   A. Increased interstitial fluid in the lung
   B. Increased intravascular pressures in the pleura
   C. Increased permeability of the capillaries in the pleura
   D. Increased pleural fluid protein levels
   E. Decreased pleural pressures
   F. Increased fluid in the peritoneal cavity
   G. Disruption of the thoracic duct
   H. Disruption of blood vessels in the thorax

2. **Decreased pleural fluid absorption, in turn, is attributed to the following factors:**
   A. Parietal pleura lymphatics obstruction
   B. Raised systemic vascular pressures
   C. Pleural aquaporin system disruption

Pathogenesis of pleural effusions

(SCORER — normally the capacity of the lymphatics to remove the pleural fluid is 0.20 mL/kg/hour = rate of fluid formation (0.01 mL/kg/hour) × 20 times).

Mechanism of pleural effusion

1. INCREASED PLEURAL FLUID FORMATION, IN TURN, IS ATTRIBUTED TO THE FOLLOWING FACTORS

-- INCREASED INTERSTITIAL FLUID IN THE LUNG

LVF - PNEUMONIA - CONSTRICTIVE PERICARDITIS - MASSIVE PULMONARY EMBOLISM - PERICARDIAL EFFUSION

-- INCREASED INTRAVASCULAR PRESSURES IN PLEURA

RVF/LVF - SUPERIOR VENA CAVA SYNDROME - CIRRHOSIS - NEPHROTIC SYNDROME - MALNUTRITION - SMALL BOWEL DISEASE

-- INCREASED PERMEABILITY OF THE CAPILLARIES IN THE PLEURA

PLEURAL INFLAMMATION - MYXEDEMA - SMALL PULMONARY EMBOLISM - RAISED VEGF

-- DECREASED PLEURAL PRESSURES

LUNG ATELECTASIS INCREASED ELASTIC RECOIL OF LUNG

-- INCREASED FLUID IN THE PERITONEAL CAVITY

ASCITES - LIVER TRANSPLANTATION - HEPATOHYDROTHORAX - PERITONEAL DIALYSIS

-- DISRUPTION OF BLOOD VESSELS IN THE THORAX

VENO-OCCLUSIVE DISEASE - SUBARACHANOID PLEURAL FISTULA - CENTRAL VENOUS OCCLUSION

-- INCREASED PLEURAL FLUID PROTEIN LEVELS

-- DISRUPTION OF THE THORACIC DUCT

---

2. CAUSES OF DECREASED PLEURAL FLUID ABSORPTION
A. Parietal pleura lymphatics obstruction
B. Raised systemic vascular pressures
C. Pleural aquaporin system disruption

Classification based on etiology

1. Transudative effusions
2. Parapneumonic effusions
3. Empyematous effusions
4. Tuberculous effusions
5. Secondary to fungal infections
6. Secondary to parasitic effusions
7. Due to HIV
8. Secondary to pulmonary embolism
9. Secondary to git diseases
10. Secondary to heart diseases
11. Secondary to obstetrical diseases
12. Secondary to collagen vascular diseases
13. Secondary to drug reaction
14. Secondary to miscellaneous diseases
15. Hemothorax
16. Chylothorax and pseudochylothorax
17. Hydropneumothorax

...

CLASSIFICATION BASED ON CAUSES ------------------------------

TRANSUDATIVE	**EXUDATIVE**
A-RAISED HYDROSTATIC PRESSURES	A-NEOPLASTIC DISEASES
B-DECREASED CAPILLARY ONCOTIC PRESSURES	B-INFECTIONS
C-TRANSMISSION FROM PERITONEUM	C-PULMONARYEMBOLISMS/INFARCTION
D-INCREASED CAPILLARY PERMEABILITY	D-GIT DISEASES
E- OTHER VENOUS/IATROGENIC CAUSES	E-COLLAGEN VASCULAR DISEASES
	F- OTHER CAUSES

Exudative pleural effusions based on etiology

1. Neoplastic	2. Infections	3. Vascular	4. GIT disorders	5. Collagen vascular diseases/immune disorders	6. Others
— Metastatic diseases — Mesothelioma — Lymphomas	— Tuberculosis — HIV — Pneumonia, abscess — Actinomycosis and nocardiosis — Fungal — Viral — Parasitic	Pulmonary embolism and infarction	— Esophageal perforations — Pancreatic diseases — Intra-abdominal abscesses — Post abdominal surgery	— Rheumatoid pleuritis — Systemic lupus erythematosus — Wegener's granulomatosis — Eosinophilic granulomatosis	— Sarcoidosis — Drug reactions — Asbestos exposure — Meigs syndrome — Yellow nail syndrome — Radiation therapy — Hemothorax — Chylothorax

Pleural effusions in special situations

1. In ICUs — 8.4% of all pleural effusions
   24.4% — transudative effusion
   42.7% — parapneumonic effusion
   32.9% — noninfectious exudates
2. Massive pleural effusions requires immediate thoracocentesis
   — There is high incidence of empyema in patients with effusion in medical ICU.
   — On doing thoracocentesis, mean PaO_2 improves for patients on mechanical ventilation.

Pleural effusion: clinical features and diagnosis

Clinical manifestations

Symptoms

1. Determined by the underlying pathological process causing pleural effusion.
2. In small effusions, the patient may be asymptomatic.
3. Chest pain
   a. Pleuritic chest pain; indicates inflammation of the parietal pleura.
   b. Dull aching chest pain; suggestive of pleural malignancy.
   c. Referred pain to the abdomen due to distribution of intercostal nerves.
4. Nonproductive cough: either due to inflammation of the pleura or contact between bronchial walls due to lung compression by the fluid.
5. Dyspnea; often due to larger pleural effusions as they cause a significant reduction in lung volumes.
   Dyspnea disproportionate to the volume of effusion is observed in the following conditions:
   a. Pleural effusion with underlying parenchymal involvement.
   b. Ventricular filling may be compromised, leading to reduced cardiac output causing dyspnea.
6. A history of cancer can be suggestive of a malignant pleural effusion (MPE). Recent leg swelling or deep vein thrombosis (DVT) may result in an effusion related to pulmonary embolism.

7. A history of recent or current pneumonia suggests a parapneumonic effusion, either complicated (empyema) or uncomplicated.
8. Previous trauma may result in hemothorax or chylothorax. Previous exposure to asbestos is common in patients who have a benign effusion related to the exposure or have mesothelioma.
9. Recent esophageal dilatation or endoscopy can result in esophageal rupture.
10. Certain medications, including amiodarone, methotrexate, phenytoin, and nitrofurantoin, can cause pleural effusions. Rheumatoid arthritis and other autoimmune conditions can also result in effusions.
11. A sign such as hemoptysis may be associated with a malignant neoplasm, pulmonary embolism, or severe tuberculosis.
12. Fever occurs in tuberculosis, empyema, and pneumonia. Weight loss can be associated with a malignant neoplasm and tuberculosis.

Signs

Inspection:

a. Limitation of movement on the affected side.
b. Enlargement of hemithorax with bulging of intercostal spaces.

Palpation:

a. Tracheal deviation and mediastinal shift to the opposite side due to large effusions. An exception is the presence of ipsilateral mass lesion causing fixing of the mediastinum.
b. Decreased or absent tactile vocal fremitus.
c. Shifting of the apex beat.

Percussion:

a. Dull to stony dull note on percussion more toward the lung bases.
b. Slow shifting dullness.
c. Hyper-resonance above the level of effusion due to compensatory emphysema.

Auscultation:

a. Decreased or absent breath sounds and vocal resonance.
b. Bronchial breathing and egophony may be heard at the superior border of the fluid due to increased conductance of breath sounds through the partially atelectatic lung compressed by the fluid.
c. Pleural rub may be present; coarse, creaking, leathery sounds most commonly heard in late inspiration or early expiration.

Diagnosis

Causes of Unilateral Exudative vs Transudative Effusion:

	Exudative effusion	Transudative effusion
Common causes	Parapneumonic effusion Tubercular Trauma Post-surgery Neoplastic / Malignant	left ventricular dysfunction / failure Hepatic failure/cirrhosis Hypoprotenemia Hypoalbuminemia
Less Common	Pancreatitis Sub diaphragmatic abscess Liver abscess Splenic abscess/infarct Pulmonary embolism Auto-immune diseases	Nephrotic Syndrome Mitral Stenosis Pulmonary Embolism Hypothyroidism
Rare causes	Uremia Chylothorax Radiotherapy	SVC obstruction Constrictive pericarditis Meig syndrome

a. For a unilateral pleural effusion evident on chest radiographs, the differential diagnosis is extensive.
b. The differential diagnosis for bilateral pleural effusions is narrower and includes causes of transudative effusions, such as cardiac, hepatic, and renal failure and hypoalbuminemia, and in rare cases, malignant neoplasm, pulmonary embolism, and rheumatoid arthritis.
c. Congestive heart failure is the most common cause of bilateral pleural effusion.

1. **Diagnostic thoracocentesis**: Thoracentesis with analysis of the fluid can quickly narrow the differential diagnosis of an effusion.

Relationship between pleural fluid appearance and causes

Fluid appearance/odor	Cause
Clear, pale yellow	Normal
Milky white	Chylothorax, pseudochylothorax
Putrid	Anaerobic empyema
Urine	Urinothorax
Bile stained	Chylothorax (biliary fistula)
Black	Aspergillus infection
"Anchovy" brown	Amoebic liver abscess
Turbid	Empyema
Food particles	Esophageal rupture
Blood stained	Trauma, pulmonary embolism, malignant neoplasm, pneumonia, after myocardial infarction, benign asbestos-related effusion

Pleural fluid laboratory parameters with their range and significance							
Protein	Lactate dehydrogenase	Albumin	Glucose	Cell cytology	ADA	PCV	pH
<3 mg/dL: Transudate **>3 mg/dL:** Exudate **Light's criteria** to differentiate exudative and transudative effusion — for an effusion to be exudate: Effusion protein/serum protein ratio greater than 0.5. Effusion lactate dehydrogenase (LDH)/serum LDH ratio greater than 0.6. Effusion LDH level greater than two-thirds the upper limit of the laboratory's reference range of serum LDH	Ratios of pleural fluid to serum LDH are useful in diagnosing exudative effusion as per Light's criteria as mentioned. Elevated LDH values are seen in tuberculosis and lymphoma. LDH values of >1,000 U/L seen in empyema	Difference of >1.2 mg/dL indicates transudate	In exudative effusions, glucose <28.8 mg/dL occur in tuberculosis, malignant neoplasm, empyema, rheumatoid arthritis, systemic lupus erythematosus, and esophageal rupture. Rheumatoid arthritis probably is not responsible for a pleural effusion if the fluid glucose level is greater than 1.6 mmol/L	*Neutrophil predominant*: Parapneumonic effusion, acute tubercular effusion, pulmonary embolism, benign asbestos-related effusion *Lymphocyte predominant*: Tubercular, sarcoidosis, rheumatoid arthritis, malignant neoplasms *Eosinophilic*: No diagnostic value, can sometimes be due to air in the pleural fluid (traumatic/iatrogenic) Other cells like reactive mesothelial cells and cells pointing toward specific malignancy can be studied. Up to three samples should be sent in consecutive aspirations for malignant cytology	Levels of adenosine deaminase >40 U/L have a sensitivity >90% and specificity of about 85% for the presence of TB, particularly in lymphocyte-predominant effusions where the specificity is 95%. Values may be normal in TB coexisting with HIV. Elevated ADA may also be present in malignant neoplasms, RA, and empyema	In frankly bloody effusions; fluid PCV > half the serum PCV indicates hemothorax	<7.2 points toward empyema Low pH can also occur in malignant neoplasms, esophageal rupture and rheumatoid arthritis

a. Microbiology: Gram staining, Ziehl Neelsen staining, and culture/sensitivity testing to look for organisms including *Mycobacteria*; however, only expected in complicated parapneumonic effusion.

b. Polymerase chain reaction (PCR): Can be used for *Streptococcus pneumoniae* infection and *Mycobacterium tuberculosis.*

The high specificity of the pleural fluid cartridge-based nucleic acid amplification test (CBNAAT) makes it an excellent test despite its low sensitivity, since it obviates the need for an invasive procedure in at least one-fourth of patients with tubercular pleural effusion. Patients having consolidation along with pleural effusion and sputum MTB detected in CBNAAT may have higher possibility of MTB detection in pleural fluid CBNAAT.

c. Tumor markers in pleural fluid may be useful in certain clinical situations, although in general, the sensitivity is quite low (<30%). In patients with adenocarcinomatous or squamous malignant effusion, the combination of pleural fluid levels of 1,000 U/mL or greater for cancer antigen 125 and 100 ng/mL or greater for cytokeratin-19 fragments 21-1 was predictive of a lower survival.

d. Complement levels in pleural fluid have traditionally been analyzed when autoimmune disease such as rheumatoid arthritis or systemic lupus erythematosus (SLE) is suspected (reduced levels of complement). However, recently, an association between transudates and low complement levels was described. In a prospective study of 135 patients with pleural effusion of known causes (cardiac failure, malignant neoplasm, parapneumonic effusion after lung transplantation, and Dressler syndrome), effusions related to congestive heart failure could differentiated from parapneumonic and postoperative pleural effusions by the low level of complement in the first type. Normal levels of complement almost unequivocally indicate that congestive heart failure is not an etiological factor.

In lung transplant recipients, normal or high levels of complement in pleural fluid may indicate that the pleural effusion is not attributable to the surgery, but to another secondary cause (e.g., parapneumonic effusions).

Pleural fluid test and suggested diagnosis

Test	Cause
Amylase	Pancreatitis / oesophageal rupture
Hematocrit / PCV (> 20 or >50% of blood PCV)	Hemothorax
NT-Pro BNP level	Heart Failure
Creatinine (if > Serum creatinine)	Urinothorax
Polymerase Chain Reaction	Tuberculosis or Streptococcus pneumoniae infection
Adenosine Deaminase (ADA)	Tuberculosis
Cholesterol and triglycerides	Chylothorax
Tumor markers- CEA, CA 15.3, CA 549 levels CYFRA 21-1 level CA 125, HER-2/ neu level SMRP (Soluble mesothelin related protein)	Breast Carcinoma Lung Carcinoma Ovarian, endometrial, breast cancers Malignant mesothelioma
Complement C4 level (lower than normal)	Rheumatoid arthritis
Plasma Cells	Multiple myeloma
ANA	Lupus Pleuritis

Pleural fluid characteristics of chylothorax and pseudo-chylothorax

Triglycerides	< 0.56 mmol/l – Pseudo-chylothorax > 1.24 – Chylothorax
Cholesterol	>5.18mmol/l – Pseudo-chylothorax < 5.18 – Chylothorax
Cholesterol crystals	Present in Pseudo-chylothorax
Chylomicrons	Present in Chylothorax

Biomarkers: routine and novel in pleural fluid

Disease condition	Biomarker
Heart failure	NT-Pro BNP > 1,500 pg/mL
Bacterial infection	• Leukocyte Esterase Reagent Strips: 42% sensitivity, 100% specificity. • Rapid Pneumococcal Antigen Test: Immunochromatographic detection of pneumococcal antigen. Plays an important role when discordant urine antigen results. 71% sensitivity and 90% specificity. • CRP: parapneumonic effusions are usually exudates, with predominantly PMNLs in more than 80% of the cases, which is also predominant in 10%, 20%, and 60% of tuberculous, malignant, and pulmonary emboli–associated pleural fluids, respectively. However, if a neutrophilic pleural fluid has CRP concentrations greater than 45 mg/L, it is most likely parapneumonic. • Novel: In decreasing order of likelihood ratios, biomarkers to differentiate nonpurulent complicated and uncomplicated parapneumonic effusions are: tumor necrosis factor α greater than or equal to 80 pg/mL (LR 6.8), myeloperoxidase greater than 3,000 μg/L (LR 5.9), matrix metalloproteinase-2 less than or equal to 343 ng/mL (LR 5.5), neutrophil elastase greater than 3,500 μg/L (LR 4.6), interleukin-8 greater than or equal to 1,000 pg/mL (LR 4.6) lipopolysaccharide-binding protein greater than or equal to 17 μg/mL (LR 4), soluble triggering receptor expressed on myeloid cell greater than or equal to 180 pg/mL (LR 3.9), pleural interleukin 1β greater than 3.9 pg/mL (LR negative 0.02), terminal complement complex SC5b-9 greater than 2,000 μg/L (LR negative 0.03), and 8-isoprostane greater than 35.1 pg/mL.

(*Continued*)

(*Continued*)

Disease condition	Biomarker
Tuberculosis	• Adenosine deaminase: >40 U/L; the reported sensitivity, specificity, positive LR, negative LR, and odds ratio of pleural fluid ADA levels in the diagnosis of pleural tuberculosis were 92%, 90%, 9, 0.10, and 110, respectively. An extremely high ADA activity in pleural fluid (>250 U/L) should raise the suspicion of empyema or lymphoma rather than tuberculosis. There are two different molecular forms of ADA: ADA1 and ADA2. The first is ubiquitous and found in many cells, whereas the second is produced mainly by monocyte/macrophages and is responsible for most of the increase in ADA activity in tuberculous pleural fluids. • IFN-γ: cytokine released by activated CD4+ T lymphocytes and increases the mycobactericidal activity of macrophages. There exist two different methods to evaluate it in the pleural fluid. The first is the measurement of unstimulated IFN-γ (most commonly by enzyme-linked immunosorbent assay [ELISA]), and the second consists of the detection of IFN-γ release by pleural fluid mononuclear cells under stimulation with specific antigens of M tuberculosis (IFN-γ–releasing assays [IGRAs]). Sensitivity, specificity, positive LR, and negative LR for pleural IGRA assays (T-SPOT-TB and QuantiFERON-TB) in diagnosing tuberculosis were 75%, 82%, 3.5, and 0.24, respectively. • Neopterin: Neopterin is produced by activated macrophages in response to interferon-gamma of lymphocyte origin. It can be used as marker of cellular immunity. Cutoff > 30 nmol/L, sensitivity 85%, specificity 93%. • Others: IL-2sRα, IP-10, IL-12p40, IL-18, TNF-α, Fas ligand, human MDC, IL-23.

(*Continued*)

Disease condition	Biomarker
Malignancy	• CEA > 50 ng/mL, CA 15-3 > 75 U/mL, CA 125 > 2,800 U/mL, CYFRA 21-1 > 175 ng/mL — cutoff limits for 100% specificity. These markers also act as independent indicators of prognosis. • Mesothelin: for detection of malignant mesothelioma. Specificity of 95% and sensitivity of 60%, making it a good marker for the detection of even early mesothelioma. • Fibulin-3: an extracellular glycoprotein that mediates cell-to-cell interactions and has variable angiogenic effects. Cutoff value > 346 ng/mL; sensitivity 84%, specificity 92%, useful for early diagnosis of mesothelioma. • Immunohistochemical markers to differentiate benign and malignant effusion: □ Markers of malignancy — positive in adenocarcinoma: EMA, GLUT-1 □ Mesothelial markers — positive in reactive mesothelial cells and mesothelioma: calretinin, CK 5/6, WT-1, mesothelin, HBME-1

2. **Radiography**

a. Chest X-ray

An erect posterior–anterior (PA) CXR should be performed wherever possible, using the lateral CXR and additional views such as the lateral decubitus film and the shoot through lateral supine film, when necessary, for the detection of small pleural effusions.

Blunting of the costophrenic angle usually occurs in the presence of approximately 200 mL of pleural fluid, although the plain film can be normal with up to 500 mL fluid.

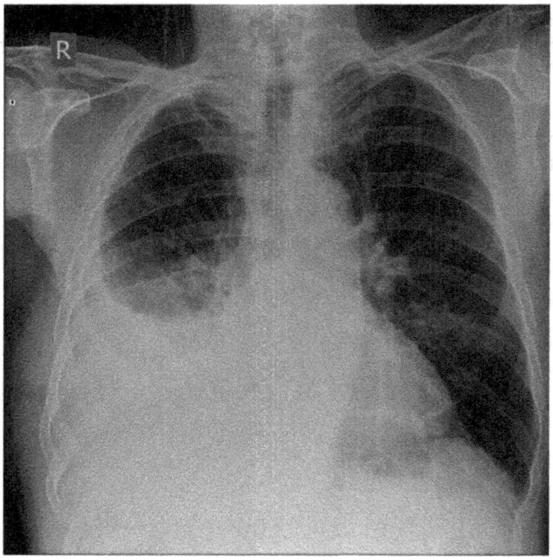

Figure 1: Moderate right sided pleural effusion with a lateral upward sloping upper margin. Pleural meniscus sign

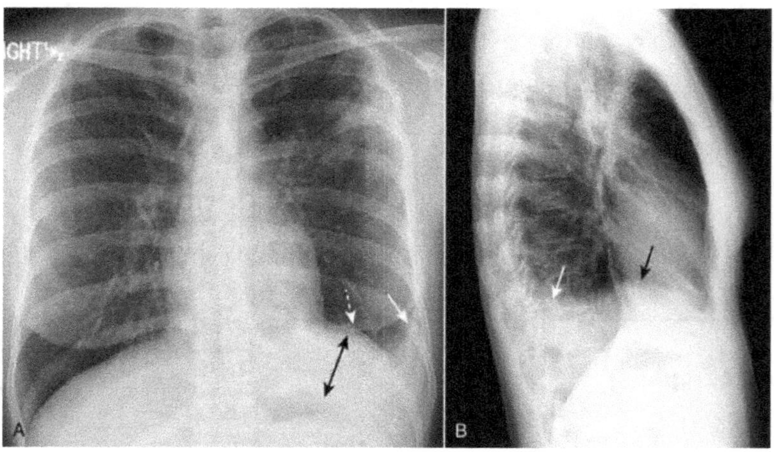

Figure 2: Sub-pulmonic effusion in the left side. A wide gap is seen between the dome of the left hemidiaphragm and the fundal gas shadow suggesting the possibility of fluid. Figure 2b: The presence of effusion is confirmed in a lateral view

Lateral decubitus films are occasionally useful as free fluid gravitates to the most dependent part of the chest wall, although ultrasound is now more commonly used.

As the effusion size increases, the characteristic meniscus becomes apparent (Figure 1). Sometimes the fluid collects between the lung and the

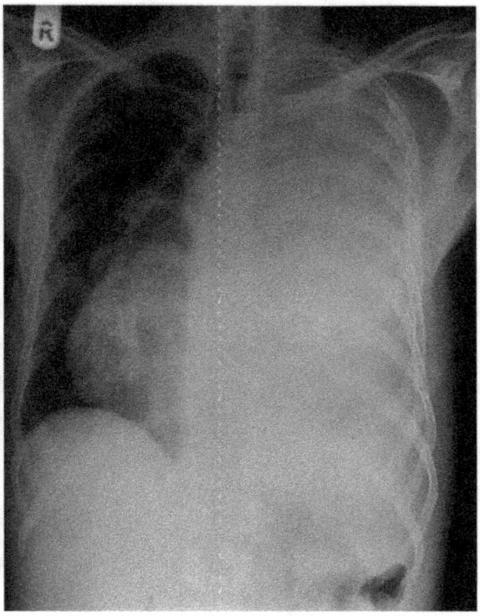

Figure 3: Radiographic failure of drainage.

dome of the diaphragm and is called as sub-pulmonic effusion, which may not be easily apparent. The left dome of the diaphragm may be elevated. There is an increased distance between the dome of the hemidiaphragm and the fundal gas shadow (Figure 2a). The subpulmonic effusion can be confirmed on a lateral view of the same side (Figure 2b).

Complete opacification of the hemithorax with contralateral mediastinal shift occurs with massive effusions although no mediastinal shift occurs if there is associated pulmonary collapse or mediastinal fixation. Large effusions can invert the ipsilateral hemidiaphragm, particularly on the left, as the liver splints the right hemidiaphragm. This inversion reverts to normal following fluid drainage causing an apparent, and sometimes puzzling, radiographic failure of drainage (Figure 3).

Subpulmonic effusions, which occur when the pleural fluid accumulates in a subpulmonic location, can be difficult to diagnose on the erect PA CXR. The diagnosis should be considered when there is apparent lateral peaking of a raised hemidiaphragm with a steep lateral slope and gradual medial slope. The lateral chest X-ray might have a flat appearance of the posterior aspect of the hemidiaphragm with a steep downward slope at the major fissure (Figure 4).

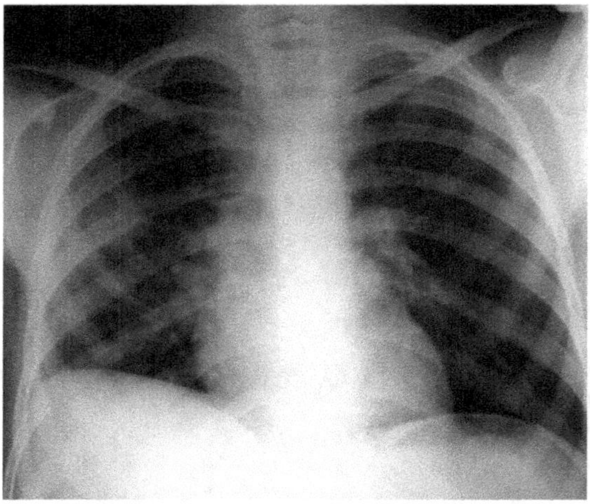

Figure 4: Right subpulmonic effusion.

The sensitivity of an upright PA view chest X-ray to detect pleural effusion has been studied to be around 82% and specificity 81%.

b. Ultrasound

Ultrasound is most frequently used to evaluate or guide aspiration and drain insertion in patients with suspected pleural effusions seen on CXR. The intercostal spaces are used as sonographic windows. A small footprint probe (either linear or phased array) allows the easiest intercostal access, and probe selection is a balance between spatial resolution and penetration.

A 7.5-MHz probe provides excellent spatial resolution of the pleural surfaces but might not provide sufficient penetration in larger patients or in large effusions. A 3.5–5.0-MHz sector transducer provides a good balance and can also be used to guide intervention.

Normal pleura are seen as an echogenic stripe comprising both parietal and visceral pleura. During normal respiration, there is a shimmering of inhomogeneities, described as "lung sliding," at the pleural stripe. There is also a "comet tail" appearance of reverberation of the ultrasound wave distal to the pleura.

Ultrasound can confirm the presence of the effusion and can be used to assess its character and guide drain placement. Pleural effusions with

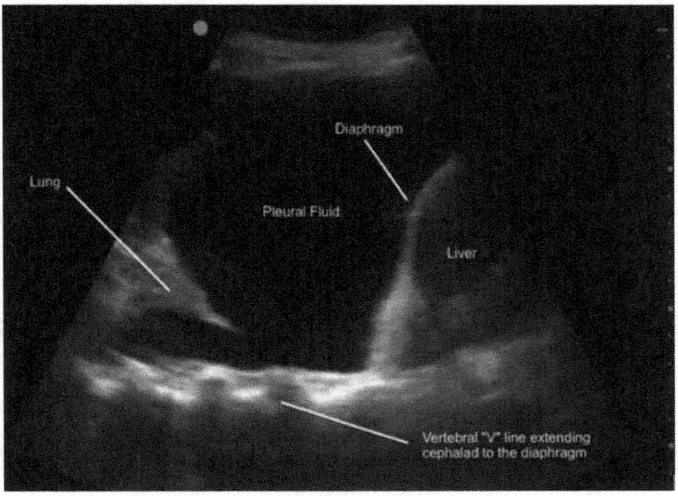

Figure 5: Homogenously echogenic.

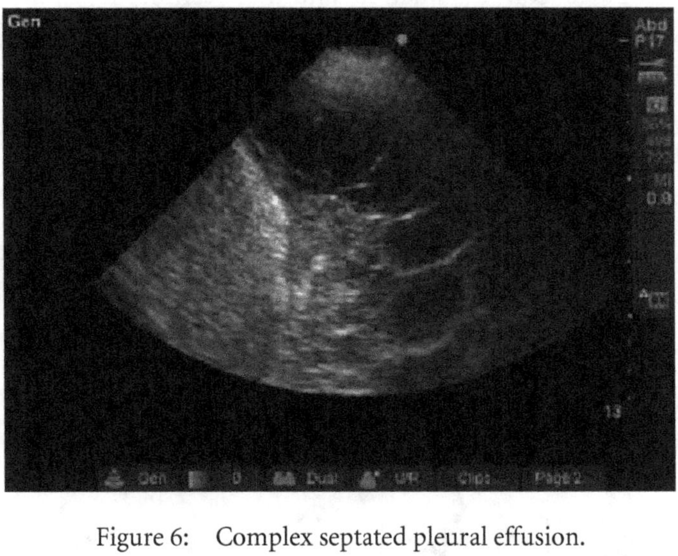

Figure 6: Complex septated pleural effusion.

complex septated, complex nonseptated, or homogeneously echogenic patterns on ultrasound are always exudates, whereas hypoechoic effusions can be either transudates or exudates even when clearly purulent. Most parapneumonic effusions and empyemas are septated on ultrasound.

The sensitivity of ultrasound to detect pleural effusion has been studied to be around 96% and specificity 93%.

c. Computed tomography

CT in pleural effusions do not have an additional role as compared to X-ray and ultrasound for preliminary diagnosis; however, it is useful to diagnose multiloculated pleural collections to assess the need for surgical management, to differentiate empyema from lung abscess, and in MPEs.

Contrast enhancement should always be used with imaging performed at 20–60 seconds to allow maximal tissue enhancement. It allows identification of associated pleural thickening, and pleural enhancement confirms that the effusion is an exudate.

Thickening of the parietal pleura and extrapleural subcostal tissues with increased attenuation of the extrapleural fat is present in parapneumonic pleural effusion (PPE) and empyema.

Loculated effusions have a lenticular shape with smooth margins and relatively homogeneous attenuation, and these can occur within fissures. A pulmonary abscess abutting the pleural surface might be difficult to differentiate from empyema. Pulmonary abscesses tend to appear rounder and have a thicker wall often forming an acute angle with the chest wall, whereas empyemas usually form an obtuse angle. Empyemas also cause

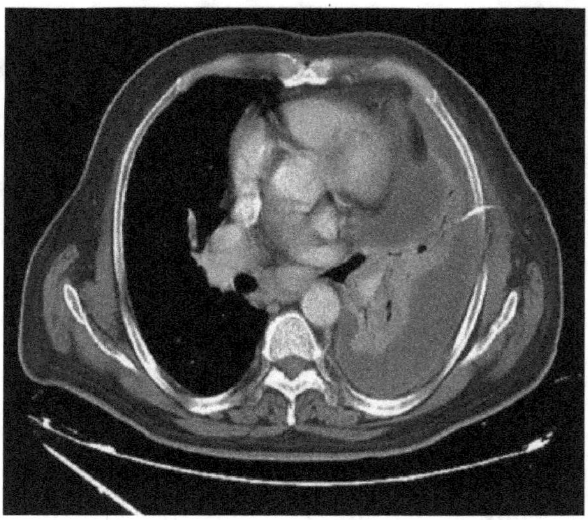

Figure 7: Loculated pleural effusion.

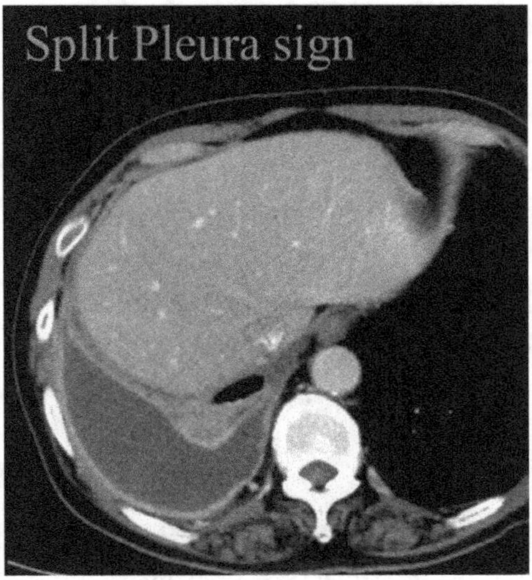

Figure 8: Split pleura sign.

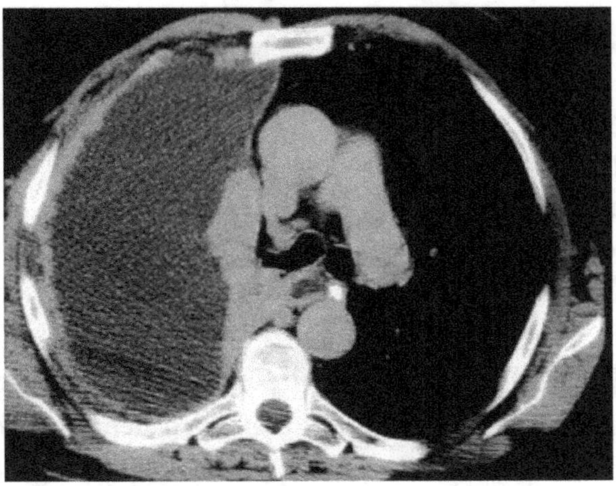

Figure 9: Axial CT images showing nodular irregular pleural enhancement following the administration of intravenous contrast medium.

passive atelectasis of the adjacent lung, a feature not seen with pulmonary abscesses. The "split pleura" sign referring to the separation of enhancing parietal and visceral pleura in empyema can also help differentiate it from an abscess.

Features of contrast-enhanced CT scanning that favor malignant disease rather than benign disease are nodular pleural thickening, mediastinal pleural thickening, parietal pleural thickening greater than 1 cm, and circumferential pleural thickening. These features have specificities of 94%, 94%, 88%, and 100%, respectively, and sensitivities of 51%, 36%, 56%, and 41%, respectively.

A CT scan should be performed before drainage of the effusion to dryness as pleural abnormalities surrounded by fluid will be more easily seen.

d. MRI

The role of MRI is unclear, but with its reduced spatial resolution and respiratory and cardiac motion artefacts, it does not at present provide better imaging information than CT scanning. Triple-echo pulse sequences on MRI can be used to differentiate transudates, simple exudates, and complex exudates, which return progressively higher signals.

Diffusion-weighted sequences have also been used to differentiate between transudates and exudates. MRI allows differentiation of effusions from parenchymal disease and from pleural tumors. The presence of hemoglobin breakdown products and chyle is also detectable on MRI.

e. PET CT

The use of PET is still being evaluated in patients with suspected malignant pleural effusions; it appears to be more useful in patients with focal or generalized pleural thickening, with one report suggesting it is of value, compared to CT, in identifying pleural malignancy. PET discriminates poorly between infective and malignant causes, and low-grade malignancy, as in patients with fibrous mesothelioma and small volume disease, it is difficult to identify.

3. Pleural biopsy

a. Closed needle biopsy

Closed pleural biopsy requires careful local anesthesia. The main complication is pneumothorax. The large calibre of the Abrams needle combined with the patient's respiratory movements can allow outside air to enter the pleural space if the device is not kept closed at all times. This is often aided by falling intrapleural pressure during evacuation of the pleural fluid.

Although a pneumothorax may be seen in up to 15% of patients undergoing biopsies, only a small minority require intervention.[1] Other complications include site pain (1%–15%), vasovagal reaction with potential syncope (1%–5%), hemothorax (<2%), and site hemorrhage with hematoma formation (<1%).

Unaided (blind) closed pleural biopsy has a diagnostic yield of less than 60% for pleural malignancy. The overall yield for malignancy over pleural fluid cytology is only increased by 7%–27%. Tuberculous granulomas are far more homogenously distributed over the pleura than is the case for malignant deposits, and unaided closed biopsies are therefore more likely to be diagnostic if TB is the underlying disease, yield being 80%–87%.

b. Image-guided closed pleural biopsies

Under transthoracic ultrasound and CT guidance, the yield is far higher, and the risk of complications is lower. The diagnostic yield of ultrasound-guided Tru-cut pleural biopsy to be as high as 87% for all pleural pathologies (77% for malignancies) irrespective of pleural thickness or nodularity.

While CT-guided pleural biopsy lacks the mobility and accessibility provided by ultrasound and needs the input of a specialist radiologist, it allows access to visualisation and guidance in areas not discernible by ultrasound. CT-guided biopsy has a sensitivity of about 87.5%, and as high as 95% when pleural thickening is present.

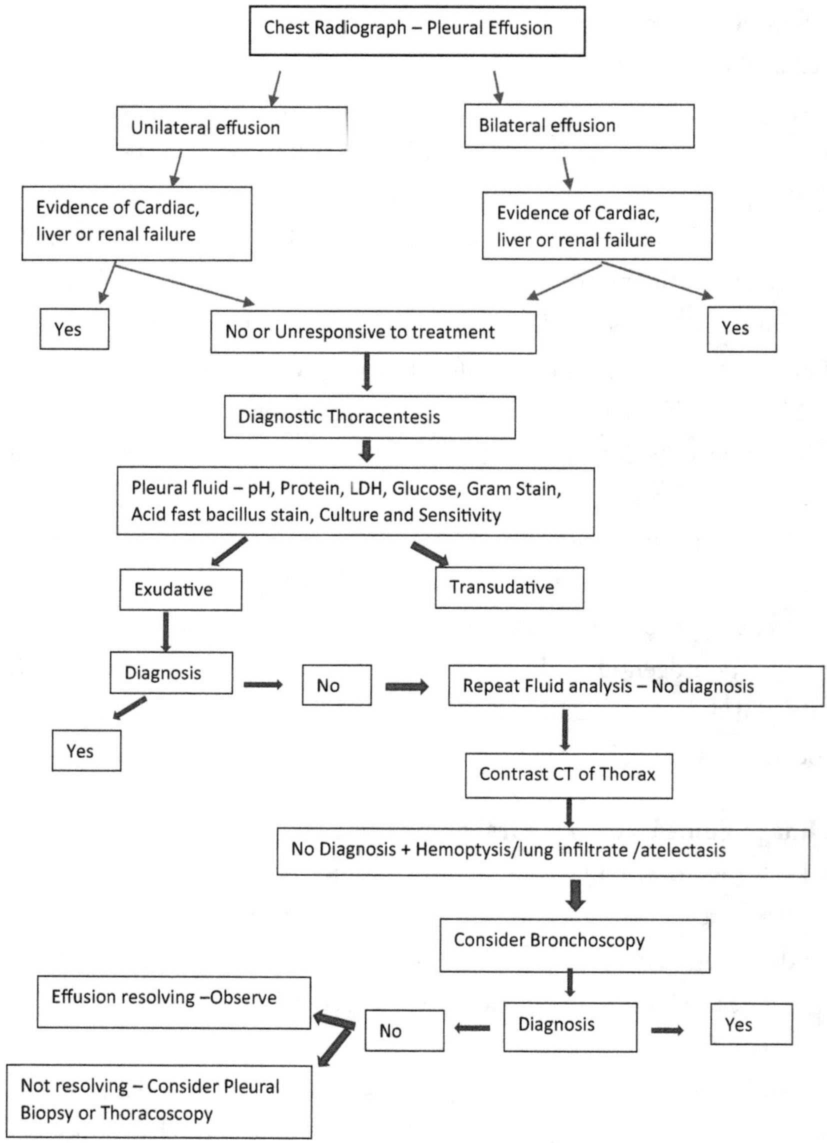

Figure 1: Diagnostic algorithm for pleural effusion:

Adapted from: Mcgrath, Emmet and Paul B. Anderson. "Diagnosis of pleural effusion: a systematic approach." *American journal of critical care: an official publication, American Association of Critical-Care Nurses* 20 2 (2011): 119–27; quiz 128.

c. **Medical/surgical thoracoscopy**

It is the gold standard investigative modality for arriving at a diagnosis for pleural effusions, especially undiagnosed exudative effusions.

Even after extensive diagnostic evaluation of a patient with pleural effusion, the etiology often remains unclear. Pleural fluid studies and blind pleural biopsy have their own limitations. It is in this context that thoracoscopy becomes an important investigation so that the pleural surface can be visualized and representative sample can easily be picked.

The 2000 American Thoracic Society statement on management of malignant pleural effusions stated that indications for performing thoracoscopy include "the evaluation of exudative effusions of unknown cause," among others, and that in cases of undiagnosed exudative effusions with a high clinical suspicion for malignancy, some clinicians may proceed directly to thoracoscopy if the facilities for medical thoracoscopy are available.

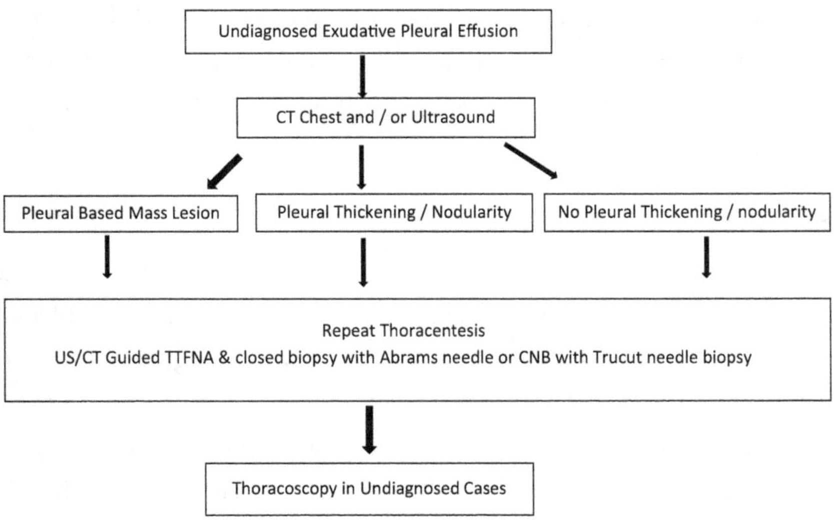

Figure 2: Evaluation of Undiagnosed Exudative Pleural Effusion

Parapneumonic effusion and empyema

Pleurisy, also known as pleuritis, is best defined as an inflammatory process of the pleura, which can be caused either by a variety of infectious micro-organisms or by other inflammatory mechanisms. It is usually associated with localized chest pain that is synchronous with the respiratory cycle and is often manifested as a pleural rub on auscultation. It may induce an exudative pleural effusion. The pain and the rub sometimes subside when an effusion develops.

A "parapneumonic effusion" is an accumulation of exudative pleural fluid associated with an ipsilateral pulmonary infection.

Uncomplicated parapneumonic effusions are not infected and do not usually need tube thoracostomy.

Complicated parapneumonic effusions are usually associated with the pleural invasion of the infectious agent and require tube thoracostomy and sometimes decortication for their resolution.

"An effusion is called an "empyema" when the concentration of leukocytes becomes macroscopically evident as a thick and turbid fluid (pus). In more than 50% of cases, it is of parapneumonic origin. Other common causes include surgical procedures (mainly thoracic surgery), traumas, and esophageal perforation.

The pleuritis sicca stage

The inflammatory process of the pulmonary parenchyma extends to the visceral pleura, causing a local pleuritic reaction. This leads to a pleural rub and the characteristic pleuritic chest pain, which originates from the sensitive innervation of the adjacent parietal pleura. A significant number of patients with pneumonia report pleuritic chest pain without developing a pleural effusion, suggesting that the involvement of the pleura may be limited to this stage in many cases of pneumonia.

The exudative stage

The ongoing inflammatory process leads to a mediator-induced increased permeability of local tissue and of regional capillaries. The subsequent accumulation of the fluid in the pleural space is probably the combined result of the influx of pulmonary interstitial fluid and of a local microvascular exudate. In the exudative stage, the fluid is usually clear and sterile, cytological specimens show a predominance of neutrophils, the pH is normal, and the lactate dehydrogenate (LDH) activity is <1,000 international units (IU).

The fibropurulent stage

This stage may develop quickly (within hours) in patients who are not receiving antibiotics, or who are treated with ineffective antibiotics. It is characterized by the deposition of fibrin clots and fibrin membranes ("sails") in the pleural space, which lead to loculations with increasing numbers of isolated collections of fluid. It is usually accompanied by (and caused by) bacterial invasion from the pulmonary parenchyma. The fluid is often turbid or frank pus. Cytology shows neutrophils and often degenerated cells, and Gram stains and bacterial cultures are usually positive. The metabolic and cytolytic activity in these effusions is high, as reflected by low pH values (<7.2) and high LDH.

The organizational stage

This final stage is characterized by the invasion of fibroblasts, leading to the transformation of interpleural fibrin membranes into a web of thick and nonelastic pleural peels. Functionally, gas exchange is often severely impaired on the side of the organizing empyema ("trapped lung"). The further course may vary from spontaneous healing with persistent defects of lung function to chronic forms of empyema with high risks for further complications, such as bronchopleural fistula (BPF), lung abscess, or "empyema necessitatis" (spontaneous perforation through the chest wall).

The finding of a purulent effusion without pneumonia may be explained as a postpneumonic empyema, in which the pulmonary infiltrates have already resolved. However, pleural empyemas are not necessarily caused by pneumonia. The majority of nonpneumonic empyemas are of iatrogenic origin, most commonly as a complication of a pneumonectomy or other thoracic surgical procedures. Thoracic surgery is responsible for about 20% of all thoracic empyemas. Around 5% occur following a thoracic trauma and 5% following an esophageal perforation (often iatrogenic). Fever, pulmonary infiltrates, and a pleural effusion are not invariably due to pneumonia or to a complication of some surgical procedure. A very important differential diagnosis, which should always be considered, is pulmonary infarction.

Management

Thoracentesis is recommended when the suspected PPE is greater than or equal to 10 mm thick on a lateral decubitus chest radiograph. Pleural fluid appearance may vary from a clear yellow liquid to an opaque turbid fluid to grossly purulent thick, viscous, foul-smelling pus. Foul-smelling fluid indicates an anaerobic infection. Pleural fluid pH (iced blood gas syringe) values of less than 7.20 are suggestive of a complicated pleural effusion. Other laboratory tests suggestive of complicated pleural effusion or empyema include (1) an LDH value of greater than 1,000 U/L, (2) a pH of less than 7.00, and (3) a glucose level of less than 40 mg/dL.

Treatment

The following classification and treatment scheme has been used to characterize parapneumonic effusions and empyema.

Category 1 (parapneumonic effusion)
Minimal free-flowing fluid, smaller than 10 mm on decubitus films; culture, Gram stain, and pH unknown; no thoracentesis needed; treatment with antibiotics alone.

Category 2 (uncomplicated parapneumonic effusion)
Larger than 10 mm fluid and less than half the hemithorax on decubitus films; Gram stain and culture negative; pH higher than 7.20; treatment with antibiotics alone.

Category 3 (complicated parapneumonic effusion)
Large free-flowing effusion, more than half the hemithorax; pH lower than 7.20; LDH level greater than 1,000 U/L and glucose level greater than 40 mg/dL; Gram stain or culture positive; treatment with tube thoracostomy and antibiotics; multiloculated effusions may require multiple tubes; thrombolytics may help resolution.

Category 4 (empyema)
Large free-flowing effusion; greater than equal to half the hemithorax; loculated effusion or effusion with thickened pleura; gross pus on aspiration; treatment with tube thoracostomy; thrombolytics may help resolution; may require decortication.

Antibiotics

The initial antibiotic selection is usually based on whether the pneumonia is community or hospital acquired and on the severity of the patient's illness. For a patient with community-acquired pneumonia, the recommended agents are second- or third-generation cephalosporins in addition to a macrolide. For patients hospitalized with severe community-acquired pneumonia, initiate treatment with a macrolide plus a third-generation cephalosporin with antipseudomonal activity. Enteric Gram-negative bacilli frequently cause pneumonia acquired in institutions (e.g., hospitals, nursing homes). Therefore, initial antibiotic coverage should include an antibiotic effective against pseudomonas. If aspiration is evident or suspected, oral anaerobic microorganism should also be covered.

Thoracoscopy

Thoracoscopy is an alternate therapy for multiloculated empyema thoracis. In patients with multiloculated PPEs, the loculations in the pleural space can be disrupted with a thoracoscope, and the pleural space can be drained completely. If extensive adhesions are present or thick pleural peel entraps the lung, the procedure may be converted to open thoracostomy and decortication.

Decortication

In decortication, all the fibrous tissue is removed from the visceral pleural peel, and all pus is evacuated from the pleural space. Decortication is a major thoracic operation requiring full thoracotomy; therefore, decortication is not tolerated by critically ill patients. Decortication is the procedure of choice for patients in whom pleural sepsis is not controlled by closed-tube thoracostomy, intrapleural thrombolytic agents, and, possibly, thoracoscopy. Mortality rates as high as 10% have been described with this procedure.

Video-assisted thoracoscopic surgery

Video-assisted thoracoscopic surgery (VATS) is preferred in incompletely drained parapneumonic effusion, because if the lung cannot be expanded, VATS can be converted to full thoracotomy. Chest CT scan provide anatomic information about the size and extent of empyema cavity and whether pleural surfaces are thickened. With VATS, the loculi in pleural space can be disrupted, pleural space can be drained completely, chest tube can be optimally placed, if the lung is trapped decortication can be attempted, incision can be enlarged so that decortication can be completed with a full thoracotomy. Patients with loculated parapneumonic effusion, a primary treatment strategy of VATS is associated with a higher efficacy, shorter hospital duration, and less cost than catheter-directed fibrinolytic therapy. VATS procedure is used to insert a chest tube. At the time that the chest tube inserted, VATS is used to irrigate the pleural space and breakdown all the fibrous strands. Chest tube through VATS has lesser hospital stay and required less decortication. Decortication can be performed with VATS or full thoracotomy. When decortication is necessary, VATS is the procedure of choice. In the acute stages of pleural infections, decortication should only be considered to control the pleural infections. Decortication cannot be performed just to remove thickened pleura because such thickening will resolve spontaneously over several months. If after 6 months, the pleura remains thickened and patients' pulmonary function is sufficiently reduced to limit activities, decortication should be considered.

Tube thoracostomy

The initial drainage modality for most patients with complicated parapneumonic effusions is tube thoracostomy. The chest tube should be positioned in a dependent part of the pleural effusion. Visceral pleura is covered with fibrinous peel; the application of negative pressure to the chest tube help expand the underlying lung and hasten the obliteration of the empyema cavity. Regular chest tube size is relatively large 28–36f; smaller tubes like 10–14f will become obstructed with thick fluid. Flushing needed if a small-bore catheter is used.

Intrapleural fibrinolytics

Drainage of complicated parapneumonic effusion is difficult if loculations are present. Pleural fluid loculations are produced by fibrin membranes that prevent the spread of the infected pleural fluid. Intrapleural fibrinolytics will destroy the fibrin membranes and facilitate drainage of the pleural fluid. The intrapleural injection of fibrinolytics facilitated pleural drainage in patients with empyema. Original articles on enzymatic debridement for loculated parapneumonic effusions used fibrinolytic and a recombinant DNAase. Administration of combination of TPA and DNAase resulted in significantly greater reduction in the pleural opacity, significant decrease in surgical referrals, and shorter hospital stay.

Tuberculous pleural effusion

Tuberculous pleurisy can occur with primary infection or as a reactivation disease. It accounts for 30%–80% of all pleural effusions in developing countries and occurs in up to 30% of patients who present with pulmonary tuberculosis.

Its prevalence is lower in developed nations accounting for 1% of all pleural effusions and occurring with pulmonary tuberculosis in only 3%–5% of patients. HIV-positive patients, however, have a higher incidence of tuberculous pleurisy presenting with underlying pulmonary tuberculosis.

Patients with tuberculous pleurisy commonly resolve their effusions spontaneously but present within 2 years with pulmonary tuberculosis.

Pleural fluid develops from an intrapleural hypersensitivity response to mycobacterial antigens released by rupture into the pleural space of a subpleural caseous focus. The number of viable acid-fast organisms in PF is insufficient to allow reliable diagnosis by standard PF staining and culture techniques.

Patients present with subacute symptoms characterized by cough, pleuritic chest pain, dyspnea, and fever, although some patients present more acutely simulating bacterial pneumonia and others more indolently with weight loss and fatigue.

Purified protein derivative skin tests are positive in only 50% of patients but usually convert to positive within 2 months.

The effusion is usually unilateral encompassing less than two-thirds of the hemothorax. Standard chest radiographs and chest CT scans detect active parenchymal tuberculosis in 20% and 80% of patients, respectively.

Any undiagnosed exudative pleural effusion should prompt consideration of tuberculous pleurisy with highest suspicion for lymphocyte-predominant effusions (>60% lymphocytes) with protein concentrations >5 g/dL. Up to 17% of patients, however, have lymphocyte percentages <50%. The PF cell differential may be neutrophil predominant within the first 2 weeks of symptom onset. PF mesothelial cell percentages are nearly always <5%. PF glucose and pH mirror the serum levels, although some patients have PD levels lower than serum.

PF staining for acid-fast organisms has a low yield except in the presence of HIV-infection wherein 20% may be smear positive. Although PF culture has traditionally been reported to have a sensitivity <50%, studies using liquid culture techniques report a sensitivity of 63%–75%. Sputum mycobacterial cultures may be positive in >50% of patients with positivity of either sputum and/or PF cultures in 79%.

Adenosine deaminase (ADA) is found in increased concentrations in tuberculous effusions and some other inflammatory and neoplastic pleural conditions. In regions with a high prevalence of tuberculosis, a PF ADA >40 IU/L in a lymphocyte-predominant effusion change confirms to has a high probability of tuberculous pleurisy, allowing a diagnosis for 90% of patients after a single thoracentesis.[2] An ADA value <40 IU/L adequately excludes the diagnosis in high-prevalence settings. In regions with low or intermediate prevalence of tuberculosis, PF ADA assay has insufficient sensitivity and specificity, and most patients with negative PF microbiologic evaluations require pleural biopsy. Although elevated ADA concentrations in the pleural space represent the ADA2 isoform, ADA2-specific PF assays provide only negligible benefits over ADA. Although several other biomarkers (interferon-gamma, interferon-gamma-induced protein of 10 kDa, and dipeptidyl peptidase [DPP] 4 levels in unstimulated PF provide similar diagnostic value as compared with PF ADA, none has comparable availability for routine use. Commercially available T-cell interferon-gamma release assays performed on both blood and PF have inadequate diagnostic accuracy as do PF nucleic acid amplification tests.

Pleural biopsy may be required in complicated settings. Tuberculous granulomata are diffusely distributed over pleural surfaces, which allows up to 70%–87% of patients to be diagnosed by closed (blind) needle biopsy using an image-guided Abrams needle technique. This approach is appropriate when the pretest probability of tuberculosis is high for an undiagnosed exudative pleural effusion. Six pleural biopsies are recommended. For other patients, thoracoscopy provides a 100% diagnostic yield. Biopsied pleural tissue must be cultured for acid-fast organisms and examined for organisms and granulomata. Microscopic-observation drug-susceptibility culture as compared with Lowenstein–Jensen culture has a higher diagnostic yield.

Drug therapy for tuberculous pleurisy is the same as for pulmonary tuberculosis with a four-drug regimen for susceptible organisms. Evidence does not support a role for adjunctive corticosteroids. When examined with chest CT after chemotherapy, nearly 70% of patients will have some degree of residual pleural thickening that may contribute to measurable pulmonary restriction. Some experts recommend therapeutic thoracentesis to prevent pleural fibrosis for moderate to large tuberculous effusions, although evidence of benefit is uncertain. Ultrasonographic detection of complex septated pleural space, CT evidence of extrapleural fat proliferation or loculated effusion, and long duration of symptoms at initiation of therapy may identify patients at greatest risk of pleural thickening 1 year later.

Management of tubercular pleural effusion

Treatment of tubercular pleural effusion have three goals:

a. To prevent the subsequent development of active TB.
b. To relieve the patient symptoms.
c. To prevent the development of a fibrothorax.

Chemotherapy

The initial phase of a 6-month regimen is a 2-month period of INH, rifampicin, pyrazinamide, and ethambutol. The second phase of the treatment is continuation phase for 4 months. DOTS is advised for such cases.

Nine-month regimen using INH and rifampicin is also effective when the organisms are fully susceptible. A study demonstrates that penetration of INH into the pleural fluid was excellent. But the penetration of pyrazinamide was poor. The penetration of rifampicin was intermediate.

Recommended doses of first-line anti-tuberculosis drugs for adults in tubercular pleural effusion

	Recommended dose			
	Daily		3 times/week	
Drug	Dose and range (mg/kg body weight)	Maximum (mg)	Dose and range (mg/kg body weight)	Daily maximum (mg)
Isoniazid	5 [4–6]	300	10 [8–12]	900
Rifampin	10 [8–12]	600	10 [8–12]	600
Pyrazinamide	25 [20–30]	—	35 [30–40]	—
Ethambutol	15 [15–20]	—	30 [5–35]	—

*Adapted from World Health Organization. Guidelines for treatment of tuberculosis, Fourth edition, 2010.

A study by S.K. Malik — ethambutol was administered in single daily dose for 9 months to 91 patients with pleural effusion and 45 patients with lymphadenitis, both of tuberculous etiology. Clinical and chest X-ray clearance of pleural effusion was successfully achieved in all cases at the end of 9 months of treatment. Follow-up of 80 cases of pleural effusion up to 9 months, in 55 cases up to 1 year, and up to 2 years in 30 cases after completion of therapy showed no recurrence. It is reasonable to include ethambutol in the treatment regimen for TPE, although it is likely that the standardized therapy without this drug would be a valid treatment option, unless there is little possibility of drug resistance. Once susceptibility to isoniazid, rifampin, and pyrazinamide has been confirmed, ethambutol can be discontinued. In young children with TPE, ethambutol is always omitted if the source of transmission is known to have drug-susceptible tuberculosis, because the toxic effects of ethambutol may be of more concern in children.

The patients with isolated tuberculous pleuritis has a small bacterial burden as most of the symptoms are due to delayed hypersensitivity therefore even less intensive regimens can be useful. In a study, even 5 mg/kg of

INH and 10 mg/kg of rifampicin daily for 6 months has reported no treatment failures among 130 cases of isolated tubercular pleuritis.

Symptoms	Duration of treatment for resolution of symptoms	Symptoms persist up to
Fever	2 weeks	2 months
Resorption of pleural fluid	6 weeks	12 weeks
Pleuritic chest pain	6 weeks	4 months

Pleural thickening associated with tubercular pleural effusion

Approximately 50% of patients with tubercular pleural effusion can develop pleural thickening at 6–12 months of initiating ATT. The incidence of pleural thickening is not related to the initial pleural fluid findings. Pleural thickening is more common if the initial fluid is loculated. Residual pleural thickening will continue to improve for at least 18 months after ATT is initiated.

— Complete removal of pleural fluid does not decrease the amount of pleural thickening.

— Intrapleural fibrinolytic administration in case of loculated pleural effusion have shown to reduce the incidence of pleural thickening. A study showed width of pleural thickening was 0.46 cm when along with antitubercular therapy urokinase was administered through pigtail starting from when the amount of pleural fluid was less than 100 mL/day and finishing when the amount of fluid was less than 50 mL/day. The controls of the study received only antitubercular therapy, and the pleural thickness in them was noted to be 1.86 cm.

— Often addition of streptokinase in loculated pleural effusion is associated with a faster radiological improvement.

Immune reconstitution inflammatory syndrome

Paradoxical worsening of the disease after anti tuberculous treatment is initiated. A study was conducted on 61 patients with tubercular pleural effusion who were started on a standard HRZE regimen for the first 2 months. In nearly 17% of the patients, the size of the effusion worsened after the initiation of the tubercular therapy. Six of these cases developed increasing dyspnea and treated with pleural aspiration and oral prednisolone with complete resolution of pleural effusion. It is suggested that such paradoxical response can be secondary to INH-induced lupus pleuritis.

The following strict criteria must be applied to diagnose tuberculosis-immune reconstitution inflammatory syndrome (TB-IRIS):

1. Initial improvement of TB-related symptoms and/or radiographic findings after adequate anti-TB treatment for a certain time;
2. Paradoxical deterioration of TB-related symptoms and/or radiologic findings at the primary or at new locations during or after anti-TB treatment;
3. Absence of conditions that reduce the efficacy of anti-TB drugs (e.g., poor compliance, drug malabsorption, drugs side effects);
4. Exclusion of other possible causes of clinical deterioration.

Pleural TB-IRIS (manifesting as a new or increased pleural effusion) happens in 16%–45% of HIV-uninfected patients with pleural, lymph node, or pulmonary TB. It generally develops within 3–19 weeks of treatment initiation.

Patients with soft-tissue abscesses or symptomatic pleural effusions often require aspiration. Systemic corticosteroid administration for 4–6 weeks improves the outcome of certain forms of TB-IRIS (symptomatic enlarging intracranial tuberculoma, endobronchial obstruction) and reduces proinflammatory cytokines.

Prednisone significantly reduced days of hospitalization and outpatient therapeutic procedures, more rapidly improving symptoms, quality-of life score, and chest radiography. For most patients, a 4-week course of prednisone reduced morbidity from TB-IRIS. There was no difference in mortality between prednisone and placebo-treated participants, even though cases with neurological involvement were excluded from the trial. Minor infections (oral candidiasis and uncomplicated herpes simplex) were more common in patients on prednisone. Most authors suggest treatment with corticosteroids for a maximum of 4–6 months.

In nearly 4 out of 29 patients who have TB-IRIS features, the pleural fluid analysis showed exudative fluid with culture positive for *M. tuberculosis*. Most of the patients had good symptomatic improvement for the same chemotherapeutic regimen.

Use of corticosteroids in tubercular pleural effusion

A study done on Role of Corticosteroids in Tubercular Pleural Effusion in Chennai published in 2021, showed that subjects with ADA higher than 50 1/U were more prone to develop pleural thickening than subjects with ADA lesser than the cutoff level. When In addition to ATT and therapeutic thoracentesis patients in were given Oral corticosteroids in the form of prednisolone 1 mg/kg/day for first 2 weeks and slowly tapered to 0.5 mg/kg/day for next 2 weeks followed by 0.25 mg/kg/day for next 2 weeks followed by 0.10 mg/kg/day for last 2 weeks and In addition to ATT fared better with only 20% of patients developing pleural thickening. Another group of therapeutic thoracentesis patients were given oral corticosteroids in the form of prednisolone 1 mg/kg/day for the first 2 weeks and slowly tapered to 0.5 mg/kg/day for next 2 days followed by 0.25 mg/kg/day for next 2 weeks followed by 0.10 mg/kg/day for last 2 weeks + 5 mg Dexamethasone was injected into the pleural cavity during every sitting of therapeutic thoracentesis and 33% of the cases developed pleural fibrosis. This study concludes that the most effective route to administer corticosteroids will be through oral route as it gave better results over intrapleural as well as oral and intrapleural combined. In this study, it was also concluded that though the level of pleural fluid ADA positivity for TB is set at 40 1/U, administering corticosteroids in patients with a pleural fluid ADA of more than 50 1/U would be beneficial as that group of patients are more prone to develop residual pleural thickening.

If a patient has severe symptoms including fever, malaise, pleuritic chest pain, malaise after a therapeutic thoracocentesis, and a definitive diagnosis has been established, steroids can be used.

Engel et al. studied the effect of corticosteroids in the treatment of pleural effusion; they concluded that corticosteroids have no effect on death of patients from any cause including respiratory or pleural adhesions.

Surgical procedures

Indication for surgery in tubercular pleurisy

Persistent dyspnea in spite of 6 months of ATT. After this period, decortication is rarely required as generally the pleural thickening resolves with ATT.

Tuberculous BPF

Usually seen in patients with old, healed TB. Such patients have varying degree of sputum production sometimes associated with superinfection with bacteria. Confirmation of fistula: instillation of methylene blue into the pleural space and observing if the dye is seen in sputum or tracheobronchial tree. Diagnosis is suggested by the presence of an air fluid level in the pleural space and often the levels fluctuates with serial chest X-rays.

a. Tubercular BPF communicates with bronchus and pleural space; therefore, entry of bacteria to pleural space and causes pleural infection.
b. Increased chances of fulminant pneumonia noted as infected material from the pleura can reach the remainder of tracheobronchial tree.
c. Tubercular bacteria is likely to be resistant to anti tubercular drugs.

Treatment of tubercular BPF

Institution of ATT along with insertion of the chest tube into the lower parts of the pleural cavity. Insertion of the chest tube is important as BPF does not heal spontaneously. The danger of contamination of the contralateral lung by infected pleural fluid is controlled. It also controls systemic toxicity from the bacterial infection. Minimum of 90–120 days of ATT is required or until the sputum becomes negative for AFB before a definitive surgical procedure is attempted.

Definitive surgical options for tubercular BPF

a. Decortication
b. Decortication with thoracoplasty — in patients where the underlying lungs are severely damaged by TB, and such a lung cannot expand to fill the pleural space.

Operative mortality can be up to 20%.

Tuberculous empyema

a. Purulent pleural fluid associated with tuberculous organisms on AFB stains.
b. Develops in fibrous scar tissue from pleurisy, pneumothorax, and thoracoplasty.
c. Rarely tuberculous empyemas can lead to empyema necessitatis, where the empyema ruptures through the chest wall.
d. CXR will show an obvious pleural effusion, most often it might be only pleural thickening.
e. CT thorax shows a thick, calcified pleural rind and rib thickening surrounding a loculated pleural effusion.
f. To establish a diagnosis of tuberculous empyema — AFB smear should be positive.

Treatment options include multiple episodes of thoracocentesis with intensive chemotherapy; surgical options including decortication, extrapleural pneumonectomy, and thoracoplasty are recommended. These procedures have substantial mortality and morbidity.

Atypical mycobacteria

— Pleural effusions due to atypical mycobacteria are rare.

Organisms	Incidence of pleural pathology
— *M. kansasii*	— 5% small pleural effusion
— *M. intracellulare*	— 5% small pleural effusion
— MAC	— 15% pleural thickening with >2 cm

In a case series analysis, it was observed that nearly 16 of the 22 patients who had pleural fluid growth of nontuberculous *Mycobacterium* had another explanations for pleural effusion. In only three, the *Mycobacterium* was responsible for the pleural effusion.

Therefore, the new conclusion is that nontuberculous *Mycobacterium* cannot be concluded as the etiology of a pleural effusion unless another tissue infection shows evidence of same organism.

Disseminated disease due to MAC is an important cause of infection in patients with AIDS. More than 50% of patients with AIDS who die have disseminated disease due to MAC. Overall, disease due to MAC accounts for a very small percentage of the pleural effusions in patients with AIDS.

Malignant pleural effusion

a. Malignant pleural effusion is the second leading cause of exudative pleural effusions (after parapneumonic effusions).
b. Malignant pleural effusion is diagnosed by detecting exfoliated malignant cells in pleural fluid or demonstrating these cells in pleural tissue obtained by percutaneous pleural biopsy, thoracoscopy, and thoracotomy.
c. Pleural effusions associated with malignancy, with no direct pleural involvement with tumor and no other cause for the effusion is found, are categorized as premalignant effusions.
d. Carcinomas of lung and breast account for approximately 65% of all malignant pleural effusions. Ovarian and gastric cancers account for approximately 5% of malignant pleural effusions. Lymphomas account for approximately 10%.

e. Etiology: Lung, breast, ovary, stomach, and lymphomas account for 80% of all malignant effusions. Metastatic ovarian carcinoma is the fourth leading cause of malignant pleural effusions. Sarcomas, particularly melanoma, account for a small percentage of malignant pleural effusions.
f. In patients of lung cancer, up to 15% have a pleural effusion.
g. During the course of the disease, at least 50% of patients with disseminated lung cancer develop a pleural effusion.
h. Pleural effusions occur with all types of lung cancers, but most frequent with adenocarcinoma and least with small cell ca (15%).

The presence of pleural effusion in a patient with lung cancer almost always indicates that the patient is not curable with surgery whether or not the cytology is positive.

Malignant mesothelioma is a primary tumor of the pleura. An early manifestation of the tumor is a pleural effusion that is reabsorbed and then replaced by tumor and fibrosis. The lung is often encased in tumor that involves both visceral and parietal pleural surfaces. Tumor never penetrates deeply into the lung parenchyma but extends into interlobar fissures. Hilar lymph nodes are involved by tumor in less than 50% of patients. Distant hematogenous metastases are unusual but found in liver, bone, adrenals, thyroid, and kidneys.

Unknown primary: Patients with a malignant pleural effusion and an unknown primary should have a further evaluation with CT scan of chest, abdomen, and pelvis. If pulmonary parenchymal abnormalities are discovered, then a bronchoscopy is indicated with special attention to the area of abnormality. Masses in the abdomen should be evaluated. If the patient has symptoms referable to a specific organ, that organ should be evaluated. If the patient is a woman, mammography and a careful pelvic examination should be performed.

Pathophysiology

Direct result

a. Pleural metastases with increased permeability.
b. Pleural metastases with obstruction of pleural lymphatic vessels.
c. Mediastinal lymph node involvement with decreased pleural lymphatic drainage.
d. Thoracic duct interruption (chylothorax).
e. Bronchial obstruction (decreased pleural pressures).
f. Pericardial involvement.

Indirect result

a. Hyponatremia.
b. Postobstructive pneumonitis.
c. Pulmonary embolism.
d. Postradiation therapy.

Clinical presentation

Dyspnea, cough, and chest pain are the most common symptoms.

The degree of dyspnea depends on the size of effusion and the patient's underlying pulmonary function.

Most common presenting symptom is chest pain in 60%–70% of patients due to the involvement of parietal pleura, ribs, or chest wall.

However, 25% were asymptomatic at the time of presentation.

Patients with malignant pleural effusions have dull chest pain, whereas benign disease have pleuritic chest pain.

Diagnosis

Chest radiograph

Pleural effusion is usually ipsilateral to the primary lesion in carcinoma of the lung.

When the primary site of cancer is elsewhere, there is no ipsilateral predilection, and bilateral effusions are common (with the possible exceptions of breast cancer).

In 75% of patients, pleural effusion is moderate to large, with volumes ranging from 500 to 2,000 mL of fluid.

Approximately 10% present with effusions of <500 mL; another 10% present with massive pleural effusions (complete opacification).

If mediastinum does not shift contralaterally in the face of a large pleural effusion (>1,500 mL), malignancy is highly likely.

The following diagnoses are then considered:

1. Carcinoma of ipsilateral mainstem bronchus resulting in atelectasis.
2. A fixed mediastinum due to malignant lymph nodes.
3. Malignant mesothelioma (the radiodensity represents predominantly tumor with only a small effusion).
4. Extensive tumor infiltration of the ipsilateral lung, radiographically mimicking a large effusion.

CT chest: Findings on CT can help distinguish benign and malignant effusions.

The following findings were suggestive of malignancy:

a. Pleural nodularity.
b. Pleural rind.
c. Mediastinal pleural involvement.
d. Pleural thickening > 1 cm.
e. Pleural calcification usually suggests a benign process.
f. Interstitial infiltrates with effusions (lymphangitic carcinomatosis) and multiple nodules with effusions also suggest malignant disease.

Pleural biopsy

Needle biopsy of pleura can establish diagnosis of a malignant pleural effusion.

Percentage of positive pleural biopsies ranges from 39% to 75%.

It has lower diagnostic yield than pleural fluid cytologic examination, as in approximately 50% of patients, costal parietal pleura is not involved.

An alternative — pleural biopsy can be obtained with CT-guided cutting-needle biopsy, where the pleura is the most thickened.

Medical thoracoscopy and VATS

Medical thoracoscopy (pleuroscopy) — advantage that it can be performed under local anesthesia or conscious sedation.

MT into VATS has allowed for an even greater range of therapeutic solutions.

MT is primarily a diagnostic procedure.

Indication

a. The evaluation of exudative effusions of unknown.
b. To rule out the cause, staging of malignant mesothelioma or lung cancer, and treatment of malignant or other recurrent effusions.
c. Talc pleurodesis.
d. Another purpose may be biopsy of the diaphragm, lung, mediastinum, or pericardium. Thoracic surgery backup should be available.

Thoracoscopy or open thoracotomy

Thoracoscopy will establish the diagnosis of malignancy in approximately 90% of patients with malignancy.

If thoracoscopy is not available, an alternative approach is to perform a thoracotomy with open biopsy of pleura.

Thoracoscopic biopsy has a high diagnostic yield for mesothelioma, approaching 100% in some series.

Characteristics of malignant pleural effusion

Malignant pleural fluid may be serous, sero-sanguineous, or grossly bloody.

Malignant pleural effusion is typically an exudate with a protein.

Concentration of about 4 g/dL.

In about one-half of malignant pleural effusions, lymphocytes predominate (50%–70% of nucleated cells).

In about one-third of patients, the pleural fluid pH is low (<7.30), ranging from 6.95 to 7.29.

In these low-pH effusions, glucose concentration is also low (<60 mg/dL), the lactate concentration is high, which frequently exceeds 600 IU/L.

Cytology is a more sensitive than percutaneous pleural biopsy.

Cytologic study of the pleural fluid establishes the diagnosis of a malignant pleural effusion ranging from 40% to 87%.

When three separate pleural fluid specimens are submitted to an experienced cytologist, it is diagnostic in 80% of patients.

Most cases of metastatic adenocarcinoma can be diagnosed by pleural fluid cytology.

With lymphoma, cytologic test is positive in approximately 25% of patients with Hodgkin's disease and in 50%–60% of patients with non-Hodgkin's lymphoma.

Management of malignant pleural effusions

The presence of malignant pleural effusions indicates that the malignancy cannot be cured by surgery. Management of such effusions centers around palliation of symptoms. Initial step is to identify the primary tumor. The main reason to identify the primary tumor is to decide whether systemic chemotherapy is indicated. Systemic chemotherapy is effective in some patients with small cell ca, breast ca, non-small cell ca, and lymphoma.

If the patient has a primary tumor that does not respond to systemic chemotherapy, then the attempt should be made to remove the pleural fluid. The following are the two primary modes of treatment to control the accumulation of pleural fluid — one by an indwelling catheter and second by pleurodesis. If the patient is not symptomatic because of pleural effusion, then removal of pleural fluid is not recommended. Before attempting the pleurodesis, the position of mediastinum should be confirmed. If shifting of mediastinum is noted, bronchoscopy is done to rule out bronchial obstruction. If the patient is dyspneic and dyspnea responds well to thoracocentesis, then the procedure of choice for patients with a strong family support and who can receive a home health care is the insertion of an indwelling catheter and periodic change of pleural fluid. If these conditions are not met, then the preferred treatment is pleurodesis with a sclerosing agent through a chest tube. If the lung is not expanded after ICD, then use of an indwelling catheter or a pleuroperitoneal shunt should be considered.

Thoracocentesis

Therapeutic thoracentesis may serve as the primary therapeutic modality in select patients. In the patient with far advanced disease, poor

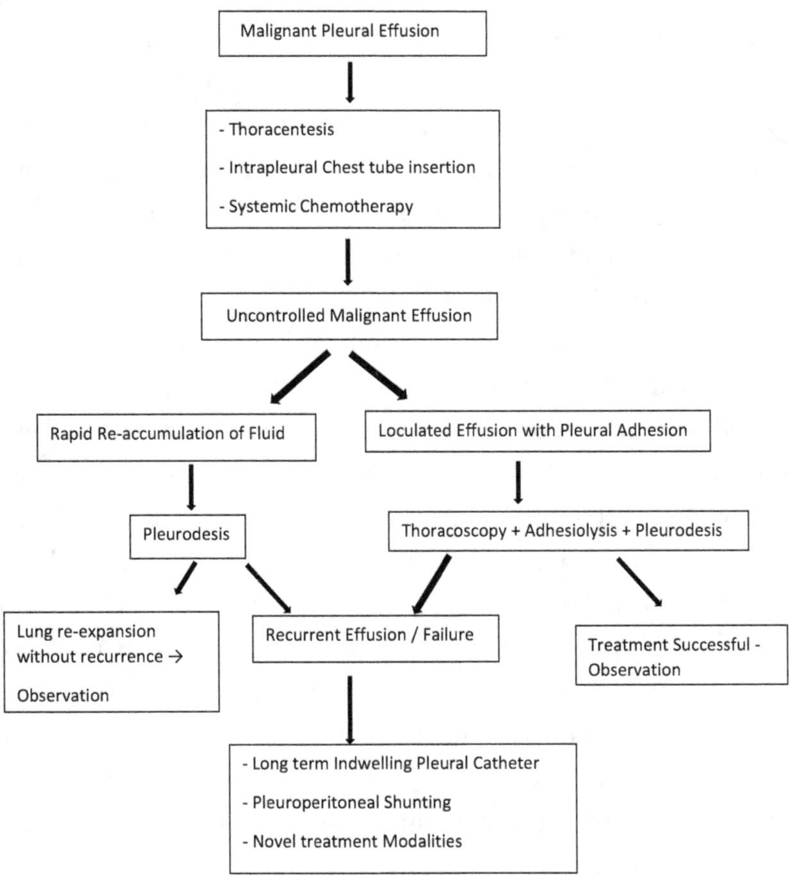

Figure 3: Management of Malignant Pleural Effusion

performance status (PS), and low pleural fluid pH (pH $\leqslant$ 7.2), relief can be provided by periodic outpatient therapeutic thoracenteses in lieu of hospitalization for more invasive and morbid procedures. After thoracentesis, total lung capacity (TLC) increases by approximately one-third the volume of fluid removed, and the forced vital capacity (FVC) increases by one-half the increase in TLC. The improvement in FVC and TLC after thoracentesis is variable and is greatest in patients with high lung compliance.

Intrapulmonary shunt is the main mechanism underlying the arterial hypoxemia associated with a large pleural effusion. Thoracentesis has short-term effects on pulmonary gas exchange. The effect on PaO_2 is variable, and it can increase, remain the same, or decreased. After therapeutic thoracentesis, there appears to be delayed lung volume re-expansion, with or without the coexistence of minimal pulmonary edema.

Removal of only 1–1.5 L of fluid at one sitting, as long as the patient does not develop dyspnea, chest pain, or severe cough is recommended. When a patient with contralateral mediastinal shift on chest radiograph tolerates thoracentesis without chest tightness, cough, or dyspnea, removal of several liters of pleural fluid is probably safe. Neither patient nor operator, however, may be aware of a precipitous decrease in pleural pressure. In patients without contralateral or with ipsilateral mediastinal shift, the likelihood of a precipitous fall in pleural pressure is increased, and either pleural pressure should be monitored during thoracentesis or only a small volume of fluid (<300 cm^3) should be removed. In the patient with ipsilateral mediastinal shift, it is unlikely that removal of pleural fluid will result in significant relief of dyspnea, because there is either mainstem bronchial occlusion or a trapped lung. Re-expansion pulmonary edema can occur after rapid removal of air or pleural fluid from the pleural space and is not necessarily related to the absolute level of negative pleural pressure. The mechanism of edema is believed to be increased capillary permeability; the injury may be related to the mechanical forces causing vascular stretching during re-expansion or to ischemia–reperfusion.

After thoracocentesis, usually rapid reaccumulation of pleural fluid is noted by 1–3 days. In addition, frequent thoracocentesis can lead to loculation of pleural fluid and thereby making subsequent pleurodesis difficult.

Systemic chemotherapy

Malignancy	Percentage of cases with complete resolution of effusion with systemic chemotherapy
Malignant breast carcinoma	32%–75%
Small cell lung ca	36%–50%
Non-small cell lung cancer (NSCLC)	38% complete resolution, 21% partial resolution

Lymphoma pleural effusions generally shows response to chemotherapy.

Non-small cell lung cancer-associated pleural effusions responds well to cisplatin, ifosfamide, irinotecan.

Recent studies showed that anti-vascular endothelial growth factor (VEGF) antibody bevacizumab, combined with standard first-line chemotherapy agents, provides survival advantage for patients with non-small cell lung cancer (NSCLC). Pleurodesis should never be attempted in patients who are receiving anti-VEGF antibody as angiogenesis is necessary for pleurodesis which is inhibited by bevacizumab.

Intrapleural chemotherapy

The heated chemotherapy is circulated for 90–120 minutes and then is removed and chest is flushed with a sterile solution. In select patients, this combination therapy is effective at slowing or preventing the recurrence of the disease and can add quality months — even years — to life. Most patients benefit from this multimodality treatment that includes surgery, HIPEC, and intravenous chemotherapy or immunotherapy.

There are very few studies that support this method of chemotherapy, as malignant pleural effusions indicate that local chemotherapy is unlikely to be useful. This method decreases the number of tumor cells in pleural space, thereby reducing the rate of pleural fluid accumulation.

1. A study recently done in patients with NSCLC
   A total of 27 patients received combination of systemic chemotherapy + intrapleural chemotherapy + radiotherapy — overall response was good with 7% complete resolution and 48% partial resolution. Median overall survival was 18 months (6 times longer than a patient with malignant pleural effusion secondary to NSCLC).
2. Therapeutic efficacy of *Staphylococcus aureus* superantigen (SSAg) in NSCLC patients — in another study 14 patients with NSCLC received the pleural instillation of SSAg 100–400 mg once or twice weekly until the pleural effusion resolved. The effusion was controlled completely in 11 patients — median survival was 7 months.
3. One report that shows intrapleural administration of increasing doses of rituximab, a monoclonal antibody against CD20, effective in controlling pleural effusions with a $CD20^+$ NHL.

The Lung Cancer Study Group evaluated intrapleural cisplatin and cytarabine in patients with malignant pleural effusions from a variety of solid tumors. Forty-six patients with cytologically proven symptomatic and previously untreated malignant pleural effusions were entered. Cisplatin, as a single dose of 100 mg/m^2, plus cytarabine 1,200 mg, were instilled into the pleural space via a chest tube that was then immediately removed. The overall response rate, complete plus partial at 3 weeks, was 49% (18/37 patients). One patient experienced reversible grade 3 renal toxic reactions, four patients had grade 3 hematologic toxic reactions, and five patients had grade 3 cardiopulmonary toxic reactions. Median length of response was 9 months for a complete remission and 5.1 months for a partial remission.

Mediastinal radiation

If the patient with malignant pleural effusion develops chylothorax, thoracic duct is usually involved by the neoplastic process. Therefore, radiotherapy is administered to the mediastinum. A study showed that chylothorax resolved in 68% of cases with lymphomas and 50% with metastatic carcinoma.

Indwelling pleural catheter (PleurX)

PleurX catheter is a 15.5 F silicone rubber catheter, 66 cm in length with fenestrations along the proximal 24 cm. Using Seldinger technique, it is inserted into the pleural space. The catheter is maintained in its place with a chest wall tunnel 5–8 cm in length. This catheter has a particular valve on its distal end. The valve prevents fluid or air from passing to either direction through the catheter. The pleural fluid is drained intermittently by inserting the access tip of the drainage line into the valve of catheter and then draining the fluid through an external tube into vacuum bottles.

Study comparing the safety and efficacy of PleurX catheter drainage and doxycycline pleurodesis through intercostal drainage tube

Parameter	PleurX catheter	Doxycycline pleurodesis
Hospitalization days (median)	1.0	6.5
Fluid drained first 24 hours (mL)	1,905 ± 916	1,500 ± 916
Recurrence of effusion post-discharge (%)	12 of 91 (13)	6 of 28 (21)
Complications (%)		
Pleural infection	1 of 91 (1)	0
Cellulitis	6 of 91 (7)	0
Obstruction of catheter	2 of 91 (3)	0
Tumor seeding of catheter tract	3 of 91 (3)	0

The presence of PleurX catheter leads to spontaneous pleurodesis in nearly 50% of patients with a median time of 28 days. Patients who developed spontaneous pleurodesis gradually have decreased the amount of pleural fluid formed daily. Spontaneous pleurodesis was common in cases of breast or gynecological malignancy, absence of chest wall irradiation, cytological positivity, and complete re-expansion of the underlying lung.

Advantages — recent advance in the treatment of malignant pleural effusion, allowing patient to be treated in outpatient basis. Repeat thoracocentesis can be avoided. Cost effective. If the patient develops spontaneous pleurodesis, significant symptomatic relief has been achieved.

Exercise improvement

The initial mean values for the resting and exercise Borg score and the dyspnea component of the Guyatt CRQ were similar among the two groups. When the Borg scores were re-evaluated after the initial treatment was completed, the mean degree of improvement both at rest and after exercise were nearly identical among the two treatment groups. The Borg scores postexercise at 30 days, 60 days, and 90 days after the initial treatment showed a trend toward greater improvement in the indwelling catheter group, which was statistically significant at 30 days ($P = 0.05$). The improvements in the Guyatt CRQ scores were similar 30 days, 60 days, and 90 days posttreatment in both groups.

Comparison of initial Borg and Guyatt scores and mean improvements from the initial score in the two treatment groups

	Borg score rest		Borg score exercise		Guyatt CRQ	
Time group	Catheter	Doxycycline	Catheter	Doxycycline	Catheter	Doxycycline
Initial	2.4 ± 1.7 (99)	2.5 ± 2.0 (44)	4.9 ± 1.9 (99)	4.9 ± 2.1 (45)	14.5 ± 4.8 (96)	15.8 ± 5.7 (44)
Change after initial Rx	1.1 ± 1.9 (93)	1.1 ± 1.8 (30)	2.5 ± 2.0 (90)	2.5 ± 1.7 (28)	—	—
Change at 30 days	0.9 ± 1.8 (62)	0.5 ± 2.1 (28)	2.2 ± 2.4 (60)b	1.0 ± 2.4 (26)	5.2 ± 7.5 (59)	5.5 ± 8.7 (27)
Change at 60 days	1.3 ± 1.2 (49)	1.3 ± 1.4 (20)	2.3 ± 2.5 (46)	1.6 ± 2.3 (20)	6.5 ± 8.5 (44)	7.8 ± 7.1 (20)
Change at 90 days	0.4 ± 2.1 (35)	0.4 ± 1.9 (21)	2.2 ± 2.3 (34)	1.3 ± 2.3 (20)	7.2 ± 7.1 (33)	6.3 ± 8.2 (21)

Complications

Morbidity is generally low; common complications include fever, pneumothorax, misplacement of the catheter, and re-expansion pulmonary edema. In a study, it was observed that 3 out of 96 patients on catheter developed tumor seeding of the catheter tract within 90 days of insertion. Local cellulitis was also noted in some cases.

Two important complications include pleural infection and obstruction of the catheter.

	Pleural space infection — empyema	Obstruction of the catheter
Incidence	2.8%	3.4%
Treatment	Broad-spectrum antibiotics and drainage of the space	Instillation of fibrinolytics into the space to restore the patency

Since in 50% of the cases spontaneous pleurodesis is not achieved, chemical pleurodesis via the catheter is attempted in patients with > 1,000 mL of fluid after catheter has been in place for a maximum of 14 days.

Pleurodesis

There are two methods of pleurodesis:

1. Chemical pleurodesis: It is done by inserting a sclerosing agent into the pleural cavity via a chest tube.
2. Mechanical/surgical pleurodesis: This is done through medical thoracoscopy, VATS, or open thoracotomy.

Patient selection:

1. Patients who are not candidates of indwelling catheter, systemic chemotherapy or have chylothorax.
2. Patients in whom systemic chemotherapy or mediastinal radiotherapy have failed.

3. If the patient is dyspneic because of pleural effusion and goes for palliative care for dyspnea.
4. If a patient's quality of life is diminished by dyspnea and he or she has a life expectancy of a few more weeks, pleurodesis can be considered as it improves the quality of life.

Evaluation before the procedure:

Position of the mediastinum should be evaluated before pleurodesis.

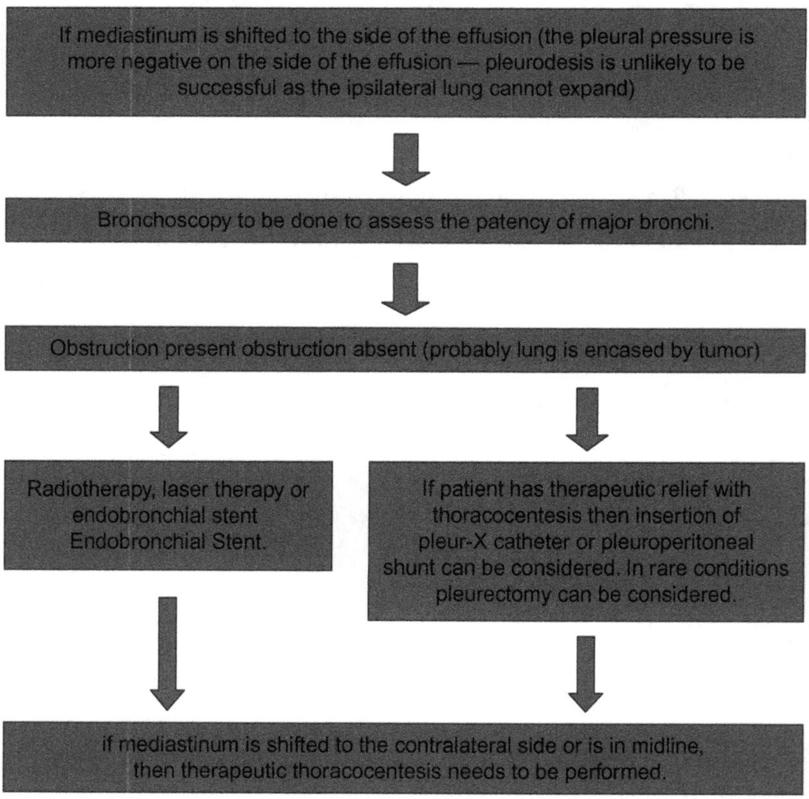

Prognosis factors for successful chemical pleurodesis:

1. pH level of the pleural fluid — if the pH is <7.2, more chances of failure with talc insufflation during thoracoscopy. Comparable reports are seen with intrapleural tetracycline.

2. Pleural fluid glucose level of less than 60 mg/dL — more chances of failure of pleurodesis noted.
3. Pleurodesis can fail if the two pleural surfaces cannot be brought into approximation. The rapid fall in pleural pressure is an indication that the underlying lung is unlikely to expand with the removal of fluid.
4. Success rate of pleurodesis also depends on the site of primary tumor — in talc pleurodesis patients with lung cancer and mesothelioma had a significantly lower complete response rate than patients with breast ca or other metastatic effusions. Similar conclusions were noted with doxycycline pleurodesis.

Mechanisms of chemical pleurodesis

1. Originally antineoplastic agents were used — including nitrogen mustard or radioisotopes in the hope that these agents would kill the tumor cells and control the effusion.
2. Effectiveness of intracavitary nitrogen mustard is greater when instillation of this agent is combined with tube thoracostomy, as the apposition of the two pleural surfaces allows the fibrotic process to obliterate the space.
3. Later, nonspecific irritants including talc, tetracycline derivatives, silver nitrate, iodopovidone and quinacrine were combined with tube thoracostomy.

Injury to the pleura is the first step in pleurodesis that often leads to an acute exudative pleural effusion that develops within 12 hours of instillation of the chemical agent.

Complex mechanism by which pleura responds to the injury — multifactorial and incompletely understood process leading to development of fibrosis if the procoagulant system dominates leading to obliteration of the pleural space.

If fibrinolytic system dominates, however, the pleurodesis will not be successful and restoration of the pleura to the normal state happens.

Transforming growth factor-beta

TGF-β is a potent fibrogenic cytokine that regulates extracellular matrix production, a study conducted in a rat lung showed significant overexpression of TGF-β that leads to marked pleural and interstitial fibrosis. Often a single injection is sufficient as TGF-β induce its own transcription. TGF-β is an ideal agent for pleurodesis; however, effectiveness and safety as an agent in humans is awaiting clinical trials.

Advantages of intrapleural injection of TGF-β for pleurodesis

a. Better and faster pleurodesis noted after intrapleural injection of TGF-β compared to doxycycline or talc.
b. Pleural fluid that results from intrapleural injection of TGF-β is noted to have low WBC count and LDH level than pleural fluid post doxycycline or talc pleurodesis.
c. Pleurodesis by TGF-β is not inhibited by corticosteroids.
d. It can lead to fibrotic reaction in the pleural space without the necessity for pleural injury.

The amount of collagen deposition (expressed as a percentage of the total area of the pleura) and the proportion of mature and immature fibers between the two groups at different time points are shown here. Significantly more total collagen, as well as mature (thick) and immature (thin) fiber depositions, were seen in the pleura of rabbits that received TGF-β_2 when compared with those that received talc ($p < 0.01$ for all three collagen groups). The amount of collagen deposition was approximately fivefold higher in the TGF-β_2 group than in the talc group consistently at all time points studied. As expected, there were more total collagen and mature and immature collagen fiber depositions ($p < 0.001$; $p < 0.05$; $p < 0.01$, respectively) at Day 7 than in the earlier time points. The proportion of mature and immature collagen fibers deposited were comparable in each group.

Pleural fluid characteristics after intrapleural administrations of TGF-β_2 and talc at 24 hours after injection*			
Effusion indices	TGF-β_2	Talc	*p* Value
Volume, mL	16.5 ± 9.0	1.8 ± 1.0	$p < 0.001$
LDH, IU/L	3,156 ± 1,426	12,733 ± 5,249	$p < 0.001$
Protein, mg/dL	2.96 ± 0.51	3.00 ± 0.46	$p = 0.89$

The pleural fluids collected at 24 hours after the injection of TGF-β_2 or talc slurry were compared. The TGF-β_2 group of rabbits produced significantly more fluid than did the talc group at 24 hours post injection. The fluid produced after TGF-β_2 injection was characterized by lower LDH levels, though the protein levels were similar in both groups. The amount of fluid produced after TGF-β_2 decreased rapidly over the following days. None of the rabbits killed at Day 4 had pleural fluid present at the time of necropsy.

Vascular endothelial growth factors

When mesothelial cells are incubated with TGF-β, the mesothelial cells produce increased amounts of VEGF. VEGF antibodies when administered had a significant effect on diminished pleural effusion; however, it prevented pleurodesis in rabbit lung model. Analysis of pleural tissue vasculature showed a close relation between amount of vasculature and pleurodesis score. Therefore, it is studied that angiogenesis is an important factor in the production of pleurodesis.

Sclerosing agents

Currently, talc (either insufflated or slurry), Tetracycline Derivatives (minocycline or doxycycline), Antineoplastic Agents (bleomycin or mitoxantrone), Silver Nitrate, and Iodopovidone are the most recommended agents.

A Cochrane database review in 2004 analyzed the efficacy of talc pleurodesis and found that comparison of successful pleurodesis:

Talc pleurodesis (74%) was more successful than tetracycline pleurodesis (57%).

Talc (79%) more successful than bleomycin (64%).

Tetracyclines and bleomycin have similar success rate of approx. 60%.

Thoracoscopic talc much better than medical talc.

(From Cochrane database of systematic reviews 2004 by Shaw p, Agarwal R)

In 2012, a preliminary study was conducted, and an article was published comparing the pleurodesis using tetracycline, erythromycin, and Aerosil [TM] 200, which is hydrophilic fumed amorphous silica, and it was concluded that Aersoil [TM] 200 with or without erythromycin was a more successful agent for pleurodesis compared to tetracycline and erythromycin alone.

It is also noted that there is no ideal sclerosing agent.

Talc:

a. Most commonly used sclerosing agent.
b. Widely available, inexpensive.
c. Can be insufflated as an aerosol (done at the time of thoracoscopy) or as slurry (suspended in saline).

A prospective study published in a European journal in 2006 confirms that intrapleural talc carries good results in the treatment of malignant pleural effusion. TP was significantly more effective than TS; both methods were safe, but TS had a higher incidence of thoracic pain during the procedure. Talc pleurodesis should be offered to every patient with MPE, apart from terminally ill ones, provided that a satisfying lung re-expansion has been achieved. TP should be performed whenever possible; otherwise, a slurry bedside procedure will be worthwhile, even in patients with low PS, though poorer results have to be expected. A careful selection is essential to define the proper technique.

Aydogmus et al. studied the factors for successful talc pleurodesis, and the conclusion of the study was success rate with talc slurry pleurodesis was significantly higher if the time period between diagnosis of effusion and administration of talc slurry was less than 30 days or spontaneous expansion was attained after chest tube drain or if the daily drainage was less than 200 mL/day before the talc slurry. The success rate was not related to the source of the primary tumor or the amount of drainage when chest tube was terminated.

Complication with talc pleurodesis:

- Most important concern is the development of acute respiratory distress syndrome (ARDS) in patients who received talc pleurodesis. Most of the reported case studies are from the United States. A study showed 4% of patients who received talc slurry and 8.1% of patients who received insufflated talc developed ARDS. Rehse et al. studied retrospectively on 78 patients who received talc pleurodesis — 7 patients (9%) developed ARDS requiring ventilator support, 1 patient succumbed.

Mechanisms of ARDS in talc pleurodesis

One hypothesis is systemic absorption of talc with subsequent development of inflammatory markers acute pneumonitis.

This is supported by large quantities of talc in bronchoalveolar lavage (BAL) fluids of most of the patients who developed ARDS secondary to talc pleurodesis as per the case reported by Rinaldo et al. A case report by Ribas Milanez de campos et al. noted the presence of talc in almost every organ including ipsilateral and contralateral kidney, lung, brain, liver, heart, and skeletal muscles.

Incidence of ARDS was noted more when smaller particles of talc were used; therefore, the recent studies suggest to avoid using talc preparations with particle size smaller than 10 μm.

a. Another complication reported from talc insufflation is pulmonary embolism. A study showed 7.4% of patients who received talc pleurodesis died within 15 days and thrombotic events were noted in nearly 30% of these cases. These patients were noted to have higher IL6 levels. It is unknown whether the same happens with talc slurry.

b. Whereas pain and fever were the most frequent complications of thoracoscopic talc insufflation, the incidence of ARDS was low. Pneumothorax, pneumonia, emphysema, prolonged air leakage, pulmonary embolism, arrythmia, re-expansion pulmonary edema, and empyema are important complications of thoracoscopic talc insufflation.

Tetracycline derivatives

a. Second most common agent used in pleurodesis.
b. Tetracycline 1,500 mg effectively controlled 94.4% of 108 malignant pleural effusion according to a study by Sherman et al.
c. As parenteral tetracyclines are no longer available, their derivatives including minocycline and doxycycline are being used.
d. Lower dose is required with doxycycline and minocycline compared to tetracycline to achieve pleurodesis.
e. Tetracycline derivatives causes a high incidence of fatal hemothoraces.
f. In animal models also, tetracycline have been showed increased incidence of hemothorax, which can be fatal.
g. Five reports with a total of 110 patients were analyzed — at 30 days — there was control of effusion in nearly 83% cases with doxycycline 500 mg.
h. Minocycline at a dose of 300–500 mg produced a complete response at 30 days in nearly 62.5% of cases. In nearly 25% of the cases, the pleural effusion got controlled that repeat thoracocentesis was not required.
i. Dikensoy et al. demonstrated that administration of combination of sclerosing agents can also be used and often their efficacy was better compared to individual agents.
j. Administration of one-half (5 mg/kg doxycycline + 200 mg/kg talc) or one-fourth (2.5 mg/kg doxycycline + 100 mg/kg talc) or the usual dose

(10 mg/kg doxycycline + 400 mg/kg talc) in rabbits resulted in a better mean pleurodesis score than usage of doxycycline or talc alone.

k. Side effect with pleurodesis — Primary side effect is severe chest pain; chest pain is noted to be more severe in cases where tetracycline derivative are given for pneumothorax compared to pleural effusion. Most severe pain is noted in malignant pleural effusion cases. Therefore, it is recommended to give lorazepam or midazolam in addition to systemic pain medications.

Incidence of chest pain and fever are more after pleurodesis with doxycycline, compared to other agents.

Sclerosing agent	Fever (%)	Chest pain (%)
Talc	16	7
Doxycycline	31	40
Tetracycline	10	14
Bleomycin	28	24

Antineoplastic agents — bleomycin, nitrogen mustard, mitoxantrone

Bleomycin

a. Is an agent that is sometimes used for malignant pleural effusion.
b. Ruckedeschel et al. studied in a randomized control trial (RCT) the success rates of bleomycin compared to tetracycline in 44 patients and noted that at 30 days success rate with bleomycin (64%) was much better than that with tetracycline (33%).
c. However, the recent studies show that bleomycin is less effective compared to talc or tetracycline derivatives in pleurodesis.
d. It was also ineffective as a pleurodesis agent in animal models.
e. The overall success rate in patients using bleomycin pleurodesis was less, and in an RCT, it was noted that the failure rate with bleomycin at 30 days was 41%, at 90 days was 59%, and at 180 days was 65%.

f. In another study, a second dose of bleomycin was administered if the output from the chest tube was more than 100 mL/day on the third day after the administration of bleomycin, and 83% of the patients responded.
g. In view of bleomycin being expensive compared to talc or tetracycline derivatives, it is not recommended.

Nitrogen mustard

a. One of the first antineoplastic agents used to treat malignant pleural effusions.
b. Effective in animal models.
c. Leininger et al. studied that administration of 10 mg of nitrogen mustard through a chest tube to 18 patients, and the treatment was effective in 17 of them.
d. Kinsey et al. studied the usage of nitrogen mustard in malignant pleural effusion cases, 92% of the pleural effusions got controlled.
e. As it is cheaper than bleomycin and effective, it is the agent of the choice if an antineoplastic agent is preferred to be used.

Mitoxantrone

a. In a study, 114 patients with malignant pleural effusions with breast carcinoma were given 40 mg mitoxantrone intrapleurally, and 53.5% of cases showed complete resolution, and 25% showed partial resolution.
b. Another study showed that by 60 days complete resolution of pleural effusion noted in all 21 cases after administering 40 mg mitoxantrone.
c. It can bind to cell membranes and therefore stays much longer in the pleural space compared to other agents.
d. Side effects include cardiotoxicity.
e. Due to similar success rates compared to other agents and increased side effects, mitoxantrone is not the preferred sclerosing agent.
f. Another agent that showed some response in the clinical trials is cisplatin. Sero et al. studied the effectiveness and found that 25 mg cisplatin in 500 mL distilled water intrapleurally in 80 patients with non-small cell carcinoma and found that nearly 34% of the patients had complete response and 49% of the cases at partial response at 4 weeks.

g. An article published in *Journal of American Geriatrics Society* in 2006 studied that pleurodesis with intrapleurally administrated carboplatin in elderly patients with MPE accompanied by advanced lung adenocarcinoma, renal insufficiency, and poor PS may be an effective palliative therapy with acceptable toxicity profiles. Observed side effects included nausea (4%), vomiting (3%), pyothorax (1%), and dyspnea (1%).

Other antineoplastic agents including doxorubicin, etoposide, fluorouracil, and mitomycin c have been evaluated for the pleurodesis; however, the response rate is unsatisfactory.

Silver nitrate

A study on the efficacy and safety of intrapleural cisplatin versus silver nitrate in treatment of malignant pleural effusion, Mohammad K. El Badrawy et al. published in *Egyptian Journal of Bronchology* volume 12, pages 98–104 (2018), showed that the success rate of pleurodesis in silver nitrate group was 90% versus 76.7% in cisplatin group, without significant difference, and chest pain was reported in 26.7% in silver nitrate group and 13.3% in cisplatin group, and fever was reported in 33.3% in silver nitrate group and 20.0% in cisplatin group. Recurrence was reported in 10% in silver nitrate group and in 23.3% in cisplatin group.

A comparison study analyzing the silver nitrate and talc pleurodesis showed that talc slurry pleurodesis was associated with more recurrent effusions compared to silver nitrate; however, more studies are required to rule out side effects of silver nitrate in pleurodesis.

Iodopovidone

Olivares-Torres et al. studied the effectiveness of betadine as a pleurodesis agent in 40 patients after thoracoscopy and 12 patients through chest tube, and it was noted that complete clearance with no reaccumulation was noted in nearly 96% of the cases. Post-procedure hypotension and severe chest pain were noted in some of the cases; however, no fatalities were reported. A comparison study analyzed the usage of insufflated talc and iodine as pleurodesis agent — higher incidence of pain was noted with betadine with similar recurrence rate with both the sclerosing agents.

50–100 mL of 2% iodopovidone can be considered.

A report from Germany showed that using approx. 200–500 mL of 10% iodopovidone led to the development of blindness. This dosage is more than 25 times the recommended dosage. None of the other studies have showed visual disturbances. It is also a reasonable alternative compared to talc and tetracycline for pleurodesis.

Other agents for pleurodesis include

a. **Dried killed *Corynebacterium parvum***, an anaerobic Gram-positive bacterium has been studied, and it is presumed that it works by being immunomodulators. It was noted to have been quite effective with an overall success rate of 76%. The availability of *C. parvum* in worldwide is limited, and this can limit its overall use.
b. **OK-432**, obtained from SU strain of *S. pyogenes*, both immunostimulatory and cytotoxic, have been used in Japan as a sclerosing agent. Response rates as high as 75% were noted.
c. **Quinacrine** has been used in some Scandinavian countries for pleurodesis in malignant pleural effusions; the intrapleural injection of quinacrine can lead to systemic inflammatory response similar to talc injection. Success rate was about 86% in a study with 98 patients of malignant pleural effusion who were treated with quinacrine.

Agent of choice

Malignant pleural effusion with tube thoracostomy	Doxycycline 500 mg, tetracycline 1,500 mg, minocycline 300 mg Alternatively: 20 mL of 0.5% silver nitrate or 100 mL of 2% iodopovidone
Malignant pleural effusion diagnosed during thoracoscopy or thoracotomy	Pleural abrasion or partial pleurectomy

Intrapleural injection of sclerosing agent

Pleurodesis is performed by injecting the sclerosing agent via the chest tube; pleurodesis needs the both layers of pleura in close proximity, if that is not achieved, then pleurodesis is unlikely to occur; hence, using chest tube for pleurodesis is preferred.

a. Success of pleurodesis does not depend on the size of the chest tube.
b. After inserting the chest tube for malignant pleural effusion, it is not advised to give negative pressure for the initial time as chronic pleural effusion, and application of negative pressure can lead to re-expansion pulmonary edema. If lung expansion has not happened in 24 hours, then negative pressure can be applied to the chest tube.
c. If the patient is on NSAIDS or corticosteroids, then pleurodesis is less likely to happen.
d. The underlying lung should be fully expanded before pleurodesis. If the underlying lung is not fully expanded, then additional thickening of visceral pleura can develop post-pleurodesis, which can further complicate the lung expansion.
e. Sclerosing agent needs to be instilled as soon as the lung is fully expanded. The duration of drainage is noted to be less in patients in whom the sclerosing agent was instilled immediately after lung expansion compared to the patients in whom sclerosing agent was instilled once the drainage was less than 150 mL/day.
f. If the patient is having a loculated pleural effusion, to inject a fibrinolytic agent intrapleurally, Hsu et al. injected urokinase, for at least 3 days in 12 patients with trapped lungs and 36 cases with loculated pleural effusion. If the lung does not expand with tube thoracostomy with or without instillation of fibrinolytics, pleural fluid can be drained on chronic basis using PleurX catheter or with a pleuroperitoneal shunt.
g. If mediastinum is shifted away from the side of effusion, one of the options to be considered.

h. Tetracycline derivatives can cause intense pleuritic chest pain and reactions. And therefore systemic medications to control the pain to be considered.
i. After the sclerosant is injected, catheter is flushed with 50–100 mL of saline and the chest tube clamped for at least 1 hour.
j. After 1–2 hours, the chest tube is unclamped and the negative pressure (–15 to –20 cm H_2O) is applied to the chest tube. Suction is maintained for at least 24 hours and until the pleural drainage is less than 150 mL/day. The chest tube is removed after 96 hours regardless of the volume of the pleural fluid.

Thoracoscopy for pleurodesis

1. **VATS with talc poudrage**

This has replaced the conventional talc slurry instillation through tube thoracostomy. Precisely, 62% of patients have no recurrence of pleural effusion for their lifetime following VATS with talc poudrage. In a study, it was noted that 8.1% developed respiratory failure and died. Froudarakis reported that patients who underwent thoracoscopy with talc insufflation had:

a. Greater temperature elevation.
b. Increased peripheral blood WBC count.
c. Increased CRP.

2. **Mechanical abrasion of the pleura**

In animal studies, mechanical abrasion of the pleura is as effective as talc for pleurodesis. A total of 44 patients were treated with mechanical abrasion for pleural effusion, and it was noted that in 6 months, there was no recurrence in 94% of the cases. It was noted that mechanical abrasion was effective in pleural effusion with pleural fluid pH being less than 7.3.

Criteria	Mechanical abrasion	Talc insufflation
Duration of hospital stay	Lesser	Longer
Duration of ICD care	Lesser	Longer
Pleural fluid PH	Effective in both less or more than 7.3	Less effective if <7.3

Therefore, it is noted that mechanical abrasion of pleura is the best method for pleurodesis in patients undergoing thoracoscopy.

Alternatives to pleurodesis and indwelling catheter

If the patient is not a good candidate for chemical pleurodesis or insertion of PleurX catheter, options, including symptomatic treatment, implantation of a pleuroperitoneal shunt, serial thoracocentesis, pleurectomy, can be considered.

Symptomatic treatment

a. The two primary symptoms of malignant pleural effusion include chest pain and shortness of breath.
b. If chest pain is present, sufficient analgesics need to be given.
c. If the primary symptom is dyspnea, the patient should be given opiates or oxygen or both, if PleurX catheter cannot be used for them.

Pleuroperitoneal shunt

This device consists of two catheters connected with a valved pump chamber. The two one-way valves in the pump chamber are positioned such that fluid can only go from pleural space to the pump chamber to the peritoneal cavity. To a positive pressure of 1 cm H_2O, these valves open. Capacity of the pump chamber is 1.5 mL.

On compression

↓

Fluid is forced from the chamber and is pushed to the peritoneal cavity.

On releasing the pump → negative pressure created in the pump chamber draws the fluid from the pleural cavity to the pump chamber.

Modification of the pump: The pump is placed exteriorly compared to the subcutaneous pocket caudal to a skin incision in the lateral part of the inframammary crease and fixed to the tissues with suture through sewing holes in the base of pump chamber. The volume of the pump is 2.5 mL rather than 1.5 mL.

Pleural catheter — inserted at the lateral and superior aspect of incision using a Seldinger-type introducer kit.

Abdominal catheter — tunnelled subcutaneously across the coastal margin and inserted through a 3 cm skin incision in the anterior abdominal wall into the peritoneal cavity through a small incision in the peritoneum.

Advantages of shunts

a. Less hospitalisation time compared to pleurodesis.
b. Amount of pain is less with chemical pleurodesis.
c. The procedure can be performed on op basis.
d. Patient can use the pump when dyspneic and thereby giving psychological help.

Disadvantages

a. Shunt becomes obstructed in some patients.
b. Insertion requires general anesthesia.
c. Shunt to be inserted by a surgeon.
d. Daily pump usage is required.

Indications

a. As an OPD therapy for malignant pleural effusion, PleurX catheter is recommended.
b. If a chylothorax is present, shunt is recommended as the nutritional status of the patient is preserved.
c. Pleuroperitoneal shunt is also preferred in patients with trapped lungs as the patient will require drainage for the rest of life.

Pleurectomy

Can be attempted in two different situations in selected patients.

1. In patients who underwent a diagnostic thoracotomy for undiagnosed pleural effusion and if malignant disease is found, an immediate parietal pleurectomy can prevent the recurrence of effusion. In such cases, parietal pleurectomy consists of stripping all the parietal pleura from the rib cage and the mediastinum.
2. Another situation is in symptomatic patients with persistent pleural effusion and trapping of the ipsilateral lung. Here, injection of sclerosing agent is contraindicated. Surgical procedure here is decortication of the trapped lung in conjunction with parietal pleurectomy.

   It controls malignant pleural effusion in nearly 90% cases; however, the mortality of this procedure is around 10%.

Drug-induced pleural disorders

Introduction

Drug-induced pleuropulmonary diseases are becoming quite increasing apparent since pulmonology has established itself as a superspeciality in medicine in developing countries. A relatively small amount of drug can induce its adverse effects on the pleura, which resolves on discontinuation of the drug but reappears when re-exposed to the same drug. The drug-induced pleural disease may occur in the form of pleuritis with or without effusion or pleural thickening/fibrosis. Where lupus-like syndrome can occur with hydralazine, nitrofurantoin may produce an eosinophilic pleural effusion. Mitomycin therapy may precipitate small pleural effusion and pleural thickening and practolol may cause pleural fibrosis. Because of the sporadic nature of many of these reactions and lack of specific markers, it is difficult to estimate true incidence of drug-induced pleural disorders.

Lupus pleuritis

Drug like chlorpromazine, isoniazid, procainamide hydralazine, phenytoin, methyl dopa, and quinidine may precipitate or exacerbate lupus-like syndrome in a patient with pre-existing SLE. Exudative pleural effusion is a usual accompanying feature of pleuritis, and lupus erythematosus cells can be demonstrated in the pleural fluid analysis. With the removal of offending drug, pleuritis often subsides.

Pleural effusion (eosinophilic)

Drugs like nitrofurantoin, dantrolene, bromocriptine, valproic acid, propylthiouracil, and isotretinoin are often associated with eosinophilic pleural effusion when administered. Pleural effusion with nitrofurantoin is often accompanied with parenchymal infiltrates, and this hypersensitivity reaction occurs within few hours of drug intake. Peripheral eosinophilia is often accompanying. Stopping of offending drug and sometimes corticosteroids help in early recovery. Chronic drug administration leads to pulmonary adverse effects such interstitial pneumonitis and fibrosis, where pleural affection is not common.

A unilateral, exudative eosinophilic pleural effusion with peripheral eosinophilia and without any pulmonary involvement is reported with chronic administration of dantrolene. Pleural fibrosis can also occur. Pleural effusion may take quite a longer duration to resolve even after total withdrawal of the offending drug.

Eosinophilic pleural effusion with peripheral eosinophilia with valproic acid and pleural effusion without peripheral eosinophilia or pulmonary infiltrates with propylthiouracil and isotretinoin have been reported.

Pleuritis, effusion, and thickening of pleura

Hypersensitivity reaction or as a result of direct toxicity certain chemotherapeutic agents such as bleomycin, methotrexate, cyclophosphamide, mitomycin, and procarbazine can produce pleuropulmonary manifestations, where pleural effusion may be accompanying a small number of patients with interstitial pneumonitis. Pleural thickening may develop as a late manifestation in cyclophosphamide therapy. Pleural thickening may occur with methotrexate when used in high dose and rarely with mitomycin therapy.

Bleomycin adverse effects are also dose-related.

Cardiovascular drugs such as minoxidil, practolol, and amiodarone are notorious to cause pleuropulmonary lung disease with pleural effusion may occur with a miodarone therapy, which may develop into pleural thickening due to chronic inflammation. Practolol can cause pleural effusion with pleural thickening and rarely pleural fibrosis. Both pericardial and pleural effusions are reported with minoxidil therapy.

Pleural effusion and fibrosis can occur with bromocriptine and methysergide treatment.

Rarely, pleural effusion may develop with the use of a variety of agents such as clozapine, simvastatin, tryptophan, absolute alcohol, recombinant interleukin-2 acyclovir, D-penicillamine, metronidazole, itraconazole, and granulocyte colony-stimulating factor.

Comments: Pleural disorders induced by drug use may manifest as pleurisy, with or without pleural effusion, thickening or fibrosis, and may occur with or without accompanying pulmonary disease. Management lies in practice. ADR reporting is important, and PR Shankar has initiated spontaneous ADR reporting service to promote ADR.

HIV disease and pleural effusion

Introduction

Pleural affection in HIV disease is not uncommon; association of pleural effusion is more with the advanced stages of HIV disease. Although etiology may remain obscure in a few cases, diagnosis can be made in most of these patients, pinpointing infective or noninfective etiology in almost one-third and two-thirds of cases, respectively.

Infective etiology of pleural effusion

Pleural effusion is present in association with AIDS, in infections causing pulmonary infiltration. Pleural effusion is present in almost one-third of cases of bacterial pneumonia in HIV disease. In 50% of cases, *S. pneumoniae* is responsible for pneumonitis; *Haemophilus influenzae*, *Mycoplasma pneumoniae*, *Legionella*, and *Nocardia asteroides* have also been implicated. Right-sided endocarditis may also lead to septic pulmonary embolization that may result in small pleural effusion; the effusions are small, ipsilateral, and exudative in nature with low nucleated cell count and rarely become empyematous, especially in parapneumonic effusions in AIDS. *S. aureus* may be responsible for life-threatening community-acquired pneumonia with parapneumonic effusion in association with HIV disease, with history of intravenous drug users.

Precisely, 2%–11% of pleural effusion in observed in cases of *Pneumocystis carinii* pneumoniae, more so in patients receiving aerosolized pentamidine therapy and is often accompanied with pleural masses or pneumothorax. The effusions are usually small, unilateral, or bilateral, serous or bloody in nature, with raised LDH levels, having a fluid-to-serum ratio more than 1.0 (i.e., exudate in nature), and without any acidosis or alteration in fluid-amylase and glucose levels. Total nucleated cell count in the fluid is low with predominant mononuclear cells. Trophozoites of *P. carinii* in the fluid can be demonstrated by Grocott silver staining; however, examination of an air-dried Diff-Quik-stained cytospin preparation is ideal. Pleural fluid demonstrates numerous vacuolated macrophages, granular eosinophilic aggregates, and scattered benign mesothelial cell clusters. Occurrence of pleural effusion does not alter the prognosis of the PCP, although occurrence of pneumothorax often means prolonged indwelling chest tube drainage.

Tuberculous pleural effusion accounts for 10% of cases with AIDS, and the effusion in usually larger one. Accompanying miliary or pulmonary parenchymal infiltration may be present. This exudative fluid has neither fluid acidosis nor low glucose levels. Nucleated cell count is low in the fluid with predominance of lymphocytes: AFB positivity in the fluid is less than 15%. Pleural biopsy reveals granulomatous lesion in almost 90% of cases. Tuberculin positivity is varying from 20% to 64%.

In *Cryptococcus neoformans* in HIV disease, pleural effusion in an isolated finding, but often it represents disseminated cryptococcal disease in AIDS patients. Fluid is exudative with low count of nucleated cells.

Cryptococcal antigen determination in the fluid is a rapid and specific test

Pleural effusion with *Histoplasma capsulatum* in AIDS patients is rare and occurs with disseminated disease, contiguous spread, hypersensitivity pleuritis, or active pericarditis. Effusion is serosanguinous with low number of nucleated cells. Wright-Giemsa staining demonstrates intracellular yeast, typical of *H. capsulatum.*

Unilateral or bilateral pleural effusion may rarely be seen in *Toxoplasma gondii* infection in late stages of AIDS. *T. gondii* trophozoites within the neutrophils can be demonstrated by Giemsa staining in the centrifuge pleural fluid.

Noninfective pleural etiology

Hypoalbuminemic pleural effusion may occur in progressive HIV disease. These are moderate-sized transudates which occur bilaterally. Nucleated cells are low in the fluid, with predominant mononuclear cells.

Isolated pleural effusion is a sole presentation of AIDS-related lymphoma, occurring in 5%–10% of cases. Thoracic involvement in AIDS-related lymphoma is uncommon with the absence of mediastinal and hilar involvement of lymph nodes. Such an effusion is unilateral and larger one, serosanguinous exudate with normal glucose contents and lymphocytic predominance.

Pleural pulmonary involvement is seen in one-fifth of cases of AIDS with Kaposi's sarcoma, and 60% of these cases have pleural effusion. Cutaneous and thoracic involvement may not correlate and pleuritic pain may be absent because of involvement of visceral pleura and sparing of parietal pleura. Unilateral or bilateral alveolar or interstitial involvement is present along with hilar or mediastinal lymphadenopathy in 25%–60% of cases. Effusions are large and predominantly bilateral. Autopsy findings reveal bilateral hemorrhagic pleural effusions, visceral pleural purplish lesions of Kaposi's sarcoma, and infiltration of lung parenchymal lymphatics and mediastinal lymph nodes. Bleeding from highly vascular visceral pleural lesions make the fluid serosanguinous that gets complicated because of impaired drainage, secondary to obstruction of lymphatics. Nucleated cell count in the fluid is low, with predominance of mononuclear cells. The fluid is exudative, pH being more than 7.4, with higher glucose contents and LDH levels varying from 111 to 3,301 U/L. Percutaneous pleural biopsy is noncontributory (because of the absence of lesion on the parietal pleura). Open lung biopsy is diagnostic in more than three-fourths of cases but not recommended for being highly risky. Bronchoscopy demonstrates diagnostic cherry-red endobronchial lesions in a patient with bilateral hemorrhagic pleural effusion in cases of Kaposi's sarcoma.

Pleural effusion due to congestive cardiac failure (CCF) may occur in AIDS patients, due to cardiomyopathy, usually caused by infectious myocarditis with toxoplasmosis, cytomegalovirus and HIV. These are small transudates, unilateral or bilateral, and usually resolve following the treatment of cardiac failure.

Management

Infection is empirically treated in intravenous drug abusers in bacterial pneumonia. PCP is managed with intravenous pentamidine, supplemented with aerosolized pentamidine. TB is treated with full-dose four-drug regimen for 9–12 months. Amphotericin B is useful in treating *C. neoformans* infection in HIV disease. *H. capsulatum* pleural effusion resolves spontaneously. Effusion with lymphoma in HIV disease responds to chemotherapy. Treatment of pleural effusion with Kaposi's sarcoma is symptomatic, and radiation may offer palliative management. Tetracycline pleurodesis is effective. Alpha interferon or combined chemotherapy gives partial relief. Transudate effusion resolves by itself when heart failure is treated.

Treatment of transudative pleural effusion

Treatment options and further management of pleural effusion depends on the type of pleural effusion.

1. **Secondary to heart failure** — Effusion secondary to heart failure can be successfully managed by treating the heart failure. Digitalis, diuretics, and

afterload reduction are the treatment strategies used to manage cardiac pleural effusions. Occasionally, large pleural effusions may lead to dyspnea in such patients; hence, removal of approximately 500–1,000 mL leads to rapid relief of dyspnea. If the effusions cannot be managed by standard therapy, use of interventions to control pleural effusion can be considered. For example, pleurodesis using a sclerosing agent. In such cases, the preferred sclerosing agent is doxycycline 500 mg through a chest tube is preferred.

An alternative method is to insert an indwelling pleural catheter or to use a pleuroperitoneal shunt. Herlihy et al. inserted indwelling catheter for five patients with pleural effusion refractory to standard therapy — after 5–15 months, two patients developed empyema and after 4 months, one patient developed loculated pleural effusion. With the PleurX, the patient connects the catheter to vacuum bottles every other day to drain the fluid.

Pleuroperitoneal shunt consists of two catheters connected with a valved pump chamber. The two one-way valves in the pump chamber are positioned such that fluid can only flow from the pleural space to the peritoneal space through the pump chamber. Because the pleural pressure is almost negative compared to the peritoneal pressure, the pumping chamber must be used to move the fluid from the pleural cavity to the peritoneal cavity. Little et al. reported that two patients with refractory pleural effusion secondary to cardiac failure were managed with pleuroperitoneal shunts successfully.

2. **Hepatic hydrothorax** — pleural effusion can be seen as a complication of cirrhosis in patients having ascites. Pleural effusion in patients with cirrhosis and ascites is usually right sided (67%) but occasionally left sided (16%) and bilateral (16%).

In patients with cirrhosis, ascites, and pleural effusions, there is a possibility of spontaneous pleural effusion analogous to spontaneous bacterial peritonitis. Also called spontaneous bacterial empyema; however, it may not look like pus. Therefore, also called spontaneous bacterial pleuritis. Diagnosis of spontaneous bacterial pleuritis can be made if they have cirrhosis along with a positive pleural fluid bacterial culture and a neutrophil count greater than 250 cells/mm^3 or if negative pleural culture and neutrophil count more than 500 cells/mm^3.

Management of pleural effusions associated with cirrhosis and ascites should be directed toward the treatment of ascites because the hydrothorax is an extension of peritoneal fluid. The patient should be put on a low-salt diet and diuretics. Best diuretic therapy in such cases is found to be combination of furosemide and spironolactone.

The starting dose of furosemide is 40 mg and spironolactone is 100 mg. Serial therapeutic thoracocentesis are not indicated due to rapid reaccumulation of the pleural fluid.

In patients who are refractory to the standard treatment, option of liver transplantation should be discussed. The presence of hepatic hydrothorax does not appear to adversely affect the results with liver transplantation.

The next best treatment is to implant a transjugular intrahepatic portosystemic shunt (TIPS). A recent RCT showed that TIPS was superior to serial thoracocentesis in patients with refractory hepatic hydrothorax. If neither TIPS or liver transplantation is feasible, the next option is videothoracoscopy with closure of diaphragmatic defects and pleurodesis.

Insertion of a chest tube in patients with hepatic hydrothorax carries significant morbidity and mortality with questionable benefits. University of Michigan series analyzed the placement of chest tubes in 17 patients with hepatic hydrothorax, and 16 had complications — AKI in 11 patients, pneumothorax in 7, empyema in 5 cases, encephalopathy in 3, pneumonia in 3, and most of the cases had multiple complications.

Another option in such cases include implantation of a peritoneojugular shunt. The explanation for the effectiveness of shunt is related to the peritoneal cavity, pleural space, and systemic veins. Because the pleural pressure is less than the central venous pressure, fluid will preferentially move to the pleural space rather than the central veins hence shunts frequently do not control the pleural effusion.

3. **Pleural effusion as a complication of percutaneous transhepatic coronary vein occlusion** — patients with bleeding esophageal varices are sometimes managed by injecting gelfoam or other materials transhepatically into the coronary veins so that the injected material will lodge in esophageal veins and stop the bleeding. For this procedure, the liver is reached by entering through the diaphragm. Pleural effusion is noted in most of the patients with ascites before the procedure. It is hypothesized to be because of iatrogenic diaphragmatic defect allowing the ascites to collect in the pleural space.

4. **Peritoneal dialysis** — in the past 30 years, there has been an increase in the use of continuous ambulatory peritoneal dialysis for the treatment of chronic renal failure. Pleural effusion can be secondary to CAPD owing to the movement of dialysate from the peritoneal cavity into the pleural cavity through a mechanism similar to that of ascites and cirrhosis. The effusion typically develops within 30 days of initiating the dialysis in 50% of the patients, but 18% had been on dialysis for more than a year before the effusion developed. Pleural effusion occurred on the right side 90% of the times, but it can also be bilateral or left side. Pleural effusion can also be as a complication of acute peritoneal dialysis. Diagnosis of cases of pleural effusion secondary to peritoneal dialysis — pleural fluid is characteristically noted to have glucose level intermediate between that of dialysate and serum, protein level below 3 g/dL, and a low LDH level <100 IU/L, which is higher than that in the peritoneal dialysate. When a patient on peritoneal dialysis develops pleural effusion, the dialysis must be stopped. It is recommended the dialysis be stopped for a period of 2–6 weeks. After this time, the peritoneal dialysis can be resumed, and approximately 50% of patients do not develop recurrence of pleural effusion. If there is recurrence of pleural effusion or such a waiting period is felt to be inappropriate, a procedure should be performed to create a pleurodesis. The approach is to insert a chest tube with instillation of a sclerosing agent — doxycycline. After this procedure, typically small-volume peritoneal dialysis can be performed for 10–14 days after the pleurodesis is performed. Recently, VATS

has been used. Halstead et al. subjected six patients to VATS during which they clipped communication in the diaphragm and performed a partial pleurectomy. At a median follow-up of 40 months, all had returned to CAPD, and there was no recurrence of hydrothorax. Another treatment strategy includes thoracoscopy with insufflation of talc allowed 17 of 18 patients to return to CAPD according to a study by Tang et al. This allows one to examine the diaphragm and clipping of the sites where leaking is noted can be attempted. Partial pleurectomy is preferred over talc pleurodesis due to the dangers of talc inducing the ARDS.

5. **Nephrotic syndrome**

In nephrotic syndrome, the pleural effusions are generally bilateral and are frequently intrapulmonary in location. The mechanism in the combination of decreased plasma oncotic pressure and increased hydrostatic pressure. In nephrotic syndrome, the patient can also develop pulmonary emboli; therefore, a lung scan or a CT angiogram is preferred in all patients with pleural effusion and nephrotic syndrome. If it is equivocal, evidence of DVT should be assessed. The treatment of pleural effusion associated with nephrotic syndrome is aimed at decreasing the protein loss in the urine to increase the plasma protein and to decrease the increased extracellular volume. Administering diuretics in conjunction with a low-sodium diet, ACE inhibitors, and using NSAID cautiously. Serial thoracocentesis is not preferred as it can further deplete the protein stores.

6. **Pulmonary veno-occlusive disease** — this disease is characterized by repeated pulmonary emboli. When a pleural effusion is noted in a patient with pulmonary artery hypertension, then diagnosis of pulmonary veno-occlusive disease has to be considered. The pleural effusion is probably related to increased interstitial fluid that results from obstruction of pulmonary veins. Diagnosis is made by surgical lung biopsy. The prognosis is bad with most patients dying within 2 years of diagnosis. The only treatment that significantly improves the prognosis of patients with pulmonary veno-occlusive disease is lung transplantation.

7. **Urinothorax** — pleural effusion can develop if there is a retroperitoneal urinary leakage secondary to urinary obstruction, trauma, retroperitoneal inflammatory or malignant processes, failed nephrostomy, or kidney biopsy. It is a rare cause of pleural effusion, and until 2006, only 58 cases have been noted. Pleural effusion typically happens within hours of the precipitating event and dissipates rapidly once the obstruction is relieved. There are two types of urinothorax: one is characteristically seen when there is bilateral obstruction of the urinary tract and the other one when there is trauma to the urinary tract.

8. **Myxedma** — pleural effusion can happen as a complication of myxedema. In one review of 128 patients with hypothyroidism in Massachusetts General Hospital and the Medical University of South Carolina, pleural effusion was noted in 28 patients. In one of them, pleural effusion was secondary to myxedematous pericardial effusion. When the pleural effusion is noted associated with a pericardial effusion, it is generally transudative. The obvious treatment is thyroid replacement.

9. **Leakage of cerebrospinal fluid into the pleura** — this is commonly seen following a ventriculoperitoneal shunting, but it can also happen when a ventriculoperitoneal shunt migrates to the pleural cavity. Other causes of subarachnoid pleural fistulas include penetrating and nonpenetrating traumas. The trauma is commonly surgery of spine. Diagnosis is made when the pleural fluid has characteristics of CSF. Fluid is clear, and protein level is very low. In case of recent trauma, the pleural fluid will be bloody.

10. **Meigs syndrome** — the diagnosis of Meigs syndrome should be made in all women with pelvic masses, ascites, and pleural effusion. If in such cases, cytological examination of the ascitic and pleural fluid is negative and exploratory laparotomy or a diagnostic laparoscopy can be performed with surgical removal of the neoplasm. The diagnosis is made when the ascitic and pleural fluid do not recur postoperatively. It is usually completely gone within 2 weeks.

11. **Pulmonary embolus** — treatment of pleural effusion secondary to pulmonary embolus is to treat the embolus. If the patient has high probability of having pulmonary embolus, then treatment should be started before the imaging studies are obtained. Low-molecular-weight heparin is preferred. With treatment, gradually the effusion resolves if there are no infiltrates. If the pleural effusion increases in size in spite of management of pulmonary embolus or if they develop contralateral pleural effusion, the patient probably has recurrent emboli or other complication including infection. On rare occasion, the administration of anticoagulants can lead to development of hemothorax. It can happen within the first week of the anticoagulant therapy. Therefore, if a patient with pulmonary embolus receiving anticoagulant therapy is having increased pleural effusion, diagnostic thoracocentesis has to be done, and pleural fluid hematocrit needs to be assessed. If hct is more than 50% of that of peripheral blood, then anticoagulation needs to be discontinued and ICD to be inserted.

12. **Sarcoidosis** — this condition is occasionally accompanied by a transudative effusion rather than an exudative effusion. Extensive thoracic involvement is noted, and they may also have extrathoracic involvement. Effusions are usually bilateral. Usually, small. The administration of corticosteroids to patients with pleural sarcoidosis can lead to symptomatic improvement and a resolution of the pleural effusion.

References and suggested readings

1. Penz E, Watt KN, Hergott CA, Rahman NM, Psallidas I. Management of malignant pleural effusion: challenges and solutions. Cancer Manag Res. 2017 Jun 23;9:229–241. doi: 10.2147/CMAR.S95663. PMID: 28694705; PMCID: PMC5491570.
2. Sundling KE, Cibas ES. Ancillary studies in pleural, pericardial, and peritoneal effusion cytology. Cancer Cytopathol. 2018 Aug;126(Suppl 8):590–598. doi: 10.1002/cncy.22021. PMID: 30156768.
3. Eccher A, Girolami I, Lucenteforte E, Troncone G, Scarpa A, Pantanowitz L. Diagnostic mesothelioma biomarkers in effusion cytology. Cancer Cytopathol.

2021 Jul;129(7):506–516. doi: 10.1002/cncy.22398. Epub 2021 Jan 19. PMID: 33465294.

4. Beaudoin S, Gonzalez AV. Evaluation of the patient with pleural effusion. CMAJ. 2018 Mar 12;190(10):E291–E295. doi: 10.1503/cmaj.170420. PMID: 29530870; PMCID: PMC5849448.
5. Cortes JE, Jimenez CA, Mauro MJ, Geyer A, Pinilla-Ibarz J, Smith BD. Pleural effusion in dasatinib-treated patients with chronic myeloid leukemia in chronic phase: identification and management. Clin Lymphoma Myeloma Leuk. 2017 Feb;17(2):78–82. doi: 10.1016/j.clml.2016.09.012. Epub 2016 Sep 17. PMID: 28082112.
6. Brogi E, Gargani L, Bignami E, Barbariol F, Marra A, Forfori F, Vetrugno L. Thoracic ultrasound for pleural effusion in the intensive care unit: a narrative review from diagnosis to treatment. Crit Care. 2017 Dec 28;21(1):325. doi: 10.1186/s13054-017-1897-5. PMID: 29282107; PMCID: PMC5745967.
7. Terra RM, Dela Vega AJM. Treatment of malignant pleural effusion. J Vis Surg. 2018 May 22;4:110. doi: 10.21037/jovs.2018.05.02. PMID: 29963399; PMCID: PMC5994464.
8. Lv Y, Han G, Fan D. Hepatic hydrothorax. Ann Hepatol. 2018 Jan–Feb;17(1):33–46. doi: 10.5604/01.3001.0010.7533. PMID: 29311408.
9. Redden MD, Chin TY, van Driel ML. Surgical versus non-surgical management for pleural empyema. Cochrane Database Syst Rev. 2017 Mar 17;3(3):CD010651. doi: 10.1002/14651858.CD010651.pub2. PMID: 28304084; PMCID: PMC6464687.
10. Ceruti P, Lonni S, Baglivo F, Marchetti G. Endoscopic diagnosis and management of pleural effusion in malignant pleural mesothelioma. J Thorac Dis. 2018 Jan;10(Suppl 2):S269–S275. doi: 10.21037/jtd.2017.09.142. PMID: 29507795; PMCID: PMC5830554.
11. Porcaro F, Procaccini E, Paglietti MG, Schiavino A, Petreschi F, Cutrera R. Pleural effusion from intrathoracic migration of a ventriculo-peritoneal shunt catheter: pediatric case report and review of the literature. Ital J Pediatr. 2018 Mar 27;44(1):42. doi: 10.1186/s13052-018-0480-2. PMID: 29587815; PMCID: PMC5870185.
12. Zeng N, Wan C, Qin J, Wu Y, Yang T, Shen Y, Wen F, Chen L. Diagnostic value of interleukins for tuberculous pleural effusion: a systematic review and

meta-analysis. BMC Pulm Med. 2017 Dec 8;17(1):180. doi: 10.1186/s12890-017-0530-3. PMID: 29216864; PMCID: PMC5721598.

13. Baenas DF, Retamozo S, Pirola JP, Caeiro F. Shrinking lung syndrome and pleural effusion as an initial manifestation of primary Sjögren's syndrome. Reumatol Clin (Engl Ed). 2020 Jan–Feb;16(1):65–68. English, Spanish. doi: 10.1016/j.reuma.2018.01.007. Epub 2018 Feb 19. PMID: 29472172.
14. Yang Y, Liu YL, Shi HZ. Diagnostic accuracy of combinations of tumor markers for malignant pleural effusion: an updated meta-analysis. Respiration. 2017;94(1):62–69. doi: 10.1159/000468545. Epub 2017 Apr 21. PMID: 28427079.
15. Zhang M, Yan L, Lippi G, Hu ZD. Pleural biomarkers in diagnostics of malignant pleural effusion: a narrative review. Transl Lung Cancer Res. 2021 Mar;10(3):1557–1570. doi: 10.21037/tlcr-20-1111. PMID: 33889529; PMCID: PMC8044497.
16. Wei XS, Wang X, Ye LL, Niu YR, Peng WB, Wang ZH, Zhang JC, Zhou Q. Pleural effusion as an indicator for the poor prognosis of COVID-19 patients. Int J Clin Pract. 2021 Jun;75(6):e14123. doi: 10.1111/ijcp.14123. Epub 2021 Mar 16. PMID: 33650234; PMCID: PMC7995219.
17. Brookes JDL, Williams M, Mathew M, Yan T, Bannon P. Pleural effusion post coronary artery bypass surgery: associations and complications. J Thorac Dis. 2021 Feb;13(2):1083–1089. doi: 10.21037/jtd-20-2082. PMID: 33717581; PMCID: PMC7947477.
18. Abou-Alfa GK, Sahai V, Hollebecque A. Pemigatinib for previously treated, locally advanced or metastatic cholangiocarcinoma: a multicentre, open-label, phase 2 study. Lancet Oncol. 2020 May;21(5):671–684. doi: 10.1016/S1470-2045(20)30109-1. Epub 2020 Mar 20. PMID: 32203698; PMCID: PMC8461541.
19. Aggarwal AN, Agarwal R, Dhooria S, Prasad KT, Sehgal IS, Muthu V. Unstimulated pleural fluid interferon gamma for diagnosis of tuberculous pleural effusion: a systematic review and meta-analysis. J Clin Microbiol. 2021 Apr 20;59(5):e02112–e02120. doi: 10.1128/JCM.02112-20. PMID: 33208475; PMCID: PMC8091832.

https://doi.org/10.1142/9789811271410_0044

44 Drug-induced pleural disorders

Introduction

Drug-induced pleuropulmonary diseases are becoming quite increasingly apparent since pulmonology has established itself as a super specialty in medicine in developing countries. A relatively small amount of drug can induce its adverse effects on the pleura, which resolves on discontinuation of the drug but reappears when reexposed to the same drug. The drug-induced pleural disease may occur in the form of pleuritis with or without effusion or pleural thickening/fibrosis. Where lupus-like syndrome can occur with hydralazine, nitrofurantoin may produce an eosinophilic pleural effusion. Mitomycin therapy may precipitate small pleural effusion and pleural thickening, and practolol may cause pleural fibrosis. Because of sporadic nature of many of these reactions and lack of specific markers, it is difficult to estimate true incidence of drug-induced pleural disorders.

Lupus-pleuritis

Drugs such as chlorpromazine, isoniazid, procainamide hydralazine, phenytoin, methyldopa, and quinidine may precipitate or exacerbate lupus-like syndrome in patient with preexisting SLE. Exudative pleural effusion is a usual accompanying feature of pleuritis and lupus erythematosus cells can be demonstrated in the pleural fluid analysis. With the removal of offending drug, pleuritis often subsides.

Pleural effusion (eosinophilic)

Drugs such as nitrofurantoin, dantrolene, bromocriptine, valproic acid, propylthiouracil, and isotretinoin are often associated with eosinophilic pleural effusion when administered. Pleural effusion with nitrofurantoin is often accompanied with parenchymal infiltrates, and this hypersensitivity reaction occurs within few hours of drug intake. Peripheral eosinophilia is often accompanying. Stopping of offending drug and sometimes corticosteroids helps in early recovery. Chronic drug administration leads to pulmonary adverse effects such as interstitial pneumonitis and fibrosis, where pleural affection is not common.

A unilateral, exudative eosinophilic pleural effusion with peripheral eosinophilia and without any pulmonary involvement is reported with chronic administration of dantrolene. Pleural fibrosis can also occur. Pleural effusion may take quite a longer duration to resolve even after total withdrawal of the offending drug.

Eosinophilic pleural effusion with peripheral eosinophilia with valproic acid and pleural effusion without peripheral eosinophilia or pulmonary infiltrates with propylthiouracil and isotretinoin has been reported.

Pleuritis, effusion, and thickening of pleura

Hypersensitivity reaction or, as a result of direct toxicity, certain chemotherapeutic agents such as bleomycin, methotrexate, cyclophosphamide, mitomycin, and procarbazine can produce pleuropulmonary manifestations, where pleural effusion may be accompanying a small number of patients with interstitial pneumonitis. Pleural thickening may develop as a late manifestation in cyclophosphamide therapy. Pleural thickening may occur with methotrexate when used in high dose and rarely with mitomycin therapy.

Bleomycin adverse effects are also dose-related.

Cardiovascular drugs such as minoxidil, practolol, and amiodarone are notorious to cause pleuropulmonary lung disease with pleural effusion may occur with amiodarone therapy, which may develop into pleural thickening due to chronic inflammation. Practolol can cause pleural effusion with pleural thickening and rarely pleural fibrosis. Both pericardial and pleural effusions are reported with minoxidil therapy.

Pleural effusion and fibrosis can occur with bromocriptine and methysergide treatment.

Rarely pleural effusion may develop with the use of a variety of agents such as clozapine, simvastatin, tryptophan, absolute alcohol, recombinant interleukin-2 acyclovir, D-penicillamine, metronidazole, itraconazole, and granulocyte colony-stimulating factor.

Pleural fluid eosinophilia	Dantrolene Isotretinoin Mesalamine Nitrofurantoin Propylthiouracil Valproic acid
Pleural fibrosis	Amiodarone Beta adrenergic blockers Practolol Oxprenolol Methysergide
Pleurisy and pleuritic chest pain 1. Cardiovascular agents	Amiodarone Minoxidil Bromocriptine Methysergide
2. Serotherapeutic agents	Sodium morrhuate/absolute alcohol
3. Chemotherapeutic agents	Bleomycin Mitomycin

4. Miscellaneous agents	Procarbazine Methotrexate Cyclophosphamide Docetaxel Acyclovir Clozapine P-penicillamine Simvastatin Mesalamine Itraconazole

Comments: Pleural disorders induced by drug use may manifest as pleurisy, with or without pleural effusion, thickening or fibrosis, and may occur with or without accompanying pulmonary disease. Management lies in practice. ADR reporting is important, and PR Shankar has initiated spontaneous ADR reporting service to promote ADR.

References and suggested readings

1. Badyal D, Bhatia RS. Adverse drug reaction. New Delhi: Pee Pee Publ. 2006:103–114.
2. Yung RI, Richardson BC. Drug induced lupus. Rheum Dis Clin North Am. 1994;20:61–85.
3. Shankar PS. Drug induced pleural diseases. Med Update; API. 2002;9:21–22.
4. Bhatia RS. Drug induced pulmonary disease. IN: Chest Medicine. Arora Publ. 2005;1:1–12.
5. Mahoney JM, Bachtel MD. Pleural effusion associated with chronic dantrolene administration. Ann Pharmocotherap. 1994;28:587–589.
6. Kanfman J. Eosinophilic pleural effusion associated with valproic acid administration. Scand Med J. 1996;88:881–882.
7. Urban C, et al. Chemical pleuritis as the cause of acute chest pain following high-dose methotrexate treatment. Cancer. 1983;1:34–37.
8. Webb DB, Whale RJ. Pleuropericardial effusion associated with minoxidial administration. PG Med J. 1982;58:319–320.

9. Gonzalez-Rothi RJ, et al. Amiodarone pulmonary toxicity presenting as bilateral exudative effusions. Chest. 1987;92:179–182.
10. Pusateri DW, Muder RR. Fever, pulmonary infiltrates and pleural effusion following acyclovir therapy for herpes zoster ophthalmicus. Chest. 1990;98:754–756.
11. Pfitzenmeyer P, et al. Pleuro-pulmonary changes induced by ergoline drugs. Eur Respir J. 1996;9:1013–1019.
12. Parikh SS, et al. Development of pleural effusion after sclerotherapy with absolute alcohol. Gastrointes Endoscop. 1993;39:404–405.
13. Huggins JT, Sahn SA. Drug-induced pleural disease. Clin Chest Med. 2004 Mar;25(1):141–153. doi: 10.1016/S0272-5231(03)00125-4. PMID: 15062606.
14. Antony VB. Drug-induced pleural disease. Clin Chest Med. 1998 Jun;19(2):331–340. doi: 10.1016/s0272-5231(05)70080-0. PMID: 9646984.
15. Rosenow EC 3rd. Drug-induced bronchopulmonary pleural disease. J Allergy Clin Immunol. 1987 Dec;80(6):780–787. doi: 10.1016/s0091-6749(87)80265-8. PMID: 3320158.
16. Tryfon S, Papadopoulou E, Saroglou M, Vlachopoulos D, Georgopoulou A, Serasli E, Ismailos G. Clinical and pathophysiological characteristics of valproate-induced pleural effusion. Clin Toxicol (Phila). 2021 Oct;59(10): 869–876. doi: 10.1080/15563650.2021.1945081. Epub 2021 Jul 14. PMID: 34259092.
17. Goldman A, Maor E, Bomze D, Liu JE, Herrmann J, Fein J, Steingart RM, Mahmood SS, Schaffer WL, Perales MA, Shouval R. Adverse cardiovascular and pulmonary events associated with chimeric antigen receptor T-cell therapy. J Am Coll Cardiol. 2021 Nov 2;78(18):1800–1813. doi: 10.1016/j.jacc.2021.08.044. PMID: 34711339; PMCID: PMC8562317.
18. Castinetti F, Albarel F, Amodru V, Cuny T, Dufour H, Graillon T, Morange I, Brue T. The risks of medical treatment of prolactinoma. Ann Endocrinol (Paris). 2021 Feb;82(1):15–19. doi: 10.1016/j.ando.2020.12.008. Epub 2020 Dec 26. PMID: 33373604.
19. Rousselot P, Mollica L, Guilhot J, Guerci A. Dasatinib dose optimisation based on therapeutic drug monitoring reduces pleural effusion rates in chronic myeloid leukaemia patients. Br J Haematol. 2021 Jul;194(2):393–402. doi: 10.1111/bjh.17654. Epub 2021 Jun 30. PMID: 34195988.

20. de Ghellinck L, Frusch N, Duysinx B. Eosinophilic pleural effusion induced by paliperidone palmitate: case report and literature review. J Acad Consult Liaison Psychiatry. 2022 Jul–Aug;63(4):394–399. doi: 10.1016/j.jaclp.2022.02.010. Epub 2022 Mar 17. PMID: 35307578.
21. Venetsanopoulou AI, Markatseli TE, Iliou C, Tziortzioti Z, Argyropoulou MI, Drosos AA, Voulgari PV. Pleural effusion in psoriatic arthritis patients: a case series and review of the literature. Clin Rheumatol. 2021 Nov;40(11):4741–4748. doi: 10.1007/s10067-021-05712-9. Epub 2021 Mar 29. PMID: 33782750.
22. Kotsiou OS, Gourgoulianis KI, Zarogiannis SG. The role of nitric oxide in pleural disease. Respir Med. 2021 Apr;179:106350. doi: 10.1016/j.rmed.2021.106350. Epub 2021 Feb 23. PMID: 33662805.

https://doi.org/10.1142/9789811271410_0045

45 Diseases of the chest wall

Introduction

Deformities and diseases involving the thoracic cage are not uncommon but have received adequate attention from pulmonologists and physician specialists. Nevertheless, these problems are considered in greater details in thoracic surgical and orthopedic specialities. Nonetheless, physicians are confronted quite often with medical disorders which involve the structures enclosed in the thoracic cage and/or the chest wall itself. These can involve the ribs, the sternum, the thoracic spine, and the tumors of the chest wall.

1. The Ribs

Congenital anomalies such as a bifid rib or fusion of two are commonly encountered on plain chest x-ray. Another common congenital anomaly is the presence of accessory cervical rib which takes its origin from the cervical seventh vertebra, and these people with accessory cervical ribs are usually asymptomatic. However, occasionally when the accessory rib is compressing the brachial plexus or the subclavian artery, the individual experiences pain in the affected arm along with weakness of muscles; radial artery pulsation on the two sides may also show differences. Thrombosis of the subclavian artery by an accessory rib, having further extension into the carotid system, has also been documented.

Notching of the inferior or superior rib margins is yet another important radiological finding, which may occur in diseases such as coarctation of thoracic aorta, Tetralogy of Fallot, pulmonary stenosis, superior vena cava obstruction, or intercostal arteriovenous fistulae. The notching of the superior rib margin is not that common but has been described in conditions such as rheumatoid arthritis, scleroderma, Marfan's syndrome, hyperparathyroidism, and sometimes in paralytic poliomyelitis. The noticing in poliomyelitis is more shallow, and perhaps it occurs secondary to uneven stresses put by the intercostal muscles on the involved ribs.

Ribs may also be involved in inflammatory diseases such as tuberculosis, fungal infections, actinomycosis, and empyema. The affected rib develops osteomyelitis that appears on a chest x-ray as an expanded lesion or may exhibit destruction and periosteal reaction.

Tietze's syndrome (costochondral osteochondritis) is a painful inflammation of costosternal or costochondral joint, usually affecting the second rib. Commonly seen in younger individuals, the condition is benign and self-limiting. Only symptomatic treatment and assurance that pain will subside is sufficient but may occasionally take a long time.

2. Sternum

Congenital defects of sternal body are frequently encountered in clinical practice. The funnel chest or pectus excavatum is common. It is a congenital defect in the body of sternum as well as associated attachments of the diaphragm. The anomaly causes variable depression of the chest wall. Funnel chest is quite commonly observed in patients with Marfan's disease, essentially causing cosmetic defect. In severe cases, the bony defect may be responsible for reduction in vital capacity and maximum breathing capacity, and thus the patient may experience exertional dyspnoea. Satisfactory treatment of the deformity is still being explored.

Pectus carinatum or pigeon chest is another frequently encountered abnormality which is characterized by marked forward protrusion of the ribs and sternum. It is commonly *seen* in patients (usually children) suffering from atrial or ventricular septal defects and *severe* bronchial asthma. Symptoms as such *due* to the deformity are minimal. Sternal infections are quite commonly encountered where microorganisms such as the tubercle bacillus, actinomycosis, *Pseudomonas aeruginosa*, and *Staphylococcus aureus* involve the sternum and produce generally a superficial abscess or ometimeseven osteomyelitis.

3. The thoracic spine

Mobility of the chest wall gets restricted in patients of ankylosing spondylitis, which usually involves young males in the second or third decades of life. Pathologically, there is synovitis and chondritis of the costovertebral joints. Loss of cartilage in the advanced stage may occur in bony ankylosis. As a result, the chest cage is held in fixed inspiratory position; secondary kyphosis of the thoracic spine is usually accompanying. Hyperinflated lung fields are seen on plain chest X-ray, and in some patients, bilateral upper lobe fibrosis may also be present. Kyphoscoliosis is a more common deformity of the thoracic spine. These cases are categorized as:

a. Congenital, such as hemivertebrae, seen frequently in association with diseases like neurofibromatosis or Marfan's syndrome.
b. Paralytic conditions of the muscles of the thoracic spine, for example, poliomyelitis.
c. Idiopathic variety.

Reduction of lung function causing disability is secondary and further varies with the severity of the deformity. On the side of the severe concavity, the affected lung is small, ribs are crowded and underventilated. Hypoxemia and carbon dioxide retention may occur in severe cases. Pulmonary arterial hypertension is a usual accompanying feature. Vital capacity is markedly reduced and death occurs because of cardiorespiratory failure.

4. Chest wall tumors

A soft tissue lipoma is a commonly encountered benign tumor of the chest wall. It may occasionally originate close to parietal pleural and projects inwards into the thoracic cavity. Malignant tumors from breast and lung may involve the ribs. Extrathoracic tumors may have secondary metastasis in the ribs and other bony structures such as clavicles, scapulae, and thoracic vertebrae.

References and suggested readings

1. Faber P, Somers J, Templeton AC. Chest wall tumors. Curr Probl Surg. 1995;32:661, 663–747.
2. Tateishi U, et al. Chest wall tumors: radiologic findings and pathologic correlation: part 1. Benign tumors. Radiographics. 2003;23(6):1477–1490.
3. Lee TJ, Collins J. MR imaging evaluation of disorders of the chest wall. Magn Reson Imag Clin N Am. 2008;16(2):355–379.
4. Elgar G, Smiley A, Latifi R. Major risk factors for mortality in elderly and non-elderly adult patients emergently admitted for blunt chest wall trauma: hospital length of stay as an independent predictor. Int J Environ Res Public Health. 2022;19(14):8729.
5. Sabanathan S, et al. Primary chest wall tumors. Ann Thorac Surg. 1985; 39(1):4–15.
6. Von Bezold M. Thoraxschmerzen [Chest pain]. Internist (Berl). 2021 Jan; 62(1):17–23. German. doi: 10.1007/s00108-020-00918-6. Epub 2020 Dec 17. PMID: 33331950.
7. Wang L, et al. Expert consensus on resection of chest wall tumors and chest wall reconstruction. Transl Lung Cancer Res. 2021 Nov;10(11):4057–4083. doi: 10.21037/tlcr-21-935. PMID: 35004239; PMCID: PMC8674598.
8. Li G, Yao J, Chen J, Cai B, Lin X, Chen Z, Chen J, Wang H, Yang S. The survival effect of chest wall with or without regional lymphatic radiotherapy for breast cancer patients with T3~4N0M0. Front Oncol. 2021 Jul 12;11:653831. doi: 10.3389/fonc.2021.653831. PMID: 34322377; PMCID: PMC8311914.
9. McKnight CL, Burns B. Pneumothorax. IN: StatPearls [Internet]. Treasure Island, FL: StatPearls Publishing. 2022 Jan–Aug 8. PMID: 28722915.
10. Fraiwan M, Fraiwan L, Khassawneh B, Ibnian A. A dataset of lung sounds recorded from the chest wall using an electronic stethoscope. Data Brief. 2021 Feb 26;35:106913. doi: 10.1016/j.dib.2021.106913. PMID: 33732827; PMCID: PMC7937981.
11. Zheng Y, Wang L, Ben S. Meta-analysis of chest CT features of patients with COVID-19 pneumonia. J Med Virol. 2021 Jan;93(1):241–249. doi: 10.1002/jmv.26218. Epub 2020 Jul 11. PMID: 32579236; PMCID: PMC7361361.

12. Łyżwa E, Siemion-Szcześniak I, Sobiecka M, Kacprzak A, Winiarska A, Szołkowska M, Karuś K, Tomkowski W. Pulmonary actinomycosis complicated by fistula of the chest wall. Adv Respir Med. 2021;89(5):532–537. doi: 10.5603/ARM.a2021.0071. Epub 2021 Jul 16. PMID: 34269403.
13. Sahu S, Halder S, Jain S, Koul RK. Undifferentiated pleomorphic sarcoma of the chest wall: a rare diagnosis. BMJ Case Rep. 2021 Oct 12;14(10):e245366. doi: 10.1136/bcr-2021-245366. PMID: 34642220; PMCID: PMC8513258.
14. Basit GY, Muraveji Q, Nazari FA. Primary hydatid disease of chest wall mimicking chest wall mass-case report. Int J Surg Case Rep. 2021 Mar;80:105602. doi: 10.1016/j.ijscr.2021.01.096. Epub 2021 Jan 30. PMID: 33601329; PMCID: PMC7898065.
15. Gideon EA, Cross TJ, Coriell CL, Duke JW. The effect of estimating chest wall compliance on the work of breathing during exercise as determined via the modified Campbell diagram. Am J Physiol Regul Integr Comp Physiol. 2021 Mar 1;320(3):R268–R275. doi: 10.1152/ajpregu.00263.2020. Epub 2020 Dec 23. PMID: 33356877.
16. Liu X, Ali MK, Dua K, Xu R. The role of zinc in the pathogenesis of lung disease. Nutrients. 2022 May 19;14(10):2115. doi: 10.3390/nu14102115. PMID: 35631256; PMCID: PMC9143957.
17. Santoshi RK, Chandar P, Gupta SS, Kupfer Y, Wiesel O. From chest wall resection to medical management: the continued saga of parapneumonic effusion management and future directions. Cureus. 2022 Jan 7;14(1):e21017. doi: 10.7759/cureus.21017. PMID: 35018275; PMCID: PMC8741136.
18. Skotsimara G, Antonopoulos A, Oikonomou E, Papastamos C, Siasos G, Tousoulis D. Aortic wall inflammation in the pathogenesis, diagnosis and treatment of aortic aneurysms. Inflammation. 2022 Jun;45(3):965–976. doi: 10.1007/s10753-022-01626-z. Epub 2022 Jan 25. PMID: 35076833.
19. Bertoglio P, Garelli E, Brandolini J, Kawamukai K, Antonacci F, Ricciardi S, Cipolli A, Bonfanti B, Forti Parri SN, Daddi N, Dolci G, Solli P. Surgical management and reconstruction of diaphragm, pericardium and chest wall in mesothelioma surgery: a review. J Clin Med. 2021 May 26;10(11):2330. doi: 10.3390/jcm10112330. PMID: 34073544; PMCID: PMC8197912.

https://doi.org/10.1142/9789811271410_0046

46 Pneumothorax

Definition: Pneumothorax is defined as air in the pleural space, or air between lung and the chest wall. Itard coined the term pneumothorax, and Laennec gave the full clinical description.

Types

1. Spontaneous: Spontaneous occur without antecedent trauma or other obvious cause
2. Traumatic: Traumatic occur from direct or indirect trauma to the chest

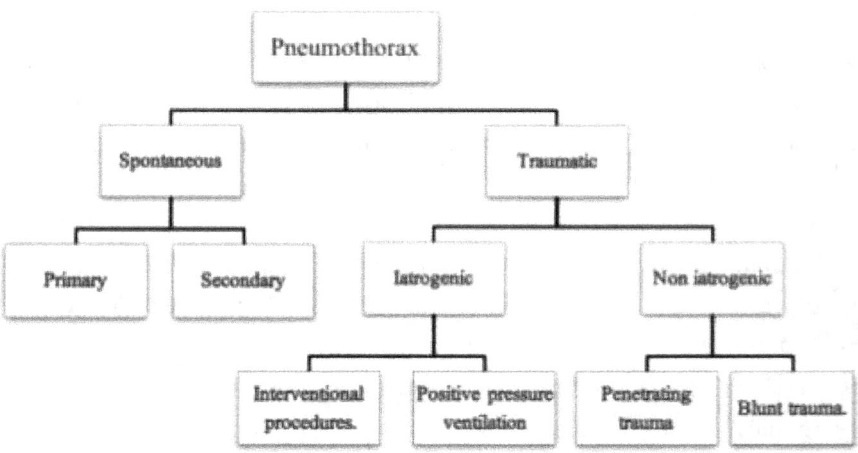

Clinical features	Signs	Etiology
• Dyspnea	• Cyanosis	• COPD:MC
• Chest pain — Pricking type — Stabbing type — Cutting type	• Chest assessment findings — Hyper-resonant note on percussion — Decreased breath sounds on auscultation — Diminished heart sounds — Tracheal shift — Subcutaneous emphysema	• Tuberculosis
• Dry cough	If symptoms and signs are severe then there are chances of tension pneumothorax	• Malignancy
		• Sarcoidosis
		• Other infections

Etio-pathogenesis of spontaneous pneumothorax and its management: current practices.

Summary

Presence of preexisting lung disease would differentiate secondary from primary pneumothorax. Apart from a wide range of causative factors, active pulmonary tuberculosis, chronic bronchitis emphysema, bronchogenic carcinoma, suppurative pneumonia, bronchiectasis, and so on, are common causes for secondary spontaneous pneumothorax. A common entity in males, spontaneous pneumothorax has smoking as high-risk factor. Chest X-ray is diagnostic; HRCT has added new dimensions to diagnostic yield. The pathological varieties, such as closed, open, and valvular types, determine the course of the disease as well as its management. The tension-type spontaneous pneumothorax is a medical emergency, and an urgent management action is rewarding. The controversy is still on between physician's conservative management and surgeon's active measures. In small closed pneumothorax of less than 20% of hemithorax, no specific treatment is required. Pneumothorax of more than 20% or with dyspnea requires active management. The ultimate choice is chest tube drainage under water seal, and if not giving good results, it has to be assisted by open thoracotomy. With video-assisted thoracoscopic surgery (VATS), recurrence prevention can be targeted, with optimal use of HRCT chest. With underlying lung disease. In case of simultaneous bilateral spontaneous pneumothorax, surgical pleurectomy should be attempted. Chemical pleurodesis using a sclerosing agent such as tetracycline hydrochloride can be of value. Outcome is good in healthy adults in the absence of preexisting pulmonary disease.

Primary spontaneous pneumothorax is common in

1: Young healthy tall, thin adults,
2: Age group of 20–40 years,[1]
3: With male to female ratio being 6:1 and incidence being 7.4 per 100,000 per year for males, with corresponding figure of 1:2 for females in United States and United Kingdom. It affects both the lungs equally.

This results from rupture of small air spaced measuring 1–2 cm in diameter (subpleural bleb) into the pleural space because of congenital weakness in connective tissue of subpleural alveoli or may arise as an interstitial emphysema.[1] This occurs almost in 90% of cases, often multiple and commonly involving the apices, possible because of mechanical stress of regional distending forces which are maximum over the apices. Relative ischemia of lung apices may also contribute. An association of smoking, high pulmonary concentration of hydroxyproline (a degradation product of collagen), and specific HLA antigen and antitrypsin ecotypes (in familial occurrence of spontaneous pneumothorax have been observe.[2] Secondary spontaneous pneumothorax occurs as a result of lung disease. Spontaneous pneumothorax occurs because of rupture of cavity of subpleural tuberculous lesion giving way into the pleural cavity.[3] 1.4% of cases of active pulmonary tuberculosis are complicated by pneumothorax, 90% of these cases are cavitary. If not treated, these cases get further complicated as empyema or bronchopleural fistula. Rarely pneumothorax may occur in acute miliary tuberculosis[4] possible mechanisms suggested are an initial pneumomediastinum with leakage of air through mediastinal pleura, rupture of caseation or necrosis of sub pleural miliary nodule through pleura, rupture of bullous lesion of miliary tuberculosis or paroxysmal cough causing forceful expiratory effort against a closed glottis causing rupture. Chronic bronchitis and emphysema significantly contribute to this type of pneumothorax. Trapped air leaks through weakened walls of dilated and distended alveoli, assisted by high intrabronchial pressure aggravated by cough. Secondary spontaneous pneumothorax can be life threatening in COPD patients.[5] In less than 1% of adults and 2.5% of children, bronchial asthma is the cause of pneumothorax. Staphylococcal pneumonia in children and Klebsiella pneumonia in adults are the infections which are commonly associated with pneumothorax. It is the multiple cystic areas (pneumatoceles) that rupture into the pleural space. A recurrent pneumothorax associated with menstruation, almost always on right side, and occurring in women over 25–30 years of age has been described by Maurer et al. in 1958 as catamenial pneumothorax.[6] About one-third of patients have associated pelvic endometriosis. Air leaks occur possibly from peritoneal cavity into the pleural space through diaphragmatic fenestrations. AIDS-related pneumothorax is frequently associated with pneumocystis carinii pneumonia. A virulent form-a necrotizing subpleural necrosis results in diffuse air leaks.[7,8] Due to age of more than 60 years, pulmonary fibrosis and increased height/weight ratio recurrence are common. Spontaneous pneumothorax is the main respiratory manifestation in Marfan's syndrome also.[9] Basic defect in collagen fiber having fewer side-to-side linkages results in increased tissue friability along with patchy abnormal alveolar elastica, that is more pronounced over the areas of emphysema. Apart from manifestation of honeycomb lung or cystic fibrosis, it can rarely be seen in bronchogenic carcinoma, sarcoidosis, hydatid cyst of lung, pulmonary alveolar proteinosis, Wegener's granulomatosis, eosinophilic granuloma of lung, and aseptic cavitating pulmonary infarction.[10–16]

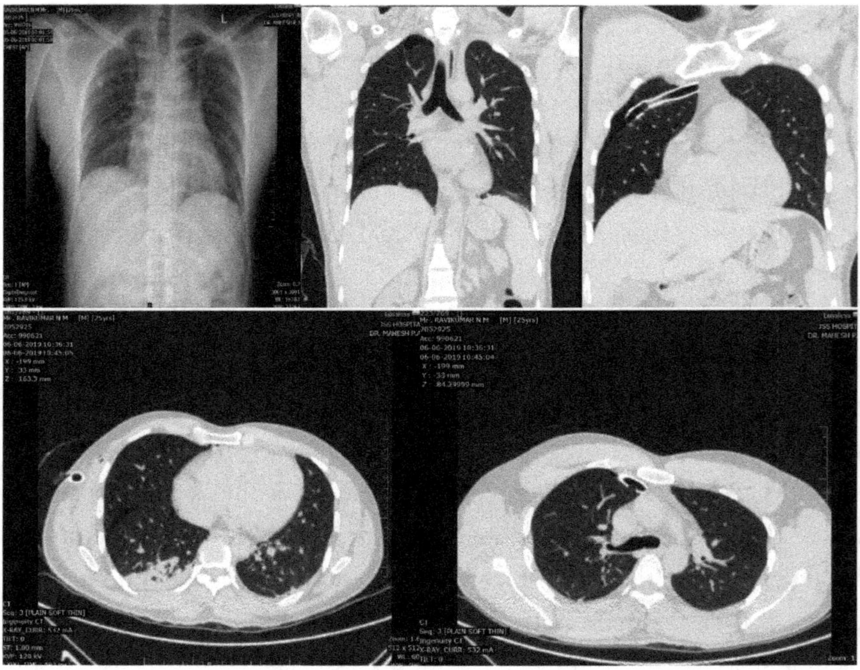

Figure 1: X-ray and CT scans of primary spontaneous pneumothorax.

Three types of pneumothorax are recognized pathologically:

1. Closed

Where the communication with the atmospheric air gets sealed off as the ruptured site closes. Air in the pleural cavity gets absorbed and the lung re-expands to its original position over a few weeks. Intrapleural pressure remains lesser than atmospheric pressure.

2. Open

Where the communication with the atmospheric air remains patent in the form of bronchopleural fistula as the ruptured site does not close. Intrapleural pressure approximates to the atmospheric pressure and not allowing the lung to re-expand. Patent bronchopleural fistula makes the pleural space susceptible to infections resulting in pyopneumothorax.

3. Tension (valvular)

Where the communication with the outside air is persistent but is small and valvular, allowing the air to enter only without permitting it to escape. This allows a large amount to air trapping in the pleural cavity. Intrapleural pressure becomes more than atmospheric pressure, resulting in mediastinal displacement toward the opposite side, consequently compressing the opposite lung.[17]

Clinical presentation and diagnosis: Small pneumothoraces can be asymptomatic and only detected as accidental radiological finding. Clinical features and functional abnormalities depend on the size of pneumothorax, amount of lung collapse, and preexisting lung disease. Its course depends on the type of pneumothorax. Sudden onset of chest pain is the most common clinical symptom, often associated with breathlessness. Pain is continuous invariably exacerbated by deep inspiration or postural change. Severe dyspnea with cardio-pulmonary compromise forms the hallmark of tension dyspnea. Restless, anxious, tachypneic patient may have cyanosis as well. Failure in rapid relief of tension may result in rapid low-volume pulse with hypotension and pulsus paradoxus.

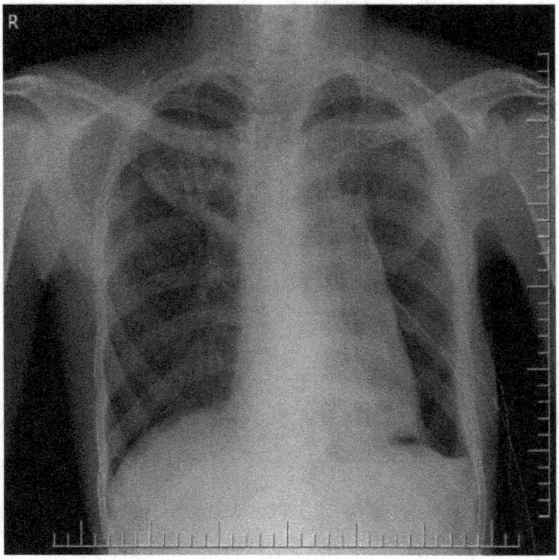

Figure 2: Pneumothorax with ICD cut emphysema.

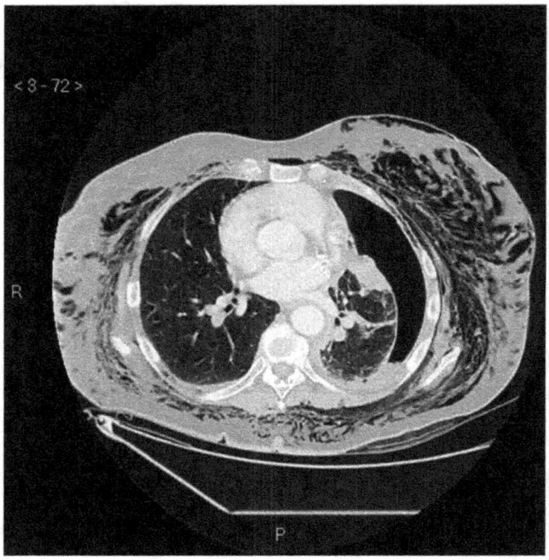

Figure 3: Pneumothorax with sub.

Small pneumothoraces are often missed on clinical examination. Otherwise clinical chest findings include prominent chest wall, the diminished respiratory movements, percussion note is hyper-resonant, coin test positive, presence of mediastinal shift to opposite side and breath sounds are diminished or absent on auscultation.[18] Succussion splash may be hard if there is hydropneumothorax. One may find a mediastinal crunch (crepitus) over the precordium that occurs due to close proximity of trapped air and the moving cardiac muscle (earlier called Hamman's sign). Mediastinal emphysema (Figure 3) may cause central chest pain simulating myocardial infarction.[19]

Diagnosis is often based on clinical findings, confirmed by chest X-ray. Classical radiological features of pneumothorax include a lucent zone devoid of lung marking with sharply defined lung edge (the lung compressed toward the hilum), with a convexity outwards. Small pneumothoraces can be detected in the expiratory film, especially in the lateral view (preferably) in children). Because of increased blood flow to the lung, exaggerated broncho-vascular markings can be seen on the opposite side. In massive compression collapse (complete pneumothorax),

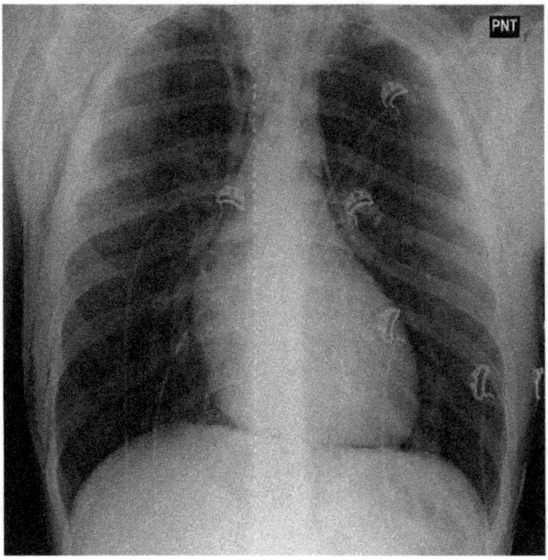

Figure 4: Pneumomediastinum.

lung is compressed toward the hilum and appears as a dense globular mass.

In tension pneumothorax, mediastinum is shifted to the opposite side. Radiological findings are characteristics of pneumomediastinum (Figure 4). If hydropneumothorax is present, a horizontal at fluid level is visualized.

A restrictive type of ventilator impairment is classically seen in pneumothorax, with reduced vital capacity, functional residual capacity, and total lung capacity. Diffusion capacity is reduced; vital capacity is reduced a little. If pneumothorax is more than 20%, hypoxemia may be present. Initial hypoxemia occurs due to collapsed lung causing lesser blood flow to the side. It improves gradually because of compensatory hypoxic vasoconstriction that corrects gross ventilation/perfusion imbalance. Cyanosis disappears later due to reduction in the perfusion of the collapsed lung. Value of HRCT adds meaningfully in diagnosing spontaneous pneumothorax, since etiological diagnosis is important for definitive treatment of any disease.[20] Also, HRCT can detect even lesions such as eosophilic granuloma

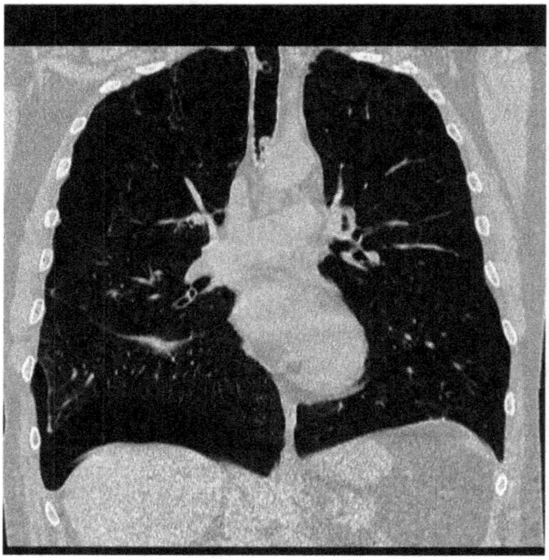

Figure 5: Secondary to bullae.

and lymphangioleiomyomatosis. I-ISCT can also diagnose pulmonary tuberculosis in patient where chest X-ray may be reported normal.[21,22] HRCT findings suggestive of active TB are

a. Centrilobular nodule with branching linear structures.
b. Tree-in-bud appearance, having more than one contiguous branching site.
c. Consolidation of cavitary nodule.
d. 5–8 mm diameter poorly defined nodules.
e. Lobular consolidation with thickening of interlobular septae.
f. Bronchial wall thickness with or without bronchiectasis.

Re-expansion pulmonary oedema can occasionally complicate decompression procedures in different lung diseases

Management

Management of pneumothorax may be conservative or active, depending upon the amount of air in the pleural cavity and the underlying physiological disturbance, for example, tension pneumothorax is taken as a medical emergency. Conservative therapy is indicated in a healthy non-dyspneic adult, having a pneumothorax of very small volume, occupying less than 20% of hemithorax. Air will get absorbed at the rate of 1.25% per day, if there is no further leak, thus allowing re-expansion of hemithorax volume at the same rate. This would help 20% of pneumothorax re-expanding within 20 days. 100% supplemental oxygen help in enhancing the air absorption by several folds, through creating a substantial fall in the total end capillary pressure nearly from 706 mmhg to 146 mmhg. 100% oxygen increases 10 times the gradient for movement of gas from capillaries in parietal and visceral pleura to air in pleural cavity of replacing nitrogen with oxygen in capillaries.[23] High oxygen concentration may be harmful in cases of COPD with carbon dioxide retention. Since relapse is common in 1/3 to 1/2 of patients, observation alone should be avoided, except in very small pneumothoraces or apical pneumothoraces. Guidelines have been laid down by British group for the management of spontaneous pneumothorax (Figure 6).[24]

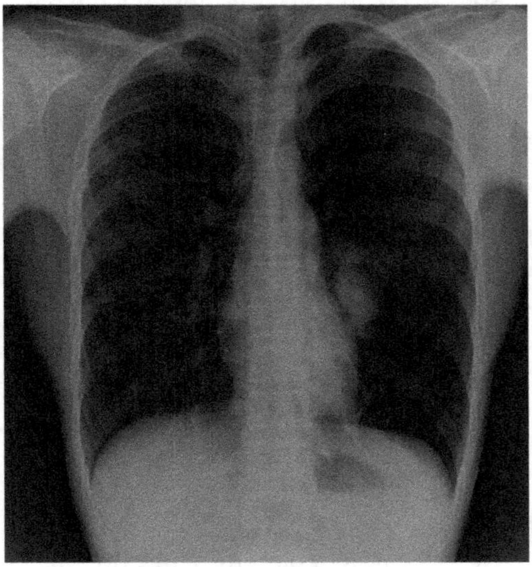

Figure 6: Spontaneous pneumothorax.

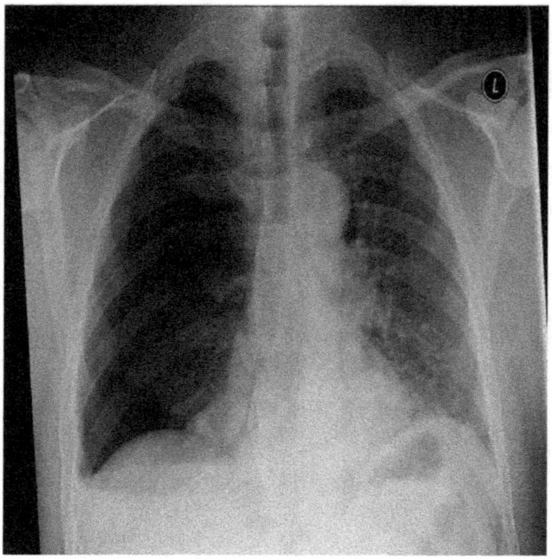

Figure 7: Traumatic pneumothorax.

Air from pleural cavity should be removed by simple aspiration or by inserting chest tube through intercostal space under water-seal device. Chest X-ray is not as effective as CT and therefore, for secondary pneumothoraces, intercostal tube drainage offers better option for those with a distance of more than 2 cms above which the volume of pneumothorax will be more than 50%.[20] Tip of the wide-bore needle has to be introduced into the pleural cavity above the rib to prevent injury to the intercostal vessels as an emergency measure, followed by replacement with intercostal catheter (connected to water seal) to prevent any injury by the needle tip to the expanding lung. Simple aspiration is safe as an initial treatment of choice in patients with normal lungs who present with spontaneous pneumothorax, irrespective of its size, and may offer short hospital stay and reduces the rate of pleurectomy with no increase in recurrence rate at one year.[25] Appropriate treatment is not just on the size of a pneumothorax on chest X-ray but, more importantly, on the clinical status of the patient.[24] Active management is indicated in tension pneumothorax, pneumothorax of more than 20% of hemithorax, with coexisting pulmonary disease, in a dyspneic patient, in a patient with previous pneumothorax in opposite lung, in an increasing (progressive) pneumothorax, in bilateral pneumothorax, and also in cases with accompanying pleural effusion or empyema.

Initial simple method includes inserting an intercostal tube connected to an underwater seal that allows re-expansion of lung. In case of failure of response, suction can be applied. Complications such as heamothorax and thromboembolism can occur. Alternatively, a Heimlich flutter valve can be connected to the tube, though it

Although it is cheap and makes the patient mobile, mechanical problems with the valve, however, restrict its use. Others have used urinary bag with a flutter valve.[26] The only drawback is that suction cannot be applied to it, in case it is required for persistent leak, although suction application has been found to be necessary.[27] Risk of lung laceration and complications such as empyema and chronic pneumothorax are commonly seen with needle aspiration. In open pneumothorax, re-expansion usually does not occur by this method. And persistent air leak following tube drainage for spontaneous pneumothorax is potentially troublesome complication. Thoracentesis can be of therapeutic value in closed spontaneous pneumothorax only in selected cases, since there are more relapses, more changes of lung laceration and empyema. In case of failure of re-expansion of lung within 7–10 days despite of good chest tube, parietal pleurectomy is carded out for a posterolateral recurrence, contralateral occurrence, bilateral simultaneous pneumothorax, persistent pleural effusion, and high-risk patients such as air-crew, divers, and sea farers.

Surgical management of 7–9 days would provide a reasonable opportunity for persistent air leak to resolve with medical treatment with normal lungs. Under thoracoscopic guidance, allowing for both the excision and closures of ruptured blebs in a fashion identical to the traditional approach with open thoracotomy can be done. With VATS, recurrence prevention can be targeted with optimal use of HRCT chest.[28] Recurrence rate of primary spontaneous pneumothorax after VATS bullectomy combined with surgical pleurodesis is in the range of 1.7%–5%.[29] Lesser shoulder dysfunction and pain medication requirements are observed with VATS as compared to post-lateral thoracotomy during post-operative period.[30] Surgical pleurectomy should be attempted early especially in simultaneous bilateral spontaneous pneumothorax, secondary to underlying lung disease. Tension pneumothorax is treated as medical emergency, urgently converting the tension pneumothorax into an open variety, by inserting any available wide-bore needle into the pleural space. Needle is then replaced by an intercostal catheter, as early as possible. Minimal invasive management is suggested for first and recurrent pneumothorax.[31] Recurrent pneumothorax, seen in about 20% of cases within a year, treatment with sclerosing agents in more effective in preventing ipsilateral recurrence than chest tube insertion alone. Although thoracotomy remains current standard treatment, chemical pleurodesis can be useful especially in patients who run risk for surgery. 1 gm tetracycline hydrochloride solution in 50 mi of norreguil saline with 10 mL of 1% lignocaine is injected into the chest tube[32] and is allowed to remain there for several hours before drainage. Due to inflammatory reaction (Chemical pleuritis), with visceral and parietal pleurae get adherent, thus leading to pleural symphysis. It is less painful and causes lesser exudation and patient has a shorter hospital stay. Catamenial hemothorax (and pneumothorax) is also effectively treated with chemical pleurodesis.[33]

Autologous blood patch pleurodesis can be used as simple, painless, and inexpensive alternative treatment in patients with persistent air leaks.[34]

An aggressive stepped care management by large bore intercostal chest tube drainage, chemical pleurodesis, and an early video-assisted talc poudrage in AIDS-related spontaneous pneumothorax as it carries high mortality.[5]

Chronic pneumothorax due to persistent bronchopleural fistula or leak through multiple congenital or emphysematous bullae needs to be treated by decortication, by stripping the parietal pleura or by suturing the fistulous tract or segmental resection of diseased lung.[35] A huge bulla associated with spontaneous pneumothorax should be an indication for VATS, since this giant bulla can itself be manifestation of lung carcinoma or a focus for recurrent infection.[36]

Table 1: Spontaneous pneumothorax

<table>
<tr><th colspan="2">Etiology of spontaneous pneumothorax</th></tr>
<tr><td>A. Primary: Apical blebs</td><td>B. Secondary:
1. Common causes
• Tuberculosis
• COPD
• Asthma
• Abscess
• Pneumonia
• Cystic fibrosis
• Carcinoma
• Bronchiectasis
2. Rare cause
• Interstitial lung diseases
• Connective tissue disorders
• Hemosiderosis
• Catamenial pneumothorax
• Hydatid disease</td></tr>
<tr><td colspan="2">C. Associated with other diseases
1. Rupture of staphylococcal pneumatocele
2. As a manifestation of
• honeycomb lung
• bronchogenic carcinoma
• coal worker's pneumoconiosis
• sarcoidosis
• silicosis
• fibrosing alveolitis
3. Bilateral spontaneous pneumothorax secondary to osteosarcoma metastasis.[38]
4. AIDS-related associated with PCP</td></tr>
</table>

Analgesics, backrest, oxygen therapy, and prophylactic antimicrobial therapy form important supportive measures. Three months follow up for one year, to detect recurrence is recommended (I).

Complications such as hemothorax, infection, and atelectasis can be treated with thoracotomy and clot evacuation, antimicrobials and physiotherapy respectively.

Prognosis is good in healthy adults without any underlying lung diseases. Tension pneumothorax may be rapidly fatal if not urgently treated. Mortality is higher in the elderly with airways obstruction. Complications like hemothorax pose a great hazard. With lowered morbidity and proven safety, VATS can be used in elderly and pediatric population.[37]

Etiology

Secondary:

1. Common causes: Pulmonary tuberculosis, chronic bronchitis and emphysema, bronchial asthma, suppurative pneumonia, lung abscess, bronchiectasis, Birt-Hogg-Dube Syndrome, bronchogenic carcinoma, and cystic fibrosis.

2. Rare causes

Cryptogenic fibrosing alveolitis, occupational lung disorders (acute silicosis), Shaver's disease), granulomatous disease (late fibrotic stage of sarcoidosis, histocytosis X, Wegener's disease), connective tissue disorders (SLE, rheumatoid disease), hemosiderosis, pulmonary alveolar proteinosis, hereditary disease (neurofibromatosis, tuberous sclerosis), inherited syndrome (Marfan's syndrome, Ehlers-Danlos syndrome, Marfanoid hypermobility syndrome), coccidioidomycosis, parasitic disease (hydatid disease), intrathoracic tumors (metastatic sarcomas, germ cell tumors, metastatic Wilms' tumor), cavitating pulmonary infarction, and catamenial pneumothorax.

Table 2: Occurrence of spontaneous pneumothorax in association with other diseases

Spontaneous pneumothorax may occur

1. As a complication of
   — bronchial asthma
   — rupture of staphylococcal pneumatocoele
2. As a manifestation of
   — honey comb lung
   — bronchogenic carcinoma
   — coal worker's pneumoconiosis
   — Sarcoidosis
   — silicosis
   — fibrosing alveolitis
3. Is precipitated during
   — corticosteroid therapy
   — positive pressure breathing (using PEEP)
   — menstruation
4. AIDS-related
   — associated with pneumocystic
5. Bilateral spontaneous pneumothorax secondary to osteosarcoma metastasis.[38]

Pneumothorax has an acute presentation with chest pain and shortness of breath which can be mimic by other conditions. table 3 list the most common differential diagnosis.

Table 3: Differential diagnosis of pneumothorax

Differential diagnosis
1. Myocardial infarction
2. Bronchial asthma
3. Pulmonary embolism
4. Perforated peptic ulcer
5. Large emphysematous bulla
6. Diaphragmatic hernia

Table 4: Spontaneous pneumothorax

Treatment options
A. Therapeutic options
(a) Conservative with oxygen supplementation
(b) Thoracentesis
(c) Chest tube thoracostomy
(d) Chest tube thoracostomy with chemical pleurodesis
(e) Surgical interventions
• Thoracostomy
• Thoracoscopy with pleurodesis

A. Therapeutic options

(a) Observations alone (conservative)

(b) Thoracentesis

(c) Chest tube thoracostomy

(d) Chest tube thoracostomy with chemical pleurodesis

(e) Surgical interventions:

- Thoracostomy
- Thoracoscopy with pleurodesis

B. Suggested methods of treatment in spontaneous pneumothorax

Type of pneumothorax	Treatment option
1. Pneumothorax of less than 20% of lung volume — Apical pneumothorax — Closed type pleural leak	Observation alone
2. Pneumothorax of more than 20% — Leak if closed type — Pneumothorax with clinical symptoms	Thoracentesis
3. Pneumothorax with open type — Pneumothorax with bronchopleural fistula	Chest tube thoracostomy

— Pyopneumothorax	
4. Tension pneumothorax	Urgent chest tube thoracostomy
5. Ipsilateral recurrent pneumothorax	Chest tube thoracostomy with chemical pleurodesis

References and suggested readings

1. Ohata M, Suzuk H. Pathogenesis of spontaneous pneumothorax with special *reference* to ultra structure of emphysematous bullae. Chest. 1980;77:771.
2. Sharpe IK, et al. Familial spontaneous pneumothorax and HLA antigens. Chest. 1980;78:264.
3. Bhatia RS. Pulmonary tuberculosis: an update. Curr Med J. 1997;3(5):19–24.
4. Narang PK, Kumar S, Gupta A. Pneumothorax and pneumomediastinum complicating acute military tuberculosis. Tubercle. 1997;58:79–82.
5. Videm V, et al. Spontaneous pneumothorax in COPD: complications, treatment and recurrences. Eur J Respir Dis. 1987;7:1365–1371.
6. Bhatia RS, Bhardwaj BL. Pulmonary changes during perimenstrual period. IN: SB Gupta, ed. Med Update; API. 2005;15:565–568.
7. Motorsky ML, Clot HG, Olson LK, Shanks TC. AIDS related spontaneous pneumothorax. Chest. 1995;408:946–951.
8. Wait MA, Dal-Nogare AR. Treatment of AIDS related spontaneous pneumothorax-a decade of experience. Chest. 1994;106:693–696.
9. Vidyasagar B, Jayan R, Ranjana SD. Recurrent pneumothorax in Marfan's syndrome. Lung India. 1998;16(1):29–31.
10. Ross RJM, Empey EW. Bilateral spontaneous pneumothorax in sarcoidosis. PG Med J. 1983;59:106.
11. Kim YI, et al. Concurrent pneumopericardium and pneumothorax complicating lung cancer. Korean J Radiol. 2000;1(2):118–120.
12. Zbar B, et al. Risk of renal and clonic neoplasms and spontaneous pneumothorax in the Birt-Hogg-Dube syndrome. Cancer Epidemiol Biomarker Preven; Am Assn Cancer Res. 2002;11:393–400.
13. Khoo SK, et al. Clinical and genetic studies of Birt-Hogg-Dube syndrome. J Med Genet. 2002;39(12):906–912.
14. Handa AK, Eggleston FC. Pneumothorax caused by hydatid cyst. Ind J Chest Dis. 1982;24:47.

15. Onell S, et al. Pneumothorax in the Ehlers-Danlos syndrome. Irish J Med Sci. 1981;150:43.
16. Jaspan T, et al. Spontaneous pneumothorax in Wegener's granulomatosis. Thorax. 1982;37:774.
17. Bhatia RS, Sibia SS. Management of spontaneous pneumothorax. IN: S. Venkataraman, ed. Med Update; API. 2004;4(14):221–226.
18. Bhatia RS. Pulmonary sounds in common lung diseases. Lung India. 1994;2:89–92.
19. Gupta S. Pneumothorax. IN: BC Bansal, ed. PG Med; API. 1997;11:334–338.
20. Baumann MG, et al. Management of spontaneous pneumothorax: an ACCP Delhi consensus statement. Chest. 2001;119:590–602.
21. IMIG, et al. Pulmonay TB; CT findings-early active disease and sequential change with ATT. Radiology. 1993;186:653.
22. Webb WR. HRCT of chest of obstructive lung disease-advances in chestradiology. RCNA. 1994;32:747. goi6ns-i-et-A-C-T-pattern-of-br-ortthietar-diseaservoliafle-iti-iflR7-1998;171.365.
23. Jindal SK, Agarwal R. Oxygen therapy. 2nd ed. Jay Pee Publ. 2008;10:157–182.
24. Mac Buff A, et al. Management of spontaneous pnumothorax: BJS pleural disease guidelines. Thorax. 2016;65:18–31.
25. Noppen M, et al. Manual aspiration vs chest tube drainage in first term episode of primary spontaneous pneumothorax. Am Respir Crit Care Med. 2002;164:1240–1244.
26. Aggarwal BK. Urinary bag with a flutter valve for management of chest drainage. Lung India. 2100;18(1):8.
27. Huan NC, Sidhu C, Thomas R. Pneumothorax: classification and etiology. Clin Chest Med. 2021 Dec;42(4):711–727. doi: 10.1016/j.ccm.2021.08.007. PMID: 34774177.
28. DeMaio A, Semaan R. Management of pneumothorax. Clin Chest Med. 2021 Dec;42(4):729–738. doi: 10.1016/j.ccm.2021.08.008. PMID: 34774178.
29. Gilday C, Odunayo A, Hespel AM. Spontaneous pneumothorax: pathophysiology, clinical presentation and diagnosis. Top Companion Anim Med. 2021 Nov;45: 100563. doi: 10.1016/j.tcam.2021.100563. Epub 2021 Jul 22. PMID: 34303864.
30. Aragaki-Nakahodo A. Management of pneumothorax: an update. Curr Opin Pulm Med. 2022 Jan 1;28(1):62–67. doi: 10.1097/MCP.0000000000000839. PMID: 34857696.

31. Tran J, Haussner W, Shah K. Traumatic pneumothorax: a review of current diagnostic practices and evolving management. J Emerg Med. 2021 Nov;61(5):517–528. doi: 10.1016/j.jemermed.2021.07.006. Epub 2021 Aug 29. PMID: 34470716.
32. Thachuthara-George J. Pneumothorax in patients with respiratory failure in ICU. J Thorac Dis. 2021 Aug;13(8):5195–5204. doi: 10.21037/jtd-19-3752. PMID: 34527359; PMCID: PMC8411185.
33. Jouneau S, Vuillard C, Salé A, Bazin Y, Sohier L, Kerjouan M, Ricard JD, Messika J. Outpatient management of primary spontaneous pneumothorax. Respir Med. 2021 Jan;176:106240. doi: 10.1016/j.rmed.2020.106240. Epub 2020 Nov 20. PMID: 33248364.
34. Porcel JM, Lee P. Thoracoscopy for spontaneous pneumothorax. J Clin Med. 2021 Aug 26;10(17):3835. doi: 10.3390/jcm10173835. PMID: 34501282; PMCID: PMC8432077.
35. Louw EH, Shaw JA, Koegelenberg CFN. New insights into spontaneous pneumothorax: a review. Afr J Thorac Crit Care Med. 2021 Mar 9;27(1). doi: 10.7196/AJTCCM.2021.v27i1.054. PMID: 34240041; PMCID: PMC8203058.
36. Agrafiotis AC, Rummens P, Lardinois I. Pneumothorax in otherwise healthy non-intubated patients suffering from COVID-19 pneumonia: a systematic review. J Thorac Dis. 2021 Jul;13(7):4519–4529. doi: 10.21037/jtd-21-208. PMID: 34422378; PMCID: PMC8339789.
37. Hallifax R. Aetiology of primary spontaneous pneumothorax. J Clin Med. 2022 Jan 19;11(3):490. doi: 10.3390/jcm11030490. PMID: 35159942; PMCID: PMC8836443.
38. Hashinokuchi A, Akamine T, Kometani T, Shikada Y, Nozoe T, Kato S. Spontaneous pneumothorax associated with cavitating pulmonary metastasis from breast cancer: a case report and literature review. Gen Thorac Cardiovasc Surg. 2021 Jan;69(1):137–141. doi: 10.1007/s11748-020-01423-1. Epub 2020 Jul 2. PMID: 32617838.
39. Athalve AU, et al. Role of HRCT chest in aetiology of spontaneous pneumothorax. Lung India. 2000;XVIII(4):116–119.
40. Mazarika B, et al. Reexpansion pulmonary oedema. The PulmoFace. 2014;14:46–48.

© 2024 World Scientific Publishing Company
https://doi.org/10.1142/9789811271410_0047

47 Pulmonary embolism

Pharmacologic management of PE involves a stratified approach in terms of initial, long-term, and extended treatment. Pharmacologic options include thrombolytics and anticoagulants.

Initial phase	to reduce mortality and recurrence in the 5–10 days after presentation	Thrombolytics
		Parenteral anticoagulants
		Oral anticoagulants
Long-term treatment	In patients whose PE was provoked, either by surgery or another risk factor	Oral or parenteral anticoagulation therapy for 3 months
	Patients with unprovoked PE	Oral or parenteral anticoagulant therapy for 3 months with reevaluation at 3 months to determine the risk versus benefit of continuing therapy
		Patients with low or moderate bleeding risk should be considered for extended anticoagulant therapy
		Patients with high bleeding risk should not be considered for continuing anticoagulation after 3 months

(*Continued*)

Extended anticoagulation	Patients with unprovoked PE with low-to-moderate bleeding risk	Extended anticoagulation therapy with frequent reevaluations for continuation
	Patients with a second unprovoked PE	Extended anticoagulation therapy if bleeding risk is low or moderate
	Patients with active cancer and cancer-associated PE	Extended anticoagulation therapy irrespective of bleeding risk

Drug name	Dose	Renal dose	CI	Initial Rx	Long-term Rx	Extended Rx	ADR
Oral anticoagulants							
Rivaroxaban	15 mg PO q12 hours for 21 days then, 20 mg PO qDay	CrCl<30 mL/minute: Avoid use		✓	✓		Anemia, dizziness, headache, eye hemorrhage, hypotension, hematoma, epistaxis, hemoptysis, gingival bleeding, GIT hemorrhage, increase in transaminases, pruritus, fever, peripheral edema, decreased general strength and energy
	10 mg od					✓	
Apixaban	10 mg bid for 7 days then, 5 mg bid	Patients with SCr>2.5 mg/dl or CrCl<25 mL/minute were excluded from clinical trials		✓			Anemia, eye hemorrhage, hypotension, epistaxis, nausea, GI hemorrhage, Rectal hemorrhage, gingival bleeding, increased GGT, hematuria, contusion
	5 mg bid or 2.5 mg bid				✓		

Drug name	Dose	Renal dose	CI	Initial Rx	Long-term Rx	Extended Rx	ADR
Edoxaban	60 mg od if >60 kg 30 mg od if <60 kg or on concomitant P-gp inhibitor after parenteral anticoagulation	CrCl 15–30 mL/minute: 30 mg od CrCl< 15 mL/minute is not recommended		✓	✓		Anemia, dizziness, headache, epistaxis, Abdominal pain, lower/upper GI hemorrhage, oral/pharyngeal hemorrhage, nausea, blood bilirubin increased GGT increased, cutaneous soft tissue hemorrhage, rash macroscopic hematuria/urethral/vaginal/pruritic site hemorrhage
Dabigatran	150 mg bid after parenteral anticoagulation	Patients with CrCl ≤30 mL/minute were excluded from clinical trials	Mechanical prosthetic valve	✓	✓		Dyspepsia and gastritis, intracranial hemorrhage, hypersensitivity

Warfarin	Patient-specific dosing based on INR requires bridging for at least 5 days and until INR is at least 2.0 for 24 hours	Monitor INR closely	Hemorrhagic tendencies, recent/potential eye/CNS surgeries, major regional lumbar block, pericarditis, bacterial endocarditis, eclampsia/pre-eclampsia, pregnancy	✓	✓	✓	Cholesterol embolus syndrome, intraocular hemorrhage, abdominal pain, flatulence, alopecia, rash, taste disturbance, tissue necrosis, headache, lethargy, dizziness, hematuria, anemia, hepatitis, respiratory tract bleeding, hypersensitivity reaction, hemorrhage, blood dyscrasias, fever, "purple toe" syndrome, increased fracture risk with long-term usage, calciphylaxis
Parenteral anticoagulants							
UFH	80 units/kg IV bolus then continuous infusion of 18 units/kg/hour	None	History of HIT, severe thrombocytopenia				Heparin-induced thrombocytopenia, possibly delayed

Drug name	Dose	Renal dose	CI	Initial Rx	Long-term Rx	Extended Rx	ADR
LMWX	Enoxaparin: 1 mg/kg SC bid or 1.5 mg/kg SC od	CrCl<30 mL/minute: 30 mg od	History of HIT in the past 100 days	✓	✓	✓	Hemorrhage, elevation of serum aminotransferases, fever, local site reactions, thrombocytopenia, nausea, anemia, ecchymosis
Fondaparinux	<50 kg: 5 mg SC od 50–100 kg: 7.5 mg SC od >100 kg: 10 mg SC od	CrCl<30 mL/minute: contraindicated	CrCl<30 mL/minute, bacterial endocarditis	✓			Anemia, fever, nausea

(*Continued*)

(*Continued*)

Thrombolytics							
Alteplase	100 mg IV infusion over 2 hours	None	Active bleed, ischemic stroke within 3 m, prior intra-cranial bleed, serious head trauma, severe uncontrolled HTN, suspected aortic dissection	✓			Intracerebral hemorrhage, bleeding from damaged blood vessels, pharyngeal hemorrhage, gastrointestinal hemorrhage, ecchymosis, urogenital hemorrhage, injection site hemorrhage

The following classes of drugs are used for the treatment of pulmonary embolism.

1. Anticoagulants

Indirect factor Xa inhibitor

Fondaparinux is a synthetic analog of the AT-binding pentasaccharide found in UFH or in the LMWHs. It exerts its anticoagulant effects by binding to AT and evoking a conformational change at the reactive site of AT, which enhances its reactivity with factor Xa. Neutralization of factor Xa interrupts the blood coagulation cascade and thus inhibits thrombin formation and thrombus development. Fondaparinux neither inactivates thrombin nor has any known effect on platelet function. At the recommended dose, fondaparinux sodium does not affect fibrinolytic activity or bleeding time.

Vitamin K antagonist

Warfarin acts indirectly through inhibition of vitamin K epoxide reductase complex 1 (VKORC1), which is an essential enzyme for activating the vitamin K available in the body. By inhibition of VKORC1, there is depletion of functional vitamin K reserves and therefore reductions in the synthesis of active coagulation factors II, VII, IX, and X as well as regulatory factors protein C and protein S.

Direct factor Xa inhibitor

Rivaroxaban competitively inhibits factor Xa and is more than 10,000-fold more selective for factor Xa than other related serine proteases, and it does not require cofactors (such as antithrombin) to exert its anticoagulant effect. Unlike indirect factor Xa inhibitors, rivaroxaban inhibits both free and clot-bound factor Xa, as well as prothrombinase activity, thereby prolonging clotting times.

Direct thrombin inhibitor

Dabigatran is a reversible, potent, competitive direct thrombin inhibitor. Unlike heparin, which can only bind free thrombin, dabigatran is capable of binding and inhibiting both free and clot-bound thrombin.

Endothelial injury results in the exposure of tissue factor which interacts with activated factor VII to initiate the coagulation cascade. Thrombin, a serine protease, enables thrombus formation by activating factors V, VIII, and XI and catalyzing the conversion of fibrinogen to fibrin. Additionally, thrombin causes platelet aggregation by activating protease-activated receptors on the platelet surface.

Thrombin also initiates fibrinolytic events, as the thrombin–thrombomodulin complex activates protein C, which subsequently inactivates factors Va and VIIIa. Antithrombin III, a serine protease inhibitor, inactivates factors Xa, IXa, XIIa, and IIa. The anticoagulative effects of antithrombin III are accelerated hundreds to thousands of times in the presence of unfractionated and low-molecular-weight heparins.

Structurally, thrombin contains three major drug-binding domains: the active (or serine protease catalytic) site and two exosites (1 and 2). Exosite 1 binds fibrin, while exosite 2 binds heparin. Heparin-bound thrombin can then bind fibrin or antithrombin. Once heparin-bound thrombin is joined to fibrin, both exosites are occupied, and the complex is relatively protected from the effects of antithrombin. As a result, heparin has little effect on fibrin-bound thrombin.

In contrast, direct thrombin inhibitors, such as dabigatran, can inhibit free, fibrin-bound, and clot-bound thrombin. Bivalent direct thrombin inhibitors, such as hirudin and bivalirudin, bind both the active site and exosite 1, while univalent direct thrombin inhibitors, like dabigatran, bind only the active site. Additionally, the direct thrombin inhibitors reduce the platelet-aggregating effects of thrombin.

Thrombin enables thrombus formation by activating multiple coagulation factors, catalyzing the conversion of fibrinogen to fibrin, and causing platelet aggregation. Dabigatran binds at the active site, thus inhibiting both free and fibrin-bound thrombin. Heparin exerts its action by increasing the affinity of antithrombin for thrombin. Heparin can only inhibit free thrombin since fibrin-bound thrombin has both exosites occupied and is relatively protected from the effects of antithrombin.

2. Thrombolytics

Alteplase is a recombinant human tissue-type plasminogen activator, a glycoprotein, which activates plasminogen directly to plasmin. When in the systemic circulation at pharmacologic concentration, it binds to fibrin, causing the conversion of plasminogen to plasmin initiating local fibrinolysis with limited systemic proteolysis.

Protein C and S deficiency

Protein C concentrate

Treating the manifestations of Severe Congenital Protein C Deficiency (SCPCD) usually involves anticoagulation and/or protein C (PC) replacement, depending on the circumstances.

The acute management of SCPCD involves PC replacement. Anticoagulants may be added concomitantly or during the transition to long-term management. Maintenance can be achieved through, oral anticoagulants or a combination of oral anticoagulants and PC replacement. Curative treatment has been achieved with liver transplantation.

PC replacement is an established method for treating purpura fulminans (PF) and warfarin-induced skin necrosis, for prophylaxis in patients with SCPCD. Replacement of PC can be achieved with infusions of fresh frozen plasma (FFP), cryoprecipitate, PC-rich prothrombin-complex concentrate or PC concentrate. FFP contains all plasma components (water, electrolytes, albumin immunoglobulins coagulation factors, and factors of the complement system) including PC in a non-concentrated form. Prothrombin-complex concentrates can consist of a combination of factors, such as factors II, VII, IX, PC, and protein S.

PCC in acute episode or short-term prophylaxis is given as initial dose of 100–120 IU/kg IV, then 60–80 International Units/kg IV q6 hours for 3 doses, thereafter 45–60 IU/kg IV BID/QID.

For long-term prophylaxis, it is given as 45–60 IU/kg IV q12 hours.

Guidelines, published by the American College of Chest Physicians for antithrombotic therapy in neonates and children, recommend the administration of either FFP or PC concentrate, when available, until the clinical lesions resolve. PC replacement therapy temporarily increases a patient's PC levels, slowing down the clotting process and preventing thrombotic events associated with excess blood coagulation.

Protein C Replacement
PC Concentrate Severe congenital PC deficiency manifestation Prophylaxis for short and long term
Cryoprecipitate Severe PC deficiency manifestation
Fresh Frozen Plasma Severe PC deficiency manifestation
PC- Rich Prothrombin rich concentrate Severe PC deficiency manifestation
Factor IX Concentrate Severe PC deficiency manifestation

Anticoagulation
Coumarin derivatives Treatment of severe PC deficiency-Long term
UFH Long term coumarin derivatives for SCPCD
Factor Xa Inhibitors Prevention of DVT and PE
LMWH Treatment of severe PC deficiency-Long term
Direct Thrombin inhibitors Treatment of severe PC deficiency-Long term

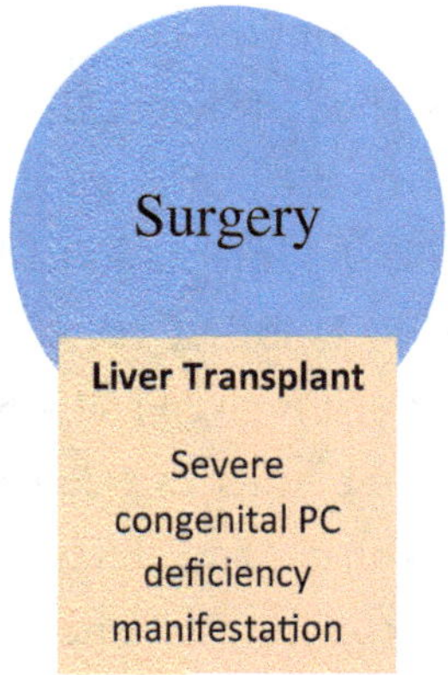

- Moderate PC deficiency

Treatment is based on the type and location of thrombotic complication. Patients with venous thrombosis, such as DVT or PE, are initially started with heparin followed by initiation of an oral anticoagulant like warfarin for 3–6 months following occurrence of the first thrombotic episode. Long-term prophylaxis against venous thrombosis can be achieved by using LMWH.

- Severe PC deficiency

Initial treatment of patients with severe PC-deficient neonates must be started immediately to prevent death. PC replacement with factor IX concentrates has been used for long-term management; however, it has an increased risk of causing thrombosis. Human vapor-heated PC concentrates might be another option which is under investigation. Neonates may be treated with FFP with the usual starting dose range of 8–12 mL/kg every 12 hours. Close monitoring for hydrocephalus, seizures, hyperproteinemia, and blind is required when frequent infusions are administered.

Treatment of hyperhomocysteinemia

Folic acid

Folic acid occurs naturally in certain foods and can also be fortified in cereals. Cereals providing 127, 299, and 665 μg of folic acid increased the plasma folate level by 30.8%, 64.8%, and 105.7%, respectively, and lowered plasma homocysteine levels by 3.7%, 11.0%, and 14.0%, respectively. The homocysteine-lowering effects of folate from supplements and from fortified foods appear to be comparable. Folic acid supplement of 450 μg/day and folate-fortified breakfast cereal of 298 μg/day could increase serum folate levels by 27 and 21 nmol/L, respectively, and decrease homocysteine levels by 21% and 24%, respectively. The Homocysteine Lowering Trialists' Collaboration21 has summarized in a meta-analysis of 12 treatment trials the use of folate for treating hyperhomocysteinemia. The conclusion was that folic acid supplementation reduced blood homocysteine levels by 25% with similar effects in the range of 0.5–5 mg folic acid daily. The reductions were greater at higher pretreatment homocysteine concentrations and at lower pretreatment serum folate concentrations.

Methyltetrahydrofolate

5-Methyltetrahydrofolate (MTHF) has also been studied as an agent to decrease homocysteine levels, but it was to be useful only in the heterozygous MTHFR mutation subjects with a reduction of only 7% in the homocysteine levels.

Vitamins B6 and B12

Vitamin B6 at a dose of 250 mg/day is able to normalize homocysteine levels in 56% of the 421 patients with post-methionine load hyperhomocysteinemia and premature peripheral or cerebral occlusive arterial disease.

Vitamin B12 does not have a significant effect on plasma homocysteine levels in healthy subjects, but has been shown to lower homocysteine levels up to 14.8% at a dose of 0.4 mg/day in patients with hyperhomocysteinemia.

Combination therapy

There have been several studies utilizing folate, vitamin B6, and vitamin B12 in various combinations to decrease homocysteine levels. However, certain studies show that combination therapies are not much different from use of folate alone.

Betaine

Several studies have shown a reduction in plasma homocysteine levels but its significance remains unclear.

References and suggested readings

1. Leibfried M, Falbum S, Palummo J. Treatment of Pulmonary Embolism. US Pharma. 2018;43(7):HS-2-HS12.
2. ARIXTRA® (fondaparinux sodium) Injection. PRESCRIBING INFORMATION. NDA 21-345/S-010

3. Patel S, Preuss C, Patel N. Warfarin. In: StatPearls 2023.
4. Samama MM. The mechanism of action of rivaroxaban--an oral, direct Factor Xa inhibitor--compared with other anticoagulants. *Thromb Res.* 2011;127(6):497-504.
5. Ganetsky M, Babu KM, Salhanick SD, Brown RS, Boyer EW. Dabigatran: review of pharmacology and management of bleeding complications of this novel oral anticoagulant. *J Med Toxicol.* 2011;7(4):281-287
6. Harter, Katherine, Michael Levine, and Sean Henderson (2015), "Anticoagulation Drug Therapy: A Review," *Western Journal of Emergency Medicine*, 16 (1), 11–17.
7. HIGHLIGHTS OF PRESCRIBING INFORMATION, Activase (alteplase) for injection, for intravenous use Initial U.S. Approval: 1987.
8. Shire - SCPCD. (n.d.). *How to Treat Severe Congenital Protein C Deficiency (SCPCD).* [online] Available at: https://www.scpcd.org/emergency-diagnosis/how-to-treat-scpcd/#
9. Shire - SCPCD. (n.d.). *Purpura Fulminans: Is it Sepsis or Severe Congenital Protein C Deficiency (SCPCD)?.* [online] Available at: https://www.scpcd.org/emergency-diagnosis/scpcd-action-tool/
10. Chan E, Fonseca VA. Management of hyperhomocysteinemia. *Metab Syndr Relat Disord.* 2003;1(2):159-170.
11. Kaptein FHJ, Kroft LJM, Hammerschlag G, Ninaber MK, Bauer MP, Huisman MV, Klok FA. Pulmonary infarction in acute pulmonary embolism. Thromb Res. 2021 Jun;202:162–169. doi: 10.1016/j.thromres.2021.03.022. Epub 2021 Apr 1. PMID: 33862471.
12. Kahn SR, de Wit K. Pulmonary embolism. N Engl J Med. 2022 Jul 7;387(1):45–57. doi: 10.1056/NEJMcp2116489. PMID: 35793208.
13. Rivera-Lebron BN, Rali PM, Tapson VF. The PERT concept: a step-by-step approach to managing pulmonary embolism. Chest. 2021 Jan;159(1):347–355. doi: 10.1016/j.chest.2020.07.065. Epub 2020 Aug 3. PMID: 32758561.
14. Wenger N, Sebastian T, Engelberger RP, Kucher N, Spirk D. Pulmonary embolism and deep vein thrombosis: similar but different. Thromb Res. 2021 Oct;206:88–98. doi: 10.1016/j.thromres.2021.08.015. Epub 2021 Aug 19. PMID: 34454241.

15. Arrigo M, Huber LC. Pulmonary embolism and heart failure: a reappraisal. Card Fail Rev. 2021 Feb 18;7:e03. doi: 10.15420/cfr.2020.26. PMID: 33708418; PMCID: PMC7926477.
16. Weinstein T, Deshwal H, Brosnahan SB. Advanced management of intermediate-high risk pulmonary embolism. Crit Care. 2021 Aug 31;25(1):311. doi: 10.1186/s13054-021-03679-2. PMID: 34461959; PMCID: PMC8406617.
17. Delcroix M, Torbicki A, Gopalan D, Sitbon O, Klok FA, Lang I, Jenkins D, Kim NH, Humbert M, Jais X, Vonk Noordegraaf A, Pepke-Zaba J, Brénot P, Dorfmuller P, Fadel E, Ghofrani HA, Hoeper MM, Jansa P, Madani M, Matsubara H, Ogo T, Grünig E, D'Armini A, Galie N, Meyer B, Corkery P, Meszaros G, Mayer E, Simonneau G. ERS statement on chronic thromboembolic pulmonary hypertension. Eur Respir J. 2021 Jun 17;57(6):2002828. doi: 10.1183/13993003.02828-2020. PMID: 33334946.
18. Kulka HC, Zeller A, Fornaro J, Wuillemin WA, Konstantinides S, Christ M. Acute pulmonary embolism–its diagnosis and treatment from a multidisciplinary viewpoint. Dtsch Arztebl Int. 2021 Sep 17;118(37):618–628. doi: 10.3238/arztebl.m2021.0226. Epub 2021 Sep 17. PMID: 34857082; PMCID: PMC8704819.
19. Sin D, McLennan G, Rengier F, Haddadin I, Heresi GA, Bartholomew JR, Fink MA, Thompson D, Partovi S. Acute pulmonary embolism multimodality imaging prior to endovascular therapy. Int J Cardiovasc Imaging. 2021 Jan;37(1):343–358. doi: 10.1007/s10554-020-01980-9. Epub 2020 Aug 30. PMID: 32862293; PMCID: PMC7456521.
20. Poor HD. Pulmonary thrombosis and thromboembolism in COVID-19. Chest. 2021 Oct;160(4):1471–1480. doi: 10.1016/j.chest.2021.06.016. Epub 2021 Jun 19. PMID: 34153340; PMCID: PMC8213519.
21. Sulimov DS, Freund A, Thiele H. Catheter-directed therapy in pulmonary embolism. Herz. 2021 Oct;46(5):399–405. English. doi: 10.1007/s00059-021-05059-6. Epub 2021 Sep 1. PMID: 34468788.
22. Yang R, Liu G, Deng C. Pulmonary embolism with chronic obstructive pulmonary disease. Chronic Dis Transl Med. 2021 Jun 24;7(3):149–156. doi: 10.1016/j.cdtm.2021.04.001. PMID: 34505015; PMCID: PMC8413125.
23. Blondon M, Martinez de Tejada B, Glauser F, Righini M, Robert-Ebadi H. Management of high-risk pulmonary embolism in pregnancy. Thromb Res.

2021 Aug;204:57–65. doi: 10.1016/j.thromres.2021.05.019. Epub 2021 Jun 7. PMID: 34146979.

24. Rousseau H, Del Giudice C, Sanchez O, Ferrari E, Sapoval M, Marek P, Delmas C, Zadro C, Revel-Mouroz P. Endovascular therapies for pulmonary embolism. Heliyon. 2021 Apr 1;7(4):e06574. doi: 10.1016/j.heliyon.2021.e06574. PMID: 33889762; PMCID: PMC8047492.

https://doi.org/10.1142/9789811271410_0048

48 Pulmonary hypertension

Introduction

Pulmonary arterial hypertension (PAH) is a common endpoint during the course of many chronic respiratory conditions such as COPD, chronic asthma with airway remodeling, ILD, and post-TB sequelae among many others. It is also seen in a host of other cardiac and systemic diseases and it is important to consider all of them before finalizing the diagnosis since the course of disease, prognosis, and survival depends on reaching a correct diagnosis. Rarely, it can be a primary pulmonary vascular disease (primary pulmonary hypertension). The PPH is three times more common in women than men and usually presents in third to fourth decades.

Definition

The earlier definitions by the experts during the WHO meeting in the 1960s were pulmonary artery pressures above 25 mmHg during rest in supine position on pulmonary artery catheterization. This has been very recently changed after a study of the pulmonary artery pressures of more than 1,000 normal cardiac catheterizations. The normal value was around 14 mmHg (SD 3.3) and a 97.5 percentile would be a value above 20 mmHg. Along with an elevated pulmonary artery pressure of above 20 mmHg, for the diagnosis of precapillary PH, the presence of increased pulmonary vascular resistance (PVR) above 3 or more Wood units is essential. For the diagnosis of PAH, it is necessary to have a pulmonary capillary wedge pressure below 15 mmHg. It is extremely important to know the cause of the PH and not just the measurement of pulmonary artery pressures.

WHO classification

Class I: Pulmonary arterial hypertension (PAH)

- Idiopathic PAH
- Heritable PAH (BMPR2, ALK1, ENG, CAV1, and other mutations)
- Drug- and toxin-induced pulmonary hypertension
- PAH associated with:
    - Connective tissue disease
    - HIV infection
    - Portal hypertension
    - Congenital heart disease
- Pulmonary veno-occlusive disease (PVOD) and/or pulmonary capillary hemangiomatosis (PCH)
- Pulmonary artery hypertension long-term responders to calcium channel blockers (new entry into group 1)

Class II: Pulmonary hypertension due to left heart disease

- Left ventricular systolic dysfunction
- Left ventricular diastolic dysfunction
- Valvular disease
- Congenital or acquired left ventricular outflow tract obstruction
- And congenital cardiomyopathies

Class III: Pulmonary hypertension due to lung disease and/or hypoxia

- Chronic obstructive pulmonary disease
- Interstitial lung disease
- Mixed obstruction and restriction
- Sleep-disordered breathing
- Chronic exposure to high altitude

Class IV: Chronic thromboembolic pulmonary hypertension

Class V: Pulmonary hypertension due to unclear multifactorial mechanisms

- Hematologic disorders: myeloproliferative disorders, splenectomy
- Systemic disorders: sarcoidosis, pulmonary Langerhans cell histiocytosis, lymphangioleiomyomatosis, neurofibromatosis, vasculitis

- Metabolic disorders: glycogen storage disease, Gaucher disease, thyroid disorders
- Others: tumoral obstruction, fibrosing mediastinitis, chronic renal failure on dialysis with arteriovenous fistula

Pathogenesis and pathology

The normal physiology of the pulmonary circulation is quite unique in the human body consisting of high-flow, low-pressure systems. Normally, the pulmonary artery pressure rarely exceeds 15 mmHg with a flow of 5–6 L/minute at rest. During strenuous exercise, when the flow increases to about 25 L/minute, there is hardly any change in the pulmonary artery pressures. There are large areas of the lung that normally do not take part in gas exchange; though there is air, there is hardly any blood supply except at the height of systole. These pulmonary vasculatures open up when there is an increase in the cardiac output and is one of the important reasons that the pulmonary artery pressure remains low, which means that the strain for the right ventricle pumping blood into the pulmonary arteries remains almost the same. The resistance of the pulmonary vasculature to the blood flow is termed as the PVR. Two of the most important influences on the PVR are hypoxia and the nitric oxide. As the vessel diameter decreases, further ongoing insults cause a greater increase in PVR. A sustained increase in PVR can lead to changes in the vessel wall that are irreversible.

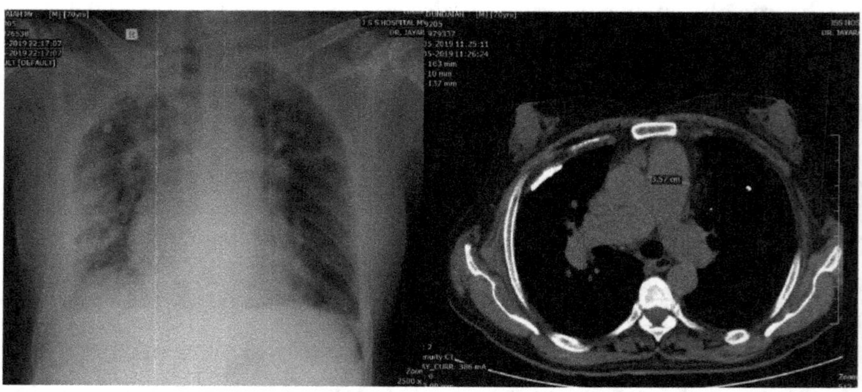

Figure 1: X-ray and CT scans of dilated pulmonary artery.

The main pathogenetic mechanisms that lead to PH are genetic predisposition, environmental influences, inflammation and autoimmune mechanisms and endothelial dysfunction. The main pulmonary artery till the sub-segmental level mainly consists of elastic arteries and the media contains plenty of elastic fibers. From the lobular level downwards, these become mainly muscular arteries and the media of the artery predominately contains smooth muscle cells. These are the main sites of involvement in various diseases that lead to PH. In the various diseases that lead to PH described in the WHO classification, there is a general imbalance among various factors such as vasodilators and vasoconstrictors and prothrombotic and antithrombotic factors. There are also disturbances in the levels of mitogenic factors, growth inhibitors, and endothelial growth factors. These disturbances cause pulmonary endothelial dysfunction as a final common pathway.

The main outcome of these various insults are vasoconstriction, pulmonary vascular remodeling, and in-situ thrombosis. Pulmonary vascular remodeling involves all the layers of the vessel including the intima (intimal thickening, fibrosis, and plexiform lesions), media (smooth muscle hypertrophy and hyperplasia and muscularization of small arterioles), and the adventitia (thickening). Intimal fibrosis and thickening due to fibroblasts, myofibroblasts, and other connective tissue cells is a common feature in PH. The thickening may be uniform and concentric or focal and eccentric. This happens mainly due to the stress originating from the vascular lumen such as an increase in pulmonary arterial pressure, endothelial damage, and shear stress. The changes can lead to either partial and in some cases complete occlusion of the vascular lumen.

Medial thickening involves both increase in the volume and the number of smooth muscle cells in the tunica media and is seen in WHO classification PH 1, 2, and 3. Thrombotic lesions or in-situ thrombosis is a common feature in many types of PH including the PVOD. Many times they get recanalized and can be seen as eccentric intimal fibrosis. These many times have multiple channels during recanalization and are called as "colander like" lesions. Another classical fibrotic lesion is called as the "onion skin" or "onion bulb" lesions due to its laminar arrangement of collagen layers. The plexiform lesions first described with idiopathic PAH have now been described with other causes of PH. It involves excessive intimal thickening causing near occlusion of the vascular lumen, channels within the intimal layer due to this thickening, and an aneurysmal dilation of the vessel wall. The key pathologic changes can involve different parts of the blood vessels including the endothelium, lamina, smooth muscles, and adventitia. Along with these structural changes there can be infiltration with various inflammatory cells, mainly mononuclear cells and fibroblasts.

Clinical features

A high degree of suspicion is needed to diagnose PH early in the course of the disease. The most common symptoms are nonspecific and are seen with many other respiratory and cardiac diseases such as unexplained dyspnea, which is usually progressive, fatigue, exertion intolerance, pedal edema, abdominal distension due to ascites, generalized edema, light headedness, syncope and chest pain. Cough is not a common symptom unless PH is secondary to pulmonary diseases such as COPD or ILD. Rare presentations include hemoptysis, arrhythmias and hoarseness of voice due to unilateral vocal cord paralysis due to compression from an enlarged pulmonary artery known as Ortner's syndrome.

The clinical findings point to right ventricular strain or failure as evidenced by elevated jugular venous pressure, prominent epigastric pulsation, hepatomegaly, splenomegaly, hepatojugular reflux, peripheral pitting pedal edema, prominent left parasternal heave, apex beat shows right ventricular lift, accentuated (loud) pulmonic component of second heart sound (P2) and pan systolic murmur at left lower sternal border (tricuspid regurgitation), pulmonary regurgitation and sometimes an S3 gallop. An initial right ventricular failure later progresses into a biventricular failure.

It is important to keep the WHO classification in mind and evaluate for all the risk factors and take a detailed relevant medical history including various connective tissue disease, personal or family history of deep vein thrombosis or pulmonary embolism, HIV infection, chronic alcoholism and cirrhosis of the liver, various cardiac and lung diseases and hypoxemia.

Diagnosis

The gold standard for the diagnosis is pulmonary artery catheterization. But it may not be possible in all the cases. There are important findings that can be obtained from noninvasive evaluation. The first test that can be easily done in most places is the ECG that shows right axis deviation, RV hypertrophy and strain pattern, RA dilatation. P pulmonale is an important finding that points to pulmonary hypertension. Chest X-rays shows enlarged bilateral hilar pulmonary arteries (if they can be measured more than 16 mm on the right side and more than 14 mm on the left side is strongly suggestive of pulmonary hypertension), enlarged cardiac silhouette (especially RV on lateral view) and in later stages biventricular enlargement and pulmonary edema. On pulmonary function testing DLCO, a reduction in diffusing capacity for carbon monoxide is the classical observation. The next investigation is the echocardiography that shows an increased RV systolic pressure, RV hypertrophy, enlarged RV and RA, and RV systolic dysfunction.

Role of different biomarkers

There is an interest regarding noninvasive biomarkers for the diagnosis and prognosis of PH. The role of various biomarkers, their cellular pathways, association, and clinical significance are discussed below in the table. The key biomarkers include markers for myocardial stress and injury, markers of inflammation, markers of endothelial dysfunction and vascular smooth muscle proliferation, markers for coagulation and platelet activation, and markers for tissue hypoxia and damage and there is some role for nonspecific markers (others).

Biomarkers	Cellular pathways	Association	Clinical significance
Markers of myocardial stress and injury			
BNP	Marker of myocardial stretch	Mortality, Hemodynamic measurements (RAP, mPAP, PVR), functional class, 6MWD	• Disease progression and therapy response • Progression in PAH • Response to PEA in CTEPH
NT-pro BNP	Marker of myocardial stretch	Pulmonary hemodynamics, survival	• Risk of PAH in high-risk groups • Disease progression and therapy response • Progression in PAH • Pressure of CTEPH after PEA • Response to PEA in CTEPH
ANP	Marker of myocardial stretch and volume overload	Cardiovascular morbidity, mortality	• Reflects RV pressure overload
Cardiac troponin isoforms	Marker of cardiac injury	Mortality, higher heart rate (indicating increased sympathetic flow), lower mixed venous saturation and 6MWD	• TnI: Risk of RHF • TnT: Progression in PAH

Markers of inflammation			
Cytokine serum levels (esp. IL-6)	Inflammatory mediators	Mortality, quality of life	• Progression in PAH
CRP	Inflammatory marker	RAP, 6MWD, poorer outcomes	• Progression in PAH • Pressure of CTEPH after PEA • Response to PEA in CTEPH
Osteopontin	Mediates cell migration, adhesion, remodeling, and survival of vascular cells	Mortality, hemodynamic measurements (RAP), functional class, 6MWD	• Risk of RHF • Progression in PAH
Adrenomedullin	Angiogenesis and inflammation regulation	Hemodynamic correlation	• Disease progression and therapy response
Markers of endothelial dysfunction and vascular smooth muscle cell proliferation			
Endothelin-1 and related molecules	Potent vasoconstrictor	Mortality, hemodynamic measurements (mPAP, PVR, CI), 6MWD	• Disease progression and therapy response

(*Continued*)

(*Continued*)

Biomarkers	Cellular pathways	Association	Clinical significance
Endostatin (ES)	Anti-angiogenic factor	Disease severity, right ventricular dysfunction, mortality	• Increased expression of ES to disease severity in PAH and demonstrate a significant relationship with adverse outcomes. Circulating ES levels can be genetically influenced, implicating ES as a genetically determined modifier of disease severity impacting on survival. These observations support serum ES as a potential biomarker in PAH with the capacity to predict poor outcomes
Circulating endothelial cells	Marker of vascular damage	Clinical response to treatment	• Noninvasive mean of accessing cells important to the pathobiology of severe pulmonary hypertension

Pentraxin	Regulates angiogenesis, inflammation, and cell proliferation	Unknown	• It is found to be elevated in patients with PAH. Plasma concentration of Pentraxin is a more reliable biomarker than BNP for PAH in particular for patients with connective tissue disorder
Angiopoietin	Angiogenic factor involved in neovascularization	Hemodynamic measurements (CI, PVR)	• Disease progression and therapy response
PIM-1	Pro-proliferative and anti-apoptotic phenotype in PAH smooth muscle cells	6MWD, cardiac index, NT-proBNP, WHO functional class, mortality	• Risk of PAH in high-risk groups
Micro RNA	Regulate gene-expression	Several types of miRNA have been identified which play a role regulation of pulmonary artery smooth muscle cells, endothelial cells, and fibroblasts	• Mi-RNA 145: Significant role to play in Hypoxia-induced PAH. Expression levels of miR-145 are higher in concentric lesions than in plexiform lesions suggesting a potential role for miRNA 145 as a diagnostic or prognostic marker in PAH

(*Continued*)

(*Continued*)

Biomarkers	Cellular pathways	Association	Clinical significance
Markers of coagulation and platelet activation			
D-Dimer	Fibrin degradation product	Hemodynamic clinical status	• Prognosis
Von-Willebrand factor	Plays a key role in homeostasis and is a marker of endothelial dysfunction	Mortality	• Progression in PAH
Markers of tissue hypoxia and tissue damage			
$PaCO_2$	Altered due to peripheral hypoperfusion	Mortality	• Disease progression and therapy response • Progression in PAH
Uric acid	Endogenous free radical scavenger protecting cells from ROS and reactive nitrogen species damage	Hemodynamic correlation	• Risk of PAH in high-risk groups • Progression in PAH • Pressure of CTEPH after PEA • Prognosis
Cystatin C	Indicator for renal filtration and is measured in patients with renal insufficiency	Correlates with RV pressure, function, and morphology	• Progression in PAH • Furthermore, cystatin C outperforms BNP

Copeptin	Mediates arteriolar vaso-constriction and diuretic effects	NYHA class, 6MWD, and kidney function	• Expression correlated with survival and disease severity
Liver function	Hyperbilirubinemia (but not other transaminases)	Associated with advanced right heart failure and reduced survival	• However, the results of the Registry to Evaluate Early And Long-term PAH Disease Management (REVEAL) registry did not confirm this finding in multivariate analysis
Others			
Serum creatinine	Marker of renal function	Mortality, hemodynamic measurements (RAP, CI)	• Progression in PAH
Serum sodium	Reflects water imbalance	Mortality	• Progression in PAH
Red cell distribution width	Unclear significance	Mortality	• A significant correlation exists between RDW and high-sensitivity C-reactive protein and the diffusing capacity of the lungs for carbon monoxide. Patients with SSc-PAH have significantly higher RDW values compared to the SSc group without pulmonary

(*Continued*)

(*Continued*)

Biomarkers	Cellular pathways	Association	Clinical significance
			disease. High RDW is considered an independent predictor of PAH in patients with SSc
Circulating fibrocytes	Contribute to organ fibrosis and extracellular matrix deposition	Unknown	• Get rid of circulating fibrocytes since the data are not conclusive about its role as a predictor of disease activity in PAH. It is exploratory at this point of time
HbA1c	Marker of metabolic dysfunction	Mortality	• Patients with pulmonary arterial hypertension (PAH) exhibit impaired glucose metabolism and increased insulin resistance. In patients with PAH, the HbA1c level at time of diagnosis is an independent predictor of long-term prognosis
HDL	Marker of vascular health	Mortality, hemodynamic measurement (PVR, CI)	• Reduced plasma levels of small HDL particles transporting fibrinolytic proteins are associated with poor outcomes in patients with idiopathic and heritable PAH

Management of pulmonary hypertension according to the WHO classification

The basic management of pulmonary hypertension depends on the cause and the likely pathways involved. The general principles of selection of management depend on the severity of the disease and have been outlined by the Canadian Medical Association.

The first step that is relevant for very early disease and limitation of daily activities involves education about the disease and risk factors, development of support groups, and exercise pulmonary rehabilitation and is applicable to all cases regardless of the cause of PH. The second step involves diuretics, oxygen, and diet that is salt restricted and oral anticoagulants and is also applicable to all cases. The third step involves testing the subjects for acute vaso-reactivity during right heart catheterization (RHC) after administration of calcium channel blockers and is applicable in subjects with familial or heritable PH, idiopathic PAH, and drug-induced PH. In subjects who are responsive to calcium channel blockers, it is a useful addition which improves the prognosis of these subjects. The fourth step involves other PH-targeted drugs and the various options include either one of these or when necessary in combination; soluble guanyl cyclase stimulators (riociguat), PDE5 inhibitors (sildenafil, tadalafil), endothelin receptor antagonists (bosentan, ambrisentan, macitentan) and prostacyclin receptor agonist (selexipag) in subjects with endogenous prostacyclin deficiency. The soluble guanyl cyclase stimulators and the PDE5 inhibitors act via the nitric oxide pathway to cause vasodilation and reduce the PH. The endothelin receptor antagonists (ERA) block the action of endothelin 1 that is known to cause vasoconstriction. Bosentan and macitentan are nonspecific endothelin A and B receptor blockers; ambrisentan and sitaxsentan are selective endothelin A blockers. The next step as the disease increases for subjects with endogenous prostacyclin deficiency is the administration of epoprostenol as an intravenous preparation and treprostinil as either an intravenous or subcutaneous preparation. The last resort in places where facilities are available is the lung or heart-lung transplant. The details of the various drugs, their indications, dose, adverse events are discussed below.

Class I

Oral anticoagulants

The high prevalence of vascular thrombotic lesions in patients with IPAH found during postmortem examination, abnormalities in coagulation and fibrinolytic pathways along with other risk factors like heart failure and immobility, warrants the need for oral anticoagulation in PAH. Patients with PAH receiving therapy with long-term i.v. prostaglandins are anticoagulated in the absence of contraindications due in part to the additional risk of catheter-associated thrombosis.

Diuretics

Diuretics are indicated in patients with fluid overload due to decompensated heart failure. The choice of diuretic must be made on clinical judgment along with appropriate monitoring of electrolytes.

Oxygen

Oxygen supplementation may be given when arterial blood O_2 pressure is consistently <8 kPa. Ambulatory O_2 may be considered when there is evidence of symptomatic benefit and correctable desaturation on exercise.

Digoxin and other cardiovascular drugs

Digoxin has been shown to improve CO acutely in IPAH, although its efficacy is unknown when administered chronically. It may be given to slow ventricular rate in patients with PAH who develop atrial tachyarrhythmias.

No convincing data are available on the usefulness and safety of angiotensin-converting enzyme inhibitors, angiotensin II receptor antagonists, beta-blockers, or ivabradine in patients with PAH.

Anemia and iron status

43% of patients with IPAH are reported to have iron deficiency anemia. Hence, appropriate iron substitution should be considered in these patients.

Calcium channel blockers

It has been increasingly recognized that only a small number of patients with IPAH who demonstrate a favorable response to acute vasodilator testing at the time of RHC do well with CCBs. The CCBs used are nifedipine, diltiazem, and amlodipine, with particular emphasis on nifedipine and diltiazem. The choice of CCB is based on the patient's heart rate at baseline, with a relative bradycardia favoring nifedipine and amlodipine and a relative tachycardia favoring diltiazem. Patients with IPAH who meet the criteria for a positive vasodilator response and are treated with CCBs should be followed closely for reasons of both safety and efficacy, with a complete reassessment after 3–4 months of therapy including RHC.

Class II and III

Prostacyclin pathway agonists

Prostacyclin, a naturally occurring prostaglandin synthesized from arachidonic acid, is a potent vasodilator with antiplatelet and antiproliferative effects. The binding of prostacyclin to its receptor triggers the activation of the G-protein and increases intracellular cAMP, which activates protein kinase A which causes inhibition of platelet aggregation, relaxation of smooth muscle, and vasodilation of the pulmonary arteries. Prostacyclin synthase, the enzyme responsible for the formation of prostacyclin, may be deficient in the pulmonary endothelium of some patients with severe PH, resulting in excessive vasoconstriction and platelet aggregation.

- Epoprostenol
- Treprostinil
- Iloprost
- Selexipag

Endothelin receptor antagonists

In patients with PAH, high plasma levels of ET_1 have been documented due to an increase in production in endothelial cells and inhibition of elimination of ET_1, primarily in the lung (clearance).

The biological action of ET_1 is mediated by two G-protein-coupled subtypes of receptors: ET_A and ET_B. ET_A receptors are expressed on pulmonary smooth muscle cells, and mediate potent vasoconstriction and promote cell proliferation. ET_B receptors are expressed predominantly on the endothelial surface of vessels, and mediate vasodilatation through the production of nitric oxide and prostacyclin; they also stimulate pulmonary clearance of circulating ET_1 to favor its elimination. ET_B receptors not only have "protective" effects but are also present in the muscle cells of vascular walls, where they have the same effects as ET_A receptors (vasoconstriction and cell proliferation). In systemic and pulmonary hypertension, expression of ET_B receptors is upregulated in the media of blood vessels, and ET_A and ET_B receptors contribute to the detrimental effects of ET_1.

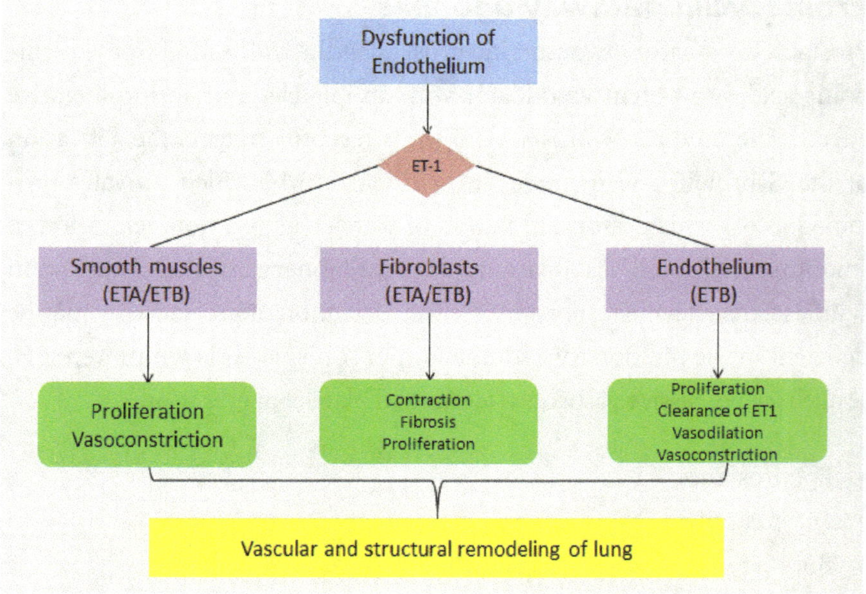

The most efficient pharmacological mechanism for antagonizing the deleterious effects of ET_1 is the use of ERAs, because they can blockade only ET_A and ET_B receptors. As such, ERAs can be distinguished into two types, based on the action on the ET receptor, with relative differences in pharmacologic effects: selective drugs (e.g., ambrisentan) and unselective (e.g., Bosentan and macitentan). If these drugs bind to ET_1 receptors, the latter cannot be activated by ET_1, which cannot exert its effects on vascular structures within the lungs. The rationale for the selective blockade of ET_A receptors is the ability to maintain the potential beneficial effects mediated by ET_B receptors (vasodilatation and ET_1 clearance) by blocking only the adverse effects (vasoconstriction and proliferation) of ET_A receptors.

- Nonselective dual action receptor antagonists — bosentan and macitentan
- Selective receptor antagonists of endothelin receptor A — ambrisentan and sitaxsentan

Nitric oxide-cGMP pathway enhancers

- PDE5 inhibitors: Sildenafil, Tadalafil

Therapies that manipulate the downstream NO signaling have revolutionized the treatment of PH.

PDE-5 inhibitors prevent the normal hydrolysis of cGMP, prolonging the NO effects on tissues. PDE-5 is mainly expressed in the pulmonary vascular bed, thus its inhibition has primarily pulmonary-specific effects. Furthermore, PDE5 is upregulated in the lung and the hypertrophied right ventricular myocardium of patients with PAH. Therefore, PDE-5 inhibitors are an ideal treatment for PAH because they decrease the right ventricular afterload and improve right ventricular inotropy, without relevant systemic hemodynamic effects.

Therapeutic strategies to increase NO effect.

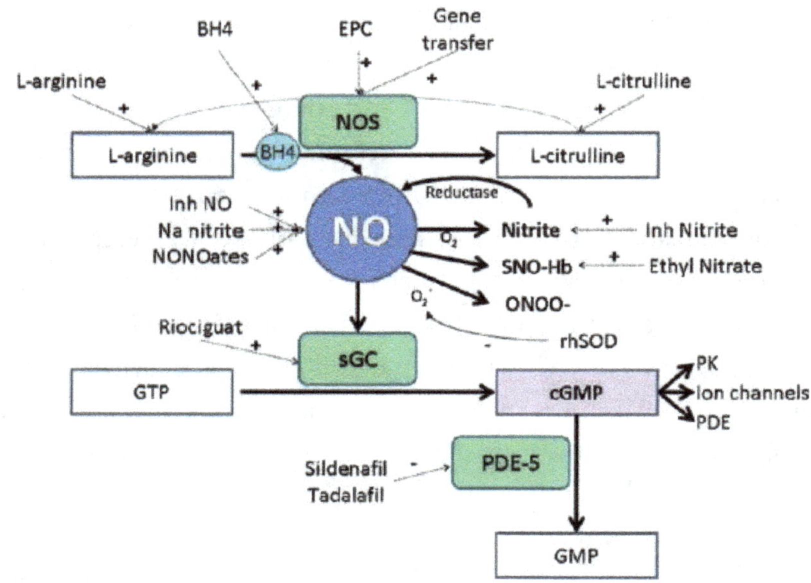

BH4, tetrahydrobiopterin; cGMP: Cyclic guanosine monophosphate; EPC: Endothelial progenitor cells; GMP: Guanosine monophosphate; GTP: Guanosine triphosphate; HMG CoA red, hydroxyl-methylglutaryl-CoA reductase; Inh, inhaled; NO: Nitric oxide; NOS: Nitric oxide synthase; $ONOO^-$, peroxynitrite; PDE: Phosphodiesterases; PK: Protein kinases; rhSOD: Recombinant human superoxide dismutase; sGC: Soluble guanylate cyclase; SNO-Hb: S-nitrosothiol — hemoglobin. L-arginine can be regenerated from L-citrulline by two enzymes (argininosuccinate synthase and argininosuccinate lyase).

- Guanylate cyclase stimulant: Riociguat

Endothelial release of nitric oxide is the initial step in vascular smooth muscle relaxation.

NOS is responsible for conversion of L-arginine to L-citrulline and the vasoactive NO. NO released from the endothelium interacts with the β-subunit of sGC, initiating a cleavage of a reduced heme moiety from a histidine residue and bioactivation of the enzyme. Activated sGC converts GTP to the intracellular second messenger cGMP within smooth muscle. Increase in cGMP concentrations results in decrease in intracellular calcium and subsequent smooth muscle relaxation.

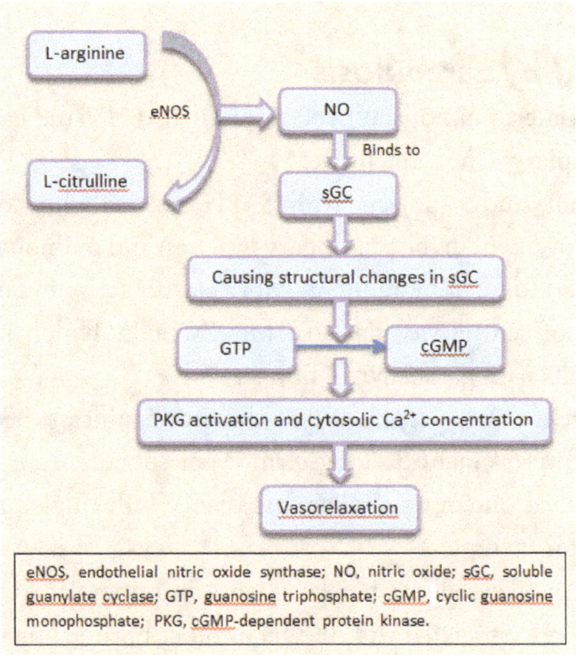

Riociguat acts by not only sensitizing sGC to endogenous nitric oxide (NO), but also directly stimulating sGC independently of NO. With this, production of cyclic guanosine monophosphate increases which leads to vasodilation and accounts for anti-inflammatory, anti-proliferative, and anti-fibrotic effects of riociguat.

Class IV

The first steps after CTEPH diagnosis should always include chronic anticoagulation and consideration of PTE surgery. For patients with CTEPH deemed inoperable due to technically distal (unreachable) disease, or for patients with residual PH following PTE, riociguat is the only approved medical therapy. It should be noted that riociguat (or any other off-label PAH-targeted medical therapy) should not be prescribed for patients with operable CTEPH.

Class V

PH caused by sarcoidosis

Sarcoid-associated pulmonary hypertension (SAPH) studies with PAH-specific therapies are not conclusive.

In a small study, subjects with SAPH treated with corticosteroid showed improvement in the pulmonary function and pulmonary pressure. They are found to be of more use in patients with active inflammation or compression of central vascular structure by bulky lymph nodes rather than in patients with parenchymal fibrosis.

Many patients with severe SAPH showed significant hemodynamic and clinical improvement on long-term IV or subcutaneous PG therapy and had survival outcomes similar to patients with moderate SAPH on oral vasodilator therapy.

Fatal pulmonary edema has been observed after IV PG therapy in patients with PH associated with PVOD or other fibrotic lung diseases.

Bosentan has been approved by the FDA for the treatment of idiopathic PAH and scleroderma-related PAH, however, needs to be studied in SAPH.

Sildenafil has also shown reductions in PVR and mPAP, more investigational studies need to evaluate its role in this category of patients.

PH in chronic hemolytic anemia

Pulmonary hypertension has emerged as a major cause of morbidity and mortality in patients with hemoglobinopathies and chronic hemolytic anemias. These hematological diseases include — but are not limited to — sickle cell disease (SCD), thalassemia, and paroxysmal nocturnal hematuria.

- SCD

Management of SCD includes administration of hydroxyurea, and chronic transfusion is recommended in patients unresponsive to hydroxyurea or are at increased risk for mortality.

Treatment of pulmonary hypertension secondary to venous thromboembolism in SCD is with indefinite anticoagulation therapy.

Studies have shown that the use of Sildenafil and Tadalafil can cause sickle cell crises; however, this being a class effect or a true sickle cell crisis needs to be evaluated. The efficacy of Bosentan in SCD with precapillary pulmonary hypertension and postcapillary pulmonary hypertension could not be evaluated due to sponsorship withdrawal. The use intravenous prostacyclin at cardiac catheterization to test reversibility of pulmonary hypertension, demonstrated acute decrease in PVR. The soluble guanylate cyclase stimulators have not yet been studied in the SCD population. A trial of targeted PAH therapy is only suggested in select patients with precapillary pulmonary hypertension as documented on RHC. In such cases, the trial of an oral endothelin receptor antagonist may be preferred over a phosphodiesterase-5 inhibitor due to better tolerance of side effects.

- Thalassemia

Chronic transfusion therapy and concomitant chelation therapy have been shown to prevent pulmonary hypertension in both forms of thalassemia.

Some small-scaled studies have shown potential benefits of targeted PH therapies in β-thalassemia patients. Sildenafil has been shown to improve NYHA functional class and echocardiographic evidence of pulmonary hypertension and 6-minute walk test

- Paroxysmal nocturnal hematuria (PNH)

Currently, there are no studies of targeted pulmonary hypertension agents used in PH secondary to PNH. However, treatment of PNH has been well established with the use of Eculizumab, an antibody that targets CD5 and inhibits complement-mediated hemolysis which dramatically reduced intravascular hemolysis, the need for transfusion, and symptoms.

PH in CKD

Due to the high prevalence of LV disorders in patients with CKD, most cases of PH in this population are WHO class II. The treatment of PH in patients with CKD has not been investigated; therefore recommendations for the treatment of WHO class II pulmonary hypertension in the general population also can be extended provisionally to patients with CKD. It is essential to treat the underlying LV disorders by optimizing body fluid volume with diuretics, reducing dietary salt intake, and/or appropriate dialysis treatment.

In a randomized trial testing epoprostenol with PH and severe LV dysfunction showed an increase in mortality. Sleep apnea, a frequent complication in patients with NDD-CKD5 and dialysis patients, is a potent trigger of pulmonary hypertension and can be reduced by correcting volume excess by peritoneal dialysis or by intensifying hemodialysis. In patients with pulmonary hypertension and high AVF flow, interventions aimed at reducing AVF flow may be considered when clinically indicated.

Class	Drugs	Dose	ADRs
Prostacyclin pathway agonists	Epoprostenol	Initial: 2 ng/kg/minute IV infusion pump over 24–48 hours Titrate by 1–2 ng/kg/minute q15 minutes or longer, until desired effect or dose-limiting pharmacologic effects occur	Infusion site reaction, headache, nausea, vomiting, diarrhea, vasodilation, jaw pain, rash, body ache, dizziness

(*Continued*)

Class	Drugs	Dose	ADRs
	Treprostinil	Initial: 1.25 ng/kg/minute continuous SC/IV infusion (0.625 ng/kg/minute if not tolerated) Titrate by no more than 1.25 ng/kg/minute qWeek × first 4 weeks, then no more than 2.5 ng/kg/minute qWeek Little experience with doses >40 ng/kg/minute	
	Iloprost	Initial: 2.5 μg inhaled, if well-tolerated, THEN 5 μg subsequent doses 6–9 times/day PRN; >q2 hours while awake Maintenance: 2.5–5 μg/dose; not to exceed 45 μg/day	
	Selexipag	Initial dose: 200 μg PO BID Increase dose by increments of 200 μg BID, usually at weekly intervals, to the highest tolerated dose; not to exceed 1,600 μg BID	

(*Continued*)

(*Continued*)

Class	Drugs	Dose	ADRs
Endothelin receptor antagonists	Bosentan	<40 kg: Maintain dose at 62.5 mg PO q12 hours >40 kg: 62.5 mg PO q12 hours for 4 weeks and then increased to maintenance dosage 125 mg PO q12 hours Discontinuation of treatment: Consider a reduction in dosage to 62.5 mg PO q12 hours for 3–7 days	Anemia, hypersensitivity reactions, headache, palpitations, flushing, hypotension, nasal congestion, abnormal liver function test, GERD, diarrhea, nasopharyngitis, bronchitis
	Macitentan	10 mg PO qDay	
	Ambrisentan	Initiate treatment at 5 mg PO qDay, with or without tadalafil 20 mg PO qDay, not to exceed ambrisentan 10 mg/day or tadalafil 40 mg/day	
PDE5 inhibitors	Sildenafil	PO: 5 mg or 20 mg 3 times daily, administered 4–6 hours apart IV: 2.5 mg or 10 mg bolus 3 times daily if patient is temporarily unable to take PO	Headache, flushing, epistaxis, dyspepsia, insomnia, erythema, diarrhea, dizziness, skin rash, myalgia, RTI, nasopharyngitis, back pain, nausea
	Tadalafil	40 mg PO once daily; dividing dose for more frequent dosing is not recommended	

(*Continued*)

Class	Drugs	Dose	ADRs
Guanylate cyclase stimulant	Riociguat	Initial dose: 1 mg PO TID; consider 0.5 mg PO TID if patient may not tolerate hypotensive effect	Dizziness, headache, dyspepsia, diarrhea, nausea, vomiting, edema peripheral

Reference and suggested readings

1. Correale M, Ferraretti A, Monaco I, Grazioli D, Di Biase M, Brunetti N. Endothelin-receptor antagonists in the management of pulmonary arterial hypertension: where do we stand? Vasc Health Risk Manag [online]. 2018;14:253–264. Available at: https://www.ncbi.nlm.nih.gov/pmc/articles/PMC6174907/ [Accessed 29 Apr 2019].
2. Dupuis J, Hoeper M. Endothelin receptor antagonists in pulmonary arterial hypertension. Eur Respir J. 2008;31(2):407–415.
3. Tonelli A, Haserodt S, Aytekin M, Dweik R. Nitric oxide deficiency in pulmonary hypertension: pathobiology and implications for therapy. Pulm Circ [online]. 2013;3(1):20–30. Available at: https://www.ncbi.nlm.nih.gov/pmc/articles/PMC3641730/ [Accessed 29 Apr 2019].
4. Lasker G, Maley J, Pankey E, Kadowitz P. Targeting soluble guanylate cyclase for the treatment of pulmonary hypertension. Exp Rev Respir Med [online]. 2011;5(2):153–161. Available at: https://www.ncbi.nlm.nih.gov/pmc/articles/PMC3108035/ [Accessed 29 Apr 2019].
5. Bolignano D, Rastelli S. Pulmonary hypertension in CKD [online]. Ajkd.org. 2013. Available at: https://www.ajkd.org/article/S0272-6386(12)01262-0/pdf [Accessed 9 May 2019].
6. Bonham C, Vij R. Prostacyclin and oral vasodilator therapy in sarcoidosis-associated pulmonary hypertension [online]. 2015. Available at: https://www.ncbi.nlm.nih.gov/pmc/articles/PMC4594624/ [Accessed 9 May 2019].
7. Diaz-Guzman E, Farver C. Pulmonary hypertension caused by sarcoidosis [online]. 2008. Available at: https://www.ncbi.nlm.nih.gov/pmc/articles/PMC2593121/ [Accessed 9 May 2019].

8. Kalantari S, Gomberg-Maitand M. Group 5 pulmonary hypertension [online]. 2016. Available at: https://www.ncbi.nlm.nih.gov/pmc/articles/PMC5391979/#R40 [Accessed 9 May 2019].
9. Kingman M, Bartlett M. Management of prostacyclin side effects in adult patients with pulmonary arterial hypertension [online]. 2017. Available at: https://www.ncbi.nlm.nih.gov/pmc/articles/PMC5841898/ [Accessed 9 May 2019].
10. Nick HK. Group 4 pulmonary hypertension: chronic thromboembolic pulmonary hypertension: epidemiology, patthophysiology, and reatment. — PubMed — NCBI [online]. Ncbi.nlm.nih.gov. 2016. Available at: https://www.ncbi.nlm.nih.gov/pubmed/27443139 [Accessed 9 May 2019].
11. Pezzuto B, Ghio S. Circulating biomarkers in pulmonary arterial hypertension: update and future direction [online]. 2015. Available at: https://www.jhltonline.org/article/S1053-2498(14)01500-9/fulltext#s0125 [Accessed 9 May 2019].
12. Preston IR, Klinger JR, Landzberg MJ, Houtchens J, Nelson D, Hill NS. Vasoresponsiveness of sarcoidosis-associated pulmonary hypertension. — PubMed — NCBI [online]. Ncbi.nlm.nih.gov. Available at: https://www.ncbi.nlm.nih.gov/pubmed/11555522 [Accessed 9 May 2019].
13. Ventura H, Silver M. Natriuretic peptides as markers of cardiovascular risk: the story continues [online]. 2011. Available at: https://www.ncbi.nlm.nih.gov/pmc/articles/PMC3228612/ [Accessed 9 May 2019].
14. Hassoun PM. Pulmonary arterial hypertension. N Engl J Med. 2021 Dec 16;385(25):2361–2376. doi: 10.1056/NEJMra2000348. PMID: 34910865.
15. Ruopp NF, Cockrill BA. Diagnosis and treatment of pulmonary arterial hypertension: a review. JAMA. 2022 Apr 12;327(14):1379–1391. doi: 10.1001/jama.2022.4402. Erratum in: JAMA. 2022 Sep 6;328(9):892. PMID: 35412560.
16. Luna-López R, Ruiz Martín A, Escribano Subías P. Pulmonary arterial hypertension. Med Clin (Barc). 2022 Jun 24;158(12):622–629. English, Spanish. doi: 10.1016/j.medcli.2022.01.003. Epub 2022 Mar 9. PMID: 35279313.
17. Sommer N, Ghofrani HA, Pak O, Bonnet S, Provencher S, Sitbon O, Rosenkranz S, Hoeper MM, Kiely DG. Current and future treatments of pulmonary arterial hypertension. Br J Pharmacol. 2021 Jan;178(1):6–30. doi: 10.1111/bph.15016. Epub 2020 Mar 23. PMID: 32034759.
18. Evans CE, Cober ND, Dai Z, Stewart DJ, Zhao YY. Endothelial cells in the pathogenesis of pulmonary arterial hypertension. Eur Respir J. 2021 Sep

2;58(3):2003957. doi: 10.1183/13993003.03957-2020. PMID: 33509961; PMCID: PMC8316496.

19. Gorelova A, Berman M, Al Ghouleh I. Endothelial-to-mesenchymal transition in pulmonary arterial hypertension. Antioxid Redox Signal. 2021 Apr 20;34(12):891–914. doi: 10.1089/ars.2020.8169. PMID: 32746619; PMCID: PMC8035923.
20. Ballard W 3rd, Dixon B, McEvoy CA, Verma AK. Pulmonary arterial hypertension in pregnancy. Cardiol Clin. 2021 Feb;39(1):109–118. doi: 10.1016/j.ccl.2020.09.007. Epub 2020 Oct 29. PMID: 33222807.
21. Lechartier B, Humbert M. Pulmonary arterial hypertension in systemic sclerosis. Presse Med. 2021 Apr;50(1):104062. doi: 10.1016/j.lpm.2021.104062. Epub 2021 Feb 3. PMID: 33548377.
22. Levine DJ. Pulmonary arterial hypertension: updates in epidemiology and evaluation of patients. Am J Manag Care. 2021 Mar;27(3 Suppl):S35–S41. doi: 10.37765/ajmc.2021.88609. PMID: 33710842.
23. Naeije R, Richter MJ, Rubin LJ. The physiological basis of pulmonary arterial hypertension. Eur Respir J. 2022 Jun 16;59(6):2102334. doi: 10.1183/13993003.02334-2021. PMID: 34737219; PMCID: PMC9203839.
24. Ramirez RL 3rd, Pienkos SM, de Jesus Perez V, Zamanian RT. Pulmonary arterial hypertension secondary to drugs and toxins. Clin Chest Med. 2021 Mar;42(1):19–38. doi: 10.1016/j.ccm.2020.11.008. PMID: 33541612.
25. Klinger JR. Novel pharmacological targets for pulmonary arterial hypertension. Compr Physiol. 2021 Sep 23;11(4):2297–2349. doi: 10.1002/cphy.c200015. PMID: 34558669.
26. Constantine A, Dimopoulos K. Pulmonary artery denervation for pulmonary arterial hypertension. Trends Cardiovasc Med. 2021 May;31(4):252–260. doi: 10.1016/j.tcm.2020.04.005. Epub 2020 May 12. PMID: 32413394.
27. Wang A, Valdez-Jasso D. Cellular mechanosignaling in pulmonary arterial hypertension. Biophys Rev. 2021 Sep 2;13(5):747–756. doi: 10.1007/s12551-021-00828-3. PMID: 34765048; PMCID: PMC8555029.
28. Vonk MC, Vandecasteele E, van Dijk AP. Pulmonary hypertension in connective tissue diseases, new evidence and challenges. Eur J Clin Invest. 2021 Apr;51(4):e13453. doi: 10.1111/eci.13453. Epub 2020 Dec 5. PMID: 33216992; PMCID: PMC7988614.

https://doi.org/10.1142/9789811271410_0049

49 Cor pulmonale

Introduction

The term "cor pulmonale," a Latin word, was coined by Paul D. White, MD, in 1931. Cor pulmonale refers to pulmonary heart disease. Cor pulmonale was classically defined as "hypertrophy of the right ventricle resulting from diseases affecting the function and/or structure of the lungs except when these pulmonary alterations are the result of diseases that primarily affect the left side of the heart".[1] Cor pulmonale can be defined as the clinical setting in which the right side of the heart, in particular the right ventricle (RV), is affected by a pressure overload that induces changes of RV function and morphology.[44]

Cor pulmonale results from GROUP 3 PH **Clinical classification of pulmonary hypertension (6th World Symposium on Pulmonary Hypertension)**[15] induced alteration in the anatomical structure and impairment in the functions of the RV. Pulmonary hypertension (PH) is the "sine qua non" of cor pulmonale. An mPAP of 20 mmHg should be considered as the upper limit of normal value.[41] According to the most recent consensus guidelines, PH is defined hemodynamically as a mean pulmonary artery pressure (mPAP) greater than 20 mmHg.[3]

Acute and chronic forms of cor pulmonale are distinguished from each other, depending on the duration of time in which the increased RV afterload is established.

Patients with cor pulmonale generally have poor prognosis and reduced survival.

Anatomy of the right heart

RV is the most anterior chamber in the normal heart residing immediately behind the sternum. The normal RV is a thin-walled structure with approximately one-sixth of the muscle mass of the LV, that is made up of RV-free wall, interventricular septum (IVS) and right ventricular outflow tract (RVOT). The RV muscle fibers are composed of two layers namely, A circumferential superficial layer and a longitudinal deeper layer. The right ventricular wall is thinner; however, it is more compliant than the left ventricle as it works against a significantly lower after load that is pulmonary vascular resistance (PVR).

The RV is in all points opposite to the left ventricle. With its sensitive systolic function[4] and a tolerant diastolic function, the RV acts as a passive crescent chamber promoting venous return from the systemic circulation to the pulmonary one.[5] Without any contractile reserve,[6] the RV has no adaptive mechanism other than its dilatation when its afterload is increased, even a little. Any ventriculo-arterial uncoupling between the RV and the pulmonary circulation leads to RV dilatation, which is responsible for LV compression on one hand and an ischemic vicious circle for itself on the other hand.

Pathophysiology

Under normal circumstances, the RV pumps against a low-resistance circuit. Normal PVR is approximately one-tenth the systemic vascular resistance. As the RV is thin walled, it is able to accommodate considerable changes in volume without significant pressure change. With increased cardiac output, there is the recruitment of under-perfused pulmonary vessels and distension of other pulmonary vessels. With increase in PVR, the pulmonary artery pressure (PAP) raises with increased RV work leading to hypertrophy and or dilatation of RV. When compensation through hypertrophy and dilatation is exhausted, it results in right ventricular failure:

Pathophysiology of chronic cor pulmonale
Chronic respiratory diseases
↓
Chronic hypoxia
↓
Pulmonary vasoconstriction
↓
Increased PVR
↓
Pulmonary hypertension
↓
Increased afterload on RV
↓
RV dilatation and hypertrophy
↓
Chronic cor pulmonale

Common conditions that lead to chronic cor pulmonale:

1. Obstructive lung diseases, chronic obstructive pulmonary disease, most common cause
2. Restrictive lung diseases, interstitial lung disease
3. Chronic thromboembolic disease
4. Sleep-disordered breathing
5. Chest wall diseases, kyphoscoliosis
6. Chronic mountain sickness

Most common cause of chronic cor pulmonale is chronic obstructive pulmonary disease (COPD),[1] The reported prevalence of cor pulmonale in COPD varies considerably from 20% to 91%, with increasing prevalence with greater severity of COPD,[3] followed by idiopathic pulmonary fibrosis (IPF) and chronic thromboembolic pulmonary hypertension (CTEPH) are the second and third most common causes of chronic cor pulmonale.[7] Commonly, these diseases induce a chronic hypoxemia and/or a remodeling of the pulmonary circulation,[8] which forces the RV to adapt in compensation for the increased mechanical work required to pump blood through the lungs.

CTEPH is a serious, progressive, and often fatal disease in which, PH occurs due to pulmonary artery obstruction from unresolved thromboembolic disease.[1,9] CTEPH is a late complication of acute pulmonary embolus and is classified as group 4 PH in WHO classification of PH (i.e., PH due to pulmonary artery obstruction).

Obstructive sleep apnea (OSA), the commonest cause of sleep-disordered breathing causes PH through hypoxia pathway with activation of vasoactive factors and hydrostatic mechanism due to increase in left atrial pressure leading to pulmonary venous hypertension. Both pathways eventually cause vascular remodeling, pulmonary arterial hypertension, and right heart dysfunction.

Some individuals residing at altitudes of 2,500 meters and higher may develop high-altitude pulmonary hypertension (HAPH) which is also influenced by genetic factors.

Clinical features of chronic cor pulmonale are predominantly related to the primary disease process causing cor pulmonale rather than the cor pulmonale itself.

Clinical manifestations of cor pulmonale are similar to those of RHF.

Symptoms

- Shortness of breath on exertion, fatigability, swelling of lower extremities
- Right upper quadrant abdominal pain resulting from passive hepatic congestion
- Syncope
- Hoarseness of voice (caused by compression of the left recurrent laryngeal nerve by dilation of the main pulmonary artery)

Clinical signs of cor pulmonale

- Resting dyspnea
- Tachypnoea
- Dependent peripheral edema
- Raised Jugular venous pressure, reflects raised atrial pressure, a specific sign of right-sided failure. Jugular venous pulsations show accentuated A waves and

  Prominent V wave indicating the presence of tricuspid regurgitation

- Cardiovascular examination shows palpable left parasternal lift/heave, accentuation of p2, pulmonary component of second heart sound sometimes may not be appreciated because of hyperinflation
- Right-sided fourth heart sound
- Murmurs of tricuspid regurgitation (may not be observed in the initial stages)
- P/A tender hepatomegaly

Management

Treatment of underlying disease is the Mainstay of treatment of cor pulmonale.

Treatment is aimed at

- Reversing hypoxemia
- Improving right ventricular contractility
- Decreasing pulmonary artery vascular resistance, and decreasing pulmonary vasoconstriction, thereby reducing PH

Investigations

ECG, Findings may be normal or show right axis deviation, right bundle branch block or RV hypertrophy classic triad of a deep S-wave in lead 1, Q-wave, and an inverted T-wave in lead 3 may be present, demonstrating evidence of RV strain and acute cor pulmonale.

Complete blood count shows increase in RBC count, increased hematocrit (secondary polycythemia resulting from chronic hypoxia)

Arterial blood gas Analysis shows decreased PaO_2 with normal or increased $PaCO_2$

Elevated BNP from RV dilation and/or hypoxia

Connective tissue disorder workup (RA FACTOR, ANA PROFILE) to exclude connective tissue disease-related pulmonary involvement.

Chest X-ray may show enlargement of the pulmonary arteries or right atrium (RA) and right ventricular dilatation or "pruning" of the peripheral vasculature.

HRCT Thorax to know the extent of pulmonary disease.

Transthoracic echocardiography

The mainstay of RV imaging in clinical practice is transthoracic echocardiography (TTE) a non-invasive, easily available most widely used tool for estimation of PAP and evaluating RV structure and function, allows the confirmation of a clinical diagnosis of cor pulmonale, assessment of the degree of PH and evaluation of RV size and systolic dysfunction. The guidelines for TTE examination of the RV recommend both qualitative and quantitative assessments.[8]

RV systolic pressure, typically calculated using the tricuspid regurgitation jet and an estimation of RA pressure based on inferior vena cava (IVC) size and collapsibility, should be reported when a complete TR Doppler velocity envelope is present. Apical four-chamber, RV-focused apical four-chamber and modified apical four-chamber, left parasternal long and short-axis, left parasternal RV inflow, and subcostal views provide the images required for a comprehensive assessment of RV size, systolic and diastolic function, and RV systolic pressures. RV dimensions are best estimated from an RV-focused apical four-chamber view obtained with either lateral or medial transducer orientation.[71]

Estimation of pulmonary artery systolic pressure

Estimation of PAP is an important component of the echocardiographic study, particularly in the evaluation of dyspnea, and in patients with evidence of cardiac pathology. The simplified Bernoulli equation, $\Delta P = 4V^2$, estimates the pressure drop between two chambers (ΔP) based on the peak velocity (V) in the presence of turbulent flow. Thus, the gradient estimated by the peak TR velocity (TRV) measured by continuous wave Doppler is equal to the systolic pressure in the RV (RVSP) minus the systolic pressure in the RA (RAP). RVSP is equivalent to pulmonary artery systolic pressure (PASP) in the absence of an RV outflow gradient (such as with pulmonic stenosis). This equation is rearranged to yield[88]:

$$\text{PASP} \approx \text{RVSP} = 4(\text{peak TRV}^2) + \text{RAP}$$

Significant elevation of right-sided filling pressure is unlikely in the presence of normal RV and RA dimensions, normal IVC size and inspiratory collapse and normal RV-free wall thickness.[42]

Echocardiography is considered the best non-invasive modality to screen for CLD-PH (GROUP 3 PH). However, the ability to determine peak tricuspid regurgitation velocity to estimate the right ventricular systolic pressure is limited in these patients.[38] Alternate echocardiographic measures including RVOT diameter, tricuspid annular plane systolic excursion (TAPSE) and qualitative assessment of right chamber structure and function has been advocated in IPF and COPD.[39,40]

In COPD, the hyperinflated lung fields obscure the standard acoustic windows leading to poor image quality thereby hampering tricuspid regurgitant jet. The sensitivity and specificity of echocardiography to predict the presence of PH range from 0.79 to 1.0 and from 0.6 to 0.98, respectively. In one of the large series of patients with advanced lung disease, a satisfactory PASP could be estimated in only 44% of patients.[10]

Three-dimensional transthoracic echocardiography (3DE)

Recent advancements allow encompassing the entire RV in a single pyramidal dataset and to perform a detailed quantitative analysis of its size, shape, and function.[8]

Cardiac magnetic resonance imaging

Is the most accurate method for the assessment of characteristics of RV including RV mass, RV volume, and systolic function. It has increasingly being used as the standard method for evaluating RV structure and function in patients with PH.

Right heart catheterization is the gold standard for estimation of PAP. It is useful in diagnosis and assessment of PH severity. Right heart catheterization reveals evidence of RV dysfunction.

Comparison between ECHO and MRI In the evaluation of cor pulmonale

Echocardiogram	Magnetic resonance imaging
Widespread availability	Lack of widespread availability
Cheaper	High cost
Shorter image acquisition time	Long image acquisition time
Long-axis view to evaluate the size of the cavity and a short-axis view to evaluate septal kinetics	Can image in any desired imaging plane
Limited by acoustic windows	Not limited by acoustic windows
Can be repeated for serial assessments during follow up	Not ideal for serial assessment

Lifestyle modification

Smoking cessation

Weight loss Sodium and fluid restriction in setting of edema from RV failure. Judicious exercise training, avoiding heavy physical exercise or isometric exercises that may cause syncope, structured rehabilitation and breathing training programs, avoidance of overexertion avoidance of pregnancy, avoidance of high altitudes.

Pharmacological treatment

Pulmonary vasodilators

The phosphodiesterase 5 inhibitor sildenafil is a specific pulmonary vasodilator and increases the effects of I NO through the cGMP pathway. It relaxes human PASMCs by inhibiting PDE 5, thereby activating large conductance calcium-activated potassium channels.[9]

Current consensus guidelines recommend treating the primary lung disease and advise against routine use of PH-targeted drugs in PH-CLD.[1]

Anticoagulation

Novel oral anticoagulants (NOAC) are used in the treatment of CTPH apixaban, dabigatran edoxaban, rivaroxaban, directly inhibit one activated coagulation factor, thromb in for dabigatran and factor Xa for apixaban, edoxaban, and rivaroxaban.

They can be administered at fixed doses without routine laboratory monitoring.

Diuretics are used to decrease the elevated RV filling volume they should be used cautiously as they can cause intravascular volume depletion that may deprive the RV of adequate preload to maintain a normal stroke volume. Moreover, accumulation of bicarbonate from diuretic therapy can worsen alveolar hypoventilation and hypercapnia. The latter can result fluid retention despite diuretic therapy.

Cardiac glycosides Digital is used only in the case of an associated left heart failure or in the case of arrhythmia.

Nonpharmacological therapy

Long-term oxygen therapy to correct hypoxemia

Long-term oxygen therapy (LTOT) refers to oxygen delivered to patients with chronic hypoxemia, in majority of the patients for the remainder of the patient's life. LTOT is usually prescribed for at least 15–18 hours/day.[3] LTOT has shown to improve survival in patients with group 3 PH with cor pulmonale. Long-term administration of oxygen reduces hypoxic vasoconstriction, RV after load, and/or pulmonary vascular remodeling the flow of oxygen is usually determined by a titration process at rest with a target SpO_2 greater than 90% or a PaO_2 of 60–80 mmHg.[11]

In stabilized hypoxemic COPD patients, LTOT for 15 hours/day prevented the progressive increase of mPAP and when used for >18 hours/day produced a slight decrease of mPAP,[43]

It has been observed that adherence to LTOT is suboptimal in many patients due to various reasons. In our practice, we have observed poor economic status and social stigma as main reasons for nonadherence to LTOT Hence, clinician should emphasize on the beneficial effects of LTOT in terms of survival and improved quality of life.

Positive airway pressure (PAP) therapy using Bi-level PAP or continuous PAP is indicated for the treatment of moderate and severe OSA (AHI > 5)

- Surgical intervention
- Lung volume reduction surgery in COPD
- Lung transplantation for end-stage COPD and IPF
- Heart-lung transplantation in end-stage chronic respiratory disease with cor pulmonale
- As the prognosis is poor in these patients, cardiopulmonary rehabilitation should be suggested for all patients with cor pulmonale to improve quality of life

Phlebotomy

Polycythemia increases the viscosity of blood, the resistance to blood flow through the pulmonary circulation and augments hypoxic pulmonary vasoconstriction by causing a local deficiency of nitric oxide (NO)[11] (Deem et al 1998) phlebotomy is indicated in patients with a severe elevation in hematocrit not responding to LTOT, yet its effects may be short lived.

Acute cor pulmonale

In the clinical setting of acute cor pulmonale, there is a rapid increase in right ventricular after load, causing dilatation and/or impairment of RV function acute cor pulmonale occurs due to rapid elevations of the PAPs, especially beyond a mean of 40 mmHg, causing RV failure and decreased cardiac output[12] acute pulmonary embolism is the commonest cause of acute cor pulmonale, where an acute obstruction of 30%–50% of the cross-sectional area of the pulmonary arterial bed, together with hypoxia-induced vasoconstriction, is responsible for the abrupt increase of PVR, which greatly affects RV function, without time for compensation.

Etiology

1. Acute pulmonary embolism
2. ARDS

Pathophysiology

Acute pulmonary embolism is commonest and most life-threatening cause for acute cor pulmonale. Patients with suspected APE should undergo risk stratification as HIGH, INTERMEDIATE and LOW risk category.

Respiratory failure in PE is predominantly a consequence of hemodynamic disturbances.[66] ventilation/perfusion mismatch, and leads to hypoxemia.

In about one-third of patients, right-to-left shunting through a patent foramen ovale can be detected by echocardiography; this is caused by an inverted pressure gradient between the RA and left atrium, and may lead to severe hypoxemia, and an increased risk of paradoxical embolization and stroke.[67]

ARDS

Pulmonary vascular dysfunction is common in acute respiratory distress syndrome secondary to several factors, including hypoxic or mediator-induced pulmonary vasoconstriction (by endothelins, thromboxane A2, or leukotrienes), mechanical compression by interstitial edema, and intravascular obstruction from endothelial swelling or thromboemboli (which are present in 95% of patients with ARDS in postmortem studies.[9,11] The increase in PAP may be ascribed to unadapted positive pressure ventilation, inducing a deleterious competition between the distending pressure of alveoli and the flow into pulmonary capillaries. Though initially acute cor pulmonale was thought to have no direct impact on prognosis of ARDS, recent studies have shown that it is associated with significant increase in resting heart rate, a decrease in systemic blood pressure, and a greater need for hemodynamic support.

Significant improvement of RV function may be achieved in all patients with ACP in severe ARDS who undergo prone-positioning incidence of ACP has decreased with improvement in ventilator management strategies. The incidence has varied between 25% and 50% in various studies.[45,46] Early identification of right heart pressure overload and ACP is crucial in order to reduce mortality.

Clinical features

Symptoms

- Dyspnea may be acute and severe in central PE; in small peripheral PE, it is often mild and may be transient in central PE
- Chest pain may have a typical angina character, possibly reflecting RV ischemia, and requiring differential diagnosis from an acute coronary syndrome or aortic dissection
- Cough Hemoptysis
- Syncope
- Clinical signs
- Tachycardia
- Tachypnoea
- Cyanosis
- Hypotension

Investigations

ECG

Electrocardiographic changes indicative of RV strain — such as inversion of T waves in leads V1–V4, a QR pattern in V1, a S1Q3T3 pattern, and incomplete or complete right bundle branch block are usually found in more severe cases of PE;[83] in milder cases, the only abnormality may be sinus tachycardia, present in 40% of patients. atrial arrhythmia, most frequently atrial fibrillation, may be associated with acute PE.

2D ECHO

According to the latest European Society of Cardiology Guidelines for the diagnosis and management of APE,[3] echocardiography plays a key role in the evaluation of patients presenting with hemodynamic instability and suspicion of APE.[13] It speeds up the diagnostic and therapeutic workup, especially in critical patients.[14] Echocardiographic examination helps in the differential diagnosis of acute dyspnea.

In some patients with suspected acute PE, echocardiography may detect increased RV wall thickness or tricuspid insufficiency jet velocity beyond values compatible with acute RV pressure overload (>3.8 m/s or a tricuspid valve peak systolic gradient >60 mmHg).[160] In these cases, chronic thromboembolic (or other) PH should be included in the differential diagnosis combination of a pulmonary ejection acceleration time (measured in the RV outflow tract) <60 ms with a peak systolic tricuspid valve gradient <60 mmHg ("60/60" sign), or with depressed contractility of the RV-free wall compared to the "echocardiographic" RV apex (McConnell sign), is suggestive of PE.[146]

Decreased TAPSE may also be present in PE patients.[148,149]

Standard indirect echocardiographic signs of acute cor pulmonale due to acute pulmonary embolism Increased RV to LV diameter ratio (RV/LV > 0.7 in PLAX or > 1 in apical four-chamber view)

Reduced TAPSE reduced RVFA

Reduced tricuspid E/A 60/60 sign (TRPG <60 mmHg or TR maximum velocity <3.9 m/s and pulmonary acceleration time <60 ms)

McConnell's sign (hypo-akinesia of the RV mid-free wall with normal motion of the apex)

Left ventricle: Abnormal or paradoxical septal motion D-shape of the LV in PSAX

Right atrium: RA dilatation interatrial septum shift toward the left atrium IVC dilatation (transversal diameter >2.1 cm), with reduced inspiratory collapse

D-dimer

Levels are elevated in plasma in the presence of acute thrombosis because of simultaneous activation of coagulation and fibrinolysis. The negative predictive value of D-dimer testing is high, and a normal D-dimer level renders acute PE or DVT unlikely. On the other hand, the positive predictive value of elevated D-dimer levels is low and D-dimer testing is not useful for confirmation of PE. D-dimer is also more frequently elevated in patients with cancer.[96,97]

Multidetector CTPA is the method of choice for imaging the pulmonary vasculature in patients with suspected PE. It allows adequate visualization of the pulmonary arteries down to the subsegmental level.[112–114] The Prospective Investigation On Pulmonary Embolism Diagnosis (PIOPED) II study observed a sensitivity of 83% and a specificity of 96% for (mainly four-detector) CTPA in PE diagnosis.[115]

Pulmonary angiography, which was earlier the GOLD standard for diagnosis or exclusion of acute PE, is now rarely performed as less-invasive CTPA offers similar diagnostic accuracy.[133]

Routine hematological investigations

- CBC
- ABG
- Renal function tests
- Liver function tests
- PRO BNP
- BNP TROPONIN I
- CHEST XRAY
- Compression ultrasonography
- V/Q scan

Management of acute cor pulmonale

Major goals of this treatment include reduction of the right ventricular afterload, a decrease of the right ventricular pressure, an improvement of the right ventricular contractility, and especially treating the cause of PH.

The goal of treatment of APE is to prevent mortality from the present embolic state and to prevent recurrence of emboli.

Acute cor pulmonale resulting from acute PE is treated with anticoagulation.

Large PE resulting in hemodynamic instability. Is treated with thrombolytics.

Catheter-based thrombectomy or surgical embolectomy are potential salvage therapies in patients with contraindication for anticoagulation or thrombolysis, or whose condition continues to deteriorate despite thrombolytics and anticoagulation.

Management of ARDS

Primary treatment involves treatment of the underlying cause of ARDS.

Acute cor pulmonale seen in cases of ARDS requires supportive treatment with low tidal volume mechanical ventilation.

Positive pressure mechanical ventilation, with lung protective ventilation strategy having low tidal volume and increased positive end expiratory pressure (PEEP). It helps to maintains alveolar ventilation through PAP, prevents premature alveolar collapse by PEEP, changes intrathoracic pressure and lung volume, and affects the RV load.

Intravenous ionotropes like dobutamine are used to support right heart contractility in decompensated right heart failure.

Reference and suggested readings

1. World Health Organization. Chronic cor pulmonale: a report of the expert committee. Circulation. 1963;27:594–598.
2. Rudski LG, Lai WW, Afilalo J, Hua L, Handschumacher MD, Chandrasekaran K, et al. Guidelines for the echocardiographic assessment of the right heart in

adults: a report from the American Society of Echocardiography endorsed by the European Association of Echocardiography, a registered branch of the European Society of Cardiology, and the Canadian Society of Echocardiography. J Am Soc Echocardiogr 2010 Jul;23(7):685–713. doi: 10.1016/j.echo.2010.05.010.

3. Mandoli GE, Sciaccaluga C, Bandera F, Cameli P, Esposito R, D'Andrea A, Evola V, Sorrentino R, Malagoli A, Sisti N, Nistor D. Cor pulmonale: the role of traditional and advanced echocardiography in the acute and chronic settings. Heart Fail Rev. 2021 Mar;26(2):263–275. doi: 10.1016/0002-9149(71)90116-0.
4. Redington AN, Rigby ML, Shinebourne EA, et al. Changes in the pressure-volume relation of the right ventricle when its loading conditions are modified. Br Heart J. 1990;63:45–49. doi: 10.1136/hrt.63.1.45.
5. Guyton AC, Lindsey AW, Abernathy B, et al. Venous return at various right atrial pressures and the normal venous return curve. Am J Physiol. 1957;189:609–615. doi: 10.1152/ajplegacy.1957.189.3.609.
6. Spruijt OA, de Man FS, Groepenhoff H, et al. The effects of exercise on right ventricular contractility and right ventricular-arterial coupling in pulmonary hypertension. Am J Respir Crit Care Med. 2015;191:1050–1057. doi: 10.1164/rccm.201412-2271OC. PubMed: 25710636.
7. Konstantinides S, Meyer G, Becattini C, Bueno H, Geersing GJ, Harjola VP, Huisman M, Humbert M, Jennings CS, Jiménez D, Kucher N. 2019 ESC guidelines for the diagnosis and management of acute pulmonary embolism development Toed in collaboration with the European Respiratory Society (ERS). Eur Heart J. 2020 Jan 21;41(4):543–603. doi: 10.1093/eurheartj/ehz405.
8. Cameli P, Barbagli E, Rottoli P. Exhaled nitric oxide is not increased in pulmonary sarcoidosis. Sarcoidosis Vasc Diffuse Lung Dis. 2016;33(1):39–40. PMID: 27055834.
9. Michelakis ED, Tymchak W, Noga M. Long-term treatment with oral sildenafil is safe and improves functional capacity and hemodynamics in patients with pulmonary arterial hypertension. Circulation. 2003;108:2066–2069. doi: 10.1161/01.CIR.0000099502.17776.C2.
10. Arcasoy SM, Christie JD, Ferrari VA, et al. Echocardiographic assessment of pulmonary hypertension in patients with advanced lung disease. Am J Respir Crit Care Med. 2003;167(5):735–740. doi: 10.1164/rccm.200210-1130OC.

11. Azarov I, Huang KT, Basu S, Gladwin MT, Hogg N, Kim-Shapiro DB. Nitric oxide scavenging by red blood cells as a function of hematocrit and oxygenation. J Biol Chem. 2005 Nov 25;280(47):39024–39032. doi: 10.1074/jbc.M509045200. Epub 2005 Sep 25.
12. Zaidi A, Knight DS, Augustine DX, Harkness A, Oxborough D, Pearce K, Ring L, Robinson S, Stout M, Willis J, Sharma V. Echocardiographic assessment of the right heart in adults: a practical guideline from the British Society of Echocardiography. Echo Res Pract. 2020 Mar 1;7(1):G19–G41. doi: 10.1530/ERP-19-0051.
13. Patel B, Shah M, Garg L, Agarwal M, Martinez M, Dusaj R. Trends in the use of echocardiography in pulmonary embolism. Medicine. 2018 Aug;97(35). doi: 10.1097/MD.0000000000012104.
14. Haddad F, Hunt SA, Rosenthal DN, Murphy DJ. Right ventricular function in cardiovascular disease, part I: anatomy, physiology, aging, and functional assessment of the right ventricle. Circulation. 2008 Mar 18;117(11):1436–1448. doi:10.1161/CIRCULATIONAHA.107.653576.
15. McGoon M, Gutterman D, Steen V, et al. Screening, early detection, and diagnosis of pulmonary arterial hypertension: ACCP evidence-based clinical practice guidelines. Chest. 2004;126(Suppl 1):14S–34S. doi: 10.1378/chest.126.1_suppl.14S.
16. Lacasse Y, Tan AY, Maltais F, Krishnan JA. Home oxygen in chronic obstructive pulmonary disease. Am J Respir Crit Care Med. 2018 May 15;197(10):1254–1264. doi: 10.1164/rccm.201802-0382CI.
17. Burrowes KS, Clark AR, Tawhai MH. Blood flow redistribution and ventilation-perfusion mismatch during embolic pulmonary arterial occlusion. Pulm Circ. 2011 Jul;1(3):365–376. doi: 10.4103/2045-8932.87302.
18. Konstantinides S, Geibel A, Kasper W, Olschewski M, Blümel L, Just H. Patent foramen ovale is an important predictor of adverse outcome in patients with major pulmonary embolism. Circulation. 1998 May 19;97(19):1946–1951. doi: 10.1161/01.CIR.97.19.1946.
19. Simonneau G, Montani D, Celermajer DS, Denton CP, Gatzoulis MA, Krowka M, Williams PG, Souza R. Haemodynamic definitions and updated clinical classification of pulmonary hypertension. Eur Respir J. 2019 Jan 1;53(1):1801913. doi: 10.1183/13993003.01913-2018.

20. Timms RM, Khaja FU, Williams GW. Hemodynamic response to oxygen therapy in chronic obstructive pulmonary disease. Ann. Intern Med. 1985 Jan 1;102(1):29–36. doi: 10.7326/0003-4819-102-1-29.
21. Boissier F, Katsahian S, Razazi K, Thille AW, Roche-Campo F, Leon R, Vivier E, Brochard L, Vieillard-Baron A, Brun-Buisson C, Mekontso Dessap A. Prevalence and prognosis of cor pulmonale during protective ventilation for acute respiratory distress syndrome. Intensive Care Med. 2013 Oct;39(10):1725–1733.
22. Lhéritier G, Legras A, Caille A, Lherm T, Mathonnet A, Frat JP, Courte A, Martin-Lefèvre L, Gouëllo JP, Amiel JB, Garot D. Prevalence and prognostic value of acute cor pulmonale and patent foramen ovale in ventilated patients with early acute respiratory distress syndrome: a multicenter study. Intensive Care Med. 2013 Oct;39(10):1734–1742.
23. Mandoli GE, Sciaccaluga C, Bandera F, Cameli P, Esposito R, D'Andrea A, Evola V, Sorrentino R, Malagoli A, Sisti N, Nistor D, Santoro C, Bargagli E, Mondillo S, Galderisi M, Cameli M. Working Group of Echocardiography of Italian Society of Cardiology (SIC). Cor pulmonale: the role of traditional and advanced echocardiography in the acute and chronic settings. Heart Fail Rev. 2021 Mar;26(2):263–275. doi: 10.1007/s10741-020-10014-4. PMID: 32860180; PMCID: PMC7895796.
24. See KC. Acute cor pulmonale in patients with acute respiratory distress syndrome: a comprehensive review. World J Crit Care Med. 2021 Mar 9;10(2):35–42. doi: 10.5492/wjccm.v10.i2.35. PMID: 33728264; PMCID: PMC7941786.
25. Spagnolo P, Kropski JA, Jones MG, Lee JS, Rossi G, Karampitsakos T, Maher TM, Tzouvelekis A, Ryerson CJ. Idiopathic pulmonary fibrosis: Disease mechanisms and drug development. Pharmacol Ther. 2021 Jun;222:107798. doi: 10.1016/j.pharmthera.2020.107798. Epub 2020 Dec 24. PMID: 33359599; PMCID: PMC8142468.
26. Elrobaa IH, New KJ. COVID-19: pulmonary and extra pulmonary manifestations. Front Public Health. 2021 Sep 28;9:711616. doi: 10.3389/fpubh.2021.711616. PMID: 34650947; PMCID: PMC8505777.

https://doi.org/10.1142/9789811271410_0050

50 Lymphangio leiomyomatosis (LAM)

Introduction

Lymphangio leiomyomatosis (LAM) is a rare pulmonary idiopathic, diffuse, progressive interstitial lung disorder, primarily affecting the women of reproductive age-group, and is characterized by an abnormal nonneoplastic proliferation of smooth-muscle-like cells called LAM cells involving the small airways, pulmonary microvasculature, and lymphatic structures leading to airways obstruction, pulmonary hemorrhages, chylous pleural effusion, and pneumothorax. Hormonal factors are suspected to play a role since the disorder primarily occurs in premenopausal young women of childbearing age. Its prevalence in the United Kingdom, France, and the United States is one per million, Asian prevalence is lower; 0.24 and 0.03 per 100,000 are revolved in Singapore and Korea, respectively.

Clinical presentation

Clinically patient presents with progressive dyspnea.[1] Recurrent, bilateral spontaneous pneumothorax can be seen in 50% of cases.[2] Those with lymphatic disruption may present with chylothorax. Often, there is an associated wasting. Hemoptysis may occur in a few. Clinical signs are not pathognomonic. There can be features of hyperinflation, pleural effusion, or pneumothorax. Chest X-ray may reveal prominent cystic changes in addition to reticulonodular markings. Clubbing is absent. Hamartomatous tumors are composed of smooth muscle, blood vessels, and adipose tissue as well as intraabdominal or pelvic masses.[3] So, extrapulmonary features include lymph node masses, chylous ascites uterine fibroids, and renal angiomyolipomas.

Pathogenesis

It is a hormone-dependent disease, featuring smooth-muscle-like cell proliferation, occurring exclusively in women, worsened by pregnancy perhaps. Lung functions slowly worsen after menopause. A marker for LAM cells is positioned on chromosome 12q 13–15.[4] Estrogens are found to accelerate the growth of the lesion. High mitotic and low apoptotic activities are seen in LAM cells with features of specific estrogen receptors.[5] Gp 100 m RNA in the lungs of LAM patients has been demonstrated by cellular and molecular studies. Gp 100 immunoreactivity in small electron-dense granules having fine lamellar structure has been seen under an electron microscope.

Pathology

Pathologically, the entire pulmonary interstitium is involved by LAM and is characterized by abnormal proliferation of atypical smooth muscle cells in the peribronchial, perilymphatic, and perivascular areas which over period of time can grow to obstruct the airways with aggregates of lymphoid cells, terminal airspaces may show diffuse cystic dilatation, the cystic walls showing lining of smooth muscle.[6] Cystic changes form the hallmark of the disease. These smooth muscle cells — LAM cells — are heterogeneous in nature. Collagen deposits are present between the muscle cells; fibrosis is, however, not seen. LAM cells may penetrate the vessel wall, secondary to which microscopic hemorrhage is common. Peribronchiolar proliferating tissue may circumstantially narrow the bronchioles. Occlusion of venules may result in pulmonary venous hypertension and hemoptysis. Chylous pleural effusion may result from the obstruction of lymphatic channels.

Diagnosis

Features of emphysema, recurrent pneumothorax, and a chylous effusion in a young woman should arouse the suspicion of LAM. Cystic nature of the disease can be demonstrated by HRCT,[7] in the form of diffuse, small thin-walled cysts and ground glass appearance. Chest X-ray may be variable,[1] depending on the presence of pneumothorax or pleural effusion, exhibiting hyperinflation with cystic dilation of airspaces. Unlike other interstitial lung diseases, lungs are hyperinflated in LAM rather than small. It is the course reticulonodular shadows that appear because of compression smooth muscle rich interstitial tissue by dilated cystic airspaces. Lymphatic obstruction may produce Keriey B septal lines on the chest X-ray. Pulmonary function tests reveal increased total lung capacity with increased residual volume, expressing an increased gas trapping. FEV and FVC *are* deceased. So, obstructive and combined obstructive–restrictive ventilatory defects with impaired gas transfer are commonly seen in patients with LAM. Pleural fluid analysis reveals the presence of chyle (giving milky appearance), having raised triglyceride levels more than 100 mg/dL and the presence of chylomicrons. Open lung or transbronchial biopsy provides sufficient characteristic histologic picture HBM 45 staining (monoclonal antibody which in the lung stains only LAM cells) which further helps in diagnosing LAM. HRCT of the thorax reveals

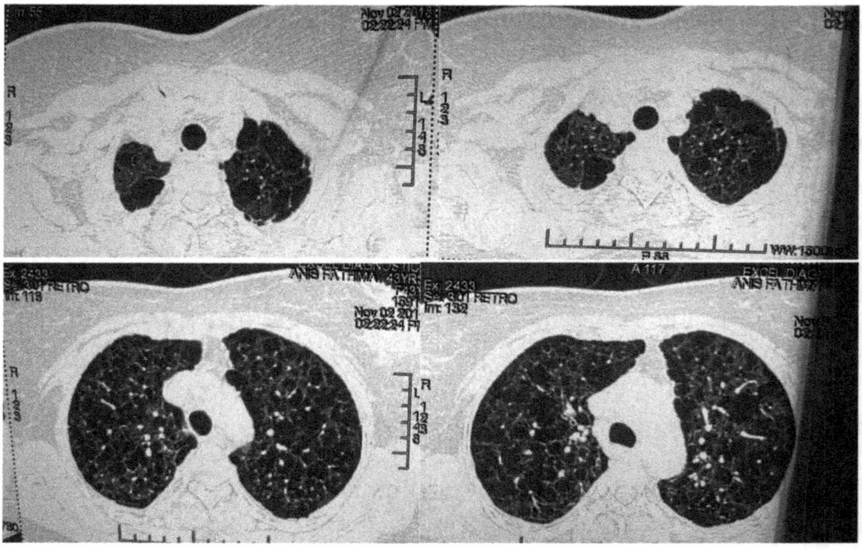

Figure 1: A 35-year-old woman with biopsy-proven lymphangio leiomyomatosis presented with respiratory failure.

thin-walled cysts of 2 mm to an almost imperceptible thickness size distributed through the lung fields with normal lung parenchyma in between. The cysts are differentiated from honeycombs due to interstitial lung disease by their diffuse distribution (sub-pleural distribution in ILDs) and the presence of normal lung parenchyma in between.

Differential diagnosis

These cysts can be differentiated from honeycombing due to ILDs by their diffuse distribution (sub-pleural location in ILDS) and the presence of relatively normal intervening parenchyma. LAM is one of the chronic interstitial lung diseases that needs to be differentiated from eosinophilic granuloma. Eosinophilic granuloma exhibits the features of multiple, thin-walled cysts in the upper and middle lobes of the lung. Stellate pattern of fibrosis with the presence of Langerhans histocytes can be demonstrated on histologic studies. Pulmonary involvement in tuberous sclerosis poses another difficult differential diagnosis. It is a congenital hamartoma of autosomal dominant inheritance,[8] commonly found in middle-aged females. Chylothorax is very rare. Idiopathic pulmonary fibrosis can be differentiated from LAM by its predilection for peripheral lung fields, with non-uniformly distributed cysts. Both leiomyoma and LAM affect females in their reproductive age and exhibit muscle-like cellular proliferation, perhaps both do share genetic origin.[9] Cystic changes with preserved lung volume *can* be seen in Langerhans cell histiocytosis, sarcoidosis, and extrinsic allergic alveolitis. In sarcoidosis, HRCT findings e linear or finely nodular interstitial shadow, ground glass opacification and segmental air space disease.

Treatment: No satisfactory treatment for LAM is available; hormonal manipulation and ovarian ablation have been tried. Oophorectomy and progesterone therapy may yield stabilization. Response is better to progesterone therapy in those having impaired lung functions. Beneficial response has been obtained with oxifen 20 mg/day[10] and analogs of luteinizing hormone-releasing hormone (LHRH). Pleurodesis has been noted for recurrent pneumothorax or pleural effusion.[11] Chylous pleural effusion should not be drained as it; to loss of proteins.

Progression of disease, as indicated by TLC > 130%, FEV, /FVC < 50%, FEW < 30%, and severe cystic disease, can consider the candidate fit for lung transplantation." However, recurrence of the disease in transplanted lung requires to continue hormonal therapy.

Prognosis

Prognosis is variable, since the rate of progression of LAM is variable. Pregnancy and the use of estrogen preparations precipitate and accelerate the disease process. Remission of disease may follow menopause. Severe cystic disease on biopsy, indicated by increased TLC and decreased FEV_1/FVC ratio, predicts poor prognosis. Respiratory failure and death express the ultimate of this slowly progressive disorder that appeared in 1937 in the literature; the etiology is still eluding us.

References and suggested readings

1. Singh A, Singh J. Sudden onset of dyspnoea in a women with skin lesions & lung cysts. Lung India. 2013;20:164–165.
2. Shankar PS. Lymphangio leiomyomatosis. Med Update. 2000;8(2):25–26.
3. Torres EU, et al. Extrapulmonary LAM and lymphangiomatous cysts in tuberous sclerosis complex. Mayo Clin Pract. 1995;70:641–648.
4. NHLBI workshop summary: report on Lymphangio-leimomatosis. Am J Respir Crit Care Med. 1999;159:679–683.
5. Usuki J, et al. Inverse correlation between markers of cell proliferation and expression of melanosomal antigens in smooth muscle melanoma cell lines (Abstract). Am J Respir Crit Care Med. 1998;157:A806.
6. Kitaichi M, et al. Pulmonary lymphangio leiomyomatosis: a report of 46 patients including a clinic opathologic study of prognostic factors. Am J Respir Crit Care Med. 1995;151:527–533.
7. Johnson SR, Tattersfields AE. Clinical experience of LAM in the UK. Thorax. 2000;55:1052–1057.
8. Castro M, et al. Pulmonary tuberous sclerosis. Chest. 1995;107:189–195.

9. Mitra S, Ghosal AG, Bhattacharya P. Pregnancy unmasking LAM. JAPI. 2004;52:828–830.
10. Verma SK, Verma SK. Pulmonary lymphangio leiomyomatosis. Lung India. 2007;24:150–152.
11. McCormack FX, et al. LAM and leiomyoma: possibility of shared genetic origins? IN: J Moss, ed. LAM and other diseases characterized by smooth muscle proliferation. New Delhi: Marcel Dekkar. 1998;373–386.
12. Trulock EP. Lung transplantation: special consideration and outcome in LAM. IN: J Moss, ed. LAM and other diseases characterized by smooth muscle proliferation. New York: Marcel Dekkar. 1998;65–78.
13. Krymskaya VP, McCormack FX. Lymphangioleiomyomatosis: a monogenic model of malignancy. Annu Rev Med. 2017 Jan 14;68:69–83. doi: 10.1146/annurev-med-050715-104245. PMID: 28099079; PMCID: PMC5663315.
14. Steagall WK, Pacheco-Rodriguez G, Darling TN, Torre O, Harari S, Moss J. The Lymphangioleiomyomatosis lung cell and its human cell models. Am J Respir Cell Mol Biol. 2018 Jun;58(6):678–683. doi: 10.1165/rcmb.2017-0403TR. PMID: 29406787; PMCID: PMC6002654.
15. Xu KF, Tian X, Ryu JH. Recent advances in the management of lymphangioleiomyomatosis. F1000Res. 2018 Jun 18;7:F1000 Faculty Rev-758. doi: 10.12688/f1000research.14564.1. PMID: 29946430; PMCID: PMC6008846.
16. Evans JF, Obraztsova K, Lin SM, Krymskaya VP. CrossTORC and WNTegration in disease: focus on lymphangioleiomyomatosis. Int J Mol Sci. 2021 Feb 24;22(5):2233. doi: 10.3390/ijms22052233. PMID: 33668092; PMCID: PMC7956553.
17. Wang X, Su F, Zhou F, Feng M. Sporadic lymphangioleiomyomatosis with multiple atypical features: a case report and literature review. Indian J Pathol Microbiol. 2018 Jan–Mar;61(1):94–97. doi: 10.4103/IJPM.IJPM_843_16. PMID: 29567892.
18. Stacker SA, Achen MG. Emerging roles for VEGF-D in human disease. Biomolecules. 2018 Jan 4;8(1):1. doi: 10.3390/biom8010001. PMID: 29300337; PMCID: PMC5871970.

https://doi.org/10.1142/9789811271410_0051

51 Rising respiratory problems: Suggested preventive measures

Introduction

Prevalence of respiratory problems has greatly increased in the past two decades. The escalation may be due to more awareness and health orientation or availability of new diagnostic facilities and specialist services in pulmonary sciences clubbed with critical care management, but there has been significant rise, especially in the nontubercular pulmonary disorders. Apart from the usual causes such as infections, tobacco-related, dietary, and constitutional factors which have been considered important etiological culprits, air pollution creating environmental issues has been attributed to be most significantly contributing to many disorders of the chest. In addition to occupational or ambient exposure to chemicals and industrial pollutants, including automobile pollutants, in recent years, AIDS-related, tobacco-induced, drug-induced iatrogenic, and traumatic pulmonary disorders have also been increasingly seen.

Respiratory diseases were earlier diagnosed in medical OPD with the help of stethoscope, assisted with routine blood tests, chest X-ray, and sputum analysis. Chest medicine in this country was considered virtually synonymous with tuberculosis. The development and growth of pulmonology in recent years into important medical subspeciality has brought forth a battalion of investigations such as bronchoscopy and BAL analysis, spectroscopy, blood gas analysis, pulmonary scintiphotography, interventional radiology, HRCT, MRI, and pleural and lung biopsy. The actual rise in respiratory disease is, therefore, partly attributed to the advancement in diagnostic facilities, availability of specialized services, and increased awareness among the physicians about the existence of certain pulmonary disorders.

Environmental pollution[1–7]

A significant part has been played by environmental pollutants in the present rise in respiratory disorders. Industrial or domestic burning of fuel and automobile exhaust pollutes the atmosphere with air pollutants such So No SPM, CO, and PO (polycyclic organic matter). Excessive and inefficient burning of fuel is leading to global warming and the greenhouse effect as reflected excess of CO_2 reduced stratospheric O_3 and increased fluctuations in climate. In addition, ladies are exposed to large scale of air pollution, in the ill-ventilated kitchens, produced from burning of poor quality of coal, wood, cow dung, and kerosene during the domestic cooking.

The hazardous occupational exposure to various pollutants in coal mine, rock crushers, silica asbestos, and cloth-making industries is responsible for acute and chronic lung disorders. More than 2,000–2,400 metric tons of air pollutants are liberated into the atmosphere in a busy city, where the automobile share is nearly 60%, industrial contribution is 30%–35%, and domestic share is 5%–10%. The synergism between these environmental pollution and undernutrition, smoking, and dusty occupation is known to contribute to a rise in respiratory diseases, aggravated by exhaustive frequent local travel through a dusty automobile exhaust-vitiated atmosphere. The United Kingdom has vowed to cut down atmosphere CO_2 by 50% in the coming decade. Kyoto treaty has not targeted sufficiently to address the problem. Wind and wave power will *be* used to achieve the target; California, USA, joins the same issue and plans to take steps for green land effect. Indian Health Interests may hopefully get a stimulus.

Diesel exhaust alters airways fluid polymorphs and delays the clearance of soot particles and lung collagen. SO_2 and NO_2 decrease the resistance to bacterial and viral infections, thereby increasing the severity and duration of the illness. In addition, SO_2 increases airway hyperreactivity, leading to airway obstruction, increased susceptibility to lung infections, and precipitation of acute asthmatic attacks. NO, possibly, causes long-term effects such as interstitial alveolitis, and high levels of SPM inhalation leads to hemorrhagic pneumonitis in animals and frequent colds and chronic productive cough in man. PAH, POM, benzene, and aldehyde absorption is increased if SPM levels are increased in the inhaling air, which in turn enhances carcinogenicity. Lung cancer is 1.5 times more with diesel fumes exposure, since the size of particles expelled after combustion is less than 1 μm in 90% of cases and causes damage in the form of epithelial metaplasia, bronchial plaques, and carcinogenesis through its toxic irritants and carcinogenic substances, CO_2, in the atmosphere is 25% more than it used to be a century ago. CO_2, level of 208 PPM in 199 to 306 PMM in 1997 is expected to reach 660 PPM in 2025 AD. If the rise in global temperature — the greenhouse effect — exceed by 10% more, it shall have deteriorating effect on the population. Power cut and the use of industrial and home generators for life comfort the release of gas used for refrigerators and air conditioners and agony to it.

Oxidants such as ozone (O_3), aldehydes, and NO induce respiratory inflammation and epithelial injury. Chronic ozone exposure leads to obstruction in small airway near centriacinar junction. Further, indoor pollution is equally responsible for sick building syndrome. Fashion of indoor games, overuse of computers, video and CD playing facilities, switch over to indoor sleeping pattern, artificial cooling facilities such as cooler and air conditioners and spending of majority of their lives indoors (the ladies), more so with the ill-ventilated kitchens have produced more of respiratory illness especially in children and ladies, as is evident from the rise in the symptoms of postnasal drip and bronchial asthma by 5%, cough in 10% chronic bronchitis in 20%–30% and dyspnea in 50% of patients. Periodic attacks of rhinosinusitis, nasobronchial allergy, and wheezing chests are commonly seen in practice where air pollution caused by thresher's use to procure grains is a precipitating factor. In younger age group, acute respiratory tract infections have shown a rising trend possibly because of indoor pollution and passive smoking, aggravated further by Vit A deficiency, low-birth-weight babies (lack of pre- and postnasal care), malnutrition (lack of health education), and improper breastfeeding (urbanizing fashion effect). A person normally inhales 10,000 L of air/day and is likely to get in contact with various irritants, allergens, and infectants. His or her right to inhale fresh air should not be vesicated by man-created pollutants. All MS study in recent past clearly reveals that an increase by 39% of acute asthma cases, 38% of other respiratory diseases ailments have increased by our times, over a period of 2 years. Delhi government has decided to run CNG buses and phasing out all diesel vehicles gradually. Also, pollution-free vehicle certificates are made mandatory.

Nearly 40,000 people die due to air pollution in America. In India, no such data are available. But, cities such as Mumbai, Kolkata, Ahmedabad, Kanpur, Nagpur, and Delhi have been facing this problem of rising air pollution, Delhi being the dirtiest. Thanks to the Delhi government for measures against automobile exhaust pollution by shifting to CNG and ordering the phased removal of diesel vehicles older than 10–15 years. Ludhiana had been declared polluted, having 893 microgram/m^3 of SPM by a report from Punjab Pollution Control Board, Patiala. Late CM immediately ordered for cutting down industrial pollution, asking for submitting a compulsory plan of prevention of water and air pollution through industrial wastes. Alas, only 626 industries could adopt accepted modes. More than 1,200 industries are still water polluting, and more than 2,200 industries are air polluting. Nearly 300 industries have been issued notices to comply with the orders, which would otherwise face closure. Political will, people's support, and professional participation are essential for success of environmental health scheme. Only recently, Deputy Commissioner, Ludhiana, has ordered to start CNG buses of public transport numbering 100, *each* bus shall be able to phase out 40–50 three-wheelers. Although 6,000 three-wheelers are permitted in the city, 25,000 are running on the roads, adding to air pollution. "Chetna Lehar" has been started to inform school children about such polluting vehicles. Whether this proves fruitful, only time will tell.

Infections

Community-acquired pneumonia has *been* one of the most common respiratory infections worldwide, one of the leading causes of hospitalization, and *one* of the most common causes of premature death. Though microbiological diagnosis is lacking in more than 50% of cases, *Streptococcus pneumoniae*, followed by other organisms such as *Mycoplasma pneumoniae*, influenza A, and haemo haemophilus influenzae, influenzae are commonly found as culprits. Less commonly implicated organisms are *Legionella pneumophila*, *Staphylococcus aureus*, and *Chlamydia psittaci*. The trend is ever rising with changing sensitivity to antimicrobials at times, requiring intensive care as chances of mortality are three to six times more, treating win a single antibiotic that must cover *S. pneumonae* till reports are awaited. Bacterial infections are responsible for acute exacerbation in 40% of cases in chronic obstructive pulmonary disease (COPD), while viral infections contribute in 30% of cases.

HIV disease'

AIDS is the great waster upon the community. The infection is dreaded, the complications are horrible, and chest infections including tuberculosis are increasingly seen in these patents. The risk of TB in HIV infection increases by 100 times in endemic areas with old infected foci due to depressed cell-mediated immunity. The most common complication in all stages of immunosuppression of HIV disease, TB is found in 70%–80% of HIV-positive cases in South Africa. In this giant pander: since 1990, the Tambaram TB sanatorium has seen 38,941 new TB cases in 1992 that grew to 1 03.635 in 2001. In a recent US report, China has been listed as a major Asian country to suffer from HIV infection due to lack of Government's commitment, improper health care and unsatisfactory preventive measure, and insufficient local resources. In North India, Punjab has been listed as leading in harboring HIV diseases, followed by Haryana and Himachal Pradesh, and thus, an alarming situation of an uprise in HIV-related opportunistic respiratory infections should send tremor signals in the health management circles.

At the term of the century, newer opportunistic infections affecting the respiratory system have also emerged, such as Rhococcusequiphernia and chlamydial pneumonia in patients with HIV disease. The end of the century has also seen zoonotic infections such as human ehrlichiosis, rodent-borne Hantavirus, and infection from nasal discharge of sick horses causing acute equine respiratory syndrome. Immunosuppressive therapy has produced complications that lead to rise in infections such as bacterial pneumonia, cytomegalovirus pneumonia, and other viral infections such as herpes simplex infection and respiratory syncytial virus infection. Candida and aspergillus fungal infections have risen in these patents, so is the increased susceptibility and occurrence of *Pneumocystis carinii* infection.

Drugs

There had been 100,000 deaths in the United States in 1988 only due to medical mistakes. Indiscriminate use of corticosteroids has led to precipitation or aggravation of various infections including respiratory infections.

Activation of pulmonary tuberculosis has been found in 6.5% of cases with the use of corticosteroids. Unsupervised usage of corticosteroids given for certain pulmonary disorders, many a times, complicates other respiratory infectious disease, thus acting as double-edged sword. This may partly be attributed to illiteracy or ignorance of the patients, that they do not report to the attending physicians and continue taking the drug for their relief, forgetting that self-medication is dangerous and may ultimately land into complication. Let us do our part of duty as physicians and use these drugs judiciously and for a required period with an educative advice to patients to come for follow-up and gradually taper off, thus working within the latest level of management.

Other drugs that may cause pulmonary disorders include antibiotic drugs, antimalarials, tranquilizers and sedatives, antiarrhythmics, antihypertensives, analgesics, anti-inflammatory drugs, etc. Recently, a rising trend of increased cough and precipitation of asthmatic bronchitis has been observed with ACE inhibitors. Reports of beta-blocker effect and aspirin-induced bronchospasm are documented. Pulmonary disorders due to cytotoxic drugs which are being used extensively in chemotherapy have also been increasingly observed in these patients being treated for a variety of malignancies.

Cases with precipitation of acute bronchial asthma with aerosol therapy have been noted where accompanying gas been found to be the culprit. Knowledge about the same shall help in an immediate stopping of using the inhaler. Penicillin and its derivative are also notorious in giving rise to such kind of drug-induced bronchial disorder. Increased use of methotrexate in various malignant and connective tissue disorders as well as in resistant bronchial asthma has been documented for an alveolar and interstitial reaction in the lungs. Same is also seen when bleomycin and busulfan are used. Increased pulmonary vascular disorders are observed due to the use of antiarrhythmic drugs in cardiology and phenytoin and carbamazepine in neurology. NFT also produces similar effects. Aspirin has been the culprit because of its significant use in routine and especially in cardiology in producing pulmonary hemorrhage that has also been observed by use of pills by females (for contraception). A lot of these cases go unnoticed, and many more remain undocumented.

Drug-induced SLE involving pleura and causing pleural fibrosis have been documented in recent years by use of protocol, methysergide, bromocriptine and ergotamine. The iatrogenic morbidity and mortality showing aall during March and April in 2000 in Israel during doctors strike should not surprise. Mediastinal pseudo lymphadenopathy has recently been recorded with the use of phenytoin and even with methotrexate. Documentation of cases of drug-induced eosinophilic lung disease has been tremendous, attributed to drugs like sulfonamides, penicillin, NFT, thiazide, and tricyclic antidepressants. Enhanced use of narcotics and opium derivatives in rural areas has led to wheezing chests, especially in adults.

Other factors

The rising trend of respiratory disorders has also been attributed to decreased body resistance to fight against infections due to undernutrition and improper dietary pattern, lack of regular exercise and changed lifestyle, and exposure to unnecessary auto-exhaust and tobacco smoke (passive effect) in cities and exposure to toxic agro-insecticides in rural areas. Even resistant bacterial chest infections have emerged, possibly because of the improper use of antimicrobials for inappropriate period, in an inadequate dose. Rise in asthma cases has been observed in these years, and a rising prevalence from 1.2% to 6.2% in adults has been recorded. An Indian data show a significant increase from 0.6% to 3.4%. Incidence of chronic bronchitis in smoking-related cases has been around 42%. Air pollution-related chronic bronchitis has risen by 2–25 times in reports from different areas, depending upon the environmental pollution. Similarly, high prevalence of cough and dyspnea patients in 13% of nonsmokers has been found in Mumbai, being attributed to the increasing industrial pollution.

Pulmonary edema due to chemicals, vegetables, drugs, or fragrance spray, humidifier lung disease due to improperly cleaned coolers, and malignant chest disorders in arsenic and nickel polish industrial workers have been observed. Various allergic inflammatory, interstitial, infective, malignant, and obstructive small airways occupational diseases are showing a rising trend. A clinical profile of chronic airflow limitation in patients attending a tertiary care center reveals that two-thirds of cases of chronic airflow limitation in a tertiary care center in India have bronchial asthma, more than 15% have COPD, less than 15% have obliterative bronchiolitis (OB), more than 5% have bronchiectasis, and more than 1% have occupational airway disease. COPD patients are tobacco inhalers, almost 85% smoke biddies, more than 90% of OB cases are postinfections, almost 80% are post tuberculosis an Indian study compared to otherwise infections and collagen disorders in India and posttransplant OB in the west fever airflow limitation is seen in more than one third of cases of COPD, almost one third of cases of bronchiectasis, more than on fifth of cases of asthma and more than half the number of cases of OB.

Almost 15% of cases of COPD, OB, and bronchiectasis develop pulmonary hypertension, while pulmonary hypertension is missing in asthma patients although two-thirds of cases of asthma have CAL, one-fifth having severe CAL. Tobacco is the common cause of CAL in COPD, while respiratory infections form an important cause of OB, where past TB–OB is commonest in almost 80% of cases.

Our own experience here in Ludhiana has found a rising trend of two-and-half times in allergic, infective, inflammatory, and airflow obstructive disorders. Even tuberculosis has a high prevalence in migrant laborers. The number of tuberculosis patients has risen from one case per month to one to four cases per week in an OPD clinic. So is the rise in MDR–TB, mostly secondary type of drug resistance. Risk of getting tuberculosis has increased from 3% in 1986 to more than 50% in 1996 and is alarmingly increasing.

Technology[8,9]

Improved diagnostic facilities have improved the diagnostic yield of non-tubercular respiratory diseases such as sarcoidosis, lung in connective tissue disorders, pulmonary metastasis, neoplastic lung disorders, and airflow obstructive pulmonary disorders. Newer diagnosis of lymphomas, malignant neurogenic tumors, and malignant thymomas of the mediastinum have been documented because of better techniques, and hence better therapeutic modalities are planned. Advancement of technology in the form of HRCT helps in determining the characteristic abnormality in fibrotic, granulomatous, and cystic lung disease and tumor and also in determining the activity of disease and optimal site for biopsy. A rising trend of 4.2–31 cases/10,000 patients admitted in a chest ward and an increase of 414 cases/annum to 658 cases/annum in just 5 years owes much to better diagnostic techniques and to some extent to a rising trend of the disease due to certain etiological factors such as smoking, air pollution, etc. Since primary lung cancer in early 60s was rare or very infrequent, a rising trend of bronchogenic carcinoma by 910 folds in average smokers and more than 20 folds in heavy smokers narrates the story by itself.

In case of sarcoidosis, which used to be a rare disease in India, 40 cases in even years in 1987, increased through diagnostic facilities by one to two cases per week at PGI, Chandigarh explains of better diagnostic facilities.

Bronchoscopy and transbronchial biopsy have shown a rise in bronchogenic carcinoma from two to three cases per month to one case per week. Increased documentation of aspergillosis through antibodies and HRCT speaks of enhanced disease awareness and improved diagnostic technology. Incidence of pickup of interstitial lung disease has increased due to easy availability of autoantibody profiles. An uncommon sarcoidosis a decade back is being diagnosed one to two cases per month with the use of transbronchial biopsy. The awareness of disease like sleep apnea has pressed for opening of sleep laboratory.

Trauma

Chest problems following chest trauma due to peronalshufie, accident, automobile collision injuries, terrorist's blasts, and police's counter-crime action injuries have *been* risingly seen during these years. The thrill in speed adds to grievous chest injuries many a times, both blunt and penetrating, requiring skilled cardiothoracic management along with the interaction of surgeons, pulmonologists, anesthetists, intensive care physicians, and physiotherapists.

In developed countries in the three Cs pattern, mortality from car accidents leads ahead coronary heart disease and cancers, as compared to developing nations, where cancers and car accidents are trying to take the side. In recent years, there is an increase in chest injuries by 25% causing pneumothorax, hemothorax, and injury to great vessels further aggravated by 10%–20% due to chest complications arising out of associated poly fracture and spinal injuries requiring early surgical intervention and ventilatory support. The potential risk of fat embolism and thromboembolism that proves fatal adds risk of 10% in mortality due to acute respiratory distress syndrome. Iatrogenic complications have also been increasingly seen due to the increased use of chest tubes being inserted in small nursing homes unlike earlier days when the insertion of intercostal chest tube was considered only the domain of hospital. Similarly, more and more number of cases of mediastinitis have been documented due to injuries and instrumental by inexperienced endoscopists. At least 10% of patients on ventilator suffer from ventilator-associated pneumonia. A rising trend in nosocomial pneumonia has been observed in the past few years.

Prevention

a) Steps for prevention of air pollution

Since none of classical pollutants with exception of particular has yet been found in influencing mortality, the strong evidence of relationship between the level of ine particulars and cardiopulmonary illnesses exists, research and prevention is directed toward its mechanism.

Catalytic converters should be used in new cars (Euro II and III models). Benzene contents to be brought down from 3% to 5% to less than 10% and sulfur content of diesel to be brought down from 0.25% to less than 0.1%

Use of four-stroke engines.

Regular check for air pollution of old vehicles, and vehicles older than 10–15 years to be phased out (government action is evident from the number of vehicles, i.e., 30–40 per month has increased to 70–90 per day for air pollution vehicles).

Legislative force to achieve goals for improved air quality.

Better traffic management through avoidance of congestion at peak hours by diversion of traffic and building of new flyovers (bridges); Delhi has taken the lead, and Ludhiana, my city, is gearing up.

Education for ventilated kitchens, safe fuel utilization, promoting outdoor games, avoiding overplaying on video games in closed, congested rooms.

Avoiding the use of toxic agro-insecticides and covered use of grain threshers.

b) Antitobacco steps

Abstinence from tobacco saves 100% from lung cancer and prevents 15%–20% of exacerbation in COPD. A separate scheme plan for tobacco-free atmosphere should be entrusted with responsibility, answerable to accountability.

Public education and implementation of the court's order for prohibition should be result-oriented and time-bound.

Government participation to mobilize other sources of more income and not from tobacco and tobacco products at the cost of public health.

The right to inhale clear air for nonsmokers should not be snatched. Supreme Court's order on tobacco ban at public places should be strictly implemented.

c) For occupational disorders

Government-suggested guidelines and safety measures to be strictly followed, all related legalities to be implemented with strict vigilance and application to prevent occupational respiratory disorders.

Regular inspection of working places, especially in silica, talc, coal, and asbestos industries; regular medical checkup of the workers; shifting of workers' place, duty hours, and even job; shifting to some other department on suspecting minimal signs of developing disease of the respiratory system. Improvement of general health through dietary supplements and educating against smoking.

Radiation-induced chest disorders can be reduced by following the guidelines strictly.

d) Infections

Timely suspecting and instituting proper antibiotic can have 10%–20% of cases of nosocomial pneumonia. Early diagnosis and urgent treatment of CAP at least prevents the exacerbation of symptoms in COPD in 50% of cases.

Proper treatment and proper use of drugs for a proper duration under medical supervision. Improving environmental sanitation and vaccination cover.

Curb should be one overue or ill-use of corticosteroids since large number of cases of dissemination of infection including tuberculosis and potential risk of development and metastasis of malignancy owe to immunosuppressive therapy.

e) HIV

Improving moral values and making people religious to cut down polygamy and educating through de addiction camps and using safe blood for transfusion to prevent the spread of HIV disease and the related chest disorders.

DOT for TB to be strictly implemented.

HAART to be given to selected patients, CD, cells>200/mm^3 in safe.

f) Trauma

Promoting humanism in police and sending message through public awareness camps to cut down terrorism and crime-related chest injuries.

Chest tube insertion and endoscopic instrumentation by experienced persons only.

Ventilator-associated pneumonia can be prevented by semirecumbent positioning, maintaining adequate endotracheal tube cuff pressures, continuous subglottic aspiration, and use of nasogastric tube to avoid gastric overdistension.

g) Lifestyle and exercise

Promotion of a healthy lifestyle through regular exercise and breathing exercise training to bring down allergic inflammatory and even infectious respiratory disorders, at least by 20%–25%. Unfortunately, in Ludhiana city, with a population of nearly 30 lakhs, one could hardly see 3,000 people going for a morning walk or exercise in parks.

Sedentary habits, excessive fatty dietary intake, and regular use of pills (in females) may be responsible for a marginal rise in peripheral vascular disease and pulmonary thromboembolism.

Early chest physiotherapy in patients with poly injuries, ventilatory support, or cardiothoracic surgery.

Accidents

Display of proper sign boards and proper roads can cut down road accidents. Unfortunately, India has 10% of the total global roads, out of which only 1% are safe. Punjab government is gearing up in this direction.

Driver's capability to drive safely, people's participation for highway traffic use of seat belts, and use of proper signals can cut down chest-injury accidents. Mobile traffic vans have recently been started by Haryana Police. Additionally, they shall help to bring out the injured from the accidental vehicle and are equipped with cutting machines, first-aid team, and mobile ambulance to take the injured to the nearby hospitals.

For anti-terrorist wave and police-created chest injuries, a peace plan, negotiation, and humanistic approach can only be requested. Medical checkup of criminals in police remand should be enforced.

Drugs:

Mushroom sale of opium and related product should be checked.

Indiscriminate use of corticosteroids should be avoided.

Drug should be judiciously used and finding an ofendant to respiratory system, should be immediately stopped, thus aiming at increasing healthy life, rather than increasing mere life expectancy. Let us all participate to curtail down the rising trend in the diseases and disorders of the chest. We are physicians with a tunnel vision, can carve a niche, and travel even in the most curved path to work together for a healthy community. After all, we are also part to it.

Summary[10–14]

A rising trend in respiratory problems has been observed in the past two decades. *The Irish Times* reported that respiratory diseases are found to 200% higher. Apart from the actual rise in diseases such as bronchial hypersensitivity, airflow obstructive disorders, and infective diseases of lungs including tuberculosis, there has been a tremendous effect on the escalation of neoplastic diseases as well. The rise in bronchitis, asthma, emphysema, respiratory infection, and lung cancer has *been* attributed to air pollution, tobacco smoke, agro-insecticides, aero-allergens, auto-exhaust, and environmental pollution from incomplete burning of fuels in houses and industries. By 2020, India alone is likely to account for 18% of the 8.4 million tobacco-related deaths. And the real tragedy of COPD is that it is preventable by cessation of tobacco smoking. Rise in infections, especially pulmonary tuberculosis, has *been* attributed to the rise in HIV disease in the past decade. Posttraumatic lung injuries have been attributed to increased terrorist activities, blasts at public places, police excesses, and automobile accidental injuries.

A variety of lung disorders have been increasingly described due to the increased knowledge about the disease since there is growth and development of pulmonology as a superspeciality as well as advancement in the diagnostic facilities in pulmonary sciences. Programs directed and preventive measures suggested toward reducing air pollution from wood firs and incomplete industrial combustion, improving the quality of diesel shaust-emission and developing cleaner modes of transport have been suggested. Preventing allergic and infective chest disorders through bringing about lifestyle changes, self-safety from modern plague (AIDS), and minimizing or initiates a chain of iatrogenic complications. Decreased body resistance and immunosuppressive effect make people more susceptible to various chest infections, including community-acquired pneumonia, in which the risk of hospitalization is aggravated if treated using an inappropriate antibiotic given at an inadequate dosage for an insufficient period. This practice is common in rural regions where people fall prey to unqualified doctors. Nosocomial infections have also been on the rise in hospitalized patients. Again, appropriate urgent measures, including appropriate antimicrobial therapy, have shown decrease in mortality by 10%–20%.

Half of what a rich man eats keeps him going, and the other half keeps the doctor going. Preventive measures start from reverting to traditional living and eating habits, regular exercise, antipollution stringent measures, clean transportation system, safe driving within rules and speed limits, safety measures applied, first aids and ambulance shift to trauma center in case of accidents, proper use of drugs, minimal hospital stay, avoidance of tobacco, check on opium products and narcotics, and restricting the use of open grain threshers and toxic agro-insecticides through education and administrative actions.

References and suggested readings

1. Raj M. Air pollution and health hazards. Envir Pollut. 2000;1:3–17.
2. Behera D, et al. Ciassive smoking, domestic fuels and lung functions in North Indian children. Ind J Chest Dis All Sci. 1998;40:89–98.
3. Bhatia RS, Vijayan VK. Tobacco and health: what can be the medical profession do? Lung India. 1994;12:178–185.
4. Juidal SK, Vij A. Health effects of air pollution. Med Update; API. 2016; 26:969–977.
5. Bhatia RS. Respiratory disease pattern in a private clinic in Ludhiana. Lung India. 1995;13:125–126.
6. Bhatia RS, Singhal M. Bronchial asthma: current trend. Med Update. 1996; 817–818.
7. Bhatia RS. Disease of small airway of lung. JIACM. 2001;2:222–224.
8. Gothi D, et al. Clinical profile of diseases causing chronic airflow limitation in a tertiary care centre in India. JAPI. 2007;55:551–555.
9. Shankar PS. HRCT of lungs. IN: BC Banal, ed. PG Med; API. 1997;11:353–359.
10. Jindal SK, Gupta D. Diagnosis and management of arcoidois: current trend. IN: BC Bansal, ed. PG Med; API. 1997;11:347–352.
11. Gupta A, Prakash C. Ind J Med Res. 2006;14:254–257.
12. Bhatia RS. Rising trend in pulmonary disorders-reasons and remedies. IN: Chest Medicine. Lucknow: Arora Publ. 2005;4:23–34.
13. Bhatia RS. Tuberculosis and AIDS. JAPI. 2000;48:613–616.
14. Udwadia ZF. The burden of undiagnosed airflow obstruction in India. JAPI. 2007;55:547–549.
15. Bhatia RS. Community acquired pneumonia: emerging aetiology with implications of therapy. IN: YP Munjal, ed. PG Med; API. 199;13:275–282.
16. Bhatia RS. HIV and TB: where we stand? IN: SB Gupta, ed. Med Update; API. 2002;12:1180–1193.

17. Vijayan VK. Drug induced resp. diseases. IN: S Chanderekhran, ed. Med Update; API. 1993;3:177–188.
18. Bhatia RS. Enalpril precipitating an attack of asthmatic bronchitis. JAPI. 1994;42:506.
19. Bhatia RS, et al. Diet, disease, drugs; has the change lead to a change? J Diab Asn India. 1996;36:31–54.
20. Bhatia RS. Humidifier disease. Lung India. 1994;12:198–200.
21. Bhatia RS. ARI in children: our exphence. IN: K Jagadeean, et al., ed. Update Med Surg. Glassgow: RCPS. 1998;162–168.
22. Klop B, Elte JW, Cabezas MC. Dyslipidemia in obesity: mechanisms and potential targets. Nutrients. 2013 Apr 12;5(4):1218–1240.
23. Csete J, et al. Public health and international drug policy. Lancet. 2016 Apr 2;387(10026):1427–1480.
24. Aydogdu MO, et al. Surface interactions and viability of coronaviruses. J R Soc Interface. 2021 Jan;18(174):20200798.
25. D'Amato G, et al. Climate change and air pollution: effects on pollen allergy and other allergic respiratory diseases. Allergo J Int. 2014;23(1):17–23.

https://doi.org/10.1142/9789811271410_0052

52 Tobacco smoking

Introduction

Smoking is a social evil, and most of the smoking (tobacco)-related lung diseases including COPD and lung cancer are dose dependent, where cumulative dose tobacco determines the risk. Pack-year (PY)-like parameters have been used to express the exposure to tobacco smoke, where PY means one packet of cigarettes or 20 g of tobacco smoked every day over a course of one year. The variability in the number of cigarettes or bodies in Indian market brings a nonuniformity, and *hence*, smoking index is used where the number of bodies or cigarettes smoked per day in relation to the number of years (duration) of smoking is accounted. Also, there is a difference among the brands in showing difference in the total particulate matter because of nonuniformity and clinical analysis of different laboratories.

Cigarette smoking is a major risk factor for CHD, stroke, lung cancer, and COPD and is even correlated with enhanced mortality from pulmonary tuberculosis. Chewing tobacco is associated with similar risks as smoking. However, it has been observed that spirometric measurements show that pulmonary physiological abnormalities such as bronchial hypersensitivity may reverse in those with higher smoking index. This is further confirmed by experimental, clinical, and epidemiological studies that a relationship exists between cigarette smoking and a wide range of respiratory diseases. Smoking not only is responsible for lung cancer but also is directly linked with enhanced morbidity and mortality from other non-neoplastic respiratory diseases such as chronic bronchitis, emphysema, cor pulmonale, and respiratory infections. The US Surgeon General's reports on smoking had, therefore, rightly concluded that cigarette smoking is the largest avoidable cause of death and disability in the United States.

Smoking effects on pulmonary anatomy and physiology

Structural changes include increased mucous formation due to hypertrophy and hyperplasia of mucous glands of large airways. Sputum production is increased, mainly because of tar contents of cigarettes. Small airways get inflamed; there is hyperplasia of goblet cells, and airways get closed because of intraluminal mucous formation. Experimental studies have demonstrated that tobacco smoke damages the tight junction of airway epithelium and facilitates epithelial permeability. This is further supported by the fact that abnormal permeability decreases after cessation of smoking. The abnormal permeability enhances absorption of inhalant toxins and other aerosols, resulting in exaggerated bronchial hyperresponsiveness to inhaled methacholine in both symptomatic and non-symptomatic smokers. The damage caused to alveolar walls by smoking leads to centrilobular emphysema. This may result in increased influx of neutrophils which release neutrophil elastase and also activate alpha-1 anti-protease.

Functional changes due to tobacco smoking result from small airway disease, manifested by an increased closing volume and closing capacity. Small airway dysfunction can occur even in asymptomatic patients. In advanced cases, expiratory flow rates are reduced, and the forced expiratory volume in one second (FEV1) can be used as a predictor of development of obstructive airway disease. Discontinuation of smoking reverses the reduction in FEV1 and it becomes similar to nonsmokers, in patients before the age of 40 years.

Chronic bronchitis and emphysema

It is now an established fact that COPD is a smoking-related disease. The pattern is similar in female smokers in the West. Prevalence of chronic bronchitis is high among Indian smokers. Various studies conducted in Mumbai, Northern India, Orissa, and Andhra Pradesh have shown similar rising trends of COPD among smokers. Airway obstruction and increased production of phlegm are commonly seen in smokers; the airway obstruction reversibility becomes difficult in susceptible smokers. For those with bronchial asthma, the response to treatment is poor among smoking patients. A steep fall in forced expiratory volume is observed in smokers with hyper-bronco reactivity.

Environmental tobacco smoke

Passive smoking or environmental tobacco smoke (ETS) is the involuntary or secondary smoking that causes impairment in lung functions and thus exposing the innocents to higher rates of respiratory illness and chronic airway disease. ETS has been associated with lung cancer and bronchial asthma in children and is also responsible for increased severity of the disease. ETS adversely affects the treatment of asthmatic patients. Airway obstruction worsens due to reflex stimulation of parasympathetic pathways by smoke particles. ETS increases bronchial responsiveness even in non-asthmatic patients, and the respiratory symptoms are more pronounced in these patients. It has been observed that wives of smokers have increased bronchial reactivity to inhaled bronchoconstrictor aerosols due to increased epithelial permeability, which starts with increased absorption of most tobacco combustion by-products that these subjects inhale in the company of smoking husbands. This would explain partially the prevalence of chronic respiratory disease and lung cancers in nonsmoking subjects, especially the women in our country.

Parental smoking badly affects and exacerbates respiratory diseases in the children. The rate of lower respiratory illness in children has been found to be linearly related to material smoking. There is twice the risk of pneumonia and bronchitis among the children of smoking parents during the first year of life. Heavy smoking during pregnancy may have a direct effect on the offspring's subsequent lung functions. Asthmatic children of smoking mothers have lower expiratory flow rates than those of nonsmoking mothers. These observations emphasize the adverse effects of exposure to ETS in children.

Exercise tolerance is reduced by smoking even in asymptomatic subjects. The effects are observed even with a single bidi or cigarette smoking. And this reduction goes further in bronchitis patients if smoking is continued due to increased levels of carboxyhemoglobin. Lung infections such as pneumonia and influenza are enhanced in smokers. Postoperative complications are more in smokers. Smoking is an important cause of spontaneous pneumothorax. In synergism also with certain occupational exposures such as coal mine dust, grain, and cotton or wool dust, smoking can produce airway obstruction following chronic bronchitis. Significant airway obstruction can be produced by tobacco smoke in silica workers. It increases the risk of lung cancer following chronic occupational exposure in these workers.

Tobacco and 'P'

Tobacco affects 5'P', that is, poverty, people, politics, policies, and professionals (medical). Although effects of tobacco are known to all and everyone, it has not been possible to eradicate this social evil because of its unique power that is enjoyed the world over. Those who favor this evil are virtually involved in its cultivation and processing. Tobacco cultivation does not require intensive irrigation and the income generated to the disciplinary operation among themselves. They must realize that their duty and contribution do not end with disease management alone; they need to extend their responsibility toward community as well as toward opinion makers of the society to create and develop a healthy atmosphere.

An epidemic of tobacco-related cancers, vascular, heart, and lung diseases including obstructive lung disorders can only be prevented by creating a national coalition of doctors, teachers, religious leaders, and opinion makers to work sincerely in this direction. Those who are afraid of political bosses for their pressure and distance experience would lose the battle by default. The political people are our people; they can be made to understand the gravity of damages caused by tobacco. They can be explained the health effect of tobacco-free environments. They need to be stressed that this can only be achieved through their help and by their action. After all, politicians are also responsible people; they are also open to arguments and pressure and suggestions which are purely based on medical facts and meant simply for the community well-being. They must be assured of the ugly heads of tobacco products which are projecting and becoming fashion of every house. They will surely confirm to lend their hand of help to save three million deaths every year that are occurring because of tobacco — the social evil. Can we dream of such a tobacco-free society where no one, not even Bollywood star, politician, or common man, would bow before these tobacco people? Let us not compromise with the health of the people at least!

References and suggested readings

1. Bhatia RS, Vijayan VK. Tobacco and health: what can medical profession do? Lung India. 1994;12:178–185.
2. Pais P, et al. Increased risk of acute myocardial infarction associated with beedi and cigarette smoking in Indians. Ind Heart J. 2001;53:731–735.
3. Bhatia RS. Smokeless tobacco: a challenging smoke. JAPI. 1994;42:344, 1995;1261.
4. Bhatia RS, Sibia SS. ST-T wave change with tobacco snuff as tooth paste. JAPI. 1993;41:668.
5. Chhabra SK, et al. Patterns of smoking in Delhi and comparison of chronic respiratory morbidity among beedi and cigarette smokers. Ind J Chest Dis All Sci. 2001;43:19–26.
6. Bhatia RS. Rise in respiratory problems and their prevention. IN: S Das, ed. Med Update; API. 2003;13:260–267.
7. Bhatia RS. Cardiopulmonary manifestations of tobacco. IN: BB Thakur, ed. Med Update; API. 2000;10716–10718.
8. Bhatia RS. Pan masala: why not ban it. JAPI. 1989;37:244.

9. Gupta BK, et al. Cardiovascular risk factors in tobacco chewer — a controlled study. JAPI. 2007;55:27–31.
10. Gothi D, et al. Clinical profile of diseases causing chronic airflow limitation in a tertiary centre in India. JAPI. 2007;55:551–555.
11. Sharma P. Nicotine quantity and packing disclosure is smoked and smokeless tobacco products in India. 2015;47:440–443.
12. Bhatia RS, Kant S. COPD. Foundation. 2014.
13. Rose MJ, et al. Role of smoking as a modifiable risk factors as a modifiable risk factor in diabetic nephropathy. JAPI. 2016;64:34–38.
14. Johi SR. Tobacco free India — save our children. JAPI. 2006;54:605–02.
15. Kant S, Bhatia RS. Lung cancer. Lucknow: JBS Foundation. 2017.
16. Fouad H, et al. Estimated and projected prevalence of tobacco smoking in males, Eastern Mediterranean Region, 2000–2025. East Mediterr Health J. 2021 Jan 23;27(1):76–82.
17. Nicolaides S, et al. The impact of tobacco smoking on treatment choice and efficacy in inflammatory bowel disease. Intest Res. 2021 Apr;19(2):158–170.
18. Thandra KC, et al. Epidemiology of lung cancer. Contemp Oncol (Pozn). 2021;25(1):45–52.
19. Baron JA, et al. Cigarette smoking and estrogen-related cancer. Cancer Epidemiol Biomarkers Prev. 2021 Aug;30(8):1462–1471. doi: 10.1158/1055-9965.EPI-20-1803. Epub 2021 May 14.
20. Haddad C, et al. Smoking and COVID-19: a scoping review. Tob Use Insights. 2021 Feb 15;14:1179173X21994612.

https://doi.org/10.1142/9789811271410_0053

53 Pathophysiological interinfluence of respiration and endocrines

Introduction

Pathophysiology of the endocrine system significantly influences the respiratory system. Pulmonary changes in metabolic disorders are fairly common since hormones play a significant role in fetal lung maturation and also affect postnatal pulmonary structures and functions.[1] All the endocrinal glands such as hypothalamus, pituitary glands, thyroid, parathyroids, pancreas, adrenals, and even genitalia both in males and females exert their influence on the respiratory system. Both hyper and hypo functions of these glands have varied forms of effects on respiratory pathophysiology.

Hypothalamus and respiratory system

Hypothalamic disorders influence lung functions in three ways, that is, by affecting the autonomic nervous system, respiratory drive, or by causing hypopituitarism. Blood flow is altered by the influence of cyclic changes that produce nasal airflow resistance through sympathetic tone, thereby modifying mucosal turgidity. Thus, central hypoventilation, depressed ventilatory response to inspired CO_2 and post-exercise hypoventilation, may result. Hypothalamic dysfunctions may produce sleep apnea in Prader–Willi and Kleine–Levin syndromes. It may be noted that human corticotropin-releasing hormone is a respiratory stimulant.[2]

Pituitary gland and respiratory system

Growth hormone has an important influence on the respiratory system. Hypopituitarism in a newborn may produce proportionate decrease in lung and thorax sizes, but without affecting the arterial blood gases. Acquired hypopituitarism in adolescence may produce underdeveloped lungs and paranasal sinuses. And adult-onset hypopituitarism does not produce clinically significant respiratory abnormality except for reduced static lung volume and disproportionate functional residual capacity. However, in Sheehan syndrome, recurrent nasal polyps have been documented.[3] Increased growth hormone levels in acromegaly may be associated with premature death which is attributed to some respiratory diseases. This occurs three times more frequently, possibly because of the upper and lower respiratory tract involvement[4] as shown in Table 1.

Acromegaly produces intra and extra thoracic airway obstruction; possibly because of macroglossia, generalized mucosal thickening and narrowing of opening between vocal cords.[5] Asymptomatic to symptomatic cases with chronic upper respiratory obstruction, with hoarseness and exertional dyspnea have been documented. Stridor is commonly observed during induction of anesthesia. Obstructive sleep apnea commonly occurs in these patients, responsible for daytime somnolence, loud snoring and life-threatening arrhythmias during sleep.[6]

Bromocriptine is the drug of choice for sleep apnea, in these patients. Possibly depressed levels of somatostatin may be responsible for altered respiratory control during sleep, octreotide therapy has successfully been tried.[2]

Thyroid and Respiratory System

In hyperthyroidism; myopathy of respiratory muscles including diaphragm, increased metabolism and enhanced central respiratory drive affect the pulmonary functions.[7] Airway resistance is not altered, lung compliance is slightly affected. An increased central respiratory drive in response to hypoxia and hypercapnia[8] is also noted. Increased bronchial

Table 1: Effect on respiratory system in hyper-secretary growth hormone dysfunction

A. Functional changes 1. Increased vital capacity and total lung capacity 2. Increased anatomic dead space 3. Small airway narrowing, without affecting large airway 4. Extra thoracic airway obstruction with normal lung compliance, elastic recoil, diffusing capacity, and lung muscles strength
B. Structural changes 1. Upper respiratory tract — Excessive pneumatization of paranasal sinuses — Macroglossia with prognathism — Excessive connective tissue deposition resulting in thickening, hypertrophy, and mucosal congestion of the upper respiratory tract — Inter-vocal cord narrowing 2. Lower respiratory tract and thorax — Periosteal bone growth resulting in thickened clavicles and ribs — Endochondral proliferation resulting in lengthening of clavicle and ribs and enlargement of the thoracic cage. Thoracic kyphosis and limited anteflexion — Lung enlargement, more in males — Lungs ossification pneumopathia osteoplastica recemosa — Narrowing of small airways

reactivity worsens bronchial asthma through unknown mechanism, possibly due to accumulation of leukotrienes and prostaglandins in the lungs.[4]

In hypothyroidism, diaphragm dysfunction and decreased breathing capacity due to muscle weakness are often encountered. Pulmonary diffusing capacity may be reduced *due* to accompanying anemia. Associated obesity and cardiac ailment may add to pulmonary dysfunction. Even bronchial reactivity is increased in normal individuals. Pulmonary function reverts to normal on administration of thyroxine.[9] Hypoxic and hypercapnic ventilation drives are depressed, and alveolar hypoventilation and lethal CO narcosis may occur in severe hypothyroidism.[10] These patients may have daytime somnolence, apathy, and lethargy, and even obstructive sleep apnea may be found in a nonobese patient. Altered permeability of pleural capillaries or extravasation of hygroscopic pleural effusions with or without pericardial effusion is also observed. Initial neutrophilic collection is seen replaced by predominant lymphocytic response of myxomatous tissue in the larynx, causing upper airway obstruction.[1]

Calcium phosphates metabolism and respiratory system

An association with hypercalcemia and apnea in infants has been documented.[11] Severe chest deformity may occur in primary hyperparathyroidism if azotemia supervenes. Acute deposits produce diffuse alveolar damage and ARDS[12] while gradual deposition causing thickening and fibrosis produces restrictive patterns of pulmonary functions. In hypoparathyroidism, hypocalcemia may induce special electrical activity in motor and sensory nerves causing titanic laryngeal spasm, causing fixing of vocal cords in the middle, producing stridor, asphyxia, and crowing respiration. Increased bronchomotor tone due to effect on autonomic ganglia may produce wheezing.

Where hyperphosphatemia has no respiratory influences, severe hypophosphatemia may precipitate acute respiratory failure due to weakness of respiratory muscles. Rickets, osteomalacia, and osteoporosis may affect thoracic cage which may indirectly produce alveolar hypoventilation and respiratory failure.

Adrenal cortex and respiratory system

Hypercortisolism as in Cushing's syndrome or *due* to oral corticosteroid therapy may produce abnormal sleep patterns and obstructive sleep apnea.[13] Even chronic respiratory failure and severe metabolic alkalosis have been documented. Exogenous corticosteroids contribute to respiratory muscle weakness,[14] apart from precipitating miliary tuberculosis, PCP, pulmonary aspergillosis, or cryptococcosis. However, it is uncommon to find bronchial asthma as a manifestation of hypocortisolism in Addison's disease.[15]

Adrenal medulla and respiratory system

Excessive catecholamines in pheochromocytoma can produce changed sleep pattern and hyperventilation, mimicking functional hyperventilation syndrome. Even pulmonary edema may occur due to left ventricular dysfunction or due to toxic effects of catecholamines. Bronchial asthma may get cured but is likely to reappear following the removal of the tumor.[4]

Female endocrine and respiratory system

Large theca lutein cysts or ovarian hyperstimulation syndrome may be produced due to hypogonadotropic caused by endogenous hydatidiform mole or chorioepithelioma or exogenous administration of gonadotropins. Massive pleural effusion with hypovolemia may be produced as a result of increased permeability due to overstimulated ovaries. Hypogonadotropic hypogonadism in prepubertal stage may give rise to small thorax with smaller lung volumes and is required to be differentiated from restrictive pulmonary disease. Exogenous estrogen may increase frequency of hay fever and pulmonary thromboembolism.

Increased progesterone (as in pregnancy) may enhance respiratory response to hypoxia and hypercapnia[16] and is useful therapeutically in treating sleep apnea syndrome. Cyclic decrease in progesterone can precipitate premenstrual bronchial asthma.

Fibroma of ovary or other tumors of ovaries may produce ascites and pleural effusion called Meig's and pseudo Meig's syndrome, respectively. Chromosomal disorders produce respiratory disorder. Shield chest and pulmonary valvular stenosis are present in ovarian dysgenesis syndrome, pulmonary valvular stenosis and pulmonary lymphangiectasis are seen in Ullrich-Noonan's syndrome, and restrictive pulmonary defects are present in Klinefelter's syndrome.

Male endocrines and respiratory system

Exogenous testosterone may produce obstructive sleep apnea. Testicular tubular disease as such has no respiratory consequences but for when both the systems are affected in Kartagener syndrome. Familiar hypogonadotropic hypogonadism as in Kallmann syndrome may have hypoplasia of the first rib. Thoracopulmonary anomalies are often associated with Klinefelter[17] and Ullrich-Noonan syndromes. Chest deformity with cystic lung disease may be associated with Marfan's syndrome.

Diabetes mellitus and respiratory system

Decreased availability of NABPH producing decreased production of superoxide anion, along with depressed respiratory burst, would contribute to impaired chemotaxis, phagocytosis, and intracellular killing of microorganisms by granulocytes and mononuclear cells in diabetes mellitus. So is the enhanced zygomycosis because of impaired ability of alveolar macrophages in inhibiting fungal spores' germination.

Pulmonary functions are altered in two-thirds of diabetic patients. Added to the agony is the influence of associates obesity, muscle weakness, and congestive cardiac failure. Lung volume may be reduced in insulin-dependent diabetes and pulmonary elastic recoil and pulmonary diffusion are impaired,[18] possibly because of pulmonary microangiopathy. Even pulmonary epithelial permeability has been found impaired.[19] Abnormal ventilatory responses to hypoxia may cause unexpected cardiorespiratory arrest in diabetic patients, possibly because of increased sleep-related breathing disorders produced as a result of autonomic neuropathy. Evidence of link between OSA and insulin independent of obesity has been documented, identifying impaired metabolism as one of the consequences of sleep loss,[20,21] suggesting the reduction in sleep duration as well as the quality of sleep that may increase with the severity of metabolic disorder, particularly diabetes mellitus.[22,23]

Cerebral edema as a result of decrease in the gradient *between* pulmonary wedge pressure and serum colloid oncotic pressure may cause neurogenic pulmonary edema, due to increased permeability during acidosis. Adult respiratory distress syndrome may also occur because of noncardio genie pulmonary edema during treatment of diabetic ketoacidosis. Alveolar hypoventilation may occur due to hypokalemia or hypophosphatemia while treating diabetic ketoacidosis because of severe muscular weakness. Diabetes mellitus and bronchial asthma rarely coexist. However, bronchospasm may get exacerbated in asthmatics in hypoglycemic conditions. Autonomic neuropathy in diabetes, however, reduces the bronchial hyperreactivity, possibly because of depressed cholinergic bronchomotor tone.[24] Diabetic neuropathy and persistent transudative pleural effusion due to left ventricular dysfunction may produce transient vocal cord paralysis. In case of diabetic ketoacidosis, dehydration may precipitate pulmonary thromboembolism.[25,26]

Diabetes can predispose to pulmonary tuberculosis 3–4 times higher than in nondiabetics and is *a* risk factor for its reactivation. Incidence is 2.2 times higher in males. Multiple loss with lower lobe predominant involvement is common in diabetics. The effect is due to low opsonic index, decreased bacterial activity, lowered tissue resistance, decreased synthesis of collagen, impaired RE cell defense, and decreased adequate substrate for antibody formation, due to disturbed protein metabolism and enhanced glycerol in tissue. Uncontrolled hyperglycemia also increases the risk for development of MDR-TB.

References and suggested readings

1. Lapex A, et al. Sleep aponea, hypothyroidism and pulmonary oedema. Chest. 1990;97:763.
2. Nink M, et al. Corticotropin releasing hormone is a respiratory stimulant in humans: a comparative study of human and bovine CRH. Life Sci. 1994;54:1793.
3. Hampal S, et al. Recurrent simple nasal polyps associated with Sheehan's syndrome. J Otolaryngol. 1992;21:368.
4. Rohatgi PK, Becker KL. Respiration and endocrinology. IN: KL Becker, ed. Principles and practice of endocrinology and metabolism. 2nd ed. Philadelphia: JB Lippincott Co. 1995.
5. Murrans NJ, Gatiand J. Respiratory problems in acromegaly. J Laryngol Otol. 1990;104:52.
6. Gustein RR, et al. Central sleep apnoea is associated with increased ventilatory response to CO, and hyeprsecretion of growth hormone in patients with acromegaly. Am J Respir Crit Care Med. 1994;150:496.

7. McElavancy GN, et al. Respiratory muscle weakness and dyspnea in thyrotoxic patients. Am Rev Respir Dis. 1990;141:1231.
8. Small D, et al. Exertional dysponea and ventilation in hyperthyroidism. Chest. 1992;102:1268.
9. Wieshamer S, et al. Effects of hypothyroidism on bronchial reactivity in non-asthmatic subjects. Thorax. 1990;45:947.
10. Gottehrer A, et al. Hypothyroidism and pleural effusions. Chest. 1990;98:1140.
11. Hartman TE, et al. Metastatic pulmonary calcification in patients with hypercalcemia: findings on chest radiographs and CT scans. Am J Roentgenol. 1994;162:799.
12. Kooh SW, Binet A. Hypercalcemia in infants presenting with apnea. Can Med Assoc J. 1990;88:369.
13. Shipley JE, et al. Sleep architecture and sleep apnoea in patients with Cushing's disease. Sleep. 1992;15:514.
14. Decramer N, et al. Corticosteroids contribute to muscle weakness in chronic airflow obstructions. Am J Respir Crit Care Med. 1994;150:11.
15. Saraclar Y, et al. Bronchial asthma and Addison's disease. Respiration. 1993;60:241.
16. Bayliss DA, Millborn DE. Central neural mechanisms of progesterone action: application to respiratory system. J Appl Physiol. 1992;73:393.
17. Morelet P, et al. Pathogenesis of lung restrictive defects of Klinefelter's syndrome. Chest. 1992;102:1550.
18. Sandler M. Is lung a target organ in diabetes mellitus? Arch Intern Med. 1990;150:1385.
19. Cancer B, et al. Impaired lung epithelial permeability in diabetics detected by technetium-99 m-DTPA aerosol scintigraphy. J Nucl Med. 1994;35:204.
20. Punabi NM, et al. Sleep disordered breathing and insulin resistance in middle aged and overweight men. Am J Respir Crit Care Med. 2002;165:677–682.
21. Ip MSM, et al. OSA is independently associated with insulin resistance. Am J Respir Crit Care Med. 2002;165:670–676.
22. Bhatia RS. Sleep apnoea syndrome. IN: LA Pathak, ed. Post Grad Med; API. 2004;18:79–83.
23. Vigg A, et al. Sleep in type 2 diabetes. JAPI. 2003;51:479–481.
24. Santos E, Fonsca CN, et al. Cholinergic bronchomotor tone and airway calibre in IDDM. Chest. 1992;101:1038.

25. Quigley RL, et al. Management of massive pulmonary thromboembolism complicating diabetic ketoacidosis. Ann Thora Surg. 1994;57:1522.
26. Bhatia RS. Metabolic disorders and lungs. IN: BB Thakur, ed. PG Med; API. 2002;16:125–129.
27. Gross I. Regulation of fetal lung maturation. Am J Physiol. 1990;259:L337.
28. Piper JM, Langer O. Does material diabetes delay lung maturity? Am Sci. 1994;54:1793.
29. Leibowitz G, et al. Improvement of sleep apnoea due to acromegaly during short-term treatment with octreotide. Intern Med. 1994;236:131.
30. Subhani AR, et al. Mitigation of stress: new treatment alternatives. Cogn Neurodyn. 2018 Feb;12(1):1–20.
31. Brunse A, et al. Co-bedding of preterm newborn pigs reduces necrotizing enterocolitis incidence independent of vital functions and cortisol levels. Front Pediatr. 2021 Apr 1;9:636638.
32. Carneiro EM, et al. Evaluation of breathing exercise in hormonal and immunological responses in patients undergoing abdominal surgery. Acta Cir Bras. 2013 May;28(5):385–390.

https://doi.org/10.1142/9789811271410_0054

54 Pleuropulmonary complications in neurosurgery

Introduction

Pleuropulmonary complications are commonly encountered following neurosurgery. Most of these occur because of interventions and infections, and even thromboembolism, since intubation, ventilation, and even tracheostomy are quite frequently done in these patients. Chest infections compounded with deep vein thrombosis (DVT) and bedsores need to pour more aggressive preventive measures in managing these pleuropulmonary complications. Atelectasis is the most commonly encountered pulmonary complication postoperatively seen following neurosurgery. This occurs because of shallow breathing and accumulation of secretions, mostly because of altered sensorium of various grades for a variable length of time often complicated by secondary infections. It has to be prevented by early mobilization, avoiding prolonged intubation during postoperative period and using spirometry. Sometimes inadvertent right main-bronchus intubation may cause whole lung collapse and hypoxemia, requiring urgent bronchoscopic clearance, correct positioning of the endotracheal tube, and vigorous physiotherapy. Ventilated patients need adequate tidal volume, preferably PEEP (5 cm) to prevent atelectasis. Additional tracheobronchial toileting is also required. Pulmonary embolism is another important non-neurological complication proving 2%–3% fatality. DVT is a frequent source, requiring prophylactic LMWH and DVT stockings, in high-risk cases such as comatosed to unambulatory cases. LMWH has short half-life and hence can be stopped few hours before surgery. Postoperative prevention of pulmonary embolism is very important, requiring early ambulation, DVT stockings, and subcutaneous LMWH which can be started within a few hours postoperatively, but, with a vigil eye not to complicate cerebral bleeding. As the acute phase is over, warfarin can be started and continued upto three months, with regular monitoring of prothrombin time. Pneumonia is yet another complication, occurring within 2–5 days of operation, presenting with fever, hypoxia, reduced breath sounds, and definitely diagnosed with sputum culture and chest X-ray. Fever may be present in case patient is on steroids. Increased total white cell count in a dehydrated patient, without any evidence of lung infiltrate, it is advisable to start empirical antimicrobial, to be modified after receiving culture and sensitivity report of sputum swab. Additional care regarding positioning for drainage, chest percussion, moisturizing the airways, and proper toileting of tracheobronchial tract whenever required forms an important part of nursing. Occasional development of drug-resistant nosocomial pneumonia often becomes difficult to manage. Management of comorbidities, especially diabetes, is equally important. Pleural effusion may result from infections, emboli, atelectasis, or heart failure. Aspiration of pleural fluid may rarely be required if large. Pneumothorax may complicate following subclavian line placement or may follow from direct chest injury and needs to be managed by a chest tube.

Respiratory arrest may occur as an emergency, pressing urgent airways clearing of obstruction, ventilation, and proficient cardiopulmonary resuscitation.

Chest complications are much more in geriatric population undergoing neurosurgical interventions. Ambulation often becomes difficult in patients with head injury and long-standing coma, and these patients are more susceptible to chest infections and bedsores. Therefore, these patients need early diagnosis and intensive therapy for better outcomes. Ventilators to prevent atelectasis and hyperventilation to treat postoperative raised intracranial tension are best utilized.

Specific complications of neurosurgery such as thoracotomy are often done; other thoracic instrumentations, and complications as a result of ventriculoperitoneal shunt may also occur, as the shunt tube traverses the anterior thoracic wall. Chest injuries along with head injury have also to be aggressively looked for and treated, which otherwise may pose serious threat to life.

Air travel, lung disease, and preventive pulmonology

Introduction

Most convenient and popular present mode of transport across the world is to travel by air. Millions of people are expected to travel by air in the coming years. The comfort, however, can get jeopardized in people with underlying lung disease, the incidence of which is almost 10%.[1] Pre-flight precautionary screening and following the guidelines can help. Physicians are often required to evaluate passengers[2] fitness to fly and need of, if any, supplemental O_2 during flight. As the plane flies higher, the pressure inside the aircraft is lowered than the atmospheric pressure at sea level and needs to be adequately pressured and supplemented with O_2 at an altitude of 5,000, 6,000, and 8,000 ft; the alveolar O_2 decreases from 75 mmHg, through 72 mmHg to SS mmHg, respectively. This fall in pressure and hypoxia results in increased respiratory ventilation, increased cardiac output, and elevated pulmonary arterial pressure due to pulmonary vasoconstriction.

Commonly faced respiratory problems during an air travel include aggravation of hypoxia in a patient with *pre*-existing lung disease such as bronchial asthma, severe COPD, bullae or may rupture giving rise to spontaneous pneumothorax or tension pneumothorax, precipitation of DVT giving rise to pulmonary embolism during or after the air travel and dissemination of infections including tuberculosis. Patients with congestive cardiac failure may worsen during air travel. The risk of these problems and preventive pulmonary medicine with the necessary precautionary measures *are* very important to know, especially in the era of increasing trend to travel by air. Use of supplemental oxygen when PaO_2 is below 50 mmHg level is suggested.

Hypoxia

Hypoxia is a very important factor in deciding for a patient to travel by air or not. Accentuation of hypoxia in a patient with underlying cardiopulmonary disorder may precipitate pulmonary edema,[3] myocardial or cerebral damage. Patients with hypercapnia, $PaCO_2 > 50$ mmHg, cyanosis, arrhythmia, and congestive cardiac failure are relative contraindications for air travel. Those with COPD should be adequately treated with bronchodilators, antibiotics for infection, and steroids as and when required and supplemented with regular O_2 supply during the travel. Even carrying one's own cylinder can be permitted. Applying three available techniques given below, clinical decision about in-flight supplemental O_2 can be made:

1. Measurement of PaO_2 inside the hyperbaric chamber.
2. Measurement of PaO_2 while breathing hypoxia gas mixture.
3. Using regression equation predicting PaO_2, 8,000 ft, based on the patient's sea level resting room PaO_2 and spirometry values.
4. PaO_2 altitude = 0.294 (PaO_2 SL) + 0.086 (FEVI% predict + 23.21.

This equation is mainly applicable to patients with COPD. For other pulmonary diseases, PaO_2 measured on the ground gives a reliable value for predicting PaO_2 at high altitudes. The patient should come forward to disclose his or her chest disease, if any. And for each passenger with lung disease who may require supplemental O_2 an interaction with the physician, a standard form of airlines to be filled up by the physician, and an advance request should be made for arrangement of adequate O_2 supply for allowing use of his own nasal prongs instead of facial masks provided by air lines. Airlines have to be informed for humidified oxygen for patients with asthma and COPD. And such an O_2-dependent person must be accompanied by a companion or spouse. Provision for pulse oximetry can also be done. The patient should get his or her seat near the toilet to have minimum exertion. Provision of wheelchair can also be requested for,[3–5] and possible precipitant irritants such as inhalant tobacco should be prohibited. So, with careful oximetric monitoring, sufficient O_2 supply, and medical escorts, most of the patients with lung disease can travel by air.[6] Airlines are all out to provide these services; what is required is to know your right and to ask for these. Pre-flight evaluation for oxygen supplementation includes 50-m walk test (often used), use of prediction equations, and the hypoxia challenge test.

Often patients of COPD with a large bullae are at higher risk of developing pneumothorax during air travel.[7] Pneumothorax forms the only absolute contraindication for air travel due to increased risk of developing respiratory distress.

Pneumothorax

During ascension, the pressure falls, and expansion of gases may result in the rupture of bullae or blebs in the lungs in patients with COPD causing an emergency and sometimes requiring diversion of air flight or forced landing of the aircraft. The same risk gets aggravated on descent for precipitation of further pneumothorax in patients with the history of pneumothorax or the presence of emphysematous bullae. The risk of spontaneous pneumothorax is 20%–50% in high-risk patients with underlying emphysematous bullae and blebs.[8] YAG laser may seal small blebs, but for those >1.5 mm, stapler suturing should be done in those who are either crew members or frequent air travelers.

DVT/pulmonary embolism lower limb edema — jet flight legs — can occur due to a drop in the cabin pressure and can be easily controlled by compression stockings. But lower limb edema can also develop due to DVT, with incidence being 0.5 per million of passengers, with an increased prevalence in females. Precipitating factors in a long air journey include immobility, cramping, dehydration, alcohol consumption, hypoxia, and underlying lung disease such as COPD.

Factors such as old age, polycythemia, obesity, minor surgery, varicose veins, hormonal therapy, lower limb recent trauma, thrombophilia, family history, malignancy, and previous history of venous thromboembolism may add to the risk. What is more important is to avoid these precipitating factors and take necessary precautions which include more facility of seat adjustment, more space for regular leg movements, space to move around in the cabin, avoidance of crossing over legs, and avoid coffee and alcohol intake. In addition, for higher-risk patients, low-dose aspirin under clinician's advice should be started (unless some contraindication exists, wearing of compression stockings and LMWH can also be started under physician's guidelines. Compression of calf muscles on regular intervals as per requirement can be done or even with an inflatable cushion device called Airogym, this can also be done. Mean duration of travel for DVT patients should not increase more than 5.4 + 2.1 hours.[9]

Pulmonary TB and other chest infections

Infections disseminate faster than love and life. And tuberculosis is the first to cross all the oceans due to immigration and travel. An air traveler with tubercular disease can easily infect four more people. Although WHO has issued guidelines for TB and air travel in 1998,[10] effectively following these guidelines is hardly observed. A long flight journey, confined space, and close proximity with very little ventilation can aggravate the rate of transmission of an infection. It will be better and safer for such a patient not to travel and postpone, atleast for 3 months, until he becomes noninfectious to others under cover of anti-tuberculosis therapy,[11] and now if he plans to travel, he should inform the authorities to get special care regarding ventilation and air filters.

Similarly, the risk of other viral and bacterial infections cannot be underrated. Individual sense of precautions and general behavior, not to disseminate infections to co-travelers should restrict him to take proper treatment and if recommended highly infectious, should postpone traveling until he is rendered noncommunicable.[12] That goes a long way in helping others and serving the community and is a step forward in prevention of spreading communicable respiratory diseases during an air travel where chances of dissemination of infections are already increased because of close proximity and limited ventilation.[13] Most of these patients complete their journey uneventfully with supplemental oxygen. Further studies to know the effects of air travel on people with lung disease would unveil new benefits.[14,15]

References and suggested readings

1. Coker RK, Partiridge MR. Assessing the risk of hypoxia in flight: the need for rational guidelines. Eur Respir J. 2000;15:128–130.
2. Vijayan VK. Air travel and chronic respiratory disase. Ind J Chest Dis All Sci. 1999;41:131–133.
3. Tyagi A. HAPO — an observational study. The Ilnd Pract. 2016;69:41–47.
4. Stoller JK. Oxygen and air travel. Respir Care. 2000;45:214–222.
5. BTS Standards of Care Committee. Managing passengers with respiratory disease planning air travel; BRITISH Thoracic Society Recommendations. Thorax. 2002;57:289–304.
6. Khilani GC, Bhatta N. Air and supplemental oxygen therapy in patients with cardiopulmonary diseases. J Assoc Physicians India. 2002 Jun;50:811–815.
7. Johnson AOC. COPD-fitness to fly with CORD. Thorax. 2003;58:729–732.
8. Bhatia RS, Sibia SS. Management of spontaneous pneumothorax-current practices. IN: S Venkataraman, ed. Med Update; API. 2004;14:221–226.
9. Kesteven PLJ. Travellers thrombosis. Thorax. 2000;55(1):532–536.
10. WHO. TB and air travel: guidelines for prevention and control to reduce transmission of the disease to the world's 1.4 billion air passengers. Press release. WHO 96/17 Dec. 1998.
11. Bhatia RS. HIV and TB: where we stand. IN: SB Gupta, ed. Med Update; API. 2002;12:1180–1183.
12. Bhatia RS. Respiratory disorders and air travel-role of physician. JAPI. 2003;51:532–533.
13. Sundram P, Joshi 1M. Lungs and air travel-problems and prevention. Med Update. 2002;9:23–26.
14. Gendreau MA, De John C. Responding to medical events during commercial airflights: current concepts. N Engl J Med. 2002;346:166–173.
15. Gulati V. Pulmonary thromboembolism-prophylaxis and management. IN: RK Singal, DG Jain, ed. Med Update; API. 2007;17:155–162.

16. Bhatia RS, Vijayan VK. Tobacco and health: what can the medical profession do? Lung India. 1994:12178–12185.
17. Murphy PB, et al. Effect of home noninvasive ventilation with oxygen therapy vs oxygen therapy alone on hospital readmission or death after an acute COPD exacerbation: a randomized clinical trial. JAMA. 2017 Jun 6;317(21):2177–2186.
18. Geerdes-Fenge HF. Pneumonien mit Reiseanamnese [Travel-associated pneumonias]. Pneumologie. 2014 Oct;68(10):685–695.
19. Kazachkov M, et al. Respiratory care in familial dysautonomia: systematic review and expert consensus recommendations. Respir Med. 2018 Aug;141:37–46. doi: 10.1016/j.rmed.2018.06.017. Epub 2018 Jun 21. PMID: 30053970; PMCID: PMC6084453.
20. Sürücüoğlu S. Seyahat ile ilişkili tüberküloz riski [Risk of travel associated tuberculosis]. Mikrobiyol Bul. 2018 Jan;52(1):96–107. Turkish. doi: 10.5578/mb.66237. PMID: 29642834.
21. Mantero M, Radovanovic D, Santus P, Blasi F. Management of severe COPD exacerbations: focus on beclomethasone dipropionate/formoterol/glycopyrronium bromide. Int J Chron Obstruct Pulmon Dis. 2018 Jul 30;13:2319–2333. doi: 10.2147/COPD.S147484. PMID: 30104872; PMCID: PMC6072677.

https://doi.org/10.1142/9789811271410_0055

55 Inhalational corticosteroids adversities on oral cavity

Abstract

Inhaled corticosteroids forms the cornerstone of treatment in airflow obstructive disorders such as asthma, small airway disease, and even chronic obstructive pulmonary disease (COPD). Asthma usually starts in childhood, and many a times, the patient has to take the inhalation therapy lifelong. On the contrary, COPD usually starts in later years, and many patients with severe airway obstruction have to take a high dose of inhalation therapy for a long duration. It is likely to exhibit several adverse effects on the oral tissues. Since the major proportion of the inhaled drug is retained in the oral cavity and oropharynx, it is likely to interfere in the normal physiology of oral tissues. The adverse influence of the inhaled corticosteroids on the oral health, including gingiva and teeth, needs timely interaction between the dentist and the attending physician to improve the safety profile of patients with airway disease.

Introduction

Asthma is a growing public health problem. Asthma is characterized by chronic airway inflammation and increased airway hyperresponsiveness, leading to symptoms such as wheezing, coughing, chest tightness, and dyspnea. It is characterized by the obstruction of airflow which varies over a short period of time and is reversible, either spontaneously or with treatment. Most asthma drugs are inhaled using various forms of inhalers or nebulizers. Inhaled corticosteroids (ICS, also known as glucocorticosteroids, glucocorticoids, or steroids) are by far the most effective controllers used in the treatment of asthma and are the only drugs that can effectively suppress the characteristic inflammation in asthmatic airways, much superior to low dose of theophylline. In both asthma and chronic obstructive pulmonary disease (COPD), ICS are commonly given as combination inhalers along with long-acting β2-agonists (LABAs). Enhanced use of corticosteroid inhalational therapy via inhalers/Rotahaler has also started showing adverse effects, especially in the buccal cavity, which, if not recognized and intervened, is likely to have deleterious consequences. Irrespective of the caste, creed, age, or sex, the drug delivery through inhalational devices in different kinds of chronic respiratory illnesses has resulted in the rising incidence of oral adverse effects, which can only be prevented through the proper use of these devices, taking all precautions to prevent these adverse events, and the timely participation of the attending physician in imparting education to the patients so as to have a positive outcome of the therapy with minimum adverse effects in these patients.

Patients are often seen visiting the dental OPD for various problems concerning oro-dental symptoms such as bad breath, distaste, candidiasis, and so forth. The role of periodontists is to create a positive atmosphere for encouraging a regular checkup in these patients, in a joint exercise with the physician or pulmonologist, so as to identify and treat and also to educate the patients to seek a physician's guidance for the proper use of these drug delivery devices in order to minimize the adverse effects of these inhalational therapies on oral health.

Mechanism of action of inhalational corticosteroids

The mechanism of action of inhalational corticosteroids and their effect on different cells is explained in Figures 1 and 2.

Pathophysiology

Prolonged use of beta-2 agonists is associated with the increased frequency of caries. It is explained on the basis of the effect of beta-2 agonist on

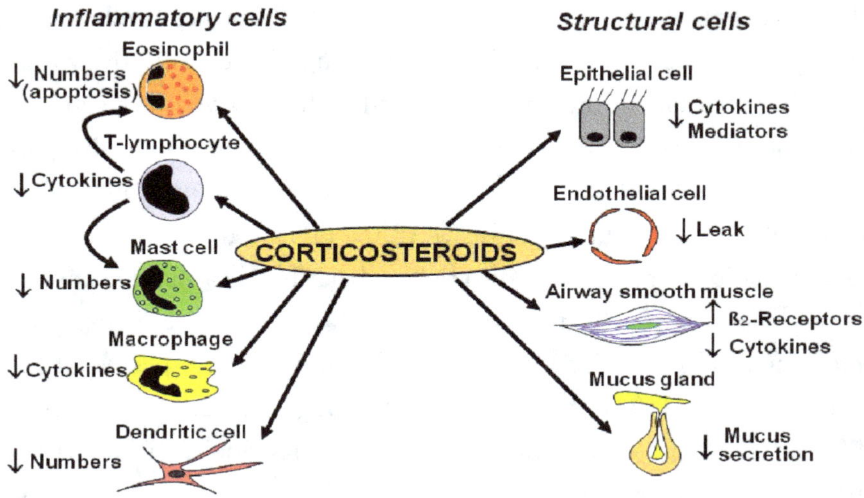

Figure 1: Cellular effect of corticosteroids.

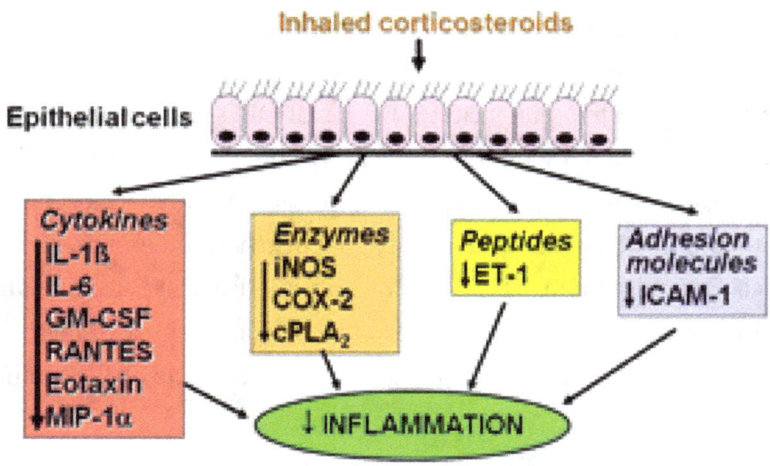

Figure 2: Inhaled corticosteroids may inhibit the transcription of several inflammatory genes in airway epithelial cells and thus reduce inflammation in the airway wall.

salivary secretion influencing the beta-2 receptors present over there, causing diminished salivary production and secretion. There is a reduction in the flow rates of whole and parotid saliva by 26% and 36%, respectively. As the reduced salivary rate is accompanied by a concomitant increase in *lactobacilli* and *Streptococcus mutans* in the oral cavity, it may be one of the major contributing factors for the increased caries rate. Normal salivary action gets further altered by the decreased availability of biologically active components like amylase, calcium ions, secretory IgA, peroxidase, and lysozyme. The decreased output of antibacterial components favors both bacterial colonization and plaque growth. Higher rate of caries may possibly occur due to inhaled drugs containing fermentable carbohydrates and sugar. ICS are themselves weak organic acids and generally are not metabolized by oral bacteria. They therefore should not pose a pH threat, except when sugar-based inhalers are used.

Oral manifestations due to ICS include

An overall reduction in the salivary output. Xerostomia is an adverse effect observed with the use of beta-2 agonists, anticholinergic inhalers, and ICS. There are symptoms of difficulty in talking or swallowing, altered taste, generalized oral discomfort, mouth soreness, burning sensation, and so forth. Xerostomia clinically manifests as oral fissuring, ulceration, and epithelial atrophy. Oral mucosa ulceration also occurs mainly due to xerostomia and immunosuppression caused by the inhaled drugs. Xerostomia produces taste changes secondary to incomplete food solubilization and also by the reduced transport of tastant molecules to the taste buds. Oral infection and xerostomia are notorious in producing bad breadth (halitosis). Children with asthma are at a greater risk of developing dental erosion. Asthma medication can place the patient at a risk of dental erosion by reducing salivary protection against extrinsic or intrinsic acids since saliva is considered to be one of the main neutralizing factors in the pathogenesis of dental erosion. The oral clearance of dietary acid is related to the rate of secretion and buffering capacity of saliva. There is a lowered salivary flow rate in asthmatic subjects treated with beta-2 adrenoceptor agonists. Drugs in current use, especially the powdered drugs, have a pH less than the critical level of 5.5 required for hydroxyapatite dissolution. Oropharyngeal candidiasis is a condition commonly associated with the use of nebulized corticosteroids. This side effect may be attributed to the topical effects of these medications on the oral mucosa, as only 10%–20% of the dose from an inhaler actually reaches the lungs, while the rest remains in the oropharynx. This opportunistic fungal infection as a local side effect is mainly observed due to immunosuppression among patients using high doses of ICS regularly. Asthmatic children have more of tooth decay (dental caries) affecting the permanent teeth. Asthma, through its disease status and its pharmacotherapy, includes some risk factors such as the decrease in the salivary flow rate and salivary pH for caries development. It was demonstrated that the duration of medication and illness has a significant influence on the risk of developing caries in asthmatics. The reason for a higher rate of caries can also be attributed to the presence of fermentable carbohydrates in asthma medications. Frequent oral inhalation of these sugar-containing drugs, combined with a decrease in the salivary flow rate, may contribute to an increased risk of caries. This risk is further enhanced in diabetic patients. An association between asthma and periodontal disease may involve the pathological activation of the immune and inflammatory process, the side effect of the asthma medications, or the interaction between the two. Periodontitis and gingivitis in asthmatic children could be explained by an altered immune response and the dehydration of alveolar mucosa due to mouth breathing. The concentration of IgE in gingival tissue is found to be elevated in patients with asthma, which can also cause periodontal destruction. Interactions between bacterial and immunological factors are found to be the main cause of destruction of the periodontal tissue. It has been suggested that children with asthma have more calculus than normal children. Higher prevalence of calculus in asthmatic children is thought to be due to an increase in the levels of calcium and phosphorous in submaxillary and parotid saliva. This can also contribute to an increase in periodontal problems in asthmatics. Regular use of conventional doses of ICS by patients with asthma can suppress the adrenal function and decrease bone density in a dose-related fashion. Systemic bone loss caused by these drugs, especially when high doses are used for a long time, may have an impact on the onset and progression of periodontal disease. Here lies the strong need of research to find anti-inflammatory drugs, replacing the corticosteroids and thus serving the community from adversities of immunosuppressants.

Conclusion

In various respiratory diseases, enhanced use of these inhalation therapies, therefore, requires a caution to must educate the patient for taking optimal oral care and using the dentist's services for adequately managing as well as preventing the adverse effects of these therapies on oral health. At present, services of dentists are being underutilized. Hence, there is a strong need of enhanced interaction between the pulmonologist and the dental surgeon. Dentists often advise for adequate oral hygiene, postmeal toothbrushing, mouth rinsing with neutral PH_4 before sleep, dietary modifications, and use of sodium fluoride as pit and fissure sealing agent. Further, salivary secretions can be enhanced by sucking a sour candy or lemon, or having frequent meals; even sugar-free chewing gum containing CPP–ACP (casein phosphopeptide–amorphous calcium phosphate or Recaldent) having a remineralizing effect has been recommended. Further research must find out replacement of corticosteroids, not with other immunosuppressants, but by developing bronchial anti-inflammatory with bronchodilatory effects.

Periodontal infections and chest

Introduction

Periodontium is a supportive tissue that connects the tooth to the bone cage. It consists of gingiva, periodontal ligament, cementum, and alveolar bone. Systemic disorders can predispose to periodontal disease and vice versa. Infective disease of the periodontal tissue, under the influence of risk factors such as local, systemic, environmental, and altered body immunity, predisposes and accelerates the inflammatory progressive destruction of periodontium which in turn may influence systemic health problem of the endocrinal, reproductive, cardiovascular, and respiratory systems.

Cardiovascular system

Atherogenesis and thrombogenesis are associated with myocardial ischemia. Key factor in promoting this hypercoagulant stage is enhanced blood viscosity that encourages thrombosis. Gram-negative bacteremia in periodontitis initiates a host response that changes the endothelial integrity and coagulability which result in atherogenic and thrombogenic changes. This is further supported by the observation that less than 10% of endocarditis has been found to be associated with periodontal and other dental disorders, even without any preceding dental procedure.

Significant vascular narrowing occlusion resulting in greater ischemia has been observed in the coexisting systemic infections. This has been noted in patients with ischemic cerepral infarction/stroke, where, in addition to higher levels of plasma fibrinogen and C-reactive protein, periodontitis is considered to be an independent risk factor for occurrence of stroke. With the coexisting hypercoagulability due to higher levels of plasma fibrinogen and C-reactive protein, periodontal infection precipitates the process that leads to atherosclerosis by contributing persistent bacterial challenge.

Respiratory system

Upper respiratory tract often gets contaminated by nasopharyngeal regional organisms. However, in nosocomial infection, the aspirated oropharyngeal potential respiratory pathogens that have colonized lead to hospital-acquired pneumonia. The dental plaque in the oral cavity serves as a reservoir, especially in critically ill patients with altered immunity and bad oral hygiene. And in the case of prolonged hospital stay, these potential respiratory pathological colonizers become a persistant source of infection.

Similarly, periodontal disease shares the pathogenic mechanism with COPD as the chronic infection challenge, along with the coexisting tobacco inhalation, results in neutrophil influx that leads to the release of oxidative and hydrolytic enzymes which cause direct tissue damage. Further release of inflammatory mediators may occur as and when monocytes and macrophages get recurited.

Important points:

— A strong correlation exists between periodontitis and cardiovascular and respiratory disease.
— Severe periodontitis goes beyond the oral cavity causing systemic inflammation and endothelial dysfunction.
— Poorer lipid control and destructive periodontal disease are observed in chronic cardiac disease.
— Periodontitis is observed in TB, *Haemophilus influenza* infection, and COPD cases.

Association of periodontal and disease	Cardiovascular risk factors
— Destruction of the tooth surface and gingiva	— Elevated WBC count
— Loss of connective tissue	— Atherosclerosis
	— Increased plasma fibrinogen
	— Coronary artery disease
— Alveolar bone erosion	— Stroke
— Tooth loss	— Myocardial infarction
	— Peripheral vascular disease
	— Abdominal aortic aneurysm

Comments: The influence of systemic disease on periodontal health and periodontal infection on systemic disease marks the existence of a two-way relationship. The possible influence of the periodontal infection on the cardiovascular and respiratory system exerts the need of increasing understanding and paying attention to organ systems while managing periodontal infective pathology. Periodontal care hence paves the path for systemic care, especially cardiopulmonary health.

References and suggested readings

1. Ryberg M, Moller C, Ericson T. Saliva composition and caries development in asthmatic patients treated with beta-2 adrenoceptor agonists: a 4-year follow-up study. Scand J Dent Res. 1991;99:212–218.
2. Godara N, Godara R, Khullar M. Impact of inhalation therapy on oral health. Lung India. 2011;28:272–275. doi: 10.4103/0970-2113.85689.
3. Ayinampudi BK, Gannepalli A, Pacha VB, Kumar JV, Khaled S, Naveed MA. Association between oral manifestations and inhaler use in asthmatic and chronic obstructive pulmonary disease patients. J NTR Univ Health Sci. 2016;5:17–23.
4. De Rossi SS, et al. Oral ulcerations in patients with severe asthma. J Am Dent Assoc. 2010;141:47–51.
5. Dugmore CR, Rock WP. Asthma and tooth erosion. Is there an association? Int J Paediatr Dent. 2003;13:417–424.
6. Kurt E, Yildirim H, Kiraz N, et al. Oropharyngeal candidiasis with dry-powdered fluticasone propionate: 500 microg/day versus 200 microg/day. Allergol Immunopathol. 2008;36:17–20.
7. Ersin NK, Gülen F, Eronat N, et al. Oral and dental manifestations of young asthmatics related to medication, severity and duration of condition. Pediatr Int. 2006;48:549–554.
8. Walker GD, Cai F, Shen P, Adams GG, Reynolds C, Reynolds EC. Casein phosphopeptide-amorphous calcium phosphate incorporated into sugar confections inhibits the progression of enamel subsurface lesions *in situ.* Caries Res. 2010;44:33–40.
9. Wactawski-Wende J. Periodontal diseases and osteoporosis: association and mechanisms. Ann Periodontol. 2001;6:197–208.
10. Konde S, Agarwal M, Chaurasia R. Effects of inhalational anti-asthmatic medications on oral health between 7 and 14 years of age. Indian J Allergy Asthma Immunol. 2018;32:70–73.
11. Oberoi SS, et al. A cross-sectional survery to study the relationship of periodontal disease with cardiovascular disease, respiratory disease and diabetes mellitis. J Ind Soc Periodon. 2016;20:446–452.

12. Rastogi T, Chowdhary Z, Krishna MK, Mehrotra S, Mohan R. Prevalence of periodontitis in patients with pulmonary disease: a cross-sectional survey in the industrial district of India. J Indian Soc Periodontol. 2019;23:269–274.
13. Jangid K, et al. Periodontitis as a risk factor for cardiovasclar diseases — hype or a fact? J Cardiovas Dis Res. 2016;6:24–27.
14. Gupta A, Verma UP, Verma AK, Choudhary SC, Sharma S, Singh N, Sharma D. Periodontal diseases: a covert focus of inflammation in pulmonary diseases. Indian J Respir Care. 2019;8:8–17.
15. Kim LHY, Saleh C, Whalen-Browne A, O'Byrne PM, Chu DK. Triple vs dual inhaler therapy and asthma outcomes in moderate to severe asthma: a systematic review and meta-analysis. JAMA. 2021 Jun 22;325(24):2466–2479. doi: 10.1001/jama.2021.7872. PMID: 34009257; PMCID: PMC8135065.
16. Doğan M, Şahiner ÜM, Ataç AS, Ballıkaya E, Soyer ÖU, Şekerel BE. Oral health status of asthmatic children using inhaled corticosteroids. Turk J Pediatr. 2021;63(1):77–85. doi: 10.24953/turkjped.2021.01.009. PMID: 33686829.
17. Durack J, et al. National Heart, Lung, and Blood Institute's "AsthmaNet". Distinct associations of sputum and oral microbiota with atopic, immunologic, and clinical features in mild asthma. J Allergy Clin Immunol. 2020 Nov;146(5):1016–1026. doi: 10.1016/j.jaci.2020.03.028. Epub 2020 Apr 13. PMID: 32298699; PMCID: PMC7554083.
18. Yorulmaz A, Yalcin B. Is inhaled glucocorticoids the only culprit in angina bullosa hemorrhagica? Indian J Pharmacol. 2018 Mar–Apr;50(2):91–93. doi: 10.4103/ijp.IJP_19_17. PMID: 30100658; PMCID: PMC6044132.
19. Horiguchi T, Kondo R. Determination of the preferred tongue position for optimal inhaler use. J Allergy Clin Immunol Pract. 2018 May–Jun;6(3):1039–1041.e3. doi: 10.1016/j.jaip.2018.01.022. Epub 2018 Feb 2. PMID: 29410307.
20. Zhang K, Liang Y, Feng Y, Wu W, Zhang H, He J, Hu Q, Zhao J, Xu Y, Liu Z, Zhen G. Decreased epithelial and sputum miR-221-3p associates with airway eosinophilic inflammation and CXCL17 expression in asthma. Am J Physiol Lung Cell Mol Physiol. 2018 Aug 1;315(2):L253–L264. doi: 10.1152/ajplung.00567.2017. Epub 2018 Apr 12. PMID: 29644894.

https://doi.org/10.1142/9789811271410_bmatter

Index

www.ingramcontent.com/pod-product-compliance
Lightning Source LLC
LaVergne TN
LVHW010833220926
848479LV00083B/92
* 9 7 8 9 8 1 1 2 7 1 4 0 3 *